Functional Nanomaterials for Regenerative Tissue Medicines

Emerging Materials and Technologies
Series Editor
Boris I. Kharissov

Advanced Materials and Technologies for Wastewater Treatment
Sreedevi Upadhyayula and Amita Chaudhary

Green Tribology: Emerging Technologies and Applications
T.V.V.L.N. Rao, Salmiah Binti Kasolang, Guoxin Xie, Jitendra Kumar Katiyar, and Ahmad Majdi Abdul Rani

Biotribology: Emerging Technologies and Applications
T.V.V.L.N. Rao, Salmiah Binti Kasolang, Guoxin Xie, Jitendra Kumar Katiyar, and Ahmad Majdi Abdul Rani

Bioengineering and Biomaterials in Ventricular Assist Devices
Eduardo Guy Perpétuo Bock

Semiconducting Black Phosphorus: From 2D Nanomaterial to Emerging 3D Architecture
Han Zhang, Nasir Mahmood Abbasi, Bing Wang

Biomass for Bioenergy and Biomaterials
Nidhi Adlakha, Rakesh Bhatnagar, and Syed Shams Yazdani

Energy Storage and Conversion Devices: Supercapacitors, Batteries, and Hydroelectric Cell
Anurag Gaur, A.L. Sharma, and Anil Arya

Nanomaterials for Water Treatment and Remediation
Srabanti Ghosh, Aziz Habibi-Yangjeh, Swati Sharma, and Ashok Kumar Nadda

2D Materials for Surface Plasmon Resonance-Based Sensors
Sanjeev Kumar Raghuwanshi, Santosh Kumar, and Yadvendra Singh

Functional Nanomaterials for Regenerative Tissue Medicines
Mariappan Rajan

Uncertainty Quantification of Stochastic Defects in Materials
Liu Chu

For more information about this series, please visit: https://www.routledge.com/Emerging-Materials-and-Technologies/book-series/CRCEMT

Functional Nanomaterials for Regenerative Tissue Medicines

Edited by

Mariappan Rajan

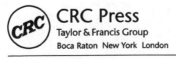

CRC Press
Taylor & Francis Group
Boca Raton New York London

CRC Press is an imprint of the
Taylor & Francis Group, an **informa** business

First edition published 2022
by CRC Press
6000 Broken Sound Parkway NW, Suite 300, Boca Raton, FL 33487-2742

and by CRC Press
4 Park Square, Milton Park, Abingdon, Oxon, OX14 4RN

© 2022 Taylor & Francis Group, LLC

CRC Press is an imprint of Taylor & Francis Group, LLC

Library of Congress Cataloging-in-Publication Data

Names: Rajan, Mariappan, editor.
Title: Functional nanomaterials for regenerative tissue medicines / edited by Mariappan Rajan.
Description: First edition. | Boca Raton : CRC Press, 2022. | Series: Emerging materials
    and technologies | Includes bibliographical references and index. | Summary: "This
    book covers nanomaterials in tissue engineering for regenerative therapies of heart,
    skin, eye, skeletal muscle, and the nervous system. It emphasizes fundamental design
    concepts and emerging forms of nanomaterials in soft and hard tissue engineering.
    This book is essential for academics and industry professionals working in tissue
    engineering, biomedicine, biopharmaceuticals, and nanotechnology. It is primarily
    intended for materials researchers (to develop the platforms related to tissue regeneration),
    as well as clinicians (to learn and apply nanomaterials in their practice) and industrial
    scientists (to develop the commercial blood substitute products)"–Provided by publisher.
Identifiers: LCCN 2021035498 (print) | LCCN 2021035499 (ebook) | ISBN 9780367690298
    (hardback) | ISBN 9780367690335 (paperback) | ISBN 9781003140108 (ebook)
Subjects: LCSH: Tissue engineering. | Regenerative medicine. | Nanotechnology.
Classification: LCC R857.T55 F85 2022 (print) | LCC R857.T55 (ebook) |
    DDC 612.028–dc23/eng/20211001
LC record available at https://lccn.loc.gov/2021035498
LC ebook record available at https://lccn.loc.gov/2021035499

ISBN: 978-0-367-69029-8 (hbk)
ISBN: 978-0-367-69033-5 (pbk)
ISBN: 978-1-003-14010-8 (ebk)

DOI: 10.1201/9781003140108

Typeset in Times
by KnowledgeWorks Global Ltd.

Contents

v

Preface

Functional Nanomaterials for Regenerative Tissue Medicines covers materials, biomaterials, and nanomaterials in tissue engineering for regenerative therapies of the heart, skin, eye, skeletal muscle, and nervous system. The advantages and limitations of nanoengineering materials are presented alongside future challenges and milestones that nanotechnology must overcome to impact biomedical applications. *Functional Nanomaterials for Regenerative Tissue Medicines* emphasizes the fundamental design concepts and emerging nanomaterials in soft- and hard-tissue engineering. Biomaterials have attracted the interest of soft- and hard-tissue engineers for the past two decades. Their unique properties make them promising for *de novo* fabrication of bio-inspired hybrid/composite materials with improved regenerative properties, including, for example, the capacity for electric conductivity and the provision of antimicrobial properties. However, so far, the use of such materials in medical applications is somewhat limited, and most of the studies have reached only the archetypical proof-of-concept stage. Therefore, *Functional Nanomaterials for Regenerative Tissue Medicines* is essential for academics and industry professionals working in tissue engineering, biomedicine, biopharmaceuticals, and nanotechnology. *Functional Nanomaterials for Regenerative Tissue Medicines* is primarily intended for materials researchers (to develop the platforms related to tissue regeneration), clinicians (to learn and apply nanomaterials in their practice), and industrial scientists (to develop the commercial blood substitute products). The book is an essential reference resource for academic and medical researchers, engineers, PhDs, MDs, MSC, postdoc students, medical staff, pharmaceutical companies, private producers and innovative companies, technological industries, biomaterials researchers, tissue engineers, dental material researchers, bioengineers, materials scientists, and anyone involved in the future development of innovative medicine that drives advancement in tuberculosis research

Editor

Mariappan Rajan, PhD, is an Assistant Professor in the Department of Natural Products Chemistry, School of Chemistry, Madurai Kamaraj University, India. He is an experienced researcher and is mainly interested in developing biodegradable polymeric nanocarrier systems, nanohydrogels, nanoparticles, nanocomposite scaffolds, bio-ceramic materials, and mineral-substituted scaffolds for drug delivery, tissue engineering, spinal cord regenerations, and wound dressing applications. Rajan has published more than 100 peer-reviewed publications, twelve book chapters, and four edited books. He has multiple editorial duties in many reputed international journals, such as *Frontiers in Cell and Developmental Biology, INNOSC Theranostics and Pharmacological Sciences, Journal of Nanoscience, Indian Journal of Applied Environmental Sciences*, and with publishers such as Cambridge Scholars Publishing.

Contributors

Sukumaran Anil
Department of Dentistry
Oral Health Institute
Hamad Medical Corporation
College of Dental Medicine
Qatar University
Doha, Qatar

Vasudha Bakshi
School of Pharmacy
Anurag University, Venkatapur, Ghatkesar
Hyderabad, India

Chinmaya Chidananda Behera
School of Pharmacy
Centurion University of Technology
    and Management
Odisha, India

Audesh Bhat
Centre for Molecular Biology
Central University of Jammu
Jammu, India

Narender Boggula
School of Pharmacy
Anurag University, Venkatapur,
    Ghatkesar
Hyderabad, India

Hemant Borase
C. G. Bhakta Institute of Biotechnology
Uka Tarsadia University
Bardoli, India

Deepika Dasari
Department of Pharmacy
Birla Institute of Technology and Sciences
Hyderabad, India

Arti Dhar
Department of Pharmacy
Birla Institute of Technology and
    Sciences
Hyderabad, India

Trupti Ghatage
Department of Pharmacy
Birla Institute of Technology and
    Sciences
Hyderabad, India

Srashti Goyal
Department of Pharmacy
Birla Institute of Technology and
    Sciences
Hyderabad, India

Gopal Jee Gopal
C. G. Bhakta Institute of
    Biotechnology
Uka Tarsadia University
Bardoli, India

Srivani Gowru
Department of Bioscience and
    Biotechnology
Banasthali University
Vanasthali, Rajasthan, India

Ohnmar Htwe
Rehabilitation Medicine Unit
Department of Orthopaedic and
    Traumatology
Faculty of Medicine
Universiti Kebangsaan Malaysia
Malaysia

Zahid Hussain
Department of Pharmaceutics
    and Pharmaceutical
    Technology
College of Pharmacy
University of Sharjah
Sharjah, United Arab Emirates

Mohammed Imran
Innatura Scientific Pvt Ltd.
Hyderabad, India

Jayant Jain
Department of Pharmacy
Birla Institute of Technology and
    Sciences
Hyderabad, India

Murugaraj Jeyaraj
National Centre for Nanoscience and
    Nanotechnology
University of Madras
Guindy Campus
Chennai, Tamil Nadu, India

Roohi Kesharwani
Department of Pharmaceutical
    Sciences
Sam Higginbottom University of
    Agriculture, Technology and
    Sciences
Prayagraj, India

Shahzeb Khan
Department of Pharmacy
University of Malakand
Chakdara, Dir Lower
Khyber Pakhtunkhwa,
    Pakistan

Gangarapu Kiran
School of Pharmacy
Anurag University, Venkapaur,
    Ghatkaser
Hyderabad, India

Vikas Kumar
Natural Product Drug Discovery
    Laboratory
and
Department of Pharmaceutical
    Sciences
Shalom Institute of Health
    Sciences
Sam Higginbottom University of
    Agriculture, Technology and
    Sciences
Prayagraj, India

Narendra Maddu
Department of Biochemistry
Sri Krishnadevaraya University
Ananthapuramu, India

Kalpana Madgula
SAS Nanotechnologies LLC
Wilmington, Delaware, USA

Sivaraj Mehnath
National Centre for Nanoscience and
    Nanotechnology
University of Madras
Guindy Campus
Chennai, Tamil Nadu, India

Sesha Subramanian Murugan
Biomaterials Research Laboratory
Yenepoya Research Centre
Yenepoya (Deemed to be
    University)
Deralakatte, India

Ashirbad Nanda
School of Pharmacy
Centurion University of Technology
    and Management
Odisha, India

Mounika Nerella
School of Pharmacy
Anurag University, Venkatapur,
    Ghatkesar
Hyderabad, India

Simanchal Panda
School of Agriculture and Bioengineering
Centurion University of Technology and
    Management
Odisha, India

Dilip Kumar Patel
Department of Pharmaceutical Sciences
Sam Higginbottom University of
    Agriculture, Technology and Sciences
Prayagraj, India

Satish Patil
School of Life Sciences
Kavayitri Bahinabai Chaudhari North
    Maharashtra University
Jalgaon, India

Venkata Sreenivas Puli
Air Force Research Laboratory
Wright Patterson Air Force Base
Ohio, USA
and
Smart Nanomaterials Solutions LLC
Orlando, Florida, USA

Nor Amlizan Ramli
Department of Pharmaceutics
Faculty of Pharmacy
Universiti Teknologi MARA
Puncak Alam Campus
Bandar Puncak Alam
Selangor, Malaysia

Bhisma N Ratha
School of Agriculture and
    Bioengineering
Centurion University of Technology and
    Management
Odisha, India

Bhairavi Rathod
C. G. Bhakta Institute of
    Biotechnology
Uka Tarsadia University
Bardoli, India

Reshma
Department of Chemistry
Osmania University
Hyderabad, India

Rai Muhammad Sarfraz
College of Pharmacy
University of Sargodha
Sargodha, Punjab, Pakistan

Gi Hun Seong
Department of Bionano
    Engineering
Center for Bionano Intelligence
    Education and Research
Hanyang University
Ansan, South Korea

S.N. Singh
Ayurvedic Services
Uttar Pradesh, India

Mohammad Sohail
Department of Pharmacy
COMSATS University
    Islamabad
Abbottabad Campus
Abbottabad, Pakistan

Hnin Ei Thu
Research and Innovation
    Department
Lincoln University College
Petaling Jaya, Selangor, Malaysia

Gouthami Thumma
Department of Pharmaceutics
University College of Pharmaceutical
    Sciences
Kakatiya University
Warangal, India

Surendra Tripathy
Northeast Frontier Railway
    Hospital
Goalpara, India

Jayachandran Venkatesan
Biomaterials Research Laboratory
Yenepoya Research Centre
Yenepoya (Deemed to be University)
Deralakatte, India

Pankaj Kumar Yadav
Department of Pharmaceutical Sciences
Sam Higginbottom University of
   Agriculture, Technology and Sciences
Prayagraj, India

1 Nanomaterials into Biological System Interactions

State of the Art

Gouthami Thumma
University College of Pharmaceutical
Sciences, Kakatiya University

Mohammed Imran
Innatura Scientific Pvt Ltd.

Srivani Gowru
Banasthali University

Reshma
Osmania University

Vasudha Bakshi and Gangarapu Kiran
Anurag University

CONTENTS

DOI: 10.1201/9781003140108-1

1.1   INTRODUCTION

Nanoscience is one of the most exciting areas of contemporary science exploration and has essential applications in physics, chemistry, and biology [1]. The main emphasis is on improving and exploring new nanomaterials' properties by changing the diameter, structure, and distribution of the particles. Nanotechnology is defined as the design, synthesis, and application of materials and systems with nanoscale size and structure [1]. Nanotechnology is a multidisciplinary field of study that plays an important role in pharmaceutical industry, particularly in drug delivery and diagnosis of disease at the biological target site. However, these are the connecting materials of physics, chemistry, and biology at the nanoscale [2]. Nanoparticles are structural components with smaller size (particularly sizes ranging from 1–100 nm) with specific characteristics including drug delivery, imaging, biosensors, microarrays and microfluidics [3, 4]. Moreover, nanotechnology employs therapeutic agents at the nanoscale range to develop effective nano-medicines [5].

The field of nanoparticles has extensive background, and many products have been discovered and marketed. Optical characteristics of nanoparticles were used in sculptures and drawings long before the 4th century AD. The Lycurgus Cup (4th century AD) is the most prominent example of a nanoparticle application [6]. This remarkable cup is the only complete historical evidence of a unique form of glass, known as dichroic glass, and it changes color when exposed to the light. When light is reflected inside, the non-transparent green cup transforms into a bright transparent color. Glass analysis showed that it contains a very tiny amount of Ag and Au metal crystals that give it unique optical properties. Earlier, ceramics from the Renaissance and Middle Ages also have distinct copper or gold-colored metallic glitter. This lustrous forming is induced by a metallic film that has been added to the translucent surface of the glazing. When the film has tolerance to ambient oxidation and other weathering, the shaping luster can be observed for an extended period [7, 8]. The luster produces copper and silver nanoparticles within the film, which are homogeneously scattered in the glassy ceramic glaze matrix. Artisans prepare such nanoparticles with the intro-duction of silver and copper salts and their oxides, such as one of ochre, vinegar, and clay on the top of the pottery that has been previously glazed. The sample is exposed to a flame and heated to 600° C in a restricted environment. The glaze softens in the fire, allowing the silver and copper ions to move through the enam-el's outer layers. Atmospheric elimination reduced the atoms down to elements, which have fused to form nanoparticles that create optical and color changes [9]. Luster methodology has demonstrated that early artisans had sophisticated scientific awareness of materials [10].

Richard Feynmann first coined the term "nanotechnology" in 1959. Inspired by this definition, K. Eric Drexler explicitly uses the word "nanotechnology" in his novel *Creation Engine: The Emerging Age of Nanotechnology* in 1980 [11]. The particle size used in nanotechnology is so tiny that it can be used in all kinds of innovative and efficient forms to address challenges we've never been able to tackle before. Nanomaterials have evolved tremendously in materials science over the past 15 years. Materials with particles consisting of at least one dimen-sion between 1–100 nm can be described as "nanomaterials." When interacting with these tiny structures, the ratio between the surface size of the device and the constituent atoms' size appears relevant [12]. The expansion of nanoscience and nanotechnology over the past few years is mostly attributed to the advancement of nanometer-scale characterization and synthetic paths. Nanotechnology is the innovation of specifications for suitable applications of all minute materials in a range of nanoscale [13]. Table 1.1 represents the timeline frame of the development of nanomaterials.

1.2 DEFINITION AND APPLICATIONS OF NANOPARTICLES AND NANOMATERIALS

Nanoscience and nanotechnology are two unusual terms that have been com-monly used these days to describe a wide variety of scientific practices around the globe. The word "nano" derives from *nanos*, the Greek term meaning "dwarf." Nanotechnology is defined as the design, synthesis, and application of materi-als and systems with nanoscale size and structure. The dimensions of these nano materials are at least one dimension within the nanometer scale range (i.e., 10^{-9}m = 1 nm) [41] (Figure 1.1).

Nanomaterials with superior properties relative to their bulk products have shown innovative uses in diverse areas. The field of nanoscience and nano-technology consists of developing modern nanoscale functional materials and modifying their physical, chemical, and biological properties with changed size, structure, shape, and morphology that make them ideal for various applications in different industrial fields. The majority of scientists also used actual mate-rial molecules to create this structure. In the various branches of materials sci-ence and engineering, such as nanobiotechnology [42], bio nanotechnology [43], quantum dots [44], surface-enhanced Raman scattering (SERS) [45], and applied microbiology [46], enormous advancement in nanotechnology has created new frontiers. In the field of information and connectivity market, nanotechnology

TABLE 1.1

Timeline Frame from the Instigation to the Current Development of Nanomaterials

Year	Inference Based on Evidence and Observations	Reference
1857	Colloid gold discovered by Michael Faraday	[14]
1905	The existence of colloids discovered by Albert Einstein	[15]
1932	Langmuir discovered atomic layers on the molecule	[16]
1958	There is "plenty of room" to work at the nanoscale by Feynman	[17]
1974	The term "nanotechnology" was first used	[18]
1981	A machine that can move a single atom around was developed by IBM	[19]
1985	A new form of carbon (C_{60}) was discovered	[20]
1990	IBM demonstrated the ability to control the position of atoms	[21]
1991	S. Iijima discovered carbon nanotubes	[22]
1993	The first high-quality quantum dot was prepared	[23]
1997	Nano transistor was discovered	[24]
1999	Discovery of nanomedicine by R. Freitas	[25]
2000	Discovery of DNA motor	[26]
2001	By using nanotubes, phototype fuel cells were made	[27]
2002	Stain-repellent trousers reach the high street	[28]
2003	Introduction of prototype nano-solar cells	[29]
2005	Nanotechnologies and nanosciences: An action plan in Europe	[30]
2006	A nanoscale car made of oligo (phenylene ethylene) with alkynyl axles and four spherical C_{60} fullerene wheels was built by James tour at Rice University.	[31]
2007	At MIT, Angela Belcher and colleagues built a lithium-ion battery with a common type of virus that was not harmful to the humans by using a low-cost and benign eco-friendly process	[32]
2008	The first official NNI strategy research was published for nanotechnology that was related to Environmental, Health, and Safety (EHS)	[33]
2009	Nadrian Seeman and colleagues created several DNA- like robotic nanoscale assembly devices at New York University	[34]
2010	Noble prize-winning development of palladium-catalyzed cross-coupling	[35]
2012	The NNI introduces two more nanotechnology signature initiatives (NSIs) and the nanotechnology knowledge infrastructure (NKI), bringing the total to five NSIs	[36]
2013	Development of first carbon nanotube computers by Stanford researchers	[37]
2014	Nobel prize-winning Nano fluorescence microscope was discovered	[38]
2015	A detailed account has been developed to control the electron charge of nanoparticle of platinum; it is an essential catalyst in the fuel cells, to maximize the efficiency of the process.	[39]
Today	Scientists discover graphene nanoparticles and are safely interacting with brain neurons, and these are precisely the controls making nanoelectronics.	[40]

reveals future importance for society [47]. It has various uses in energy and food technology, cosmetics, drugs, and medical products, textiles, coatings, and primarily used to eliminate contaminants to the atmosphere [48]. Apart from this, other microscopic and computer engineering systems made by humans have evolved micro and nanoscale sensing systems, but they are all related to

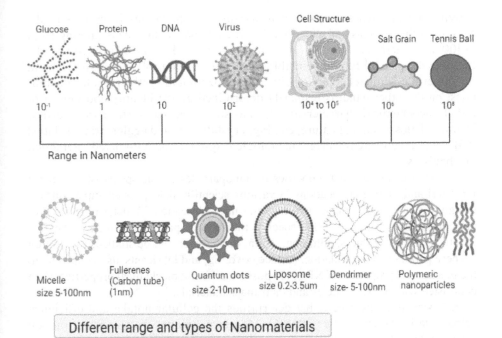

Different range and types of Nanomaterials

FIGURE 1.1 The different types of nanomaterial's and their range of various nanoparticles.

biomedical applications [49]. Nowadays, several scientists are using many ultra-thin layer magnetic nanoparticles to create sophisticated data storage systems [50]. Furthermore, nanoparticles act as an imaging tool and drug delivery system to target site specific and also serve as nano vehicles [51] (AuNps, iron oxide NPs, quantum dots, liposomes, dendrimers, micelles, and mesoporous silica NPs) by improving therapeutic and biological features of anti-carcinogenic agents (prostate, ovarian, and breast cancer). FDA-approved lipid systems, such as liposomes or micelles, are of first-generation nanoparticles [52] like DaunoXome (liposomal daunorubicin). Myocet (non-pegylated liposomal doxorubicin), a drug used to treat breast cancer, has undergone two randomized trials. Genexol-PM and Nanoxel-PM are micellar formulations used in breast, ovary, lung, and cancer cell lines. Nanoparticles have wide capacity to cross the blood brain barrier due to their small size; they have also satisfied control drug outcomes at the cellular level and in chemotherapeutic drugs. The ability of NPs to deliver drugs directly to tumor cells is their most distinguishing feature [53]. In this chapter we have summarized the biological interaction of NPs and their mechanistic actions. We have also provided detailed discussion on physicochemical properties of NPs, applications of NPs, and their status in clinical trials.

1.3 PHYSICOCHEMICAL PROPERTIES OF NANOPARTICLES

Nanotechnology has produced several types of materials at the nanoscale level. NPs possess various physicochemical properties. For instance, a more significant surface area, greater mechanical robustness, chemical reaction, and optical activity of nanoparticles makes them useful for applications in various fields. NPs are a diverse class of materials that include particulate sizes ranging from 1–100 nm, increased specific area, and specialized surface properties. NPs improve drug stability and solubility, allowing for controlled drug delivery at the target site while reducing toxicity. Internalization of synthetic molecule moieties, on the other hand, is primarily determined by the identity and impact of NP physicochemical characteristics such as structure, size, surface area, surface characteristics, chemical nature, coating, crystallinity, and agglomeration status. [55] These factors are important in biological systems and NP-related interaction mechanisms.

The various mechanical properties of nanoparticles enable specialists to search for novel and unique applications in various scientific fields, for example, surface design, tribology, nano-manufacturing, and nanofabrication. To determine the precise mechanical nature of NPs, specific mechanical parameters such as flexible modulus, stress, hardness, adhesion, strain, and erosion can be studied. In addition to these parameters, coagulation, surface covering, and lubricants also contribute to the mechanical properties of NPs. NPs possess different mechanical properties when contrasted with micro particles and their mass materials.

NPs size is a key factor that determines the cellular uptake and efficiency of particle in the endocytic path [56]. Moreover, smaller the size faster the ion release rate and increased level of interactions with cell membranes. Larger particles shows reduced level of cellular uptake than smaller particles at the equal concentrations and easily enter in to the human system and it has been noted that, NPs with 100nm size show high cellular uptake than NPs with 1 μm diameter. A report showed that NPs with 50 nm via intravenous injection interacted with all tissues faster than those above 100 nm NPs. However, size of the NPs specifies the pharmaceutical behavior; that is, NPs of less than 10 nm in size exhibit rapid clearing from the tissue circulation via renal clearance [57, 58]. In contrast, NPs greater than 15 μm particle size will not reach to tumor cells because of the restricted diffusion into extracellular space due to the EPR effect. A study by Sonavane et al., [59] demonstrated that NPs with smaller size stay in circulation longer and accumulate to increased amount in all organs. Moreover, the size of NPs can also influence other cellular internalization mechanisms, including macro pinocytosis, clathrin or caveolar mediated endocytosis, and phagocytosis [60]. Another important feature of NPs is shape. NPs have variety of shapes, such as rod-like, tubular, fibrous, spherical, planar, filament-like, spherical, and plate-shaped (Figure 1.2). NPs' shape plays a key role in affecting the pharmacokinetic property, internalization, elimination, and bio distribution. In addition, NPs' shape can make them more effective in the membrane wrapping processes in phagocytosis and endocytosis. A study of spherical NPs with smaller size showed faster internalization by endocytosis than rod-shaped NPs. Another study shown that endocytosis of spherical shaped NPs exhibits faster than NPs with a tubular shape. In addition, NPs with spherical shapes exhibit low toxicity.

Besides the NPs' size and shape, one more factor plays a significant role in NPs with cell interactions: solubility depends on the magnitude of the surface charges of NPs [60]. Moreover, surface coating of NPs modification can alter the

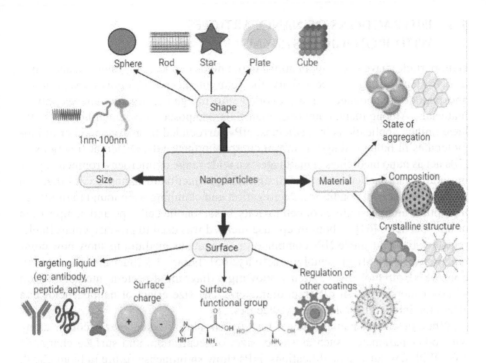

FIGURE 1.2 Physicochemical properties of nano particles.

chemical, electrical, optical, and magnetic properties. This affects the cytotoxic properties by influencing bio distribution, pharmacokinetics and accumulation. In addition, solubility, stability, colloidal behavior, and plasma protein binding are determined by the nature of surface charges. Negatively charged NPs have greater cellular absorption compared to NPs with neutral and positive charge due to resistance through plasma proteins [61]. These NPs result in platelet aggregation, hemolysis, and finally toxicity. The surface of NPs can affect absorption of biomolecules and ion levels, which leads to modification of the cellular response. Moreover, surface charge governs the colloid behavior, which means the response of the organism is to cause NPs change size and shape in the form of cellular accumulations. The effect of NPs' surface chemistry on red blood cells and immune cells have studied by both in vitro and in vivo models. For instance, a study demonstrated that the effect of surface charge of SiNPs on cell lines decreases the adenosine triphosphate (ATP) for negative hydrophobic and hydrophilic charge compared to hydrophilic positively charged amino altered surfaces. This implied that the way cells interact with NPs is largely determined by the NPs' surface. The developed NPs interaction with cells might interfere with cell adhesion, thus altering cellular properties, including cytoskeleton, morphology, and proliferation [62]. However, the surface of NPs plays a crucial role in cell adhesion. Alteration of NPs' surface chemistry is a significant usage in biomedical applications to reduce toxicity, enhance stability, and regulate internalization [63].

1.4 INTERACTIONS OF NANOPARTICLES WITH BIOLOGICAL SYSTEMS

Nanoparticles have wider applications in the fields of chemistry, biology, and physics. NPs have strong surface activity; they can interact with biopolymers, proteins, and peptides. Nanomaterials are divided into inorganic, organic, and composite materials. Among them, composite materials composed of NPs and biomolecules have unique applications in medicines. NPs surrounded by a large number of biomolecules in biological systems form composite materials. Different functions of NPs act as nano medicines. This suggests a wide range of microenvironments, posing additional challenges for the design and production of nanoparticles that can work in a variety of conditions. Aggregation and clumping were found to influence the uptake and possibilities of cell toxicity based on the cell type and composition of nanoparticles [64]. A bottom-up base method was used to produce controllable, reproducible, and stable NPs combined in an aqueous medium to show how combined silver NPs affect hemolytic activity [65]. Figure 1.3 illustrates the interactions of NPs in biological systems, showing a diagram of protein interaction with silicon nanoparticles of different diameters. The size effect of nanoparticles can affect the interactions of protein molecules.

When designing nanomedicine, toxicity should be taken into account, along with other parameters such as shape, size, concentration, and surface charge of NPs. With few surface modifications, NPs show an immense future in biomedical, clinical, and diagnostic applications, such as cancer imaging using magnetic resonance imaging (MRI) and identification of genetic mutation. Most of the NPs' surface interacted with nucleic acids and proteins at different binding points through specific or non-specific interactions [66–68]. In immune-biocompatibility, a vital role and various applications of nanomaterial proteins have been seen on nucleic acids as a result of their physicochemical stability, easy accessibility, mechanical

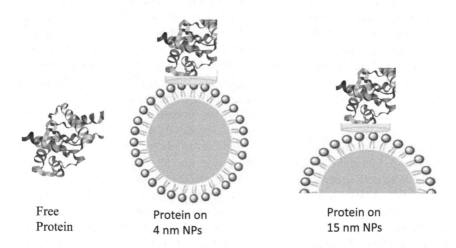

| Free | Protein on | Protein on |
| Protein | 4 nm NPs | 15 nm NPs |

FIGURE 1.3   Interaction of nanoparticles in biological systems.

rigidity, and high sensitivity of base pairing, which acts as a suitable interaction for molecular nano construction [69].

1.4.1 INTERACTION MECHANISMS

The surface of nanomaterials would be covered by protein corona upon their entrance to a biological medium. Therefore, the properties of NPs for interaction must be studied [70]. Centi et al., and Tatini et al., explained the importance of gold nanorods (GNRs) in the biomedical area [71, 72]. On the basis of particle size, coating, and shape, GNRs exhibit characteristic optical properties, which are elongated along one direction, and also usefulness in biological applications like polyethylene glycol (PEG) conjugation, also their size and shape is critical to modulate cellular penetration, intracellular localization, and biodistribution [73]. Nanoparticles have a wide range of applications in the field of drug delivery systems for targeting cancer tissues. Most targeted NPs carry drugs with an intracellular target and need to be taken into the cell by endocytosis. NPs enters into the cell by an endocytosis mechanism which is mediated by clathrin mediated endocytosis, phagocytosis, macro pinocytosis, and caveolin mediated endocytosis. Once NPs enter the cell it interacts with lysosomes, rough endoplasmic reticulum, and golgi apparatus.

1.5 NPs IN CLINICAL TRIALS

NP-based therapeutics are gaining popularity in medical field due to high efficacy, reduced toxicity, and increased solubility compared to normal medications [74, 75]. Moreover, nano-based formulation alter the drug properties, including biochemical, magnetic, optical, and electronic, which leads to endless therapeutic uses [4, 76, 77]. However, NP-based therapeutics consist of organic materials (polymers, liposomes, micelles, metals, or metal oxides), nano crystals, and inorganic materials (gold NPs, quantum dots, magnetic, polystyrene). In the past three decades, there has been a significant progression in clinical trials on nano-based therapeutics. So far, 80 clinical trials have been conducted for the treatment of various diseases, including various cancers [78], skin disorders such as atopic dermatitis [79], bacterial infections [80, 81], rheumatoid arthritis, pneumonia [82], fibrosis, Parkinson's Disease, and Alzheimer's Disease [83]. Through those, approximately 50 nano formulations have been approved and used in clinical practices, while 60 nano formulations are undergoing investigation [84, 85]. Among those, 50 nano formulations were approved; 10 are from liposomal, 15 from nanocrystal, 15 from polymer NPs, 5 from Inorganic, 1 from micelle, and 2 from protein. And in investigating 60 formulations, 33 are from liposomal, 11 from polymer, 2 from inorganic, 2 from nanocrystals, 9 from micelles, 1 from proteins, 2 from dendrimers. In fact, various nano-based drugs are now in different clinical development stages (Table 1.2). A phase-III clinical drug, ThermoDox, has been used to treat breast cancer and hepatocellular carcinoma (HCC). Similarly a phase I and II clinical trial drug, TKM - 080,301, has been used as a chemotherapy drug against HCC. A recent phase-1 clinical trial

TABLE 1.2

Current NP-Based Therapeutics in Clinical Trials and Stages

S. No.	Drug Name	Type of NP Particle in Formulation	Type of Disease	Clinical Stage	Clinical Trial Identifier No.
1.	CPX-1	Irinotecan (Liposomal NPs)	Colorectal cancer	Phase-II	NCT00361842
2.	Lipoplatin	Cisplatin (Liposomal NPs)	Non-small lung cancer, breast cancer, Gastric cancer	Phase-III	NCT02702700
3.	Aroplatin	NDDP-bis neodecanoat-o-trans-R,R-1,2-diamine cyclohexane platinum(II) (Liposomal NPs)	Refractory colorectal cancer, malignant pleural mesothelioma	Phase-II	NCT0081549
4.	NKTR-102	Irinotecan (Pegylated liposome NPs)	Metastatic solid tumors viz., breast, colorectal, and ovarian cancers	Phase-III	NCT01492101 NCT02915744
5.	Atragen	(Tretinoin Liposome NPs)	Kidney cancer	Phase-II	NCT00003656
6.	NK105	Paclitaxel (Polymeric NPs)	Breast cancer, metastatic recurrent	Phase-III	NCT01644890
7.	Oncoprex	Fus1(TUSC2) Encapsulate Liposome NPs	Lung cancer	Phase-I & II	NCT01455389
8.	Lipusu	Paclitaxel (Polymeric micelles)	Lung squamous cell carcinoma	Phase IV	NCT02142790
9.	CRLX 101	CRLX 101 drug (Polymeric conjugate)	Rectal cancer	Phase-II	NCT02769962
10.	XMT1001 (fleximertm)	Camptothecin (Polymeric conjugate)	Small-cell lung cancer and NSCL cancer	Phase-I	NCT00455052
11.	Targomirs	Microrna mimic (Crystalline NPs)	Malignant pleural mesothelio, a non-small cell lung cancer	Phase-I	NCT01946867
12.	NC6004	Cisplatin (Micelles NPs)	Head and neck cancers	Phase-II	NCT03771820
13.	Dendrimer-conjugated AZD4320	AZD0466 (Dendrimer NPs)	Advanced solid tumors, lymphoma, multiple myeloma, hematologic malignancies	Phase-I	NCT04214093

(*Continued*)

TABLE 1.2 (*Continued*)
Current NP-Based Therapeutics in Clinical Trials and Stages

S. No.	Drug Name	Type of NP Particle in Formulation	Type of Disease	Clinical Stage	Clinical Trial Identifier No.
14.	Aurimmune (CYT-6091)	TNF-α bound to colloidal Gold NPs (Metal NPs)	Adenocortical carcinoma, breast, colorectal, gastro intestinal, kidney, liver, ovarian, and pancreatic cancers; sarcoma and melanoma	Phase-I	NCT04214093
15.	Magnable Iron NPs	Magnetic NP Injection (Crystalline NPs)	Prostate cancer	Early Phase-I	NCT02033447
16.	Abraxane	Albumin bound paclitaxel (Protein NPs)	Breast cancer, non-small cell lung and pancreatic cancers	FDA 2005	Application No.021660
17.	Depocyte	Cytarabine (Liposomal NPs)	Lymphomas or leukemia with meningeal spread add neoplastic meningitis	First approved in 1999 by FDA and 2007	Application No:21-041
18.	Oncaspar	Pegaspargase (mpeg asparaginase) (Nanoemulsions)	Acute lymphocytic leukemia	EMA 2016	EMEA/ H/C/003789
19.	Vyxeos (MM-398)	Duanorubicin and cytarabine (Liposomal NPs)	Atopic dermatitis	FDA 2017	Application No-209401
20.	Eligard	Leuprolide acetate (Polymeric NPs)	Advanced prostate cancer	FDA 2016	NDA 2134/S33

micelle formulation nano-based product, IT-141, has been used to treat advanced stages of cancer.

1.6 APPLICATIONS OF NANOPARTICLES

Nanoparticles have a variety of advantages in various fields. Some of the advantages are given below.

1.6.1 DRUGS AND MEDICINES

Inorganic nanoparticles are complex in nature, with different physicochemical properties. These nanoparticles represent the importance of developing nanodevices. These can be used for various physical, chemical, and biological applications.

Nanoparticles have drawn greater interest in delivering drug substances at different dosage levels with greater therapeutic efficiency, lower side effects, and increased patient compliance. Some nanoparticles, such as supramagnetic iron oxide, are reported for in vivo applications such as tissue repair, MRI contrast enhancement, detoxification of biological samples, immunoassay, and cell separation [86]. All of these medical applications require nanoparticles in small size (less than 100 nm), high magnetic values, and lower particle-size distribution. In comparison to industrial delivery methods, nano-drug deliveries have potential as targeting product carriers because of their innovative advantages, such as the potential to shield the product material from harm, the place of action at the target, and decreased side effects and other noxiousness [87].

1.6.2   MATERIALS AND MANUFACTURING

Nanomaterials are trending substances in material sciences because of their various properties in bulk substance depending on their size. Synthesized nanoparticles have physicochemical properties that possess unique mechanical, electrical, imaging, and optical properties that are extremely helpful for specific applications in commercial, medicinal, and ecological divisions [88]. The potential benefits have been reported by many manufacturing and pharmaceutical industries for marketable products, such as microelectronics and aerospace products. Among all nanoparticles, healthcare products play a significant role, followed by computers, electronics, and garden and home products. It has to be the next revolutionary technology, including the food and packing industries [89].

1.6.3   ENVIRONMENTAL APPLICATIONS

However, the usage of nanoparticles in household and industrial applications is very severe and could cause an enormous amount of materials to be released into the environment. Therefore, it is necessary to understand the reactivity, mobility, toxicity, and persistence of nanoparticles. Mainly, the structured nanoparticle could have higher concentration in soil and groundwater, which consists of the most significant disclosure assessment of environmental risk [90, 91]. Natural nanoparticles play a crucial role in solid-water partition contaminants caused by high surface-to-mass ratio. The contaminates can be absorbed to the NPs' surface and cause co-precipitation during formation or trapping of aggregated NPs surface adsorbed the contaminants. The interaction between the nanoparticles and contaminants depends on the different characteristics such as composition, shape, morphology, aggregation/disaggregation, porosity, and aggregate structure. Nanoparticles have potential advantages. These are sustainable environmental products, remediation for contaminant materials, and hazardous substances; removal of heavy metals from natural water, viz., lead, mercury, thallium, cadmium, and arsenic [92].

1.6.4   ELECTRONICS APPLICATIONS

Nanoparticles have many applications in printed electronics in the past few years because printed electronics have an attractive technique, are cost-effective, and are flexible for larger devices such as sensors, thin film transistors, and supercapacitors.

Printed electronics possess different functional inks with NPs, such as organic-electronic molecules; metallic NPs, ceramics NPs, and CNTs are some that have been used for the production of a new variety of electronic equipment [93].

The structural, electrical, and optical characteristics of metal and single-dimensional semiconductors help make essential structures for the new generation electronic, photonic, and materials. The electronics sector is the best model for scientific discovery and development of the new semiconducting material discoveries—from vacuum tubes to transistors and diodes, and finally to miniature chips. The main characteristics of nanoparticles are reversible assembly, and facile manipulation allows NPs to be effective in electronic, electric, or optical devices [54].

1.7 NANOPARTICLES IN THERAPIES

Nanoparticles have a size range of 1–100 nm, leading to the pioneering of nanomedicines including microfluidics, drug delivery to the targeted site in controlled manner [75, 94], and involvement of microarray tests in tissue engineering [95, 96]. Currently NPs are involved in multitherapeutic agents such as chemotherapy immunotherapy, biological agents, imaging [97], neurodegenerative agents, skin disorders such as atopic dermatitis, anti-inflammatory agents, improved antibacterial diagnosis, disease prevention, and nano dimensional agents like nanorobotics [98], nano sensors [99] for diagnosis and sensory purposes, and delivery systems [100]. For instance, most drugs lose their efficacy when they enter the gastrointestinal region, and it is hard to get to the target site; with the help of NPs drug delivery system, the drugs will be sparingly water soluble and reach the target site, exhibiting higher bioavailability as the NPs undergo an uptake mechanism known as absorptive endocytosis.

Five characteristics NPs in therapy of cancer (Figure 1.4):

   i. They accumulate large volumes of drug substances and protect them against degradation. (E.g., A 70nm NP can load around 2000 small RNA(si-RNA) interfering molecules while antibody conjugates can load lower than ten molecules [101].)
   ii. They are sufficiently large to hold the different types drug moieties.
   iii. NPs contains different types of targeting ligands which results in multivalent binding to cell surface receptors [102]
   iv. The drug molecules released from NP can be adjusted pharmacokinetically for the mechanism of action [103].
   v. NPs have the potential to bypass the multidrug resistance mechanism that is involved in cell-surface protein pumps (like p-glycoprotein) as they enter cell via endocytosis.

Figure 1.3 illustrates the interactions of NPs in biological systems by targeting specific tumor cells (e.g., breast tumor in mice), minimizing the toxic effects, causing the death of the tumor cell, and providing adequate drug loading capacity due to its great surface capacity [100]. One of the advantages of NPs in drug delivery system is that they deliver the drug at the target site without distributing the drug throughout the body.

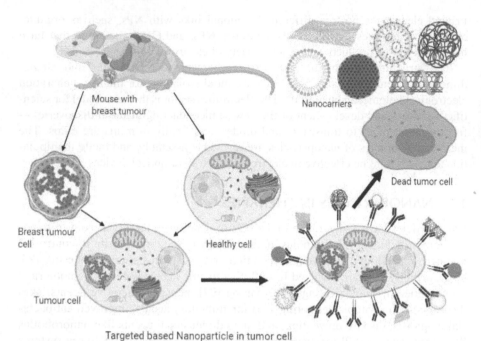

Mouse with breast tumour

Nanocarriers

Dead tumor cell

Breast tumour cell

Healthy cell

Tumour cell

Targeted based Nanoparticle in tumor cell

FIGURE 1.4   Role of nanoparticles in drug delivery systems.

1.7.1 ALZHEIMER'S DISEASE (AD)

Nanomaterials have been used to treat and diagnose chronic dementia-related neurodegenerative diseases [104]. The usage of nanocarriers for transferring bioactive to treat neurodegenerative disorders shows promising therapeutic effect compared to conventional therapies and are helpful in entering into the brain by crossing the blood-brain barrier [105–107]. Cellular signaling pathways in AD pathophysiology lead to neurotransmission damage and dysfunction. Bilal highlighted the nanocarriers applications viz. magnetic nanoparticles (MNPs), carbon nanotubes (CNTs) [108, 109], polymeric nano capsules, quantum dots, multifunctional liposomes [110] and nano emulsions [111] in the treatment of CNS disorders like AuNPs encapsulation with anthocyanin [112] and peptide inhibitors. Gold nanoparticles and PEG-coated AuNPs are very effective in preventing neurodegenerative disorders [113]. The carbon CNTs and graphene are widely used in biosensor production for the evaluation of AD biomarkers [114, 115].

1.7.2 GASTRIC CANCER

NPs with lipids such as hyaluronic acid combined with sorafenib and cisplatin are used for gastric cancer (GC) treatment [116]. Cysteine-gold NP conjugated transferrin is a novel diagnostic agent to target the tumor site and shows strong interactions with the receptor. Encapsulation of gold NPs with cysteine using purified transferrin has been targeted against gastric cancer cells [117]. NPs carried out an important role in multifunctional multimodal imaging and drug delivery carriers (Figure 1.4). Recent studies show that the techniques of NP-aided imaging can help to diagnose cancer and the possibility of metastases using advanced methods with precision.

1.7.3 Colorectal Cancer (CRC)

Transrectal ultrasound detects incursion levels and has been successfully grouped between gut wall layers but is less effective for finding the lymph node involving CRC [118]. In CRC patients, NPs can provide incredible imaging, screening, and early detection solutions. By using florescence endoscopy, early-stage small-sized CRC is detected by using peanut agglutinin (PNA). Co-encapsulating curcumin and doxorubicin (DOX) at 1:167 molar ratios in hybrids with a long circulating liposome (LCL) and PEGylated surface, which exhibits huge EPR impact, leads to a higher accumulation of the CRC site curcumin [119].

1.7.4 Liver Cancer

In order to diagnose non-invasive tumors and hepatic tumors [120] super paramagnetic iron oxide NPs coated with dextrans [121] are mostly recommended and were used as imaging agent in MRI. Recently fluorescence imaging–based MRI for hepatocellular carcinoma (HCC) is done by fucoidan-coated ultra-small zinc oxide NPs attached with iron oxide for the prognosis of advanced HCC perfusion MRI is used as biomarker [122]. NIR irradiation combination with multifunctional Iron(III) oxide-gold (Fe2O3@Au) core shell NPs results in complete inhibition of tumor growth [123]. In chitosan-coated doxurubicin NPs, the promising targeted system for drug delivery stimulates DNA and G2/M cell cycles via the pathway P53/PRC1 in HCC cells (Figure 1.4) [124].

1.7.5 Atopic Dermatitis

Atopic dermatitis is an inflammatory and immunologically dermatosis associated to ineffective skin barrier and reduced skin hydration [125]. Topically applied nanoparticles serve as an occlusive, humectant, bioactive, skin lipids, and free fatty acids. Solid liquid nanoparticles, hydrogels, and polymeric nanoparticles improve drug delivery to the dermis and epidermis [126]. Fucoidan associated with chitosan NPs delivering methotrexate into the inflamed skin results in reducing the release of pro-inflammatory cytokines (IL1-, IL-6 and TNF-α) [127]. Encapsulation of immuno-suppressants like tacrolimus and cyclosporin leads to decrease of pro-inflammatory cytokines, including IL-2 results in activation of T-cell pathways.

1.7.6 Interaction of NPs with Viral Infection

Due to their small size, NPs enter the body through inhalation, leading to pulmonary inflammation; oxidative stress results in allergic fibrosis and granuloma formation. Mechanism of NPs is by activation of pattern recognition receptors (PRRs) and related signaling pathways, modulation of lipid signaling networks, production of oxidative stress, mitochondrial dysfunction [4, 117]. For example, carbon nano dots prepared with 4-aminophenylboronic acid HCl stop the entry of herpes virus into both A549 and Vero cells [128].

1.8 ADVANTAGES AND DISADVANTAGES OF NANOMATERIALS

1.8.1 ADVANTAGES

Nanomaterial's have many advantages in the development of products in electronic, energy, IT, and medical sectors [129]. Nanotechnology is often called the technology of the future, with its impressive possibilities. For many years, our nanomaterials have already found their way into our daily life, with sports socks of silver ions, sun creams of titanium and zinc particles, or car tires with silicon and soot particles [130]. Food packaging, or even food itself, is also included in future areas of application. Nanomaterials are manufactured as consumer products, especially in sports equipment, car paints, cosmetics, textiles, and packaging.

Nanotechnology has many advantages in electronic and energy, medical, agriculture, and environmental fields. Nanotechnology will increase the economy of solar power by reducing the costs of building solar panels and the equipment involved. Nanotechnology will revolutionize the field of electronics. Quantum dots are small light-producing cells, for example, that can be used for illumination or for screens. Nanotechnology can bring significant progress in the field of medicine. By using the nanotechnology the diagnosis and treatment of heart blocks could be achieved very easily [131]. Nanobots could be sent to the arteries of a patient to clear blockages. Nanotechnology may also be used to refine drug production and molecularly tailor drugs to improve their efficacy and to reduce side effects.

1.8.2 DISADVANTAGES

Apart from the many advantages of nanomaterial, it also has several risks to environment and health. Devices or products made with nanomaterials pose risks during the disposal of the nanomaterial, as these are nano in size and may enter the environment and contaminate natural resources. Experts determined that these NPs could enter into humans and animals via the respiratory tract [132]. Nanotoxicology is a new scientific discipline that involves the safety assessment of engineered nanomaterials and nano devices. Above all, there are concerns that nanoparticles can enter the blood via the lungs or gastrointestinal tract and cause health damage. The NPs can even also cross the blood-brain barrier. These NPs have a negative effect on human health if released particles get into the body, where they can be distributed and accumulate in various organs. This can be useful for the targeted administration of drugs, but the possible negative consequences of an unintentional entry into the central nervous system have not yet been researched [133].

1.9 CONCLUSION

Nanoparticles are one aspect of nanomaterials that play and important role in biological research. The size of NPs have at least one dimension less than 100 nm in length and are smaller than red blood cells but larger than hydrogen atoms. This chapter explained the importance of nanomaterials in biological system interactions. Nanomaterials interact with a wide range of different barriers in living organisms, viz., membranes, immune cells, and mucus. Nanoparticles have tremendous potential for nanomedicine and theranostic applications, particularly in drug delivery and delivery of imaging agents at the target site. NPs have huge variation in physicochemical properties viz., size, shape, surface charge, and coatings, and these will show high drug delivery at specific target site. They also show fewer toxic effects and act as bio imaging agents in the diagnosis of various diseases. In this chapter authors have summarized the biological interaction of NPs and their mechanistic actions. Further, we also emphasized the detailed discussion on physicochemical properties on NPs, applications of NPs, and status in clinical trials. In summary, we have done a thorough literature review in the area of nanoparticles interactions with biological system, and we have explained the role of nanoparticles in medicine and theranostic applications.

ABBREVIATIONS

ATP	adenosine triphosphate
CRC	colorectal cancer
FDA	Food and Drug Administration
HCC	hepatocellular carcinoma
LCL	long circulating liposome
MRI	magnetic resonance imaging
NPs	nanoparticles
SiNPs	silica nanoparticles

REFERENCES

1. H. Liu, Z. Huang, S. Wei, L. Zheng, L. Xiao, Q. Gong, Nano-structured electron transporting materials for perovskite solar cells, Nanoscale, 8 (2016) 6209–6221.
2. J.C. Davies, Nanotechnology oversight, Washington, DC: Project on Emerging Nanotechnologies, (2008).
3. A.M Saeed, S. Najma, Q. Faiza, Nanoparticles in delivery of cardiovascular drugs, Pakistan Journal of Pharmaceutical Sciences, 20 (4), (2007) 340–348.
4. J.K. Patra, K.-H. Baek, Green nanobiotechnology: factors affecting synthesis and characterization techniques, Journal of Nanomaterials, 2014 (2014).
5. C. Binns, Introduction to nanoscience and nanotechnology, John Wiley & Sons, (2010).
6. D.J. Barber, I.C. Freestone, An investigation of the origin of the colour of the Lycurgus Cup by analytical transmission electron microscopy, Archaeometry, 32 (1990) 33–45.
7. S. Horikoshi, N. Serpone, Microwaves in nanoparticle synthesis: fundamentals and applications, John Wiley & Sons, (2013).
8. V. Klimov, A. Mikhailovsky, S. Xu, A. Malko, J. Hollingsworth, A.C. Leatherdale, H.-J. Eisler, M. Bawendi, Optical gain and stimulated emission in nanocrystal quantum dots, Science, 290 (2000) 314–317.

9. G. Reiss, H. Koop, D. Meyners, A. Thomas, S. Kämmerer, J. Schmalhorst, M. Brzeska, X. Kou, H. Brückl, A. Hütten, Magnetic Tunneling Junctions—Materials, Geometry and Applications, Magnetic Nanostructures, Springer, (2007), pp. 147–165.

10. F.A. Khan, Biotechnology fundamentals, CRC Press, (2011).

11. J.R. Antonio, C.R. Antônio, I.L.S. Cardeal, J.M.A. Ballavenuto, J.R. Oliveira, Nanotechnology in dermatology, Anais brasileiros de dermatologia, 89 (2014) 126–136.

12. S.L. Brock, Nanostructures and nanomaterials: synthesis, properties and applications by Guozhang Cao (University of Washington), London: Imperial College Press (distributed by World Scientific), (2004). xiv+ 434 pp. $78.00. ISBN 1-86094-415-9, Journal of the American Chemical Society 126 (2004): 14679–14679.

13. N.M.de S. Cameron, Nanotechnology and the human future: policy, ethics, and risk, Annals of the New York Academy of Sciences, 1093 (2006) 280–300.

14. J. Turkevich, Colloidal gold. Part II, Gold bulletin, 18 (1985) 125–131.

15. A. Brann, The effect of dissolved substances on the velocity of crystallization of water. III. Further evidence that the existence of hydrates in solution explains the retarding effect of the solute on the velocity of crystallization of water, Journal of the American Chemical Society, 40 (1918) 1168–1184.

16. J. Jorgensen, M. Avdeev, D. Hinks, J. Burley, S. Short, Crystal structure of the sodium cobaltate deuterate superconductor $Na_x CoO_2 \cdot 4_x D_2 O$ ($x \approx 1\ 3$), Physical Review B, 68 (2003) 214517.

17. K.E. Drexler, Molecular engineering: an approach to the development of general capabilities for molecular manipulation, Proceedings of the National Academy of Sciences, 78 (1981) 5275–5278.

18. D. Whitehouse, Nanotechnology instrumentation, Measurement and Control, 24 (1991) 37–46.

19. W. Fahrner, Nanotechnology and nanoelectronics, Springer, (2005).

20. A.J. Steckl, J.H. Park, J.M. Zavada, Prospects for rare earth doped GaN lasers on Si, Materials Today, 10 (2007) 20–27.

21. H.-W. Fink, Mono-atomic tips for scanning tunneling microscopy, IBM Journal of Research and Development, 30 (1986) 460–465.

22. E.T. Thostenson, Z. Ren, T.-W. Chou, Advances in the science and technology of carbon nanotubes and their composites: a review, Composites Science and Technology, 61 (2001) 1899–1912.

23. A. Mews, A. Eychmüller, M. Giersig, D. Schooss, H. Weller, Preparation, characterization, and photophysics of the quantum dot quantum well system cadmium sulfide/mercury sulfide/cadmium sulfide, The Journal of Physical Chemistry, 98 (1994) 934–941.

24. A. Svizhenko, M. Anantram, T. Govindan, B. Biegel, Nano-transistor modeling: two dimensional Green's function method, Device Research Conference. Conference Digest (Cat. No. 01TH8561), IEEE, 2001, pp. 167–168.

25. R.A. Freitas Jr, Medical nanorobotics: the long-term goal for nanomedicine, Nanomedicine design of particles, sensors, motors, implants, robots and devices, Norwood MA: Artech House, (2009) 367–392.

26. S. Myong, I. Rasnik, C. Joo, T.M. Lohman, T. Ha, Repetitive shuttling of a motor protein on DNA, Nature, 437 (2005) 1321–1325.

27. A.L. Dicks, The role of carbon in fuel cells, Journal of Power Sources, 156 (2006) 128–141.

28. T.G. Jaenson, A. Lindström, K. Pålsson, Repellency of the mosquito repellent MyggA (N,N-diethyl-3-methyl-benzamide) to the common tick Ixodes ricinus (L.)(Acari: Ixodidae) in the laboratory and field, Entomologisk Tidskrift, 124 (2003) 245–251.

29. Z. Pan, H. Rao, I. Mora-Seró, J. Bisquert, X. Zhong, Quantum dot-sensitized solar cells, Chemical Society Reviews, 47 (2018) 7659–7702.

30. R. Fries, A. Gazsó, Research projects on EHS aspects of nanotechnology in the 7th Framework Program of the EU (NanoTrust Dossier No. 030en–May 2012).

31. P. Simon, Y. Gogotsi, Materials for electrochemical capacitors, Nanoscience and Technology: a Collection of Reviews from Nature Journals, (2010) 320–329.
32. A. Yoshino, The birth of the lithium-ion battery, Angewandte Chemie International Edition, 51 (2012) 5798–5800.
33. National Research Council, Small wonders, endless frontiers: A review of the National Nanotechnology Initiative, Washington, DC: The National Academies Press (2002).
34. L. Qian, E. Winfree, J. Bruck, Neural network computation with DNA strand displacement cascades, Nature, 475 (2011) 368–372.
35. T.J. Colacot, The 2010 Nobel Prize in chemistry: palladium-catalysed cross-coupling, Platinum Metals Review, 55 (2011) 84–90.
36. P. Genther-Yoshida, M. Casassa, R. Shull, G. Pomrenke, I. Thomas, R. Price, B.V. DOE, R. John, A. Lacombe, E. Murphy, National Science and Technology Council Committee on Technology The Interagency Working Group on Nanoscience, Engineering and Technology September 1999, Washington, DC: About the National Science and Technology Council, (1999).
37. M. Rafiee, J. Yang, S. Kitipornchai, Thermal bifurcation buckling of piezoelectric carbon nanotube reinforced composite beams, Computers & Mathematics with Applications, 66 (2013) 1147–1160.
38. K.J. Thompson, C.M. Harley, G.M. Barthel, M.A. Sanders, K.A. Mesce, Plasmon resonance and the imaging of metal-impregnated neurons with the laser scanning confocal microscope, Elife, 4 (2015) e09388.
39. T.C. Johnstone, K. Suntharalingam, S.J. Lippard, The next generation of platinum drugs: targeted Pt (II) agents, nanoparticle delivery, and Pt (IV) prodrugs, Chemical Reviews, 116 (2016) 3436–3486.
40. S. Nasir, M.Z. Hussein, Z. Zainal, N.A. Yusof, S.A.M. Zobir, I.M. Alibe, Potential valorization of by-product materials from oil palm: a review of alternative and sustainable carbon sources for carbon-based nanomaterials synthesis, BioResources, 14 (2019) 2352–2388.
41. G.M. Whitesides, Nanoscience, nanotechnology, and chemistry, Small, 1 (2005) 172–179.
42. M. Moo-Young, Comprehensive biotechnology, Elsevier, (2019).
43. E.S. Papazoglou, A. Parthasarathy, BioNanotechnology, Synthesis Lectures on Biomedical Engineering, 2 (2007) 1–139.
44. S.Y. Lim, W. Shen, Z. Gao, Carbon quantum dots and their applications, Chemical Society Reviews, 44 (2015) 362–381.
45. P.L. Stiles, J.A. Dieringer, N.C. Shah, R.P. Van Duyne, Surface-enhanced Raman spectroscopy, Annual Review of Analytical Chemistry, 1 (2008) 601–626.
46. M. Rai, A. Ingle, Role of nanotechnology in agriculture with special reference to management of insect pests, Applied Microbiology and Biotechnology, 94 (2012) 287–293.
47. S.M. Rhodes, Electrically conductive polymer composites, University of Akron, (2007).
48. R.J. Peters, H. Bouwmeester, S. Gottardo, V. Amenta, M. Arena, P. Brandhoff, H.J. Marvin, A. Mech, F.B. Moniz, L.Q. Pesudo, Nanomaterials for products and application in agriculture, feed and food, Trends in Food Science & Technology, 54 (2016) 155–164.
49. P.M. Tiwari, K. Vig, V.A. Dennis, S.R. Singh, Functionalized gold nanoparticles and their biomedical applications, Nanomaterials, 1 (2011) 31–63.
50. Y. Gogotsi, Nanomaterials handbook, CRC press, (2017).
51. M.A. Gatoo, S. Naseem, M.Y. Arfat, A. Mahmood Dar, K. Qasim, S. Zubair, Physicochemical properties of nanomaterials: implication in associated toxic manifestations, BioMed Research International, (2014).
52. X. Shi, K. Sun, J.R. Baker Jr, Spontaneous formation of functionalized dendrimer-stabilized gold nanoparticles, The Journal of Physical Chemistry C, 112 (2008) 8251–8258.

53. M. Rahman, S. Beg, A. Ahmed, S. Swain, Emergence of functionalized nanomedicines in cancer chemotherapy: recent advancements, current challenges and toxicity considerations, Recent Patents on Nanomedicine, 3 (2013) 128–139.
54. I. Khan, K. Saeed, I. Khan, Nanoparticles: properties, applications and toxicities, Arabian Journal of Chemistry, 12 (2019) 908–931.
55. G. Nichols, S. Byard, M.J. Bloxham, J. Botterill, N.J. Dawson, A. Dennis, V. Diart, N.C. North, J.D. Sherwood, A review of the terms agglomerate and aggregate with a recommendation for nomenclature used in powder and particle characterization, Journal of Pharmaceutical Sciences, 91 (2002) 2103–2109.
56. A. Nel, T. Xia, L. Mädler, N. Li, Toxic potential of materials at the nanolevel, Science, 311 (2006) 622–627.
57. D.E. Owens III, N.A. Peppas, Opsonization, biodistribution, and pharmacokinetics of polymeric nanoparticles, International Journal of Pharmaceutics, 307 (2006) 93–102.
58. R.A. Petros, J.M. DeSimone, Strategies in the design of nanoparticles for therapeutic applications, Nature Reviews Drug Discovery, 9 (2010) 615–627.
59. G. Sonavane, K. Tomoda, K. Makino, Biodistribution of colloidal gold nanoparticles after intravenous administration: effect of particle size, Colloids and Surfaces B: Biointerfaces, 66 (2008) 274–280.
60. B. Yameen, W.I. Choi, C. Vilos, A. Swami, J. Shi, O.C. Farokhzad, Insight into nanoparticle cellular uptake and intracellular targeting, Journal of Controlled Release, 190 (2014) 485–499.
61. V. Forest, J. Pourchez, Preferential binding of positive nanoparticles on cell membranes is due to electrostatic interactions: a too simplistic explanation that does not take into account the nanoparticle protein corona, Materials Science and Engineering: C, 70 (2017) 889–896.
62. D. Hühn, K. Kantner, C. Geidel, S. Brandholt, I. De Cock, S.J. Soenen, P. Rivera_Gil, J.-M. Montenegro, K. Braeckmans, K. Mullen, Polymer-coated nanoparticles interacting with proteins and cells: focusing on the sign of the net charge, ACS Nano, 7 (2013) 3253–3263.
63. L. Shang, K. Nienhaus, G.U. Nienhaus, Engineered nanoparticles interacting with cells: size matters, Journal of Nanobiotechnology, 12 (2014) 1–11.
64. A. Albanese, W.C. Chan, Effect of gold nanoparticle aggregation on cell uptake and toxicity, ACS Nano, 5 (2011) 5478–5489.
65. J.M. Zook, R.I. MacCuspie, L.E. Locascio, M.D. Halter, J.T. Elliott, Stable nanoparticle aggregates/agglomerates of different sizes and the effect of their size on hemolytic cytotoxicity, Nanotoxicology, 5 (2011) 517–530.
66. C.M. Niemeyer, Nanoparticles, proteins, and nucleic acids: biotechnology meets materials science, Angewandte Chemie International Edition, 40 (2001) 4128–4158.
67. I. Firkowska-Boden, X. Zhang, K.D. Jandt, Controlling protein adsorption through nanostructured polymeric surfaces, Advanced Healthcare Materials, 7 (2018) 1700995.
68. A. Arsalan, H. Younus, Enzymes and nanoparticles: modulation of enzymatic activity via nanoparticles, International Journal of Biological Macromolecules, 118 (2018) 1833–1847.
69. S. Saallah, I.W. Lenggoro, Nanoparticles carrying biological molecules: recent advances and applications, KONA Powder and Particle Journal, 35 (2018) 89–111.
70. Z. Zhao, A. Ukidve, V. Krishnan, S. Mitragotri, Effect of physicochemical and surface properties on in vivo fate of drug nanocarriers, Advanced Drug Delivery Reviews, 143 (2019) 3–21.
71. S. Centi, F. Tatini, F. Ratto, A. Gnerucci, R. Mercatelli, G. Romano, I. Landini, S. Nobili, A. Ravalli, G. Marrazza, In vitro assessment of antibody-conjugated gold nanorods for systemic injections, Journal of Nanobiotechnology, 12 (2014) 1–10.

72. F. Tatini, I. Landini, F. Scaletti, L. Massai, S. Centi, F. Ratto, S. Nobili, G. Romano, F. Fusi, L. Messori, Size dependent biological profiles of PEGylated gold nanorods, Journal of Materials Chemistry B, 2 (2014) 6072–6080.

73. J. Pérez-Juste, I. Pastoriza-Santos, L.M. Liz-Marzán, P. Mulvaney, Gold nanorods: synthesis, characterization and applications, Coordination Chemistry Reviews, 249 (2005) 1870–1901.

74. H. Jahangirian, E.G. Lemraski, T.J. Webster, R. Rafiee-Moghaddam, Y. Abdollahi, A review of drug delivery systems based on nanotechnology and green chemistry: green nanomedicine, International Journal of Nanomedicine, 12 (2017) 2957.

75. P.-L. Lam, W.-Y. Wong, Z. Bian, C.-H. Chui, R. Gambari, Recent advances in green nanoparticulate systems for drug delivery: efficient delivery and safety concern, Nanomedicine, 12 (2017) 357–385.

76. M.S. Arayne, N. Sultana, F. Qureshi, Nanoparticles in delivery of cardiovascular drugs, Pakistan Journal of Pharmaceutical Sciences, 20 (2007) 340–348.

77. R.R. Joseph, S.S. Venkatraman, Drug delivery to the eye: what benefits do nanocarriers offer?, Nanomedicine, 12 (2017) 683–702.

78. D. Cross, J.K. Burmester, Gene therapy for cancer treatment: past, present and future, Clinical Medicine & Research, 4 (2006) 218–227.

79. G. Damiani, R. Eggenhöffner, P.D.M. Pigatto, N.L. Bragazzi, Nanotechnology meets atopic dermatitis: current solutions, challenges and future prospects. Insights and implications from a systematic review of the literature, Bioactive materials, 4 (2019) 380–386.

80. B. Ouattara, R.E. Simard, R.A. Holley, G.J.-P. Piette, A. Bégin, Antibacterial activity of selected fatty acids and essential oils against six meat spoilage organisms, International Journal of Food Microbiology, 37 (1997) 155–162.

81. G. Sharma, K. Raturi, S. Dang, S. Gupta, R. Gabrani, Combinatorial antimicrobial effect of curcumin with selected phytochemicals on Staphylococcus epidermidis, Journal of Asian Natural Products Research, 16 (2014) 535–541.

82. H. Chen, S.T. Humes, N.B. Saleh, J.A. Lednicky, T. Sabo-Attwood, Nanomaterial Effects on Viral Infection, Interaction of Nanomaterials with the Immune System, Springer, (2020), pp. 167–195.

83. M. Bilal, M. Barani, F. Sabir, A. Rahdar, G.Z. Kyzas, Nanomaterials for the treatment and diagnosis of Alzheimer's disease: an overview, NanoImpact, (2020) 100251.

84. H.A. Havel, Where are the nanodrugs? An industry perspective on development of drug products containing nanomaterials, The AAPS Journal, 18 (2016) 1351–1353.

85. H. Havel, G. Finch, P. Strode, M. Wolfgang, S. Zale, I. Bobe, H. Youssoufian, M. Peterson, M. Liu, Nanomedicines: from bench to bedside and beyond, The AAPS Journal, 18 (2016) 1373–1378.

86. G. Goya, V. Grazu, M.R. Ibarra, Magnetic nanoparticles for cancer therapy, Current Nanoscience, 4 (2008) 1–16.

87. M.I. Biggs, M.I. Dalby, S.I. Wind, Cellular response to nanoscale features, The Nanobiotechnology Handbook, (2012) 461.

88. M. Veith, S. Mathur, P. König, C. Cavelius, J. Biegler, A. Rammo, V. Huch, H. Shen, G. Schmid, Template-assisted ordering of Pb nanoparticles prepared from molecular-level colloidal processing, Comptes Rendus Chimie, 7 (2004) 509–519.

89. Z. Shi, Y. Zhang, G.O. Phillips, G. Yang, Utilization of bacterial cellulose in food, Food Hydrocolloids, 35 (2014) 539–545.

90. P.C. Ray, H. Yu, P.P. Fu, Toxicity and environmental risks of nanomaterials: challenges and future needs, J Environ Sci Health C Environ Carcinog Ecotoxicol Rev, 27 (2009) 1–35.

91. R.K. Ibrahim, M. Hayyan, M.A. AlSaadi, A. Hayyan, S. Ibrahim, Environmental application of nanotechnology: air, soil, and water, Environmental Science and Pollution Research, 23 (2016) 13754–13788.

92. F.D. Guerra, M.F. Attia, D.C. Whitehead, F. Alexis, Nanotechnology for environmental remediation: materials and applications, Molecules, 23 (2018) 1760.
93. A. Kamyshny, J. Steinke, S. Magdassi, Metal-based inkjet inks for printed electronics, The Open Applied Physics Journal, 4 (2011).
94. J.P. Martins, G. Torrieri, H.A. Santos, The importance of microfluidics for the preparation of nanoparticles as advanced drug delivery systems, Expert Opinion on Drug Delivery, 15 (2018) 469–479.
95. O.V. Salata, Applications of nanoparticles in biology and medicine, Journal of Nanobiotechnology, 2 (2004) 1–6.
96. C. Cunha, S. Panseri, S. Antonini, Emerging nanotechnology approaches in tissue engineering for peripheral nerve regeneration, Nanomedicine: Nanotechnology, Biology and Medicine, 7 (2011) 50–59.
97. E. Smyth, M. Verheij, W. Allum, D. Cunningham, A. Cervantes, D. Arnold, Gastric cancer: ESMO clinical practice guidelines for diagnosis, treatment and follow-up, Annals of Oncology, 27 (2016) v38-v49.
98. Y. Saadeh, D. Vyas, Nanorobotic applications in medicine: current proposals and designs, American Journal of Robotic Surgery, 1 (2014) 4–11.
99. M. Holzinger, A. Le Goff, S. Cosnier, Nanomaterials for biosensing applications: a review, Frontiers in Chemistry, 2 (2014) 63.
100. W.H. De Jong, P.J. Borm, Drug delivery and nanoparticles: applications and hazards, International Journal of Nanomedicine, 3 (2008) 133.
101. E. Song, P. Zhu, S.-K. Lee, D. Chowdhury, S. Kussman, D.M. Dykxhoorn, Y. Feng, D. Palliser, D.B. Weiner, P. Shankar, Antibody mediated in vivo delivery of small interfering RNAs via cell-surface receptors, Nature Biotechnology, 23 (2005) 709–717.
102. S. Hong, P.R. Leroueil, I.J. Majoros, B.G. Orr, J.R. Baker Jr, M.M.B. Holl, The binding avidity of a nanoparticle-based multivalent targeted drug delivery platform, Chemistry & Biology, 14 (2007) 107–115.
103. Y. Pommier, Camptothecins and topoisomerase I: a foot in the door. Targeting the genome beyond topoisomerase I with camptothecins and novel anticancer drugs: importance of DNA replication, repair and cell cycle checkpoints, Current Medicinal Chemistry-Anti-Cancer Agents, 4 (2004) 429–434.
104. R.N. Rosenberg, D. Lambracht-Washington, G. Yu, W. Xia, Genomics of Alzheimer disease: a review, JAMA Neurology, 73 (2016) 867–874.
105. N.J. Abbott, A.A. Patabendige, D.E. Dolman, S.R. Yusof, D.J. Begley, Structure and function of the blood–brain barrier, Neurobiology of Disease, 37 (2010) 13–25.
106. S.A. Pathan, Z. Iqbal, S. Zaidi, S. Talegaonkar, D. Vohra, G.K. Jain, A. Azeem, N. Jain, J.R. Lalani, R.K. Khar, CNS drug delivery systems: novel approaches, Recent Patents on Drug Delivery & Formulation, 3 (2009) 71–89.
107. C. Saraiva, C. Praça, R. Ferreira, T. Santos, L. Ferreira, L. Bernardino, Nanoparticle-mediated brain drug delivery: overcoming blood–brain barrier to treat neurodegenerative diseases, Journal of Controlled Release, 235 (2016) 34–47.
108. V. Georgakilas, K. Kordatos, M. Prato, D.M. Guldi, M. Holzinger, A. Hirsch, Organic functionalization of carbon nanotubes, Journal of the American Chemical Society, 124 (2002) 760–761.
109. A. Fabbro, M. Prato, L. Ballerini, Carbon nanotubes in neuroregeneration and repair, Advanced Drug Delivery Reviews, 65 (2013) 2034–2044.
110. N. Dimov, E. Kastner, M. Hussain, Y. Perrie, N. Szita, Formation and purification of tailored liposomes for drug delivery using a module-based micro continuous-flow system, Scientific Reports, 7 (2017) 1–13.
111. J. Provenzale, G. Silva, Uses of nanoparticles for central nervous system imaging and therapy, American Journal of Neuroradiology, 30 (2009) 1293–1301.

112. M.J. Kim, S.U. Rehman, F.U. Amin, M.O. Kim, Enhanced neuroprotection of anthocyanin-loaded PEG-gold nanoparticles against $A\beta$1-42-induced neuroinflammation and neurodegeneration via the NF-KB/JNK/GSK3β signaling pathway, Nanomedicine: Nanotechnology, Biology and Medicine, 13 (2017) 2533–2544.

113. H. Kim, J.U. Lee, S. Song, S. Kim, S.J. Sim, A shape-code nanoplasmonic biosensor for multiplex detection of Alzheimer's disease biomarkers, Biosensors and Bioelectronics, 101 (2018) 96–102.

114. A. Mars, M. Hamami, L. Bechnak, D. Patra, N. Raouafi, Curcumin-graphene quantum dots for dual mode sensing platform: electrochemical and fluorescence detection of APOe4, responsible of Alzheimer's disease, Analytica Chimica Acta, 1036 (2018) 141–146.

115. J. Oh, G. Yoo, Y.W. Chang, H.J. Kim, J. Jose, E. Kim, J.-C. Pyun, K.-H. Yoo, A carbon nanotube metal semiconductor field effect transistor-based biosensor for detection of amyloid-beta in human serum, Biosensors and Bioelectronics, 50 (2013) 345–350.

116. D. Cui, C. Zhang, B. Liu, Y. Shu, T. Du, D. Shu, K. Wang, F. Dai, Y. Liu, C. Li, Regression of gastric cancer by systemic injection of RNA nanoparticles carrying both ligand and siRNA, Scientific Reports, 5 (2015) 1–14.

117. M. Shahzad Lodhi, Z. Qadir Samra, Purification of transferrin by magnetic nanoparticles and conjugation with cysteine capped gold nanoparticles for targeting diagnostic probes, Preparative Biochemistry and Biotechnology, 49 (2019) 961–973.

118. R. Bor, A. Fábián, Z. Szepes, Role of ultrasound in colorectal diseases, World Journal of Gastroenterol, 22 (2016) 9477.

119. L.R. Tefas, B. Sylvester, I. Tomuta, A. Sesarman, E. Licarete, M. Banciu, A. Porfire, Development of antiproliferative long-circulating liposomes co-encapsulating doxorubicin and curcumin, through the use of a quality-by-design approach, Drug Design, Development and Therapy, 11 (2017) 1605.

120. Q. Zhou, Y. Wei, For better or worse, iron overload by superparamagnetic iron oxide nanoparticles as a MRI contrast agent for chronic liver diseases, Chemical Research in Toxicology, 30 (2017) 73–80.

121. C.E. Sjögren, C. Johansson, A. Nævestad, P.C. Sontum, K. Briley-Sæbø, A.K. Fahlvik, Crystal size and properties of superparamagnetic iron oxide (SPIO) particles, Magnetic Resonance Imaging, 15 (1997) 55–67.

122. M. Campos, I. Candelária, N. Papanikolaou, A. Simão, C. Ferreira, G.C. Manikis, F. Caseiro-Alves, Perfusion magnetic resonance as a biomarker for sorafenib-treated advanced hepatocellular carcinoma: a pilot study, GE-Portuguese Journal of Gastroenterology, 26 (2019) 260–267.

123. Z. Abed, J. Beik, S. Laurent, N. Eslahi, T. Khani, E.S. Davani, H. Ghaznavi, A. Shakeri-Zadeh, Iron oxide–gold core–shell nano-theranostic for magnetically targeted photothermal therapy under magnetic resonance imaging guidance, Journal of Cancer Research and Clinical Oncology, 145 (2019) 1213–1219.

124. B.-l. Ye, R. Zheng, X.-j. Ruan, Z.-h. Zheng, H.-j. Cai, Chitosan-coated doxorubicin nanoparticles drug delivery system inhibits cell growth of liver cancer via p53/PRC1 pathway, Biochemical and Biophysical Research Communications, 495 (2018) 414–420.

125. E.V. Ramos Campos, P.L.D.F. Proença, L. Doretto-Silva, V. Andrade-Oliveira, L.F. Fraceto, D.R. de Araujo, Trends in nanoformulations for atopic dermatitis treatment, Expert Opinion on Drug Delivery, 17 (2020) 1615–1630.

126. F.F. Sahle, C. Gerecke, B. Kleuser, R. Bodmeier, Formulation and comparative in vitro evaluation of various dexamethasone-loaded pH-sensitive polymeric nanoparticles intended for dermal applications, International Journal of Pharmaceutics, 516 (2017) 21–31.

127. A.I. Barbosa, S.A.C. Lima, S. Reis, Development of methotrexate loaded fucoidan/chitosan nanoparticles with anti-inflammatory potential and enhanced skin permeation, International Journal of Biological Macromolecules, 124 (2019) 1115–1122.

128. A. Barras, Q. Pagneux, F. Sane, Q. Wang, R. Boukherroub, D. Hober, S. Szunerits, High efficiency of functional carbon nanodots as entry inhibitors of herpes simplex virus type 1, ACS Applied Materials & Interfaces, 8 (2016) 9004–9013.
129. P.S. Aithal, & S. Aithal, Nanotechnology innovations and commercialization–opportunities, challenges & reasons for delay. International Journal of Engineering and Manufacturing (IJEM), 6 (2016): 15–25.
130. K. Aschberger, H. Rauscher, H. Crutzen, K. Rasmussen, F.M. Christensen, B. Sokull-Klüttgen, H. Stamm, Considerations on information needs for nanomaterials in consumer products, European Commission Joint Research Centre Institute for Health and Consumer Protection, Brussels, (2014).
131. E.S. Kawasaki, A. Player, Nanotechnology, nanomedicine, and the development of new, effective therapies for cancer. Nanomedicine: Nanotechnology, Biology and Medicine, 1(2), (2005) 101–109.
132. P.J. Borm, D. Robbins, S. Haubold, T. Kuhlbusch, H. Fissan, K. Donaldson, & E. Oberdorster, The potential risks of nanomaterials: a review carried out for ECETOC, Particle and Fibre Toxicology, 3(1), (2006) 1–35.
133. S.K. Sahoo, S. Parveen, J.J. Panda, The present and future of nanotechnology in human health care, Nanomedicine: Nanotechnology, Biology and Medicine, 3(1), (2007) 20–31.

2 Nanoengineered Biomaterials for Tissue Regeneration
Properties Overview

Kalpana Madgula
SAS Nanotechnologies LLC

Venkata Sreenivas Puli
Air Force Research Laboratory
Smart Nanomaterials Solutions LLC

CONTENTS

DOI: 10.1201/9781003140108-2

2.1   INTRODUCTION

Nanoscale materials are produced in single dimension or in multidimensions [1, 2]. Materials such as metals, ceramics, and naturally occurring or synthetic biopolymers that are porous and exist in nanodimensions or contain nanostructured surface morphologies are known to interact with tissues and organs of human body. These material classes, due to their resemblance to native cellular matrices in terms of structure, chemical properties, cell interactions, and inherent ability to blend, can help in generating cells and tissues. Nanoengineered biomaterials are mainly utilized for repair, replacement, and treatment of various ailments, including cancer, cardiovascular abnormalities, ocular aging, and inflammatory and infectious diseases [3, 4].

Tissue engineering (TE) as a part of regenerative medicine has drawn attention as it has provided innovative tools for repairing organs that fail or to replace tissues that get damaged [5] and can help develop novel design or strategies for organs or tissue repair [6]. Among the number of therapies available to fix or replace organs or tissues, one of the most common is the use of biomaterials as building blocks in advanced repair in tissues of skin, heart, nervous system, and cornea[7]. Biomaterials can be prepared to integrate into the body with special characteristics that can facilitate the contact (or compatibility) with human cells, tissue, and organs to avoid the body's rejection. The therapies can include cell therapy (i.e.., with stem cell, that are immature and can potentially mature or produce any vital tissue or cell). Bioengineering explores the applicability of biomaterials, whereas regenerative medicine uses medications, practices, and treatment by drugs. Recent progress either combines new methods or improves existing ones, with new strategies to repair damaged organs or tissue that was previously thought impossible.

Biomaterials have improved significantly since their discovery and now are created from various materials. For example, natural components found in the body (e.g., collagen [8]) or in sea weed (e.g., alginate [9]) or synthetic materials or combinations, such as metals and ceramics [10]. The earliest biomaterials did not interact with body but they do have physical properties similar to the organs or tissue they were repairing or replacing in the body. For example, prosthetics, or artificial body parts, in limbs or heart are used to replace damaged parts but often get rejected. Today's biomaterials are aimed at interacting with cellular components to stimulate healing and regeneration. "Bioactive" means to interact and communicate with the body by forming chemical bonds with tissues. For example, hip implants [11] could help in promoting bone growth that could stimulate the formation of a calcium layer (also known as hydroxyapatite, HA) to grow on the implant. Similarly, the third or next generation biomaterials [12] are allowed to interact with body to elicit a specific response from cells in the body, and they can also replicate the body's native 3D structure and could stimulate tissue regeneration (re-growth) or biocompatibility (i.e., no significant cell damage and good cell growth and attachment), and implants can allow the body to heal itself. The tremendous improvement in the biomaterials is now aimed to continuously improve or change the material properties for their effective operation in patients' bodies.

Even though biomaterials can take different forms or be made from different materials, ideally they should have "porous" structure' [13] that should allow gases, liquids, or even cells to move through them, and they should resemble the organ or tissue they are intended to repair. The pores on the material also can be loaded with the cells or drugs with the aim of repairing the damaged tissue, and also the biomaterial helps to retain the new cells that promote the healing. In addition, the porous structure imitates "extracellular matrix"(ECM), which is like a scaffolding that cells "hold on to" in the body. Biomaterials themselves can be directly used in the body or as "carriers" to deliver cells or drugs [14] to repair the damaged organ or tissue. For example, the biomaterial can be used to help heal and repair the damage done to the heart due to a heart attack. For this it can be used alone or carry cells (stem cells, which can be differentiated into other cells, including heart cells or cardiomyocytes) [15]. The biomaterials can be designed and tuned to get degraded or broken down after they heal or made to release certain medications that can help healing. Future developments are aimed to propose new therapies and artificial organs to eliminate long waiting lists for organ transplants [16].

2.2 NANOENGINEERED BIOMATERIALS: "MEETING OF BIO WITH NANO" AT THE INTERFACE

2.2.1 "BIOMATERIALS CAN BE ENGINEERED TO HELP HEAL THE NON-HEALING TISSUES OR ORGANS"

Organs fail for many different reasons, frequently due to a combination of factors. One of the most common organs to fail and difficult to heal is heart. The term "cardiovascular disease" (CVD) [17] refers to illness caused to the heart and blood vessels, and patients with CVD always have a risk of heart attack, which can cause significant damage to the heart and lead to the death of heart cells. The damage can further damage or cause loss of heart muscle, which is made up of beating cells called "cardiomyocytes." The loss of cardiomyocytes will reduce the heart's ability to pump blood throughout the body, and it is believed that it is not possible to regenerate the cardiomyocytes [18].

As we are still in the process of understanding the potential regenerative capabilities of the human body, many organs, such as the heart, are slow to heal; this can lead to the damage that poses challenges to heal or treat. Transplantation is an option for replacing a damaged tissue or organ. However, there is a severe shortage of organs available for transplant [19]. As an alternative to organ transplantation, regenerative medicine is showing promise as a therapy to repair the heart and other slow-healing organs.

2.2.2 Significance of Nano-dimensions and Implants for Regeneration

The beginning of this century [20] witnessed enormous growth in regenerative medicine due to the combined efforts of material scientists, biologist, and physicians. The properties of nanostructured materials, nanoparticles (NPs), nanotubes (NTs), nanofibers, surfaces, or assemblies in nanodimensions are functionalized by biomolecules such as peptides and growth factors (GFs), or biocompatible/bioactive platforms are used to improve cellular activities and interactions. These interactions are not only limited to cell adhesion, proliferation, and differentiation but also to promote tissue regeneration. Thus, to carry out all cell functions, nanoengineered materials are equipped with suitable mechanical properties – superior bioactive functions with enhanced cellular activity. In addition, nanodimensions provide enhanced specific surface area and behavior tuned with controlled release that could facilitate the mechanism to fabricate bio-mimic constructs that could simplify construction and complete regeneration [21].

Tissue engineering repairs or regenerates the tissue by the culture of cells reaped from the body of a donor or the patient. This culture is placed onto a suitable material and, after regeneration, is implanted back into patient's body at the appropriate anatomical location [22]. After successful delivery to the targeted site, the cells are believed to consolidate with tissue at the location, and gradual degradation of the scaffold will follow. Alternatively, in vivo tissue regeneration can be triggered where the direct implantation of scaffold will be performed into the patient's body; this can trigger endogenous cells to mature and proliferate on the template or scaffold [23] along with other surrounding tissue. Both of these methods have the advantage of utilizing biomaterials from natural biological molecules, synthetic polymers, composites, or ceramics, and different combinations of all these materials have a major role to play in tuning the physico/bio/chemical attributes to achieve the desired clinical result [24].

2.2.3 Significance of Extracellular Matrix (ECM): Its Interaction with Cells and Cellular Function

It is very challenging and intricate phenomenon to be able to develop and retain huge amounts of viable, functional cells and also to attain the precise control of a device that is implanted, control cell phenotype and other functionalities of the cell. Factors that can control the cell behavior can be exogenous, endogenous mechanical forces, surface chemistry or environment of the biomaterial, and other pharmacological indicators that exist in soluble state [25]. Stem cell biology offers examples to understand the transition of stem cells into mature tissue cells on exposure to ECM; its properties such as matrix structure, composition, or elastic ability are able to influence the above-mentioned forces that a cell can apply on its matrix. These biophysical signals are converted into biochemical signals that bind the cell to a precise lineage through mechanosensitive avenues [26]. ECM properties such as matrix composition, chemistry, and biochemical and mechanical signals develop in harmony. Cell–ECM interactions are well studied [27–31] in stem cells as well as in adult cells. In vitro stimuli – sensitive adult cells and the signals associated with them can further induce the change in forces generated by the cells, or in turn these forces can also influence the cell properties. Innovative material combinations have enabled recreation of morphology or stimuli conditions of in vitro to suit the in vivo conditions.

2.3 TYPES OF BIOMATERIALS, BIOMATERIAL SYNTHESIS, AND FABRICATION SUITABLE FOR TISSUE ENGINEERING APPLICATIONS

The success of biomaterials for engineering and repairing tissue depends on their interaction at the site of implantation and their ability to influence the biological activity necessary for tissue regeneration. Different kinds of biomaterials have been used for scaffold production, such as ceramics and polymers, naturals and synthetics, metals, composites, and hydrogels. Table 2.1a [32] lists and compares various biomaterials that are commonly used in TE with benefits and limitations, and Table 2.1b [33–58] provides examples of biomaterial combinations with their chemical composition displaying unique features.

TABLE 2.1a
Types of Biomaterials with Benefits and Limitations

	Advantages	Disadvantages	Clinical Uses
Ceramics	Hard surface, high mechanical stiffness, chemical-physics refractoriness, high biocompatibility, osteoconductivity	Brittleness, slow degradation, processing difficulties	Hip prosthesis, dental prosthesis, bone and cartilage
Natural Polymers	Biocompatibility, bioactivity	Poor mechanical properties, Fast biodegradation	Bone and cartilage, tendon and ligament reconstruction (e.g. collagen)
Synthetic Polymers	Possibility of modulating porosity and mechanical properties during the synthesis process	Low biocompatibility: possible release of ions and other residual particles of polymerization, low mechanical strength	Sutures, catheters, cardiovascular prostheses, bone cements
Metals	Good mechanical properties: high elastic module, yield strength, and high ductility	Reduced cell adhesion to their surface, possible corrosion mediated by biological fluid	Dentistry and orthopedic prostheses
Composites	Biocompatibility, good mechanical properties	Processing difficulties	Hard and soft tissues
Hydrogel	Biocompatibility, controlled biodegradation in vivo, possibility to modulate their parameters [cross-linking density, porosity, pore size and interconnectivity]		Hard and soft tissues

Source: Adapted with Permission from Ref [32]; copyright 2019; CC BY 4.0 http://dx.doi.org/10.5772/intechopen.83839

TABLE 2.1b
Illustrating Biomaterial Combinations with Their Chemical Composition Displaying Unique Features

Type, Chemical Composition, or Formula	References	Remarks
Ceramics	33–40	Bioglass can be made by polymer
1. CaP, calcium phosphates, including hydroxyapatite (HA) ($Ca_{10}[PO_4]_6[OH]_2$), beta-tricalcium phosphate (BTF) ($Ca_3[PO_4]_2$), biphasic calcium phosphate (mixture of hydroxyapatite and beta-tricalcium phosphate) 2. Bioglass, e.g., 45 wt% SiO_2, 24.5 wt% CaO, 24.5 wt% Na_2O, and 6.0 wt% P_2O_5 (Ref – Hench) 3. Alumina (Al_2O_3), and (4) zirconia oxide (ZrO_2).		foam replication, thermal bonding of particles or fibers, and sol-gel processing
Natural polymers or biological polymers Collagen, alginate, proteoglycans, chitin, and chitosan	41–46 (collagen 47, 48 (chitin, chitosan and alginate)	Chitin, chitosan and alginate – used for both hard- and soft-tissue generation Physical forms – fibers, films, hydrogels
Synthetic polymers – polystyrene (PS) Thermoplastic aromatic polymer with a linear structure; **polylactic acid (PLA)**, hydrophobic polymer with slow degradation rate due to microorganisms; polyglycolic acid (PGA), hydrophilic polymer with good mechanical properties and fast degradation; poly-lactic-co-glycolic acid (PLGA), biocompatible copolymers with fast degradation rate; and polycaprolactone (PCL), highly hydrophobic polymer with good permeability	49	Low biocompatibility and mechanical strength and show in vivo toxicity due to the release of ions and other residual particles of polymerization. bio-erodible – polymers undergo surface degradation with production of nontoxic low molecular weight compounds. PGA and PLA and their copolymers are natural polyesters normally present in the organism and therefore well tolerated.
Metals Stainless steel (SS): iron-based alloys with a low content of carbon and a high content of chromium Cobalt (Co): cobalt-based alloys 1. cobalt/chromium (Cr)/molybdenum(Mo) alloy – casting/melting 2. cobalt/nickel/chromium/molybdenum alloy worked by forging Titanium alloys: *alpha, beta, or alpha/beta* biphasic 1. alpha-alpha stabilizers such as aluminum and gallium – good strength, hardness, resistance sliding 2. *Beta* alloys stabilizers such as vanadium, niobium, and tantalus molybdenum – good ductility 3. *Alpha/beta* biphasic alloys show a mix of *alpha/beta* stabilizers – quite ductile even if little resistant to high temperatures (e.g., Ti_6Al_4V).	50, 51	SS – due to carbide formation, their scaffold is subject to corrosion in a biological environment. Co-based alloys – high level of Cr and Mo – it is typical of these alloys to increase granule size and improve mechanical properties.

(Continued)

TABLE 2.1b (*Continued*)
Illustrating Biomaterial Combinations with Their Chemical Composition Displaying Unique Features

Type, Chemical Composition, or Formula	References	Remarks
Composites 1. natural or synthetic polymers (PGA, PLA, gelatin, chitin, and chitosan) 2. ceramics (hydroxyapatite and beta-tricalcium phosphate or bioglass) and metals	52–55	Technological, industrial, and applicative importance as they combine biocompatibility, biodegradation, and appreciable mechanical strength. Scaffolds could be applied for both hard- and soft-tissue regeneration and greatly mimic tissue architecture being composed of cells and extracellular matrix.
Hydrogels Hydrophilic polymers with polar functional groups: carboxyl, amide, amino, and hydroxyl groups 1. natural (made of polypeptides and polysaccharides) 2. synthetic (obtained by traditional polymerization) 3. semi-synthetic 4. amorphous or semi-crystalline structure –cationic, anionic, neutral, or ampholytic 5. smart hydrogels – ease of modifying their structure and mechanical properties in response to environmental stimuli, pH or temperature	56–58	Crosslinked, ability to absorb large amounts of water or biological fluids, swell without dissolving Biodegradable – degrade into oligomers and eliminated from the body Controlled in vivo degradation, biocompatibility Parameters can be modified suitable for cell proliferation and colonization Hydrogels modified at the surface by peptides or growth factor, which can promote cell attachment and differentiation process **Natural hydrogels** are less toxic and more tolerated (e.g., natural cellulose-hydroxyapatite hybrid hydrogel for bone tissue engineering). **Synthetic hydrogels** – limitations in the biocompatibility, but they offer the possibility to modulate their mechanical features and rate of degradation in biological environment. Biodegradable oligo [(poly(ethylene glycol)fumarate] hydrogel to deliver demineralized bone matrix (DBM) in a rat bone defect.

2.3.1 Brief Note on Biomaterial Hydrogels

Hydrogels are regarded as dynamic systems made up of semi solid hydrophilic polymer materials (or backbone) with rich polar groups such as carboxyl, hydroxyl, amine, and amide that are held together by chemical links or physical links (intermolecular or intramolecular). They have the unique ability to swell when they absorb massive amounts of water or biological fluids without dissolving. Hydrogels with features on the order of one dimension in the range of micrometers to a few tens of nanometers are called micro-engineered hydrogels. These hydrogels are characterized by high resolution in space, engineered for special functions, and are usually fabricated by the technique's emulsification, photolithography, microfluidic synthesis, and micro-molding [59–62] (Table 2.1c).

Based on their origin and preparation methods, they can be classified into natural (prepared from polypeptides and polysaccharides), synthetic (conventional polymerization techniques), and semi-synthetic. Further, they can be amorphous or semi crystalline (cationic, anionic, neutral, or ampholytic). The second generation of hydrogels [63] are called stimuli-responsive hydrogels (or smart hydrogels) and further divided into physical-responsive hydrogels (temperature-responsive hydrogels, photo/light-responsive hydrogels, electro- and magnetic- responsive hydrogels), and chemical-responsive hydrogels (pH-responsive hydrogels, glucose-responsive hydrogels, and biological/biochemical-responsive hydrogels). The hydrogels can be prepared by chemical means (free radical polymerization), by physical means to transform solid to gel, or by crosslinking by irradiating the polymer precursors; and they can be fabricated by number of approaches, including freeze-drying methods or lyophilization, electrospinning, conventional sol-gel, leaching of porogens, or advanced techniques like 3D printing (or bio-inks) and photolithography

The structural and mechanical properties of hydrogels can vary depending upon the type of precursor used for preparation and the function for which they are intended to be utilized. The hydrogels constitute strong chemical crosslinks and weak physical association, and the elastic modulus can range from kilopascals to megapascals (Kpa to MPa). The properties tuned to allow cell viability in the hydrogel structure dependent on stiffness of the gel to allow cells to orient and migrate (e.g., in the case

---

TABLE 2.1c
List of Smart Hydrogels and Their Applications in Tissue Engineering Medicine

Hydrogel	Application
Temperature-responsive hydrogels	Skin-tissue engineering, wound covering, cell carriers
Light-responsive hydrogels	Drug delivery, microfluidic devices
Electro-responsive hydrogels	Membrane- and implant-based drug delivery
Magnetic-responsive hydrogels	Drug delivery, tissue repair, targeted MRI for disease diagnosis
pH-responsive hydrogels	Drug and protein delivery, 3 D cell culture
Glucose-responsive hydrogels	Immuno-isolation devices
Biochemical-responsive hydrogels	Smart sensors and actuators
Collagen-based hydrogels	Corneal, tendon-tissue engineering
Injectable hydrogels	Bone, cartilage, and meniscus tissue engineering, drug delivery, osteoarthritis therapy

Source: Adapted with permission from Ref [63]; copyright 2019, MDPI; an open access article distributed and licensed by MDPI, Basel, Switzerland (CC BY 4.0).

of wound healing hydrogels [64]). They are also characterized by unique rheology (e.g., temperature-dependent viscosity). Controlled surface and tuned degradation profile and hydrogels with enhanced physical properties like conductivity, stress-bearing, or chemical resistance are also being studied by blending functional polymers (e.g., conducting polymers) during fabrication.

In addition, hydrogels are characterized by microscopic techniques, (SEM or Cryo), swelling studies/elastic moduli or water content, thermal- or pH-responsive behaviors, crosslinking degree, porosity and permeation capability, and assessment of in vitro antimicrobial activity.

2.4 BIOMATERIALS THAT MIMIC THE ECM AND ACT AS SCAFFOLDS

Extracellular matrix (ECM), controls cellular functions with an extensive network of molecules and comprises primarily glycosaminoglycan, glycoconjugate, and proteins components. These components, along with receptors that help in adhesion of cell, could result in a crosslinking framework for cells or tissues to reside in the matrix. The significance of ECM in tissue remodeling has been studied for neuronal regeneration and wound healing mechanisms in the presence of human umbilical mesenchymal conditioned medium (HU-MSCM) [65]. It is possible to predict cell performances by in vitro studies based on the generated biophysical parameters of biomaterials made by using micro or nanoengineering strategies. However, for in vivo study, which is controlled by multi-parameters and a three-dimensional cell microenvironment, it is important to understand the functional role of cell microenvironment interactions in regulating cellular functions [66].

Current efforts are aimed at the development and design of integrated (micro/nano) engineered functional biomaterials for use in varied fields, including regenerative medicine, drug delivery, cellular biology, and disease diagnosis/progression. Various biomaterials have been engineered to create a local cell micro environment for in vitro study. The matrices are further utilized to study a mechanism that converts mechanical stimulus into electrochemical activity (i.e., mechano-sensitive and responsive cellular behaviors). The parameters that are of major influence in TE and regeneration are:

- Nano-dimensional moieties that boost the cell adhesion, proliferation and differentiating properties; Nanoengineered biomaterials are comparable to ECMs in terms of physical structure and chemical composition.
- Nanomaterials can be reinforced into synthetic or natural biomaterials (or to form scaffolds) to provide mechanical strength analogous to natural ECM.
- Nanoengineered materials can be used for the encapsulation of growth factors or bioactive systems for the slow or on demand release at the projected site, thus facilitating enhanced interaction of scaffolds or nanoengineered matrices with cells or proteins that further improve their bioavailability and biocompatibility.

Moreover, ECM is topographically characterized by materials such as collagen and elastin nanofibers in the 10–300 nm diameter range, giving rise to a groovy, ridged, pitted, porous, and fibrillar network of nano morphologies that suggests the role of surface morphology in regulating and expressing biochemical signals by cell inter-action. To control cell functionalities, these scaffolds are engineered at the scale of micro or nanosizes to result in reactions that are highly precise, to the scale of cellular and molecular dimensions. The cell behavior and formation of tissue is con-trolled by the pattern of the scaffold that contains specific chemical and structural info. Thus, the nanoscale geography provides greater control over behavior of a cell, which was further illustrated by [66–68] focusing on nanoengineered biomaterials for vascular (heart) tissue, skin, and cartilage tissue engineering and regeneration. Nanomaterials also found applications for other biomedical avenues such as drug or bioactive compounds delivery and controlled release of therapeutics, which are discussed in the number of other reviews [69, 70] in the literature.

2.4.1 SCAFFOLD ASSEMBLY AND FABRICATION

The coupling of porous structure with the nano (or micro) structured substrate offers a powerful platform to manufacture regenerative tissue as the scaffold mimics the ECM dimension, topography, and conditions. Most of the fabrication strategies used to arrive at such scaffolds included electrospinning, phase-separation, and self-assembly approaches [71, 72]. For example, fabrication of nanofibers from electrospinning of materials [73] such as silk fibroin, collagen, polyurethanes, and polyesters etc., can help control the parameters such as thickness, composition, and varying porosity in nanofibers and moreover these nanofibers can be allowed to form interconnections using a simple experimental setup. Further the composition of each class (synthetic or natural polymers) is tuned to suit the desired properties (e.g., biodegradable/non-biodegradable), blends (wide range of mechanical and biological properties) or size (a few micrometers to nanometers (3nm)) with predictable large surface areas and porosities (above 90%) with a range of pore sizes from a few microns to tens of micron to allow permeation of cells and efficient, active transport of nutrients and waster products in and out of the cells. ECM proteins and/or bioactive components can be functionalized on the nanofibers to obtain a scaffold that mimics the bio/chemical and physical features of ECM structure and functional capabilities (where cells can be nurtured to grow, adhere, proliferate, migrate, and differentiate) [74–76].

Scaffolds with complex geometries, or porosities (above 98%), are fabricated by the simple phase-separation method (resembling 3D porous scaffold structures) that involves thermodynamic mixing of a homogenous polymer solution (into the phase of polymer rich and polymer poor), and separation is achieved by either forming insoluble phase or by cooling. Tuning fabrication conditions such as polymer con-centration and/or molecular weight or viscosity results in varying properties for both synthetic and natural polymer materials [77]. (For example, if the viscosity is high, it results in low porosity and an increase in mechanical properties of the scaffold.) Another technique such as molecular self-assembly is the reorganization of various intermolecular forces covalent bonds that are hydrophobic (e.g., alkyl tails), Van der Waals, electrostatic and hydrogen bonding (e.g., disulfide bonds, ligands, or amphi-philes that are cell adhesive) in nature to form stable energy conformational, ordered structures with manifold dimensions or scales of scaffold structures with varying concentration or pH or temperature and introducing the metal ions [78, 79].

2.4.2   SCAFFOLD MATERIAL PROPERTIES THAT INFLUENCE TE APPLICATIONS (PORE SIZE, POROSITY, AND INTERCONNECTIVITY)

In design of the scaffolds, important structural, functional, and mechanical features play a major role. Again, the structural properties that influence can be macro, referred as short-lived crosslinked 3D constructs that imitate the native ECM to allow cell differentiation or micro features that influence porosity in scaffolds, shape, and size of pores and the interconnections within the matrix. On the other had mechanical strength and stiffness influence the mechanical properties in biomaterial-based scaffolds. These two properties balance to maintain integrity between mechanical strength and porosity to produce scaffolds or implants in tissue engineering.

Another parameter that can influence the performance of biomaterial scaffolds in TE applications is pore size as well as pore shape of the porous scaffolds. Pore shape with pore interconnectivities can determine the unique properties like – cell penetration into scaffolds, essential vascularization that help form new blood capillaries which can help to improve or supply essential oxygen or nutrients for viability and survival of cells. To achieve these unique features, pore sizes can be large to allow the movement and penetration of cells or sufficiently small to allow the binding of cells in critical numbers for efficient expression. For example, pores can be in the size range of micro (0.1 to 2 nm), meso (2 to 50 nm) or macro (more than 50 nm), based on dimensions; most of the scaffolds have precise pore sizes and macroporous structures as functional for the supporting tissue of the host [80]. For soft-tissue healing applications, as in hepatocyte and growth of fibroblasts, pore size of 20 microns and dimension of 20–150 microns are needed, whereas to heal the bone tissue, the size range of pores may vary from 200 to 400 microns [81]. The unique sizes of pores or porosity of the scaffolds biomaterials and composites are fabricated by various methods such as gas foaming, salt leaching, phase separation, sintering, and freeze-drying [82].

Mechanical properties such as integrity or strength of scaffold and its stiffness play a major role to support the implant or scaffold till the tissue is completely healed or remodeled. The mechanical strength depends on the bonds that hold the integrity of the scaffold, avoiding the deformation of the scaffold while loading the cells or handling the scaffolds. Another feature, stiffness measured by Youngs modulus, allows the cells respond to stiffness by various mechanisms such as ion channels activation or unfolding of the proteins that affect the differentiation and proliferation of cells. For example, increasing the stiffness of free-floating collagen matrices increases cell proliferation rates in human dermal fibroblasts [83], as reported in the literature.

Figure 2.1 illustrates the 3D mineralized cell-laden porous scaffolds with optimized stiffness and are fabricated from bio-ink prepared using unmodified polymers of alginate and gelatin combining hMSCs [84]. These bioink printed 3D scaffolds reported by Zhang et al used varying mineral content to achieve soft (0.8% alg) and stiff (1.8% alg) type gels and varying cell densities. They further combined in vitro micro-CT–based imaging with 3D bioprinting and a bioreactor system, which mimics the in vivo conditions, and then investigated the mineral formation over time lapse. The time-lapsed reconstruction of micro-CT over 42 days confirmed that the cells' soft scaffolds are better proliferated and osteogenically differentiated compared to the stiffer ones. As shown in the figure, similar morphology of the cell is

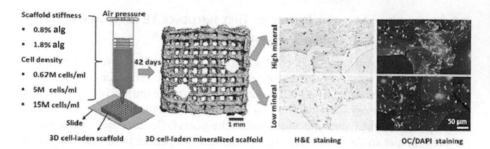

FIGURE 2.1 Exemplifying the effect of mechanical properties on cell function. Optimization of the stiffness and cell density in a 3D-printed cell (hMSCSs) laden scaffolds with varying alginate/gelatin amounts. (1) 3D bioprinting of cell-laden scaffolds—soft (0.8% alg) and stiff (1.8% alg) with varying cell densities. (2) 3D cell mineralized scaffold – reconstruction of micro-CT on day 42 – culturing in osteogenic media for 42 days, more mineralized in soft than in stiff scaffolds (3) Investigating the nuclei and osteocalcin protein expression by immunostaining of same cryosection for high mineral and low mineral regions – increased osteocalcin expression for both the groups. Adapted with permission from Ref [84]; Copyright 2020; Attribution 4.0 International (CC BY 4.0).

observed in low- and high-mineral areas of both the groups of cell-laden scaffolds, but more cells are spread for soft gels than stiff gels, and expressed osteocalcin was observed with higher amounts of mineralized ECM in both groups.

2.4.3 Engineering the Micro/Nanoscale Surface Topography

The dimensions of surface topography in cell-ECM interface ranging from tens (i.e., fibrillar collagens in the ECM of connective tissue) to a few nanometers (i.e., fibronectin fibrils) are shown in Table 2.2 [85–94]. Similarly, cell adhesion systems, or

---

TABLE 2.2

Effect of Surface Morphology and Nanoscale Characteristics of Various Substrates (e.g., Nanoengineered Biomaterials as Compared to Metallic Biomimetic Nanostructures) on the Behavior of Cells and Cell Interations

Substrate (Biomaterials or Composite) Used for Scaffolds	Cell Type	Nanoscale Feature and Size	Properties or Modifications	Reference
PEG	Primary cardiomyocytes	Array of pillars (150 nm wide and 400 nm high)	Improved cellular adhesion and retained their conductive and contractile properties	[85]
Ti	hMSC	Surface protrusions 15 nm in height, 28 nm wide and 40 nm spacing	Improved cellular adhesion and spreading	[86]

(Continued)

TABLE 2.2 (*Continued*)

Effect of Surface Morphology and Nanoscale Characteristics of Various Substrates (e.g., Nanoengineered Biomaterials as Compared to Metallic Biomimetic Nanostructures) on the Behavior of Cells and Cell Interations

Substrate (Biomaterials or Composite) Used for Scaffolds	Cell Type	Nanoscale Feature and Size	Properties or Modifications	Reference
PS and poly (4-bromostyrene)	EC	Islands 13 nm, 35 nm and 95 nm in height	Improved cellular adhesion and spreading	[87]
PMMA	hMSC	Pits 100 nm deep and 120 nm in diameter in both ordered and disordered arrays	Increased cellular adhesion and function on disordered array	[88]
PEG	Neonatal rat ventricular myocytes	Grooves 50 nm wide, 200 nm high and a ridge of 150 nm	Increased cellular adhesion, spreading and function	[89]
TiO$_2$ (a material used for clinical titanium implantations for the purpose of bone, joint, or tooth replacements)	HSC	Pits of 15 nm wide, 1.5 m deep and 15 nm spaced	Increase in cellular adhesion, proliferation, migration, and differentiation	[90]
Al$_2$O$_3$	SMC	200 and 10 nm pores	No response in cell adhesion, an alteration in cell morphology. But increase in cell proliferation for cells grown on 200-nm pore surfaces than on 20-nm pore surfaces	[91]
PCLLGA	Human vSMC	Microchannels 160 m long, 300 m wide with gaps of 40 m	Cells proliferate well initially, indicative of synthetic phenotype, but change to a contractile phenotype upon confluence	[92]

Abbreviations: PEG: polyethylene glycol; PGS: polyglycerol sebacate; Ti: Titanium; PMMA: poly (methyl methacrylate); TiO$_2$: titanium dioxide; Al$_2$O$_3$: alumina; PCLLGA: poly(Ɛ-caprolactone-r-l-lactide-r-glycolide); HSC: hematopoietic stem cells; EC: Endothelial cells; hMSC: Human mesenchymal stem cells; SMC: Smooth muscle cells; vSMCs: Vascular smooth muscle cells.

focal adhesions (Fas), also have a broad range of 10 nm to 10 μm, suggesting that the adherent cells may sense and respond to micro/nanoscale ECM topographical signals through cell-ECM adhesive interactions and subsequent adhesion mediated signaling. Innovative fabrication methods have been utilized to arrive at different synthetic surfaces based on various functional biomaterials to create regular, short-range order and completely random distributed topographies to elicit desired cellular behaviors. The master, or primary, scaffold materials would be hard (except the case of glass and quartz), brittle, and opaque and are not cyto-compatible or cannot be complied by bio-imaging approaches. Hence, transparent or intermediate materials, called stamps, are used (e.g., replica molding and related molding techniques, such as a simple organic polymer casting procedure to masters followed by thermal or UV or photo curing). A soft lithography technique has been utilized to create regular nano, microscale patterns from stamps to secondary synthetic surfaces/substrates like PDMS, gold, and hydrogel [95–97]. Polydimethyl siloxane (PDMS), an elastic, transparent, and biocompatible material, works well in the range of 500 nm or more [97]. Mechanical stiffness is the ability of ECM to resist deformation in response to a continual mechanical force acting on it. Thus, the mechanical properties of tissues that are pathological are altered greatly compared to native tissues under normal conditions [98, 99].

The stiffness of the substrate and/or the specific shape of the cell is altered by surface modification and is mostly regulated by myosin motor proteins, which can produce traction forces against the matrix; further, these forces can be restricted by pharmacological interventions that can block differentiation of the cells. The various mechanisms that define these mechanical forces responsible for rigid/stiffness of the matrix can be explained by conformational changes of proteins that are force sensitive (existing in focal adhesion points) or within the matrix, changes in activity of surface receptors (e.g., cell surface receptors or other molecule that function by activation of Rho) and calcium channels activating the stretch among others. For example, a heart attack can create a rigid scar in the muscle, which can inhibit the differentiation of MSC (mesenchymal stem cell) into muscle, instead it may induce trans differentiation to give rise to bone-like lesions in the muscle. Thus, the diseased tissues often overexpress ECM components, making the tissue more rigid, which could inhibit a cell's contractile ability [100, 101]

2.5 ILLUSTRATIVE DISCUSSION ON FEATURES OF NANOENGINEERED BIOMATERIALS UTILIZED FOR APPLICATIONS IN TISSUE ENGINEERING

Rodriguez et al. [102] synthesized magnetic core–shell nanostructures consisting of a polymeric (acrylic) core, a first shell of magnetic iron oxide nanoparticles, and an additional layer of polyethylene glycol (PEG). These composites were prepared with the aim of being used as the magnetic phase in novel magnetic field-responsive tissue substitutes or Poly@Mag@PEG composites. As prepared Poly@Mag@PEG composites were combined or blended with fibrin-agarose hydrogels (FAH) containing human oral mucosa fibroblasts to obtain magnetic field-responsive tissue substitutes. Here the magnetic properties were tuned by varying the precursor concentration. As compared to bare or solid magnetic NPs (MNPs) with the same sized core shell, the prepared composited were having higher magnetic response and increase in the response was noticeable as the magnetic shell became thinner. This low-density polymer core further helped in stabilizing the core-shell particles against gravitational settling. Here, the outer layer of PEG offered biocompatibility and nanocomposites (Poly@Mag@PEG) when loaded into fibrin-agarose hydrogels (mimic the tissue constructs) promoted the interaction of cells, and therefore both nanocomposites and magnetic tissue constructs showed increased in vivo stability and metabolic activity towards the cells, in both the cases i.e., subcutaneous injection and implantation.

These MNPs were composed by a polycrystalline magnetite core coated with methyl methacrylate co-hydroxyl ethyl methacrylate-co-ethylene glycol dimethacrylate (MMA-co-HEMA-co-EGDMA). The MagNP-OH particles were prepared for analyses following previously described procedures. Figure 2.2.1 A to C shows that the magnetic nanoparticles (MNPs) are polycrystalline aggregates with polymeric matrix coating and surrounding each aggregate; MagNP-OH (hydroxy functionalized MNPs) reveals the soft ferromagnetic character in correlation with

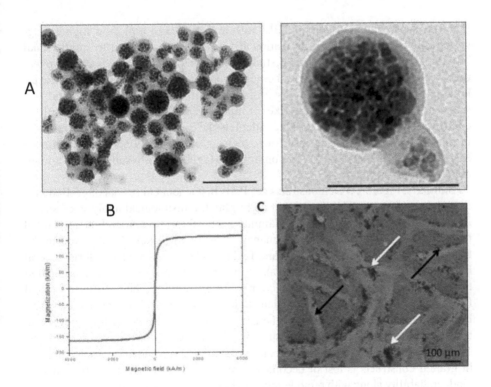

FIGURE 2.2.1 **Magnetic NPs composed by a polycrystalline magnetite core coated with methyl methacrylate co-hydroxyl ethyl methacrylate-co-ethylene glycol dimethacrylate (MMA-co-HEMA-co-EGDMA).** The in vitro characterization of the MagNP-OH particles used in this study. (A) Transmission electron microscopy ultrastructural analysis of MagNP-OH particles. Scale bar: 200 nm (left) and 100 nm (right). (B) Magnetization curve of MagNP-OH particles. (C) Phase contrast microscopy image of human fibroblasts cultured with MagNP-OH particles. Cells are labeled with black arrows, and MagNP-OH particles are highlighted with white arrows. MagNP-OH particles were prepared for analyses following previously described procedures. Adapted with permission from Ref [103].

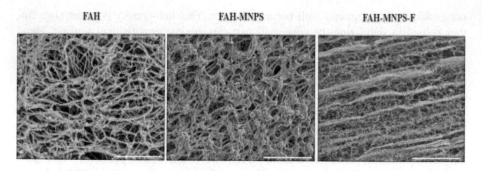

FIGURE 2.2.2   SEM analysis of materials used in this study. FAH: fibrin-agarose hydrogels; FAH-MNPs: FAH containing MagNPOH; FAH-MNPs-F: FAH containing MagNP-OH subjected to a magnetic field during gelation. Scale bar 10 μm. Adapted with permission from Ref [103].

literature where the multidomain NPs (>50nm, here 70±18 nm) show higher magnetic response (saturated magnetization 161 ± 7 kA/m compared to small (usual 30–40nm) particles [103]. In vitro studies of MagNP-OH particles could reveal that these are cytocompatible with homogeneous distribution around the extracellular space, and when co-cultured with human cells the viability and unmodified shapes (typical elongated spindle-like) of human fibroblasts similar to the positive control in the experiment. Figure 2.2.2 depicts the SEM analysis of materials used in this study where FAH: fibrin-agarose hydrogels; FAH-MNPs: FAH containing MagNP-OH; FAH-MNPs-F: FAH containing MagNP-OH are subjected to a magnetic field during gelation.

Similarly, Figure 2.3 Demonstrates the Perls histochemical results of grafted biomaterials and injected MNPs. It also highlights the histological analysis of site of implantation, where there is mild inflammatory local reaction around the implanted materials, without causing any malignancy in the other places. As observed in the figure, the particles of FAH-MNPs and FAH-MNPs-F group tend to form several independent nuclei (during five weeks), as in the MNP-INJ group. When compared the MNPs that are introduced by injection to the grafted one, the results are favored for MNPs in grafting with more efficient control, contained with improved encapsulation (connective tissue capsule) in the grafted mass in a single nucleus preventing further infiltration of connective tissue and disaggregation or dispersion of grafts. The structural integration of grafted constructs, alignment, and orientation of MNPs in grafted constructs is lost or becomes weak after five weeks, suggesting in vivo biodegradability along with remodeling, and host immune cell infiltration (e.g., macrophages). The three-dimensional orientation of biomaterials is one of the goals of current tissue engineering, since most human tissues are characterized by nonlinear and anisotropic mechanical behavior due to the non-random distribution of components, and this distribution is essential for its proper in vivo function. The use of FAH-MNPs-F could contribute to obtaining MNP-based bioartificial tissues with defined alignment with added value for use in regenerative medicine as shown in Figure 2.3.

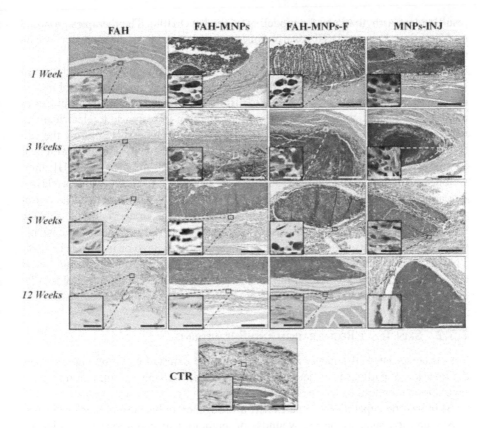

FIGURE 2.3 Perls histochemical results of grafted biomaterials and injected MNPs at 1, 3, 5 and 12 weeks in vivo. CTR: control animals; FAH: fibrin-agarose hydrogels; FAH-MNPs: FAH containing MagNP-OH; FAH-MNPs-F: FAH containing MagNP-OH subjected to a magnetic field during gelation; MNPs-INJ: MNPs injected subcutaneously. The inserted images correspond to higher magnifications of the same images. Scale bars: 300 μm (large images) and 20 μm (inserts). Adapted with permission from Ref [103]. Copyright 2021; Mat Sci Engg C.

2.5.1 A SPECIAL NOTE ON CONDUCTING POLYMER-BASED MATERIALS FOR MUSCLE TISSUE REGENERATION AND ENGINEERING

Among the various tissues, muscle tissue [104], which controls the generation of force, locomotion of the body, and functions related to the internal organs, plays a vital role since it comprise 50% of body mass. It is a soft tissue and vulnerable to injury that can lead to dysfunction or disorder of movement or organ, leading to heavy burden and pain. The skeletal muscle tissue has the capability to regenerate in mild injuries [105, 106], but major injuries, where loss of mass exceeds 20%, lead to fibrosis and scars due to the lack of regeneration by endogenesis, with most of the severe injuries requiring reconstruction by surgery, which is further limited by low rates of survival, donor morbidity, or lack of donors [107]. Among the muscle tissue, injury to the cardiac muscle is complex, due to its limited regeneration capacity, replacement by fibroblast resulting into arrhythmia, and remodeling of the heart [108]. The therapies proposed by Vacanti and Langer [109] have promising applications in tissue engineering and repair as applied to nerve, bone, and skin tissues [109–111].

Tissue engineering involving muscle tissue repair follows the therapeutic use of scaffolds, cells, and growth factors alone or in combination, and biomaterial matrix utilized in the therapy plays a vital role to mimic the extracellular matrix. For example, the characteristics like contraction, or conduction in response to electrical signals, promoting the growth of electrically responding cells that will allow the cell differentiation and proliferation, is therapeutically useful for the biomaterial matrices utilized to promote nerve cells [109] bone cells [110] muscle cells [111] interaction. In this aspect, conductive biopolymers belonging to three different classes – conducting polymers (e.g., PAni, PPy or PDMS etc.), carbon nanomaterials (graphene, carbon nanotubes, etc.), or metallic (e.g., TiO_2) – alone or in combination in various forms (such as films, nanofibers, or hydrogels), and three-dimensional porous scaffolds have lot of promising applications in ex vivo or in vivo [113–121]. They have been employed in various morphological forms as films [122], nanofibers [123, 124], hydrogels [125–127], and three-dimensional (3D) porous scaffolds [128, 129] to enhance communication among cells and porous scaffolds.

2.5.2 SKIN TISSUE REGENERATION AND ENGINEERING

Skin protects internal organs of the body from the external environment and from the invasion of pathogens by acting as a barrier. Skin also helps to maintain thermal regulation and retain moisture [130–133].

Skin has the capability to repair itself and regenerate because of stem cells, and thus scenarios such as burns, wounds, or pathological conditions (e.g., diabetic ulcer) limit the skin's ability to repair itself. Tissue engineering utilizes methods that restore the morphology (from sources or from stem cells), structural integrity, and physiology of skin or provides skin substitutes/synthetic ECMs. Tissue engineering scaffolds for skin regeneration and repair involve either cells delivered directly or delivered by combining with functionalized biomaterial matrices to help replace or repair the dermis or epidermis [134]. Tissue substitutes for skin should have characteristics such as quicker adherence, good physical and chemical properties along with nonantigenic nature. For example, for designing tissue, engineering scaffolds for wound healing requires knowledge of wound healing events and mechanisms, a complete pathological profile of patients (e.g., diabetic), and ideal or combination of dressings. There is a range of functional biomaterials [135–137] – natural ones, collagen, hydroxyapatites, alginates, chitin, cellulose, fibronectin, chitosan, hyaluronan, gelatin, polypeptides, and glycosaminoglycan with the capabilities of low toxicity, high biocompatibility, and low possibility for chronic inflammation; synthetic biomaterials like poly(lactide-co-glycolic) acid (PLGA), poly(ε caprolactone) (PCL), polylactic acid (PLA), and polyglycolide can provide ease of characterization, and can be custom-made with specific properties, but they lack the efficiency toward cell interactions and are less stable or fast degrading [138].

On the other hand, innovative approaches used to design a combination of nanomaterials with the biomaterials include nanocomposites, hydrogels, scaffolds, and dressings that offer unique characteristics such as faster wound closure and healing, control of fluid loss, strengthening of healed tissue, and histocompatibility. Nanomaterials added in small quantities to the polymeric matrix can offer unprecedented characteristics because of their unique size (e.g., high aspect ratio and mechanical properties) and improved interaction with the biological targets along with the enhanced physicochemical properties. Polymeric, inorganic, and carbon-based nanomaterials have been studied extensively for wound healing and skin regeneration. Nano silver (Ag Nano), as compared to conventional Ag or Ag ion, has been effective against a broad spectrum of microbes, and thus being used in antimicrobial dressing, to treat infection/scar free healing of burn wounds, incisions, and skin excision of acute as well as chronic wounds, including diabetic foot ulcers [139, 140]. AgNps are responsible to alter the structure of fibroblasts by suppressing the proliferation of fibroblasts, differentiating them into myofibroblasts, and reducing the expression of collagen type-1. Further they also promote quick contraction of the wound with eventual re-epithelialization [141, 142] for use in antimicrobial dressings.

A few examples from literature on such engineered materials are mentioned in the following descriptions. Kakkar et al. [142] studied in vitro susceptibility of microorganisms causing diabetic foot ulcers (disposed to severe infection) in a series of case studies of the wound ulcers of five diabetic patients; swabs were collected and cultured, and the microbes were identified (WHO recognized antibiotic-resistant microorganisms i.e., E Coli, Klebsiella pneumoniae etc.) [143] toward polyvinyl alcohol (PVA) composites. PVA and melamine formaldehyde (MFR) resin composite serve as both films and coatings; they are prepared and incorporated with AgNPs to form a PVA-MFR-Ag composite that showed significant antimicrobial efficiency toward the lab-cultured microbes as well as the cultured samples collected in case studies. Further, these antimicrobial composites were tested and compared for their activity as films, foams, and coated on Whatman paper; antimicrobial efficacy was stable over time and can be used after being stores for eight months; and it was also found to be reusable after washing, with slightly reduced efficacy. In another study by Santos et al. [144] PVA and multiwalled CNTs (MWCNTs) were conjugated to glucose oxidase and reported to be active scaffolds for wound healing. Similarly, kaolin-cellulose nanocomposites were investigated for wound healing by Wanna et al. [145], where Kaolin acted for the short term due to its blood-clotting potency and nanocellulose acted for the long term as a potential material for water absorbability. Polymeric materials act as scaffolds for tissue repair owing to their ability to be bioactive and degradable and to form a 3D, highly porous structure with high surface-to-volume ratio (NPs) that facilitates the site of nucleation for the collagen attachment and in turn promotes tissue growth [146]. In addition, tendency to retain moisture (bacterial cellulose), fibroblasts proliferation (chitosan NPs loaded on to calcium alginate hydrogels), increased antibacterial activity, rapid skin wound healing and re-epithelialization, and efficient loading with controlled-release (gelatin NPs loaded with doxocetal drug, gelatin controls the fluids loss and release the drug by enzymatic action) are some more benefits [147, 148, 150, 151] by respective bioengineered materials. Polymeric materials encapsulating bioactive components are also utilized in skin tissue engineering. For example, as compared to pure curcumin (which has the limitation of poor antioxidative and antimicrobial activity) curcumin-loaded NPs or curcumin-loaded chitosan NPs in collagen alginate scaffolds/ nanoscaffolds helped in rapid wound healing and granulation tissue formation when tested in diabetic mice [149, 152].

2.5.3 CORNEAL TISSUE REGENERATION AND ENGINEERING

For corneal regeneration, synthetic (or hydrolytically degradable) polymers rather than natural ones are preferred due to their superior mechanical properties and controlled degradation rates. Moreover, synthetic materials with inherent characteristics can be well-suited and biocompatible, due to specificity, in terms of molecular weight, soluble nature, hydrophilicity/hydrophobicity or water absorption, surface energy, lubricant ability, and degradation. For specific applications, biologically inert or custom-made materials with predictable properties [153–159] have been researched.

For example, Ozcelik et al. [160] fabricated ultrathin hydrogel films from PEG and chitosan composites and loaded them with collagen type 1. These composites with Chitosan are reported to be efficient corneal tissue regeneration materials with improved properties as compared to PEG only films. The varying PEG content helped to improve tensile and moduli properties as well as cell adhesion and proliferation ability in sheep cells. Similarly, PVA hydrogel-impregnated nanocellulose whiskers were studied by Tummala et al. [161] for use in disposable contacts lenses and as implants for corneal regeneration owing to their unique characteristics high elasticity, transparency level, and water content (PVA) retainability (90%). The composite showed superior properties such as viscoelastic and rubber-like mechanical properties (cellulose nano-whiskers) with good permeability to oxygen along with good wetting (high water content) and biocompatible properties; it was utilized for corneal epithelial cell cultivation. Furthermore, hybrid polymer networks are expected to be synergetic blends that combine bioactive merits of natural materials (e.g., collagen) and physical attributes of synthetic materials along with biological, optical functionalities, and tailorable mechanical strengths as desired for use in tissue regeneration scaffolds. Table 2.3 lists some of the biomaterial combinations utilized for corneal tissue engineering applications.

According to the global survey conducted [162, 163] and based on recent press reports, the demand for vision restoration through healing or repairing corneal damage is a persistent global challenge. The 80 eye banks in the United States recover, prepare, and provide enough donor corneas to meet national demand; for example 48,229 corneal transplants were performed up until 2013. An additional 21,000 corneas collected by the Eye Bank Association of America were sent overseas to nations who are unable to meet demands for corneal tissue. Since 1961, one million Americans between 9 days old and 100 years, have had vision-restoration transplants and procedures, with a success rate of 95 to 99 percent. A recent press release (April, 2021) from the University of Pittsburgh school of Medicine reported [164] successful healing of damaged corneas to restore vision in mice by their own stem cells. This procedure is being tested on humans in pilot studies conducted on 10 patients with scarred corneas at L V Prasad Eye Institute, Hyderabad, India. The stem cells are collected from a biopsy procedure or undamaged portion in the eye of the mice and replicated in the laboratory. These stem cells are further incorporated in the biomaterials matrix or gel of a fibrin (a protein that exists in blood clots and a common surgical adhesive), and the gel was spread on the damaged part of the cornea; it regenerated in few weeks with promising results to heal scars. Promising results are expected

TABLE 2.3
Hybrid Polymer Material and Morphologies for Corneal Scaffolds and Tissue Regeneration

Component 1	Component 2	Morphology of the Scaffold	Replaced Cornea Layer	Cell Line	Refs
Chitosan	PCL	Cast membranes	Corneal endothelium	Growth and differentiation of corneal endothelial cells (CECs)	[154]
Chitosan	Rat collagen type I, hydroxypropyl cellulose, and elastin	Hydrogel membranes	Corneal epithelium	Human corneal epithelial and limbal epithelial cells	[155]
Bombyx mori silk fibroin	Aloe barbadensis Miller gel	Cast film	Full cornea/ stroma	Rabbit CECs	[156].
Bombyx mori silk fibroin	Chitosan	Cast lamellar films	Corneal stroma	Primary rabbit corneal epithelial and stromal cells	[157]
Bombyx mori silk fibroin	Gelatin and poly (N-isopropyl acrylamide)	Direct-write assembled films	Corneal stroma bioequivalent	Goat corneal stromal cells	[158]
Poly (glycerol sebacate)	PCL	Electrospun nanofibers	Corneal endothelium and stroma	HCECs, conjunctival epithelial cells	[159]

Source: Adapted with Permission from Refs [154–159].

because the stem cell procedure is non-surgical with few rejections from the host body. However, this new procedure still requires stringent regulations and approvals from the United States Food and Drug Administration (USFDA) for clinical translation.

2.5.4 VASCULAR AND CARDIAC TISSUE ENGINEERING

Vascular-tissue regeneration is focused on endothelial cells (ECs) [165] that are part of blood vessel lining as they are in direct contact with flowing blood and can control vascular tone, vessel permeability, and anticoagulant properties. Further, ECs mediate efficient response toward uncontrolled or pathology-related conditions (inflammation, angiogenesis) during wound healing and tumor treatments (tumorigenesis, hypertension), etc. Moreover, ECs experience several forces or stresses due to shear and pressure from external surrounding tissues that invade the vessels by contraction (mediated by muscles) or input mechanical force or stiffness by local ECM. These mechanical forces that are generated by cells, either exogenously (forces imposed on cells) or endogenously (forced generated and imposed by cells), could provide key signals to connect cell responses between normal and disease conditions from tissue to molecular level. For one of the most important organs in the human body, the heart, it is difficult to promote or regenerate new cells due to unique characteristics such as tissue complexity, or hetero-geneity, and thus when damaged (by CVD) it heals slowly and poses challenges to treat or to replace with implants [19]. Hence, to maintain the structural integrity and cellular dynamics, nanoengineered biomaterials are being proposed and considered for mature cardiovascular tissue regeneration using 2D and 3D scaffolds.

Table 2.4 demonstrates [166] synthetic/natural biomaterial combinations from the recent literature that are being reported as cardiac tissue scaffolds, patches, or surfaces coated with other (conducting) polymers or nanomaterials to

TABLE 2.4
Biomaterials and Composites for Cardiac-Tissue Engineering Applications [Engineered Heart Tissue (EHT), RGD Peptide]

Source	Scaffold	Type	Advantage
Natural	Fibronectin	2D surface coating	Improved cell attachment, actin filaments development, and cell stiffness
Natural	Fiboblast-derived ECM	2D surface coating	Improved cell adhesion, cytoskeleton development, and contractility
Natural	Decellularized ECM	2D surface coating	Improved cardiac cell differentiation
Synthetic	Peptide-acrylate surface (PAS)	2D surface coating	Chemically defined and xeno-free materials
Synthetic	PLA with (poly(poly(ethylene glycol)methacrylate) and poly[N-(3-aminopropyl) methacrylamide]	2D Surface Coating	Increased cell attachment and contractility
Synthetic/Natural	poly(ethylene glycol)diacrylate with thiolated-hyaluronic acid (HA)	2D Surface Coating	Increased stiffness of hydrogels and cell maturation
Synthetic/Natural	Conductive polypyrrole (PPY) with chitosan (CHI)	2D Surface Coating	Increased Ca^{2+} transient and contractility
Synthetic	PEG with RGD peptide	Surface patterning	Improved cell organization and structural development
Synthetic/Natural	Poly(ethylene glycol) with Matrigel and fibronectin	Surface patterning	Improved cell alignment
Synthetic	Electrically conductive silicon nanowires (e-SiNW)	Spheroids	Improved synchronized beating and structural maturation
Natural	Fibrin gel	Patterned patch	Improved sarcomere development, maturation, and synchronization

(Continued)

TABLE 2.4 (*Continued*)

Biomaterials and Composites for Cardiac-Tissue Engineering Applications [Engineered Heart Tissue (EHT), RGD Peptide]

Source	Scaffold	Type	Advantage
Natural	Collagen type I	Patterned patch	Improved synchronized beating and maturation
Natural	Atelocollagen	Fibrous patch	Improved biocompatibility
Synthetic/Natural	PCL in gelatin-chitosan hydrogel	Patch	Improved mechanical properties
Synthetic/Natural	PPY nanoparticles, gelatin-methacrylate, poly(ethylene glycol) diacrylate	Patch	Improved synchronized beating and maturation
Synthetic/Natural	Gold nanorod-incorporated gelatin methacrylate	Patch	Improved cell adhesion, viability, metabolic activity, and maturation
Natural	Collagen	Rod-shaped EHT	Improved myofibrillogenesis and sarcomeric banding
Natural	Fibrin gel	Rod-shaped EHT	Improved sarcomere organization and number of mitochondria
Natural	Alginate hydrogel	Bio ink	Improved cell viability and expression of cardiac transcription factor
Natural	Hyaluronic acid/gelatin	Bio ink	Improved cardiac differentiation
Natural	Decellularized ECM	Bio ink	Improved alignment and complex structure
Synthetic	PCL with carbon nanotube	Bio ink	Improved mechanical properties
Synthetic	Gold nanorods-GelMa	Bio ink	Increased cell adhesion and synchronized contraction
Synthetic	PCL with PEDOT:PSS-PEO conductive fibers	Bio ink	Improved conductivity, cell adhesion and synchronized beating
Natural	Decellularized hydrogel with gelatin	Bio ink	Increased formation of a complex structure
Synthetic/Natural	Carbon nanotube with gelatin-chitosan hydrogel	3D scaffold	Improved electrical coupling and synchronized beating
Synthetic/Natural	Chitosan-carbon composite	3D scaffold	Improved electrical properties and porosity
Synthetic	Polyvinyl alcohol with carbon fibers	3D scaffold	Improved conductivity and elastic modulus

Source: Copyright 2020, adapted with permission from [166] MDPI.

enhance cell adhesion and interactions and to favorably respond to cardiac tissue mechanisms. First-generation biomaterials [167] were intended to generate immune response and provide functional support; subsequent generations also pointed at tailoring the needs specially to suit the individual applications. The scaffolds made from biomaterials for tissue generation [168] provide a physical space (or surface) and porosity that promotes cells to attach, migrate, proliferate, and differentiate. Furthermore, the 3D architecture helps in various functions – maintaining the appropriate cell phenotype, regulating the space available for cells to grow, providing mass transport via diffusion, and providing mechanical properties of the scaffold and interaction of cells with substrate. Tissue formation and further function depends on the cellular response, which is significantly affected by the surface morphology or topography of the biomaterial scaffolds [169]. Nanomaterial scaffolds for cardiovascular tissue regeneration are particularly focused on vascular, heart valve, and myocardium regeneration [170].

2.5.5 BONE TISSUE ENGINEERING AND REGENERATION

Bone in its natural form has a structure composed of combination materials – organic, mainly collagen fibers of tropocollagen, and inorganic hydroxyapatite (HA) crystals of calcium (Ca) and Phosphorous (P) as well as other materials, including sodium, potassium, magnesium, fluoride, chlorine, carbonate with trace elements like silicon, and iron, that give strength to the bone. Structurally it is multiscale with two types – cortical bone (99% Ca and 90% phosphate in the body, dense and strong with low porosity, located at the surface) and cancellous bone (20 wt % of the human body with high porosity and with the 20 times the specific surface area as that of cortical bone, with spongy texture and the tissue distributed inside the bone). These unique compositions and structures endow bone with superior properties to accomplish a variety of functions [171, 172] as displayed in the Figure 2.4, representing natural bone with multiscale structures and chemical composition. However, based on inherent characteristics such as the defect site, genetic inheritance, age, and the patient's living conditions, the composition and structure of bone may vary and thus pose varied challenges in bone implants. This creates continuous demand to develop ideal biomaterials of bone that can satisfy all characteristics in repairing the bone [173].

Commonly studied bone biomaterials can be categorized as bioceramics, polymers, and biomedical metals. Bioceramics are brittle, with weak mechanical properties, and hence the composites with bioceramics and polymers have been used for weight-bearing applications to avoid bone failures and help in repair. Along with strength, they have other features such as biodegradability and bioactivity to enable short time retention [174]. Bioactive ceramics are limited to applications where less or no load bearing is required; hence, to expand their applicability and mechanical properties, they are reinforced with secondary phase of nanoscaled materials [175] or coated on their surfaces [176] or various methods of self-tightening [177]. One-dimensional or multidimensional nanomaterials in the form of particles, fibers, and tubes due to their high surface to volume ratio can reinforce and enhance the mechanical properties of

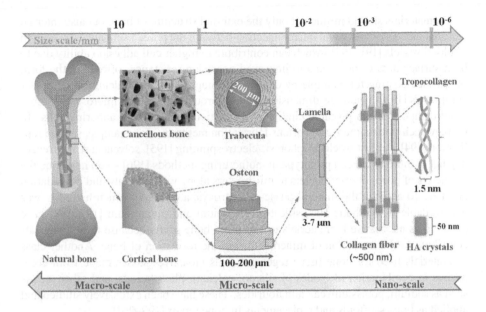

FIGURE 2.4 Natural bone with multiscale structures and chemical composition. Adapted with permission from Ref [172]; Copyright Bone research 2017. https://doi.org/10.1038/boneres.2017.59 Attribution 4.0 International (CC BY 4.0).

bioceramic bone materials by various mechanisms [178] such as inhibiting abnormal growth of ceramic grains, can act as fillers or nuclei to be wrapped in matrix to increase resistance to fracture and other properties. For example, commonly used nanotubes and nanosheets that include carbon nanotubes (CNTs) and graphene [178–181], and boron nitride nanotubes (BNNTs) when added to ceramic hydroxyapatite (HA) have improved mechanical properties by bridging crack or sword-in sheath mechanisms [182].

Similarly, synthetic or natural polymers also can be blended with bone nano/biomaterials to further enhance their strength. The combination of HA with other biopolymers can improve the properties attachment, proliferation, and differentiation in osteoblast cells. Nie et al. [183] reported HA/PLGA matrix for improved cell adhesion. PDLLA/HA composites were studied by Cui et al. [184] to form in situ and firm bonding at the interface. Most of the composites favor the formation of apatite and improved cell-attachment properties [185] along with possible tuned degradation capabilities based on the ratio of biomaterial blends used as bone implants [186–188]. For example, Bhardwaj et al. [189] have reported porous polymer composites made of chitosan-silk fibroin to tune the controlled degradation of these materials by efficient physical interactions [190]. In addition, fabrication or modification of chitosan with nanomaterials of HA and metallic nanoparticles like silver (Ag), zinc (Zn), and copper (Cu) can increase the strength, no toxicity towards osteoblasts and bestowed with antimicrobial properties.

Biomaterials should mimic not only the external structure of bone but also internal features such as porosity and interconnection between the pores to enhance the growth of blood vessels [191, 192], which can contribute to higher cell adhesion ability due to high surface area of pores and to improved corrosion resistance offered in the form of surface coating for example by depositing magnesium and calcium in nano HA composites [193]. The three-dimensional multiporous nanoscale to microscale biomaterial composites can promote binding and functional abilities for adhering cells. To prepare such porous matrices, various fabrication methods – for example, sponge replication [194], deposit by electrophoresis/electrospinning [195], solvent casting, freeze-drying, or more advanced prototype manufacturing methods [196] – can help tune the diameters of pores in micrometers to millimeters along with porosity and degradation abilities. To activate the mineral phase of hydroxyapatite (HA), which naturally was not available in synthetic Has, silicates of calcium and magnesium [197, 198] have emerged as alternative biomaterials to substitute bone grafts because these materials contribute to the formation of minerals during the formation of bone. Another class of materials used for bone tissue regeneration is bioactive glasses made from composites in combination of oxides of silicon, calcium, phosphorous, and other metals such as sodium, potassium, calcium flourides. These have been extensively studied and applied as bone scaffolds and replacements in bone repair [199–201].

2.5.6 OVERVIEW OF TISSUE ENGINEERING APPLICATIONS FOR VARIOUS ORGANS

Table 2.5 highlights nanoengineered material combinations with their properties for tissue-engineering application for various organs as reported in reviewed research articles.

2.6 LIMITATIONS AND CHALLENGES

One of the challenges with nanoengineered biomaterials used for generating new tissue (or to heal or repair) is developing tissue vasculature to supply required nutrients and oxygen until the new blood vessels are formed. It is necessary to integrate these micro-vasculatures into the host body after implantation and fabricate these controlled structures that function after implantation. Cell–cell interactions and their further interaction with the tissue architecture is another challenging area. Cells can self-assemble and establish communication with each other, but the interaction will be permanently lost during isolation of tissue and seeding processes. Uniform distribution of cells throughout the scaffolds or uniform seeding is another challenge to be considered while generating functional tissue constructs.

Biomaterials are screened for lot of promising applications for developing therapy or *in vitro,* but their full potential is yet to be explored. Some of the limitations they pose relate to how they interact with the patient's body or *in vivo.* Even though they mimic the 3D microenvironment of the organ or tissue they are repairing, they are still different from the actual organ, which can limit their regeneration. For example, biomaterial intended to repair or heal the heart should be able to contract with the heart beating; otherwise it may lead to irregular heartbeats. Moreover, they are able to repair only a part that is quarter the size of the heart; that's why in the case of damage by huge heart attack that damages a larger part of the heart, biomaterials may not be as useful.

TABLE 2.5

Various Nanoengineered Material Combinations with Their Properties for Tissue Engineering Application of Various Organs

Tissue Engineered Organ	Nanoengineered Bio Materials Blends	Properties	Ref
Bone	Carbon dot (C dot) decorated hydroxyapatite (HA) nanohybrid	Exhibited excellent cytocompatibility, cell proliferation, and alkaline phosphatase activity against MG 63 osteoblast	[202]
	Electrospun chitosan nanofibrous scaffolds with hydroxyapatite NPs and genipin	Supported adhesion, proliferation, and osteogenic differentiation of mouse 7F2 osteoblast-like cells	[203]
	Silver-doped hydroxyapatite– PVA composite nanofibers	Exhibited antibacterial activity and were hemocompatible	[204]
	MWCNTs/ chitosan / β-glycerophosphate (BGP) scaffolds	Improved electrical conductivity, mechanical properties and higher alkaline phosphatase activity; promoted osteogenic differentiation of bone marrow MSCs; provided therapeutic effect in treating chronic osteomyelitis with bone defects in rabbit model	[205] [206]
	Electrospun silk fibroin/ nanohydroxyapatite/BMP-2	Growth factor-loaded composites enhanced cell proliferation and early differentiation of osteoblast-like cells	[207] [208]
	Levofloxacin-loaded mesoporous silica microspheres/ nanohydroxyapatite/polyurethane composite scaffold		
	Hydroxyapatite (HA) layers deposited upon non-mulberry silk fibroin (from Antheraea mylitta) grafted PCL nanofibrous scaffolds		
Skin	Copper-containing mesoporous bioactive glass (MG) and nanofibrillated cellulose (NC)	Showed a profound angiogenic effect and promoted chronic wound healing	[209]
	Nanocomposites of PVA/ functionalized MWCNTs conjugated with glucose oxidase (GO) Scaffolds	Possessed better mechanical properties, antibacterial activity, degree of swelling, and cytocompatibility of skin wound healing; Enhanced wound healing activity in Wistar Albino rats	[144]
	Copper oxide NPs Fenugreek-incorporated silk fibroin nanofiber (SFNF)	Accelerated wound healing with complete re-epithelialization and enhanced collagen deposition	[210] [211]

(Continued)

TABLE 2.5 (*Continued*)
Various Nanoengineered Material Combinations with Their Properties for Tissue Engineering Application of Various Organs

Tissue Engineered Organ	Nanoengineered Bio Materials Blends	Properties	Ref
Cartilage	Hydroxypropyl methylcellulose (HPMC) interlinked with mesoporous silica nanofibers (MSNF)	These could act as reservoirs for bioactive molecules for cartilage engineering	[212]
	Electrospun chitosan (EC)/PVA reinforced with CaCO3 NPs	Found to provide the most suitable environment for cell growth and serves as alternative for artificial cartilage	[213]
	PCL scaffold with peptide RAD16-I	Self-assembling nanofibers provided important mechanical requirements and biomimetic microenvironment to re-establish the chondrogenic phenotype of human-expanded articular chondrocytes for cartilage replacement	[214]
	Electrospun gelatin (EG)/PCL nanofibers	Led to differentiation of bone marrow MSCs into chondrocyte-like cells	[215] [216]
	Magnetic nanocomposite hydrogel (MNH)	Increased the adhesion density of bone marrow MSCs for cartilage engineering	
Neural	Conjugation of neural cell adhesion molecule (L1) peptide and thiolated polyethylene glycol with AuNPs	Promoted neurite outgrowth, survival of neurons from the central and peripheral nervous systems and stimulated formation and proliferation of Schwann cells	[217] [218] [219]
	PHBV/collagen nanofibers		
	Electrospun blends of PCL and CNFs	Proliferation of nerve cells, and elongated cell morphology, with bipolar neurite extensions for nerve regeneration	[220]
	Nanocomposite fibers of gelatin/ cerium oxide NPs	Provided more favorable surfaces for attachment and proliferation of Schwann cells	[221]
	Graphene nanosheets-sodium alginate/PVA	Showed strong antioxidant properties and beneficial multicue effects for neurite development and alignment.	
	Fibrous scaffold	Provided attachment and spreading of PC12 cells, exhibited better electrical property and promoted cell proliferation	

(*Continued*)

TABLE 2.5 (*Continued*)
Various Nanoengineered Material Combinations with Their Properties for Tissue Engineering Application of Various Organs

Tissue Engineered Organ	Nanoengineered Bio Materials Blends	Properties	Ref
Cornea	Silver NPs	Fabrication of corneal implants and lenses for cornea replacements.	[222]
	A combination of lipofection with silica iron oxide magnetic NPs	Resulted in high transfection efficiency in human corneal endothelial cells and explanted human corneas for corneal therapy	[223]

There are three major concerns. The first one is underlying causes of diseases; as scientists continue to learn about these, they will be able to develop new biomaterials to treat more diseases. In addition, biomaterials themselves are still advancing, which will hopefully lead to materials that can successfully treat a wide range of illnesses. The second and most important challenge is ethical concerns and laws on use of biomaterials, with respect to type of materials and where they come from (origin) and whether it is ethical to use materials from other human beings or animals (organ transplants or implants). The third one is safety: regulating biomaterial for safe use in a patient's body because the combination of materials or components should repair the body and regenerate the organs or tissue, not cause further damage to other organs or tissue or severe infection. Limitations exist because of unclear understanding in controlling the pore diameters, or porosities, of material combinations to achieve favorable cell binding or differentiation properties. In order to develop new materials and more effective therapies, it is necessary for the scientists to continue learning about the interactions between the human body (tissues, organs and cells) and biomaterials.

2.7　DECLARATION OF COMPETING INTEREST

The authors declare that they have no known competing financial interests or personal relationships that could appear to influence the work reported in this paper. The views expressed are solely research and individual based, not those of the organizations represented by the authors.

ACKNOWLEDGMENTS

One of the authors, VSP, acknowledges for National Research Council Senior Research Associate Fellowship (National Academy of Science, Washington, DC, USA and Energy Directorate, Air Force Research Laboratory, Kirtland Air Force Base, NM and Materials and Manufacturing Directorate, Air Force Research Laboratory, Wright Patterson Air Force Base, OH, USA. KM acknowledges the support of her supervisor, Sumedh P Surwade, CEO and Founder, SAS Nantoechnologies LLC for working toward polymer nanocomposite self- healing materials.

ABBREVIATIONS

3D	three dimensional
AgNPs/ Nano silver/ Ag Nano	silver nanoparticles
Al_2O_3	alumina
BNNTs	boron nitride nanotubes
$Ca_{10}[PO_4]_6[OH]_2$	beta-tricalcium phosphate (BTF)
$Ca_3[PO_4]_2$	biphasic calcium phosphate (mixture of hydroxyapatite and beta-tricalcium phosphate)
CaO	calcium oxide
CaP	calcium phosphates
CNT	carbon nanotube
Co	cobalt
Cr	chromium
CTR	control animals
CVD	cardiovascular disease
Cu	Copper
EC	endothelial cells
ECM	extracellular matrix
FAH	fibrin-agarose hydrogels
FAH-MNPs	FAH containing MagNP-OH
FAH-MNPs-F	FAH containing MagNP-OH subjected to a magnetic field during gelation
GFs	growth factors GFs
HA	hydroxyapatite
hMSC	human mesenchymal stem cells;
HSC	hematopoietic stem cells.
HU-MSCM	human umbilical mesenchymal conditioned medium
MagNP-OH	hydroxy functionalized MNPs
MMA-co- HEMA-co- EGDMA	methyl methacrylate co-hydroxyl ethyl methacrylate-co-ethylene glycol dimethacrylate
MNPs	magnetic NPs (MNPs)
MNPs-INJ	MNPs injected subcutaneously
Mo	molybdenum
MWCNTs	multiwalled CNTs
Na_2O	sodium oxide
NP	nanoparticles
NTs	nanotubes
P_2O_5	phosphorous pentoxide
PAni	Polyaniline
PCL	poly(ε caprolactone)
PCLLGA	poly($\mathcal{E}$-caprolactone-r-l-lactide-r-glycolide)
PDLLA	Poly(DL-lactide)
PDMS	polydimethylsiloxane

PEG	polyethylene glycol
Perls or	histochemical stain used to demonstrate the distribution
Prussian Blue	and amount of iron deposits in liver tissue
Staining	
Protocol	
PGA	polyglycolic acid
PGS	polyglycerol sebacate
PLA	polylactic acid
PLGA	poly(lactide-co-glycolic) acid
PLGA/	
PLG	poly-dl-lactic-co-glycolic acid
PMMA	poly (methyl methacrylate)
PPy	polypyrrole
ps	polystyrene
pva	polyvinyl alcohol
pva/mfr	polyvinyl alcohol-melamine formaldehyde resin blend
pva-mfr-ag	polyvinyl alcohol-melamine formaldehyde – nanosilver
rgd	arginylglycylaspartic acid
sem	scanning electron microscopy
sio$_2$	silicon dioxide
SMC	smooth muscle cells
vSMCs	vascular smooth muscle cells
ss	stainless steel
te	tissue engineering
Ti	titanium
Ti$_6$Al$_4$V	alpha-beta titanium alloy
TiO$_2$	titanium dioxide
WHO	World Health Organization
Zinc	(Zn)
ZrO$_2$	zirconia oxide

REFERENCES

1. Lombardo, D., Kiselev, M. A., and Caccamo, M. T. (2019). Smart nanoparticles for drug delivery application: Development of versatile nanocarrier platforms in biotechnology and nanomedicine. J Nanomater. 2019, Article ID 3702518, 1–26. https://doi.org/10.1155/2019/3702518

2. Mclaughlin, S., Podrebarac, J., Ruel, M., Suuronen, E. J., McNeill, B, and Alarcon, E. I. (2016). Nano-engineered biomaterials for tissue regeneration: What has been achieved so far? Front Mater. 3:27. DOI: 10.3389/fmats.2016.00027

3. Cross, L. M., Thakur, A., Jalili, N. A., Detamore, M., and Gaharwar, A. K. (2016). Nanoengineered biomaterials for repair and regeneration of orthopedic tissue interfaces. Acta Biomaterialia. 42:2–17

4. Mozafari, M., Rajadas, J., and Kaplan, D. L. (2018). An Introduction to Nanoengineered Biomaterials. In: Mozafari, M., Rajadas, J., and Kaplan, D. (eds), Nanoengineered Biomaterials for Regenerative Medicine: A Volume in Micro and Nano Technologies, 1st Edition. Elsevier. eBook ISBN: 9780128133569, 1–11.

5. Steinhauser, M. L., and Lee, R. T. (2011). Regeneration of the heart. EMBO Mol Med. 3:701–712. doi: 10.1002/emmm.201100175

6. Chaudhuri, R., Ramachandran, M., Moharil, P., Harumalani, M., and Jaiswal, A. K. (2017). Biomaterials and cells for cardiac tissue engineering: Current choices. Mater Sci Eng C. 79:950–957. DOI: 10.1016/j.msec.2017.05.121

7. Bhat, S., and Kumar, A. (2013). Biomaterials and bioengineering tomorrow's healthcare. Biomatter. 3:e24717. DOI: 10.4161/biom.24717

8. Radhakrishnan, S., Nagarajan, S., Bechelany, M., and Kalkura, S. N. (2020). Collagen Based Biomaterials for Tissue Engineering Applications: A Review. In: Frank-Kamenetskaya O., Vlasov D., Panova E., Lessovaia S. (eds) Processes and Phenomena on the Boundary Between Biogenic and Abiogenic Nature. Lecture Notes in Earth System Sciences. Springer, Cham. https://doi.org/10.1007/978-3-030-21614-6_1

9. Liberski, A., Latif, N., Raynaud, C., Bollensdorff, C., and Yacoub, M. (2016). Alginate for cardiac regeneration: From seaweed to clinical trials. Glob Cardiol Sci Pract. 2016(1):e201604. https://doi.org/10.21542/gcsp.2016.4

10. Ha, T. L. B., Quan, T. M., Vu, D. N. and Si, D. M. (2013). Naturally Derived Biomaterials: Preparation and Application. In: Andrades J.A. (ed) Regenerative Medicine and Tissue Engineering. IntechOpen, DOI: 10.5772/55668

11. Zhang, B. G., Myers, D. E., Wallace, G. G., Brandt, M., and Choong, P. F. (2014). Bioactive coatings for orthopedic implants-recent trends in development of implant coatings. Int J Mol Sci. 15(7), 11878–11921. https://doi.org/10.3390/ijms150711878

12. Hench, L. L. and Polak, J. M. (2002). Third-generation biomedical materials. Science. 295 (5557):1014–1017. DOI: 10.1126/science.1067404

13. Ahumada, M., Jacques E., Calderon, C., and Martínez-Gómez F. (2019). Porosity in Biomaterials: A Key Factor in the Development of Applied Materials in Biomedicine. In: Martínez, L., Kharissova, O., Kharisov B. (eds) Handbook of Ecomaterials. Springer, Cham. https://doi.org/10.1007/978-3-319-68255-6_162

14. Langer, R., and Tirrell, D. A. (2004). Designing materials for biology and medicine. Nature. 428(6982):487–492.

15. Samak, M., and Hinkel, R. (2019). Stem cells in cardiovascular medicine: Historical overview and future prospects. Cells. 8:1530. https://doi.org/10.3390/cells8121530

16. Lewis, A., Koukoura, A., Tsianos, G.-I., Gargavanis, A. A., Nielsen, A. A., and Vassiliadis, E. (2021). Organ donation in the US and Europe: The supply vs demand imbalance. Transplant Rev. 35(2):100585. https://doi.org/10.1016/j.trre.2020.100585

17. Courtesy by https://www.mayoclinic.org/tests-procedures/heart-transplant/about/pac-20384750

18. Eschenhagen, T., Bolli, R., Braun, T., Field, L. J., Fleischmann, B. K., Frisén, J., Giacca, M., Hare, J. M., Houser, S., Lee, R. T., Marbán, E., Martin, J. F., Molkentin, J. D., Murry, C. E., Riley, P. R., Ruiz-Lozano, P., Sadek, H. A., Sussman, M. A., and Hill, J. A. (2017). Cardiomyocyte Regeneration: A consensus statement. Circulation. 136(7):680–686. https://doi.org/10.1161/CIRCULATIONAHA.117.029343

19. Lazurko, C., Harden, S., Suuronen, E. J., and Alarcon, E. I. (2019). Biomaterials for organ and tissue repair. Front. Young Minds. 7:8. doi: 10.3389/frym.2019.00008

20. Chaurasia, S. S., Lim, R. R., Lakshminarayan, R., and Mohan, R. R. (2015). Nanomedicine approaches for corneal diseases. J Funct Biomater. 6:277–298.

21. Greiner, A., Wendorff, J. H., Yarin, A. L., and Zussman, E. (2006). Biohybrid nanosystems with polymer nanofibers and nanotubes. Appl Microbiol Biotechnol. 71:387–393

22. Leszczynski, J. (2010). Nano meets bio at the interface. Nature Nanotech. 5:633–634.

23. Mozafari, M., Rajadas, J., and Kaplan, D. (eds). (2018). Nanoengineered Biomaterials for Regenerative Medicine. Elsevier. eBook ISBN: 9780128133569, 516.

24. Langer, R., and Vacanti, J. P. (1993). Tissue engineering. Science. 260:920–926.
25. von der, M. K., Park, J., Bauer, S., and Schmuki, P. (2010). Cell Tissue Res. 339:131; M. J. Webber, J. A. Kessler, and S. I. Stupp, J. Intern. Med. 267, 71 (2010).; K. M. Stroka and H. Randa-Espinoza, FEBS J. 277, 1145 (2010).
26. Reilly, G. C., Engler, A. J., and Reilly, G. C. (2010). Intrinsic extracellular matrix properties regulate stem cell differentiation. J Biomech. 43:55–62.
27. Butcher, D.T., Alliston, T., and Weaver, V.M. (2009). A tense situation: Forcing tumour progression. Nat. Rev. Cancer. 9:108–122.
28. Geiger, B., Bershadsky, A., Pankov, R., and Yamada, K. M. (2001). Transmembrane crosstalk between the extracellular matrix–cytoskeleton crosstalk. Nat Rev Mol Cell Biol. 2:793–805.
29. Nelson, C. M., and Bissell, M. J. (2006). Of extracellular matrix, scaffolds, and signaling: Tissue architecture regulates development, homeostasis, and cancer. Annu Rev Cell Dev Biol. 22:287–309; Schwartz, M.A., 2001.
30. Schwartz, M. A., and DeSimone, D. W. (2008). Integrin signaling revisited. Trends Cell Biol. 11:466–470.
31. Nicolas J., Magli S., Rabbachin L., Sampaolesi S., Nicotra F., and Russo L. (2020). 3D Extracellular Matrix Mimics: Fundamental Concepts and Role of Materials Chemistry to Influence Stem Cell Fate. Biomacromolecules. 21(6):1968–1994.
32. Dolcimascolo, A., Calabrese, G., Conoci, S., and Parenti, R. (2019). Innovative Biomaterials for Tissue Engineering. In: Barbeck, M., Jung, O., Smeets, R. and Koržinskas, T. (eds) Biomaterial-supported Tissue Reconstruction or Regeneration. IntechOpen, DOI: http://dx.doi.org/10.5772/intechopen.83839
33. Albee, F., and Morrison, H. (1920). Studies in bone growth. Ann Surg. 71:32–38.
34. Lagers R. Z. (2002). Properties of osteoconductive biomaterials: Calcium phosphates. Clin Orthop Relat Res. 395:81–98.
35. Ray, R. D., Ward, A. A. (1952). A Preliminary Report on Studies of Basic Calcium Phosphate in Bone Replacement. In: Surgical Forum, American College of Surgeons, 1951. WB Saunders Co, Philadelphia. pp. 429–434.
36. Calabrese, G., Giuffrida, R., Fabbi, C., Figallo, E., Furno, D. L., Gulino, R., et al. (2016). Collagen-hydroxyapatite scaffolds induce human adipose derived stem cells osteogenic differentiation in vitro. PLoS One. 11(3). DOI: 10.1371/journal.pone.0151181
37. Calabrese, G., Giuffrida, R., Forte, S., Salvatorelli, L., Fabbi, C., Figallo, E., et al. (2016). Bone augmentation after ectopic implantation of a cell-free collagen-hydroxyapatite scaffold in the mouse. Sci Rep. 6:36399. DOI: 10.1038/srep36399
38. Calabrese, G., Giuffrida, R., Forte, S., Fabbin, C., Figallo, E., Salvatorelli, L. et al. (2017). Human adipose-derived mesenchymal stem cells seeded into a collagen-hydroxyapatite scaffold promote bone augmentation after implantation in the mouse. Sci Rep. 7(1):7110. DOI: 10.1038/s41598-017-07672-0
39. Calabrese, G., Forte, S., Gulino, R., Cefalì, F., Figallo, E., Salvatorelli, L. et al. (2017). Combination of collagen-based scaffold and bioactive factors induces adipose-derived mesenchymal stem cells chondrogenic differentiation in vitro. Front Physiol. 8(50). DOI: 10.3389/fphys
40. Calabrese, G., Gulino, R., Giuffrida, R., Forte, S., Figallo, E., Claudia Fabbi, C., et al. (2017). In vivo evaluation of biocompatibility and chondrogenic potential of a cell-free collagen-based scaffold. Front Physiol. 8:984. DOI: 10.3389/fphys.2017.00984
41. Vagaská, B., Bacáková, L., Filová, E., and Balík, K. (2009). Osteogenic cells on bio-inspired materials for bone tissue engineering. Physiol Res. 59(3):309–322.
42. Deponti, D., Di Giancamillo, A., Gervaso, F., Domenicucci, M., Domeneghini, C., Sannino, A. et al. Collagen scaffold for cartilage tissue engineering: The benefit of fibrin glue and the proper culture time in an infant cartilage model. Tissue Eng Part A. 20(5–6):1113–1126. DOI: 10.1089/ten.TEA.2013.0171

43. Hoyer, M., Drechsel, N., Meyer, M., Meier, C., Hinüber, C., Breier, A., et al. (2014). Embroidered polymer-collagen hybrid scaffold variants for ligament tissue engineering. Mater Sci Eng C Mater Biol Appl. 43:290–299. DOI: 10.1016/j.msec.2014.07.010

44. Aravamudhan, A., Ramos, D. M., Nip, J., Harmon, M. D., James, R., Deng, M., et al. (2013). Cellulose and collagen derived micro-nano structured scaffolds for bone tissue engineering. J Biomed Nanotechnol. 9(4):719–731.

45. Schneider, R. K., Puellen, A., Kramann, R., Raupach, K., Bornemann, J., Knuechel, R., et al. (2010). The osteogenic differentiation of adult bone marrow and perinatal umbilical mesenchymal stem cells and matrix remodeling in three-dimensional collagen scaffolds. Biomaterials. 31(3):46780. DOI: 10.1016/j.biomaterials.2009.09.059

46. Lu, H., Kawazoe, N., Kitajima, T., Myoken, Y., Tomita, M., Umezawa, A., et al. (2012). Spatial immobilization of bone morphogenetic protein-4 in a collagen-PLGA hybrid scaffold for enhanced osteoinductivity. Biomaterials. 33(26):6140–6146. DOI: 10.1016/j.biomaterials.2012.05.038

47. Costa-Pinto, A. R., Correlo, V. M., Sol, P. C., Bhattacharya, M., Charbord, P., Delorme, B. et al. (2009). Osteogenic differentiation of human bone marrow mesenchymal stem cells seeded on melt based chitosan scaffolds for bone tissue engineering applications. Biomacromolecules. 10(8):2067–2073. DOI: 10.1021/bm9000102

48. Bi, L., Cheng, W., Fan, H., and Pei, G. (2010). Reconstruction of goat tibial defects using an injectable tricalcium phosphate/chitosan in combination with autologous platelet rich plasma. Biomaterials. 31: 3201–3211. DOI: 10.1016/j.biomaterials.2010.01.038

49. Eğri, S., and Eczacıoğlu, N. (2017). Sequential VEGF and BMP-2 releasing PLA-PEG-PLA scaffolds for bone tissue engineering: I. Design and in vitro tests. Artif Cells Nanomed Biotechnol. 45(2):321–329. DOI: 10.3109/21691401.2016.1147454

50. Wohlfahrt, J. C., Monjo, M., Rnold, H. J., Aass, A. M., Ellingsen, J. E., and Lyngstadaas, S. P. (2010). Porous titanium granules promote bone healing and growth in rabbit tibia peri-implant osseous defects. Clin Oral Implants Res. 21:165. DOI: 10.1111/j.1600-0501.2009.01813.x

51. Zuchuat, J., Berli, M., Maldonado, Y., and Decco, O. (2018). Influence of chromium-cobalt-molybdenum alloy [ASTM F75] on bone ingrowth in an experimental animal model. J Funct Biomater. 9(1):2. DOI: 10.3390/jfb9010002

52. Qian, J., Xu, W., Yong, X., Jin, X., and Zhang, W. (2014). Fabrication and in vitro biocompatibility of biomorphic PLGA/nHA composite scaffolds for bone tissue engineering. Mater Sci Eng C Mater Biol Appl. 1(36):95–101. DOI: 10.1016/j.msec.2013.11.047

53. Sekiya, N., Ichioka, S., Terada, D., Tsuchiya, S., and Kobayashi, H (2013). Efficacy of a poly glycolic acid (PGA)/collagen composite nanofibre scaffold on cell migration and neovascularisation in vivo skin defect model. J Plast Surg Hand Surg. 47(6):498–502. DOI: 10.3109/2000656X.2013.788507

54. Wu, C., Zhou, Y., Xu, M., Han, P., Chen, L., Chang, J., et al. (2013). Copper-containing mesoporous bioactive glass scaffolds with multifunctional properties of angiogenesis capacity, osteostimulation and antibacterial activity. Biomaterials. 34(2):422–433. DOI: 10.1016/j.biomaterials.2012.09.066

55. Oughlis, S., Lessim, S., Changotade, S., Bollotte, F., Poirier, F., Helary, G., et al. (2011). Development of proteomic tools to study protein adsorption on a biomaterial titanium grafted with poly(sodium styrene sulfonate). J Chromatogr B. 879:3681–3687. DOI: 10.1016/j.jchromb.2011.10.006

56. Wichterle, O., and Lim, D. (1960). Hydrophilic gels for biological use. Nature. 185:117–129. DOI: 10.1038/185117a0

57. Pasqui, D., Torricelli, P., De Cagna, M., Milena Fini, M., and Barbucci, R. (2014). Carboxymethyl cellulose—Hydroxyapatite hybrid hydrogel as a composite material for bone tissue engineering applications. J Biomed Mater Res A. 102a(5):1568–1579. DOI: 10.1002/jbm.a.34810

58. Kinard, L. A., Dahlin, R. L., Lam, J., Lu, S., Lee, E. J., Kasper, F. K., et al. (2014). Synthetic biodegradable hydrogel delivery of demineralized bone matrix for bone augmentation in a rat model. Acta Biomaterialia. 10(11):4574–4582. DOI: 10.1016/j. actbio.2014.07.011

59. Fan, C., and Wang, D. A. (2017). Review- macroporous hydrogel scaffolds for three-dimensional cell culture and tissue engineering. Tissue Eng Part B Rev. 23(5):451–461.

60. Khandan, A., Jazayeri, H., Fahmy, M.D., and Razavi, M. (2017). Hydrogels: Types, structure, properties, and applications. Frontiers in Biomaterials. Bentham Science, Sharjah, UAE. pp. 143–169.

61. Zhu, J., Marchant, R. E. (2011). Design properties of hydrogel tissue-engineering scaffolds. Expert Rev. Med. Devices. 8(5):607–626. Doi: 10.1586/erd.11.27.

62. Hoffman, A. S. (2002). Hydrogel biomedical articles. Adv Drug Deliv Rev. 54:3–12. Doi: 10.1016/S0169-409X(01)00239-3

63. Mantha, S., Pillai, S., Khayambashi, P., Upadhyay, A., Zhang, Y., Tao, O., Pham, H. M., and Tran, S. D. (2019). Smart hydrogels in tissue engineering and regenerative medicine. Materials (Basel, Switzerland). 12(20):3323. https://doi.org/10.3390/ma12203323

64. Khademhosseini, A. and Langer, R. (2007). Review – Micro-engineered hydrogels for tissue engineering. Biomaterials. 28 (34): 5087–5092. https://doi.org/10.1016/j. biomaterials.2007.07.021

65. Kusindarta, D. L. and Wihadmadyatami, H. (2018). The Role of Extracellular Matrix in Tissue Regeneration. In: Hussein Abdel hay El-Sayed Kaoud (eds). Tissue Regeneration. IntechOpen.

66. Guilak, F. et al. (2009). Control of stem cell fate by physical interactions with the extracellular matrix, Cell Stem Cell. 5:17; Daley, W. P., Peters, S. B., and Larsen M. (2008). Extracellular matrix dynamics in development and regenerative medicine. J. Cell Sci. 121:255.

67. Lutolf, M. P. and Hubbell, J. A. (2005). Synthetic biomaterials as instructive extracellular microenvironments for morphogenesis in tissue engineering. Nat Biotechnol. 23:47–55.

68. de, M. A., Jell, G., Stevens, M. M. and Seifalian, A. M. (2008). Biofunctionalization of biomaterials for accelerated in situ endothelialization: a review. Biomacromolecules. 9:2969; Zhu J. (2010). Bioactive modification of poly(ethylene glycol) hydrogels for tissue engineering. Nat. Biotechnol. 31:4639.

69. Wan, W. K., Yang, L. and Padavan, D. T. (2007). Use of degradable and nondegradable nanomaterials for controlled release. Nanomedicine. 2:483.

70. Huang, B., Chen, F., Shen, Y., Qian, K., Wang, Y., Sun, C., Zha, X., Cui, B., Gao, F., Zeng, Z. and Cui, H. (2018). Advances in targeted pesticides with environmentally responsive controlled release by nanotechnology. Nanomaterials (MDPI). 8:102. DOI: 10.3390/nano8020102

71. Van de Voorde, K. M., Pokorski, J. K. and Korley, L. T. J. (2020). exploring morphological effects on the mechanics of blended poly (lactic acid)/poly(ε-caprolactone) extruded fibers fabricated using multilayer coextrusion. ACS Macromolecules. 53:5047–5055.

72. Hedegaard, C. L. and Alvaro, Mata. (2020) Integrating self-assembly and biofabrication for the development of structures with enhanced complexity and hierarchical control. Biofabrication. 12:032002

73. Sell, S. A., McClure, M. J., Garg, K., Wolfe, P. S., and Bowlin, G. L. (2009). Electrospinning of collagen/biopolymers for regenerative medicine and cardiovascular tissue engineering. Adv. Drug Deliv. Rev. 61:1007.

74. Zhang, Y., Lim, C. T., Ramakrishna, S., and Huang, Z. M. (2005). Recent development of polymer nanofibers for biomedical and biotechnological applications. J Mater Sci Mater Med. 16:933.

75. Thorvaldsson, A., Stenhamre, H., Gatenholm, P., and Walkenstrom, P. (2008). Electrospinning of highly porous scaffolds for cartilage regeneration. Biomacromolecules. 9:1044; Ishii, O., Shin M., Sueda T., and Vacanti, J. P., Thorac. J. (2005). In vitro tissue engineering of a cardiac graft using a degradable scaffold with an extracellular matrix–like topography. Cardiovasc. Surg. 130:1358.

76. Dhandayuthapani, B., Krishnan, U. M., and Sethuraman, S. (2010). Fabrication and characterization of chitosan-gelatin blend nanofibers for skin tissue engineering. J Biomed Mater Res B Appl Biomater. 94:264; Zhang, K., Mo, X., Huang C., He, C., Wang, H. (2010). Electrospun scaffolds from silk fibroin and their cellular compatibility. J. Biomed. Mater. Res. A. 93:984.

77. Liu, X. and Ma, P. X. (2009). Biomimetic nanofibrous gelatin/apatite composite scaffolds for bone tissue engine. Nat. Biotechnol. 30: 4094.

78. Przybyla, D. E. and Chmielewski, J. (2010). Metal-triggered collagen peptide disk formation, J Am. Chem. Soc. 132:7866; Niece, K. L., Hartgerink, J. D., Donners, J. J., and Stupp, S. I. (2003). Self-assembly combining two bioactive peptide-amphiphile molecules into nanofibers by electrostatic attraction, J. Am. Chem. Soc. 125:7146.

79. Hartgerink, J. D., Beniash, E., and Stupp, S. I. (2002). Peptide-amphiphile nanofibers: A versatile scaffold for the preparation of self-assembling materials. Proc Natl Acad Sci USA. 99:5133; Ye, Z. et al. (2008). Temperature and pH effects on biophysical and morphological properties of self-assembling peptide RADA16-I. J. Pept. Sci. 14:152.

80. Perez, R. A., and Mestres, G. (2016). Role of pore size and morphology in musculoskeletal tissue regeneration. Mater Sci Eng C Mater Biol Appl. 61:922–939.

81. Pina, S., Ribeiro, V. P., Marques, C. F., Maia, F. R., Silva, T. H., Reis, R. L., and Oliveira, J. M. (2019). Review scaffolding strategies for tissue engineering and regenerative medicine applications. Materials. 12:1824; doi:10.3390/ma12111824

82. Haider, A., Haider, S., Rao Kummar, M., Kamal, T., Alghyamah, A.-A. A., Jan Iftikhar, F., Bano, B., Khan, N., Afridi, M. A., Soo Han, S., Alrahlah A., and Khan, R. (2020). Advances in the scaffolds fabrication techniques using biocompatible polymers and their biomedical application: A technical and statistical review. J Saudi Chem Soc. 24(2):186–215.

83. Hadjipanayi, E., Mudera, V., and Brown, R. A. (2009). Close dependence of fibroblast proliferation on collagen scaffold matrix stiffness. J Tissue Eng Regen Med. 3(2):77–84. DOI: 10.1002/term.136

84. Zhang, J., Wehrle, E., Adamek, P., Paul, G. R., Qin, X.-H., Rubert, M., and Müller, R. (2020). Optimization of mechanical stiffness and cell density of 3D bioprinted cell-laden scaffolds improves extracellular matrix mineralization and cellular organization for bone tissue engineering, Acta Biomaterialia. 114:307–322.

85. Kim, D. H. et al. (2006). Guided Three-Dimensional Growth of Functional Cardiomyocytes on Polyethylene Glycol Nanostructures. Langmuir. 22:5419.

86. Guillemette, M. D. et al. (2010). Combined technologies for microfabricating elastomeric cardiac tissue engineering scaffolds. Macromol Biosci. 10(11):1330–1337

87. Sjostrom, T. et al. (2009). Fabrication of pillar-like titania nanostructures on titanium and their interactions with human skeletal stem cells. Acta Biomater. 5:1433

88. Dalby, M. J., Riehle, M. O., Johnstone. H. J. H., Affrossman, S., Curtis, A. S. G. (2002). Polymer-demixed nanotopography: control of fibroblast spreading and proliferation. Tissue Engineering. 8(6):1099–1108.

89. Dalby, M. J., Gadegaard, N., Tare, R. (2007). The control of human mesenchymal cell differentiation using nanoscale symmetry and disorder. Nature Materials. 6(12):997–1003.

90. Kim D-H et al. (2010). Nanoscale cues regulate the structure and function of macroscopic cardiac tissue constructs. Proc Natl Acad Sci USA. 107:565.

91. Lu, J., Rao, M. P., MacDonald, N. C., Khang, D., and Webster, T. J. (2008). Improved endothelial cell adhesion and proliferation on patterned titanium surfaces with rationally designed, micrometer to nanometer features. Acta Biomater. 4:192.
92. Park, J. et al. (2009). TiO2 nanotube surfaces: 15 nm--an optimal length scale of surface topography for cell adhesion and differentiation. Small. 5:666.
93. Nguyen, K. T., Shukla, K. P., Moctezuma, M., and Tang, L. (2007). Cellular and molecular responses of smooth muscle cells to surface nanotopography. J Nanosci Nanotechnol. 7:2823.
94. Cao, Y. et al. (2010). Regulating orientation and phenotype of primary vascular smooth muscle cells by biodegradable films patterned with arrays of microchannels and discontinuous microwalls. Nat Biotechnol. 31:6228.
95. Kim, D. H., Seo, C. H., Han, K., Kwon, K. W., Levchenko, A., and Suh, K. Y. (2009). Guided Cell Migration on Microtextured Substrates with Variable Local Density and Anisotropy, Adv Funct Mater. 19:1579. [PubMed: 20046799].
96. Kim, D. H., Han, K., Gupta, K., Kwon, K., Suh, K. Y., and Levchenko, A. (2009). Mechanosensitivity of fibroblast cell shape and movement to anisotropic substratum topography gradients, Biomaterials. 30:5433. [PubMed: 19595452]
97. Odom, T. W., Love, C. J., Wolfe, D. B., Paul, K. E., and Whitesides, G. M. (2002). Improved pattern transfer in soft lithography using composite stamps, Langmuir. 18:5314.
98. Discher, D. E., Janmey, P., and Wang, Y. L. (2005). Tissue cells feel and respond to the stiffness of their substrate. Science. 310:1139–1143.
99. Vogel, V., and Sheetz, M. (2006). Local force and geometry sensing regulate cell functions. Nat. Rev Mol Cell Biol. 7:265–275.
100. Berry, M. F., Engler, A. J., Woo, Y. J., Pirolli, T. J., Bish, L. T., Jayasankar, V., Morine, K. J., Gardner, T. J., Discher, D. E., Sweeney, H. L.(2006). Mesenchymal stem cell injection after myocardial infarction improves myocardial compliance. American Journal of physiology. Heart and Circulatory Physiology. 290(6):H2196--203. DOI: 10.1152/ajpheart.01017.2005
101. Breitbach, M., Bostani, T., Roell, W., Xia, Y., Dewald, O., Nygren, J. M., Fries, J. W., Tiemann, K., Bohlen, H., Hescheler, J., Welz, A., Bloch, W., Jacobsen, S. E., Fleischmann, B. K. (2007). Potential risks of bone marrow cell transplantation into infarcted hearts. Blood. 110:1362–1369.
102. Rodriguez-Arco, L., Rodriguez, I. A., Carriel, V., Bonhome-Espinosa, A. B., Campos, F., Kuzhir, P., Duran, J. D. G., and Lopez-Lopez, M. T. (2016). Biocompatible magnetic core–shell nanocomposites for engineered magnetic tissues. Nanoscale. 8:8138. DOI: 10.1039/C6NR00224B
103. Campos, F., Bonhome-Espinosa, A. B., Carmona, R., Durán, J. D. G., Kuzhir, P., Alaminos, M., López-López, M. T., Rodriguez, I. A., and Carriel, V. (2021). *In vivo* time-course biocompatibility assessment of biomagnetic nanoparticles-based biomaterials for tissue engineering applications. Mater Sci Eng C Mater Biol Appl. 118:111476
104. Dong, R., Ma, P. X., and Guo, B. (2020). Conductive biomaterials for muscle tissue engineering. Biomaterials. 229:119584. https://doi.org/10.1016/j.biomaterials.2019.119584
105. Brack, A. S., and Rando, T.A. (2012). Tissue-specific stem cells: Lessons from the skeletal muscle satellite cell. Cell Stem Cell. 10(5):504–14. https://doi.org/10.1016/j.stem.2012.04.001
106. Relaix, F., and Zammit, P.S. (2012). Satellite cells are essential for skeletal muscle regeneration: The cell on the edge returns centre stage. Development. 139(16):2845–56. https://doi.org/10.1242/dev.069088.
107. Garg, K., Corona, B.T. and Walters, T.J. (2015). Therapeutic strategies for preventing skeletal muscle fibrosis after injury. Front Pharmacol. 6:87. https://doi.org/10.3389/fphar.2015.00087

108. Klinkenberg, M., Fischer, S., Kremer, T., Hernekamp, F., Lehnhardt, M., and Daigeler, A. (2013). Comparison of anterolateral thigh, lateral arm, and parascapular free flaps with regard to donor-site morbidity and aesthetic and functional outcomes. Plast Reconstr Surg. 131(2):293–302. https://doi.org/10.1097/PRS.0b013e31827786bc

109. Langer, R., and Vacanti, J. P. (1993). Tissue Engineering, Science. 260(5110):920–6. https://doi.org/10.1126/science.8493529.; J.P. Vacanti, R. Langer, Tissue engineering: the design and fabrication of living replacement devices for surgical reconstruction and transplantation, Lancet, 354 Suppl 1 (1999), SI32–4. https://doi.org/10.1016/s0140-6736(99)90247-7

110. Hu, J., Kai, D., Ye, H., Tian, L., Ding, X., Ramakrishna, S. et al. (2017). Electrospinning of poly(glycerol sebacate)-based nanofibers for nerve tissue engineering. Mater. Sci. Eng. C. Mater. Biol. Appl. 70(Pt 2):1089–1094. https://doi.org/10.1016/j.msec.2016.03.035; Mohamadi, F., Ebrahimi-Barough, S., Reza Nourani, M., Ali Derakhshan, M., Goodarzi, V., Sadegh Nazockdast, M. et al. (2017). Electrospun nerve guide scaffold of poly(epsilon-caprolactone)/collagen/nanobioglass: an in vitro study in peripheral nerve tissue engineering. J. Biomed. Mater. Res. A. 105(7):1960–1972. https://doi.org/10.1002/jbm.a.36068

111. Pati, F., Song, T. H., Rijal, G., Jang, J., Kim, S. W., and Cho, D.W. (2015). Ornamenting 3D printed scaffolds with cell-laid extracellular matrix for bone tissue regeneration. Biomaterials. 37:230–41. https://doi.org/10.1016/j.biomaterials.2014.10.012

112. Zhao, X., Wu, H., Guo, B.L., Dong, R.N., Qiu, Y.S., and Ma, P.X. (2017). Antibacterial antioxidant electroactive injectable hydrogel as self-healing wound dressing with hemostasis and adhesiveness for cutaneous wound healing. Biomaterials. 122:34–47. https://doi.org/10.1016/j.biomaterials.2017.01.011.

113. Mihic, A., Cui, Z., Wu, J., Vlacic, G., Miyagi, Y., Li, S. H. et al. (2015). A conductive polymer hydrogel supports cell electrical signaling and improves cardiac function after implantation into myocardial infarct. Circulation. 132(8):772–784. https://doi.org/10.1161/CIRCULATIONAHA.114.014937

114. Wang, Y. Q., Shi, Y., Pan, L. J., Ding, Y., Zhao, Y., Li, Y., et al. (2015). Dopant-enabled supramolecular approach for controlled synthesis of nanostructured conductive polymer hydrogels. Nano Lett. 15(11):7736–7741. https://doi.org/10.1021/acs.nanolett.5b03891

115. Baheiraei, N., Yeganeh, H., Ai, J., Gharibi, R., Ebrahimi-Barough, S., Azami, M. et al. (2015). Preparation of a porous conductive scaffold from aniline pentamer-modified polyurethane/PCL blend for cardiac tissue engineering. J Biomed Mater Res A. 103(10):3179–3187. https://doi.org/10.1002/jbm.a.35447.

116. Guo, B., Qu, J., Zhao, X., and Zhang, M. (2019). Degradable conductive self-healing hydrogels based on dextran-graft-tetraaniline and N-carboxyethyl chitosan as injectable carriers for myoblast cell therapy and muscle regeneration. Acta Biomater. 84:180–193. https://doi.org/10.1016/j.actbio.2018.12.008.

117. Mu, J., Hou, C., Wang, G., Wang, X., Zhang, Q., Li, Y. et al. (2016). An elastic transparent conductor based on hierarchically wrinkled reduced graphene oxide for artificial muscles and sensors. Adv Mater. 28(43):9491–9497. https://doi.org/10.1002/adma.201603395.

118. Chun, K.Y., Hyeong Kim, S., Kyoon Shin, M., Hoon Kwon, C., Park, J.,Tae Kim, Y. et al. (2014). Hybrid carbon nanotube yarn artificial muscle inspired by spider dragline silk. Nat Commun. 5:3322. https://doi.org/10.1038/ncomms4322.

119. Lee, J., Ko, S., Kwon, C. H., Lima, M. D., Baughman, R. H., and Kim, S. J. (2016). Carbon nanotube yarn-based glucose sensing artificial muscle. Small. 12(15):2085–2091. https://doi.org/10.1002/smll.201503509.

120. Shevach, M., Fleischer, S., Shapira, A., and Dvir, T. (2014). Gold nanoparticle-decellularized matrix hybrids for cardiac tissue engineering. Nano Lett. 14(10):5792–5796. https://doi.org/10.1021/nl502673m

121. Ravichandran, R., Sridhar, R., Venugopal, J. R., Sundarrajan, S., Mukherjee, S., and Ramakrishna, S. (2004). Gold nanoparticle loaded hybrid nanofibers for cardiogenic differentiation of stem cells for infarcted myocardium regeneration. Macromol Biosci. 14(4):515–525. https://doi.org/10.1002/mabi.201300407

122. Chen, J., Dong, R., Ge, J., Guo, B., and Ma, P. X. (2015). Biocompatible, Biodegradable, and electroactive polyurethane-urea elastomers with tunable hydrophilicity for skeletal muscle tissue engineering. ACS Appl Mater Interfaces. 7(51):28273–28285. https://doi.org/10.1021/acsami.5b10829.

123. Wang, L., Wu, Y. B., Hu, T. L., Guo, B. L., Ma, P. X. (2017). Electrospun conductive nanofibrous scaffolds for engineering cardiac tissue and 3D bioactuators. Acta Biomater. 59:68–81. https://doi.org/10.1016/j.actbio.2017.06.036.

124. Ostrovidov, S., Shi, X., Zhang, L., Liang, X., Kim, S. B., Fujie, T. et al. (2014). Myotube formation on gelatin nanofibers - multi-walled carbon nanotubes hybrid scaffolds, Biomaterials. 35(24):6268–6277. https://doi.org/10.1016/j.biomaterials.2014.04.021

125. Ahadian, S., Yamada, S., Ramon-Azcon, J., Estili, M., Liang, X., Nakajima, K. et al. (2016). Hybrid hydrogel-aligned carbon nanotube scaffolds to enhance cardiac Journal Pre-proof58 differentiation of embryoid bodies. Acta Biomater. 31:134–143. https://doi.org/10.1016/j.actbio.2015.11.047

126. Wang, L., Wu, Y. B., Guo, B. L., and Ma, P. X. (2015). Nanofiber yarn/hydrogel core–shell scaffolds mimicking native skeletal muscle tissue for guiding 3D myoblast alignment, elongation, and differentiation. ACS Nano. 9(9):9167–9179. https://doi.org/10.1021/acsnano.5b03644

127. Wu, Y.B., Wang, L., Guo, B. L., and Ma, P. X. (2017). Interwoven aligned conductive nanofiber yarn/hydrogel composite scaffolds for engineered 3D cardiac anisotropy. ACS Nano. 11(6):5646–5659. https://doi.org/10.1021/acsnano.7b01062

128. Martins, A. M., Eng, G., Caridade, S. G., Mano, J. F., Reis, R. L., Vunjak-Novakovic, G. (2014). Electrically conductive chitosan/carbon scaffolds for cardiac tissue engineering. Biomacromolecules. 15(2):635–643. https://doi.org/10.1021/bm401679q

129. Chaudhuri, B., Bhadra, D., Moroni, L., and Pramanik, K. (2015). Myoblast differentiation of human mesenchymal stem cells on graphene oxide and electrospun graphene oxide–polymer composite fibrous meshes: Importance of graphene oxide conductivity and dielectric constant on their biocompatibility. Biofabrication. 7(1). https://doi.org/10.1088/1758-5090/7/1/015009

130. Mordorski, B., Rosen, J., and Friedman, A. (2015). Nanotechnology as an innovative approach for accelerating wound healing in diabetes. Diabetes Manag. 5:329–332.

131. Rai, M., Yadav, A., and Gade, A. (2009). Silver nanoparticles as a new generation of antimicrobials. Biotechnol Adv. 27:76–83.

132. Tocco, I., Zavan, B., Bassetto, F., and Vindigni, V. (2012). Nanotechnology-based therapies for skin wound regeneration. J Nanomater. 4:1–11.

133. Kaler, A., Mittal, A. K., Katariya, M., Harde, H., Agrawal, A. K., Jain, S., and Banerjee, U. C. (2014). An investigation of in vivo wound healing activity of biologically synthesized silver nanoparticles. J Nanopart Res. 16:2605–2614.

134. Snyder, D., Sullivan, N., Margolis, D., and Schoelles, K. (2020). Skin Substitutes for Treating Chronic Wounds [Internet]. Rockville (MD): Agency for Healthcare Research and Quality (US). PMID: 32101391.

135. Mir, M., Ali, M. N., Barakullah, A., Gulzar, A., Arshad, M., Fatima, S., and Asad, M. (2018). Synthetic polymeric biomaterials for wound healing: A review. Prog. Biomater. 7(1):1–21. https://doi.org/10.1007/s40204-018-0083-4

136. Suarato, G., Bertorelli, R., and Athanassiou, A. (2018). Borrowing from nature: Biopolymers and biocomposites as smart wound care materials. Front Bioeng Biotechnol. 6:137. https://doi.org/10.3389/fbioe.2018.00137

137. Alven, S., and Aderibigbe, B. A. (2020). Review chitosan and cellulose-based hydrogels for wound management. Int J Mol Sci. 21:9656. doi:10.3390/ijms21249656
138. Homaeigohar, S., and Boccaccini, A. R. (2020). Antibacterial biohybrid nanofibers for wound dressings. Acta Biomaterialia. 107:25–49. https://doi.org/10.1016/j.actbio.2020.02.022
139. Liu, J., Sonshine, D. A., Shervani, S., and Hurt, R. H. (2010). Controlled release of biologically active silver from nanosilver surfaces. ACS Nano. 4:6903–6913.
140. Kakkar, R., Sherly, E. D., Madgula, K., Devi, D. K., and Sreedhar, B. (2012). Synergetic effect of sodium citrate and starch in the synthesis of silver nanoparticles. J Appl Polym Sci. 126(S1):E154–E161. doi:10.1002/app.36727;
141. Kakkar, R., Madgula, K., Saritha Nehru, Y. V., Shailaja, and R. M., Sreedhar, B. (2014). Polyvinyl alcohol - melamine formaldehyde resin composite and nanocomposites with Ag, TiO$_2$, ZnO nanoparticles as antimicrobial films, coatings and sprays. Eur Chem Bull. 3(10–12):1088–1097. DOI: http://dx.doi.org/10.17628/ecb.2014.3.1088-1097
142. Kakkar, R., Madgula, K., Saritha Nehru, Y. V., and Kakkar, J. (2015). Polyvinyl alcohol -melamine formaldehyde films and coatings with silver nano particles as wound dressings in diabetic foot disease. Eur Chem Bull. 4(1–3):98–105.
143. The Diabetic Foot & Wound Care Clinic, https://savelegs.com/ and; ePoster presentation in the International Conference European wound management Association (EWMA 2016), Bremen, Germany on research on the treatment and management of chronic wounds and diabetic foot problems, https://ewma.conference2web.com/#resources/nanosilver-coated-polymer-for-treatment-of-foot-infections-in-this-era-of-resistance-c9e43b05-5b2c-4042-a6f3-a6ccd87f4ded
144. Santos, J. C. C., Mansur, A. A., Ciminell, V. S., and Mansur, H. S. (2014). Nanocomposites of poly(vinyl alcohol)/functionalized-multiwall carbon nanotubes conjugated with glucose oxidase for potential application as scaffolds in skin wound healing. Int J Polym Mater Polym Biomater. 63:185–196.
145. Wanna, D., Alam, C., Toivola, D. M., and Alam, P. (2013). Bacterial cellulose–kaolin nanocomposites for application as biomedical wound healing materials. Adv Nat Sci Nanosci Nanotechnol. 4:045002
146. Berthet, M., Gauthier, Y., Lacroix, C., Verrier, B., and Monge, C. (2017). Nanoparticle-based dressing: The future of wound treatment? Trends Biotechnol. 35:770–784.
147. Patel, H., Bonde, M., and Srinivasan, G. (2011). Biodegradable polymer scaffold for tissue engineering. Trends Biomater Artif Organs. 25(1):20–29.
148. Wen, X., Zheng, Y., Wu, J., Wang, L.N., Yuan, Z., Peng, J., and Meng, H. (2015). Immobilization of collagen peptide on dialdehyde bacterial cellulose nanofibers via covalent bonds for tissue engineering and regeneration. Int J Nanomedicine. 10:4623–4637.
149. Wang, T., Zheng, Y., Shen, Y., Shi, Y., Li, F., Su, C., and Zhao, L. (2017). Chitosan nanoparticles loaded hydrogels promote skin wound healing through the modulation of reactive oxygen species. Artif Cells Nanomed Biotechnol. 46:1–12.
150. Patel, A.K. (2017). In vitro and in vivo assessment of gelatin nanoparticles loaded doxocetal scaffolds. Int J Pharm Biol Sci Arch. 8:40–51.
151. Cardoso, A. M., De Oliveira, E. G., Coradini, K., Bruinsmann, F. A., Aguirre, T., Lorenzoni, R., Barcelos, R. C. S., Roversi, K., Rossato, D. R., Pohlmann, A. R., and Guterres, S. S. (2018). Chitosan hydrogels containing nano-encapsulated phenytoin for cutaneous use: Skin permeation/penetration and efficacy in wound healing. Mater Sci Eng C. 96:205–217.
152. Krausz, A. E., Adler, B. L., Cabral, V., Navati, M., Doerner, J., Charafeddine, R. A., Harper, S. (2015). Curcumin-encapsulated nanoparticles as innovative antimicrobial and wound healing agent. Nanomed: Nanotechnol Biol Med. 11:195–206.

153. Wicklein, V. J., Singer, B. B., Scheibel, T., and Salehi, S. (2019). Nanoengineered biomaterials for corneal regeneration. In: Nanoengineered Biomaterials for Regenerative Medicine. 379–415. doi:10.1016/b978-0-12-813355-2.00017-x

154. Wang, T.-J., Wang, I.-J., Lu, J.-N., and Young, T.-H. (2012). Novel chitosan-polycaprolactone blends as potential scaffold and carrier for corneal endothelial transplantation. Mol Vis. 18:255–264.

155. Grolik, M., Szczubiałka, K., Wowra, B., Dobrowolski, D., Orzechowska-Wylęgała, B., Wylęgała, E., and Nowakowska, M. (2012). Hydrogel membranes based on genipin-cross-linked chitosan blends for corneal epithelium tissue engineering. J Mater Sci Mater Med. 23:1991–2000.

156. Kim, D. K., Sim, B. R., and Khang, G. (2016). Nature-derived aloe vera gel blended silk fibroin film scaffolds for cornea endothelial cell regeneration and transplantation. ACS Appl Mater. Interfaces. 8(24):15160–15168.

157. Guan, L., Ge, H., Tang, X., Su, S., Tian, P., Xiao, N., Zhang, H., Zhang, L., and Liu, P. (2013). Use of a silk fibroin-chitosan scaffold to construct a tissue-engineered corneal stroma. Cells Tissues Organs. 198(3):190–197.

158. Nara, S., Chameettachal, S., Midha, S., Singh, H., Tandon, R., Mohanty, S., and Ghosh, S. (2015). Strategies for faster detachment of corneal cell sheet using micropatterned thermoresponsive matrices. J Mater Chem B. 3(20):4155–4169.

159. Salehi, S., Czugala, M., Stafiej, P., Fathi, M., Bahners, T., Gutmann, J. S., Singer, B. B., and Fuchsluger, T. A. (2017). Poly (glycerol sebacate)-poly(ε-caprolactone) blend nanofibrous scaffold as intrinsic bio- and immunocompatible system for corneal repair. Acta Biomater. 50:370–380.

160. Ozcelik, B., Brown, K. D., Blencowe, A., Daniell, M., Stevens, G. W., and Qiao, G. G. (2013). Ultrathin chitosan-poly (ethylene glycol) hydrogel films for corneal tissue engineering. Acta Biomater. 9(5):6594–6605.

161. Tummala, G.K., Joffre, T., Lopes, V.R., Liszka, A., Buznyk, O., Ferraz, N., Persson, C., Griffith, M., and Mihranyan, A. (2016). Hyperelastic nanocellulose-reinforced hydrogel of high water content for ophthalmic applications. ACS Biomater Sci Eng. 2(11):2072–2079.

162. Gain, P., Jullienne, R., He, Z., Aldossary, M., Acquart, S., Cognasse, F., and Thuret, G. (2016). Global survey of corneal transplantation and eye banking. JAMA Ophthalmol. 134(2):167–173. DOI: 10.1001/jamaophthalmol.2015.4776. PMID: 26633035.

163. Lambert, N. G., and Chamberlain, W. D. (2017). The structure and evolution of eye banking: A review on eye banks' historical, present, and future contribution to corneal transplantation. Journal of Biorepository Science for Applied Medicine. 5:23–40. https://doi.org/10.2147/BSAM.S114197 and https://restoresight.org/cornea-donation/faqs/

164. https://www.post-gazette.com/news/health/2015/01/13/University-of-Pittsburgh-research-uses-stem-cells-from-the-eye-to-repair-damaged-corneas/stories/201501200003

165. Califano, J. P., and Reinhart-King, C. A. (2010). Exogenous and endogenous force regulation of endothelial cell behavior. J. Biomech. 43:79.

166. Jang, Y., Park, Y., and Kim, J. (2020). Engineering biomaterials to guide heart cells for matured cardiac tissue. Coatings. 10:925. doi:10.3390/coatings10100925

167. Chen, Q.Z. et al. (2008). Biomaterials in cardiac tissue engineering: Ten years of research survey. Materials Science and Engineering R, Elsevier. 59:1–37. doi: 10.1016/j.mser.2007.08.001

168. Majid, Q. A., Fricker, A., Gregory, D. A., Davidenko, N., Hernandez Cruz, O., Jabbour, R. J., Owen, T. J., Basnett, P., Lukasiewicz, B., Stevens, M., Best, S., Cameron, R., Sinha, S., Harding, S. E., and Roy, I. (2020). Natural biomaterials for cardiac tissue engineering: A highly biocompatible solution. Front Cardiovasc Med. 7:554597. https://doi.org/10.3389/fcvm.2020.554597

169. Curtis, A., Dalby, M., and Gadegaard, N. (2006). Cell signaling arising from nanotopography: implications for nanomedical devices, Nanomed. 1:67; Gjorevski, N. and Nelson, C. M. (2009). Bidirectional extracellular matrix signaling during tissue morphogenesis, Cytokine Growth Factor Rev. 20:459.

170. Ahmed, M., Yildirimer, L., Khademhosseini, A., and Seifalian, A. M. (2012). Nanostructured materials for cardiovascular tissue engineering. J Nanosci Nanotechnol. 12:4775–4785.

171. Kargozar, S., Milan, P. B., Baino, F., and Mozafari, M. (2019). Nanoengineered Biomaterials for Bone/Dental Regeneration. In: Nanoengineered Biomaterials for Regenerative Medicine: Micro and Nano Technologies. 13–38. https://doi.org/10.1016/B978-0-12-813355-2.00002-8

172. Gao, C., Peng, S., Feng, P. et al. (2017). Bone biomaterials and interactions with stem cells, Bone Res. 5:17059. https://doi.org/10.1038/boneres.2017.59

173. Hanson, M. A., and Gluckman, P. (2014). Early developmental conditioning of later health and disease: Physiology or pathophysiology? Physiol Rev. 94:1027–1076.

174. Webber, M. J., Appel, E. A., Meijer, E. et al. (2016). Supramolecular biomaterials. Nat Mater. 15:13–.26; Windhagen H, Radtke K, Weizbauer A et al. Biodegradable magnesium-based screw clinically equivalent to titanium screw in hallux valgus surgery: short term results of the first prospective, randomized, controlled clinical pilot study. Biomed Eng Online 2013; 12: 62.

175. Levandowski, N., Camargo, N. H., Silva, D. F. et al. (2014). Characterization of different nanostructured bone substitute biomaterials. Adv Mater Res. 936:695–700. 94

176. Ching, H. A., Choudhury, D., Nine, M. J. et al. (2014). Effects of surface coating on reducing friction and wear of orthopaedic implants. Sci Technol Adv Mat. 15:014402.

177. Li, Z., Munroe, P., Jiang, Z. et al. (2012). Designing super hard, self-toughening CrAlN coatings through grain boundary engineering. Acta Mater. 60:5735–5744

178. Vila, M., Cicuéndez, M., Sánchez-Marcos, J. et al. (2013). Electrical stimuli to increase cell proliferation on carbon nanotubes/mesoporous silica composites for drug delivery. J Biomed Mater Res A. 101:213–221.

179. Tatarko, P., Grasso, S., Chlup, Z. et al. (2014). Toughening effect of multi-walled boron nitride nanotubes and their influence on the sintering behaviour of 3Y-TZP zirconia ceramics. J Eur Ceram Soc. 34:1829–1843.

180. Wu, C., Xia, L., Han, P. et al. (2015). Graphene-oxide-modified β-tricalcium phosphate bioceramics stimulate in vitro and in vivo osteogenesis. Carbon. 93:116–129.

181. Zeng, X., Ye, L., Yu, S. et al. (2015). Facile preparation of superelastic and ultralow dielectric boron nitride nanosheet aerogels via freeze-casting process. Chem Mater. 27:5849–5585.

182. Lahiri, D., Singh, V., Benaduce, AP. Et al. (2011). Boron nitride nanotube reinforced hydroxyapatite composite: Mechanical and tribological performance and in-vitro biocompatibility to osteoblasts. J Mech Behav Biomed. 4:44–56.

183. Nie, H., and Wang, C-H. (2007). Fabrication and characterization of PLGA/Hap composite scaffolds for delivery of BMP-2 plasmid DNA. J Control Release. 120:111–121.

184. Cui, W., Li, X., Chen, J. et al. (2008). In situ growth kinetics of hydroxyapatite on electrospun poly (DL-lactide) fibers with gelatin grafted. Cryst Growth Des. 8:4576–4582.

185. Wu, F., Wei, J., Liu, C. et al. (2012). Fabrication and properties of porous scaffold of zein/PCL biocomposite for bone tissue engineering. Composites Part B. 43:2192–2197.

186. Govindaraj, D., Rajan, M. (2018). Coating of bio-mimetic minerals-substituted hydroxyapatite on surgical grade stainless steel 316L by electrophoretic deposition for hard tissue applications. IOP Conf Ser.: Mater Sci Eng. 314(1):012029.

187. Govindaraj, D., Rajan, M., Hatamleh, A. A., Munusamy, M. A., Alarfaj, A. A., Sadasivuni, K. K.S., and Kumar, S. (2017). The synthesis, characterization and in vivo study of mineral substituted hydroxyapatite for prospective bone tissue rejuvenation applications. Nanomed: Nanotechnol Biol Med. 13(8):2661–2669.

188. Govindaraj, D., Govindaraj, C., and Rajan, M. (2017). Binary functional porous multi mineral–substituted apatite nanoparticles for reducing osteosarcoma colonization and enhancing osteoblast cell proliferation. Mater Sci Eng C Mater Biol Appl. 79:875–885

189. Bhardwaj, N., and Kundu, S. C. (2011). Silk fibroin protein and chitosan polyelectrolyte complex porous scaffolds for tissue engineering applications. Carbohydr Polym. 85:325–333.

190. Saravanan, S., Nethala, S., Pattnaik, S. et al. (2011). Preparation, characterization and antimicrobial activity of a bio-composite scaffold containing chitosan/nano-hydroxyapatite/nano-silver for bone tissue engineering. Int J Biol Macromol. 49:188–193.

191. Qi, Y. M., Yang, L. J., and Wang, L. L. (2012). Finite-element analysis and optimization for gradient porous structure of artificial bone. Appl Mech Mater. 271–272:922–926.

192. Qiu, L. L., and Choong, C. (2013). Three-dimensional scaffolds for tissue engineering applications: Role of porosity and pore size. Tissue Eng Part B Rev. 19:485–502.

193. Gao, J. H., Guan, S. K., Chen, J. et al. (2011). Fabrication and characterization of rod-like nano-hydroxyapatite on MAO coating supported on Mg-ZnCa alloy. Appl Surf Sci. 257:2231–2237.

194. Tripathi, G., and Basu, B. (2012). A porous hydroxyapatite scaffold for bone tissue engineering: Physico-mechanical and biological evaluations. Ceram Int. 38:341–349.

195. Ma, J., Wang, C., and Peng, K. W. (2003). Electrophoretic deposition of porous hydroxyapatite scaffold. Biomaterials. 24:3505–3510.

196. Campbell, I., Bourell, D., and Gibson, I. (2012). Additive manufacturing: Rapid prototyping comes of age. Rapid Prototyping J. 18

197. Venkatraman, S. K., and Swamiappan, S. (2020). Review on calcium- and magnesium-based silicates for bone tissue engineering applications. J Biomed Mater Res A. 108(7):1546–1562. DOI: 10.1002/jbm.a.36925.

198. Koons, G. L., Diba, M. and Mikos, A. G. (2020). Materials design for bone-tissue engineering. Nat Rev Mater. 5:584–603. https://doi.org/10.1038/s41578-020-0204-2

199. Fu, Q., Saiz, E., Rahaman, M. N., and Tomsia, A. P. (2011). Bioactive glass scaffolds for bone tissue engineering: State of the art and future perspectives. Mater Sci Eng C Mater Biol Appl. 31(7):1245–1256. https://doi.org/10.1016/j.msec.2011.04.022

200. Balasubramanian, P., Büttner, T., Pacheco, V. M., and Boccaccini, A. R. (2018). Boron-containing bioactive glasses in bone and soft tissue engineering. J Eur Ceram Soc. 38(3):855–869.

201. Erol-Taygun, M., Unalan, I., Idris, M. I. B., Mano, J. F., and Boccaccini, A. R. (2019). Bioactive glass-polymer nanocomposites for bone tissue regeneration applications. Adv Eng Mater. 21:1900287 DOI: 10.1002/adem.201900287

202. Gogoi, S., Kumar, M., Mandal, BB., and Karak, N. (2016). A renewable resource-based carbon dot decorated hydroxyapatite nanohybrid and its fabrication with waterborne hyperbranched polyurethane for bone tissue engineering. RSC Adv. 6:26066–26076.

203. Frohbergh, M. E., Katsman, A., Botta, G. P., Lazarovici, P., Schauer, C. L., Wegst, U. G., and Lelkes, P. I. (2012). Electrospun hydroxyapatite-containing chitosan nanofibers crosslinked with genipin for bone tissue engineering. Biomaterials. 33:9167–9178.

204. Anjaneyulu, U., Priyadarshini, B., Grace, A. N., and Vijayalakshmi, U. (2016). Fabrication and characterization of Ag doped hydroxyapatite-polyvinyl alcohol composite nanofibers and its in vitro biological evaluations for bone tissue engineering applications. J Sol-Gel Sci Technol. 81(3):750–761.

205. Gholizadeh, S., Moztarzadeh, F., Haghighipour, N., Ghazizadeh, L., Baghbani, F., Shokrgozar, M. A., and Allahyari, Z. (2017). Preparation and characterization of novel functionalized multiwalled carbon nanotubes/- chitosan/β-Glycerophosphate scaffolds for bone tissue engineering. Int J Biol Macromol. 97:365–372.

206. Niu, B., Li, B., Gu, Y., Shen, X., Liu, Y., and Chen, L. (2017). In vitro evaluation of electrospun silk fibroin/nano-hydroxyapatite/BMP-2 scaffolds for bone regeneration. J Biomater Sci Polym Ed. 28:257–270.

207. Wang, Q., Chen, C., Liu, W., He, X., Zhou, N., Zhang, D., and Huang, W. (2017). Levofloxacin loaded mesoporous silica microspheres/nanohydroxyapatite/polyurethane composite scaffold for the treatment of chronic osteomyelitis with bone defects. Sci Rep. 7:41808–41820.

208. Bhattacharjee, P., Naskar, D., Maiti, T. K., Bhattacharya, D., and Kundu, S. C. (2016). Investigating the potential of combined growth factors delivery, from non-mulberry silk fibroin grafted poly(ε-caprolactone)/hydroxyapatite nanofibrous scaffold, in bone tissue engineering. Appl Mater Today. 5:52–67.

209. Wang, X., Cheng, F., Liu, J., Smatt, J. H., Gepperth, D., Lastusaari, M., and Hupa, L. (2016). Biocomposites of copper-containing mesoporous bioactive glass and nanofibrillated cellulose: Biocompatibility and angiogenic promotion in chronic wound healing application. Acta Biomater. 46:286–298.

210. Sankar, R., Baskaran, A., Shivashangari, K. S., and Ravikumar, V. (2015). Inhibition of pathogenic bacterial growth on excision wound by green synthesized copper oxide nanoparticles leads to accelerated wound healing activity in Wistar albino rats. J Mater Sci Mater Med. 26:1–7.

211. Selvaraj, S., and Fathima, N. N. (2017). Fenugreek incorporated silk fibroin nanofibers: A potential antioxidant scaffold for enhanced wound healing. ACS Appl Mater Interfaces. 9:5916–5926.

212. Buchtova, N., Rethore, G., Boyer, C., Guicheux, J., Rambaud, F., Valle, K., and Le Bideau, J. (2013). Nanocomposite hydrogels for cartilage tissue engineering: Mesoporous silica nanofibers interlinked with siloxane derived polysaccharide. J Mater Sci Mater Med. 24:1875–1884.

213. Sambudi, N. S., Sathyamurthy, M., Lee, G. M., and Park, S. B. (2015). Electrospun chitosan/poly(vinyl alcohol) reinforced with CaCO3 nanoparticles with enhanced mechanical properties and biocompatibility for cartilage tissue engineering. Compos Sci Technol. 106:76–84.

214. Recha-Sancho, L., Moutos, FT., Abella, J., Guilak, F., and Semino, C. E. (2016). Dedifferentiated human articular chondrocytes redifferentiate to a cartilage-like tissue phenotype in a poly(ε-caprolactone)/selfassembling peptide composite scaffold. Materials. 9:472–489.

215. He, X., Feng, B., Huang, C., Wang, H., Ge, Y., Hu, R., and Zheng, J. (2015). Electrospun gelatin/polycaprolactone nanofibrous membranes combined with a coculture of bone marrow stromal cells and chondrocytes for cartilage engineering. Int J Nanomedicine. 10:2089–2099.

216. Zhang, N., Lock, J., Sallee, A., and Liu, H. (2015). Magnetic nanocomposite hydrogel for potential cartilage tissue engineering: Synthesis, characterization, and cytocompatibility with bone marrow derived mesenchymal stem cells. ACS Appl Mater Interfaces. 7:20987–20998.

217. Schulz, F., Lutz, D., Rusche, N., Bastus, N. G., Stieben, M., Holtig, M., and Loers, G. (2013). Gold nanoparticles functionalized with a fragment of the neural cell adhesion molecule L1 stimulate L1-mediated functions. Nanoscale. 5:10605–10617.

218. Prabhakaran, M. P., Vatankhah, E., and Ramakrishna, S. (2013). Electrospun aligned PHBV/collagen nanofibers as substrates for nerve tissue engineering. Biotechnol Bioeng. 110:2775–2784.

219. Junka, R., Valmikinathan, C. M., Kalyon, D. M., and Yu, X. (2013). Laminin functionalized biomimetic nanofibers for nerve tissue engineering. J Biomater Tissue Eng. 3:494–502.

220. Marino, A., Tonda-Turo, C., De Pasquale, D., Ruini, F., Genchi, G., Nitti, S., and Ciofani, G. (2017). Gelatin/nanoceria nanocomposite fibers as antioxidant scaffolds for neuronal regeneration. Biochim Biophys Acta. 1861:386–395.
221. Golafshan, N., Kharaziha, M., and Fathi, M. (2017). Tough and conductive hybrid graphene-PVA: Alginate fibrous scaffolds for engineering neural construct. Carbon. 111:752–763.
222. Alarcon, E. I., Vulesevic, B., Argawal, A., Ross, A., Bejjani, P., Podrebarac, J., and Griffith, M. (2016). Coloured cornea replacements with anti-infective properties: Expanding the safe use of silver nanoparticles in regenerative medicine. Nanoscale. 6484–6489.
223. Czugala, M., Mykhaylyk, O., Bohler, P., Onderka, J., Stork, B., Wesselborg, S., and Fuchsluger, T. A. (2016). Efficient and safe gene delivery to human corneal endothelium using magnetic nanoparticles. Nanomedicine. 11:1787–1800.

3 Patterning Nanomaterials for the Delivery of Growth Factors for Tissue Repair/ Regeneration

Sivaraj Mehnath and Murugaraj Jeyaraj
University of Madras

CONTENTS

DOI: 10.1201/9781003140108-3

3.1 INTRODUCTION

Over recent years, regenerative medicine techniques have merged the life science and engineering process for regulating the biological environment. It needs the intensive efforts of bioengineers, researchers, and clinical technicians to rebuild the structure and improve tissue activity. Current treatment technique for tissue repair/regeneration is transplantation, such as allografts, xenografts, substituents, synthetic devices, and delivery of stem cells at damaged region. Unfortunately, these strategies fail in many cases because of some drawbacks like a tedious surgical process, immune rejection, poor clinical prediction, chronic inflammation, and shortage of tissue/organ donors. An example of this is the surgical grafting of autologous skin to support a burn wound. The procedure is painful, difficult, and high cost, which may result in poor efficiency for affected people. An alternative approach for regulating tissue construction and its action is by reproducing the microenvironment and activating signal transduction pathways to enhance the regeneration process. This process is attained by a combination of biomaterials and GF to induce vital regeneration pathways involved in tissue growth. This chapter discusses various GFs and their role in the tissue repair/regeneration process. Direct GF delivery has some clinical limitation. So patterning of nanomaterial for effective GF delivery, different types of substrate, and strategies for immobilization and delivery technique are discussed.

3.2 GROWTH FACTORS

GFs are soluble polypeptides produced by cells that have the ability to control various regeneration process such as cell differentiation, proliferation, and migration. So controlled delivery of GF to the patients for accelerating the above process leads to improved self-healing capacity. It also serves as a vital factor for transferring signals among the cell population during regeneration and subsequently accelerates the restoration of damaged tissue. As in Figure 3.1, GF regulates the cell activity

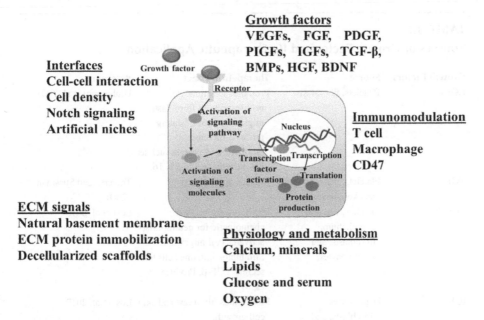

Growth factors
VEGFs, FGF, PDGF,
PIGFs, IGFs, TGF-β,
BMPs, HGF, BDNF

Interfaces
Cell-cell interaction
Cell density
Notch signaling
Artificial niches

Immunomodulation
T cell
Macrophage
CD47

ECM signals
Natural basement membrane
ECM protein immobilization
Decellularized scaffolds

Physiology and metabolism
Calcium, minerals
Lipids
Glucose and serum
Oxygen

FIGURE 3.1 Mechanism of GF to bind on the respective receptors on the surface of cells. The binding initiates a signaling pathway to activation of signaling molecules. It regulates the transcription and activates the different cellular responses such as growth, invasion, differentiation, migration.

by binding to the specific transmembrane receptors that are present on the target cells' surface. The binding of GF to its respective receptor is highly specific, which delivers a signal to the target cells. The GF-binding signals trigger the receptor to transduce the secondary signals, which activate intracellular signaling pathways like cytoskeleton phosphorylation, ion fluxes, gene expression, and protein synthesis. So the delivery of GF is a crucial step for tissue regeneration and repair (Yamakawa and Kenji 2019; Fathi-Achachelouei et al. 2019; Talebian et al. 2019). GFs involved in repair mechanisms of different tissue types are presented in Table 3.1. Some examples include VEGFs, FGF, PDGF, and PIGF, which are involved in angiogenesis in cases such as diabetic foot ulcers, periodontal regeneration, and cervical spinal cord injury (Martino and Briquez 2015; Fei et al. 2013; Okonkwo and DiPietro 2017). IGFs, TGF-β, BMPs, mainly BMP-2, BMP-4, BMP-7, are extensively used for new bone formation. HGF is used for liver cirrhosis, and BDNF is used in spinal cord injury (Losi et al. 2010; Losi et al. 2013; Zhang et al. 2006; Wang et al. 2006; Theiss et al. 2010).

3.2.1 Clinical Limitations of GFs

Accordingly, fewer clinical trials have been approved for GF on tissue regeneration applications and commercial aspects because it shows limited application. The major

TABLE 3.1

Sources of Growth Factor and Its Therapeutic Application

Growth Factors	Source	Therapeutic Effect	Reference
EGF	Platelets, fibroblasts	Promotes keratinocyte, proliferation of fibroblasts, migration during healing process. Increases production of protein such as FN, keratins K6 and K 16.	Ulubayram et al. 2001
TGF	Platelets, macrophages, and keratinocytes	Induces angiogenesis.	Traversa and Sussman 2001
PDGF	Platelets, vascular endothelium, fibroblasts, and keratinocytes.	Proliferates fibroblast, chemotactic for neutrophils, activates cell migration. Stimulates immune cells to secrete TGF-β. Produce ECM.	Losi et al. 2013
IGF	Hepatocytes, fibroblasts, and macrophages,	Proliferates fibroblast and skin cell growth.	Losi et al. 2010
VEGF	Platelets, and keratinocytes.	Multiplication and migration of endothelial cell. Stimulates angiogenesis of lymph.	Traversa and Sussman 2001
FGF	Fibroblasts, macrophages, and endothelial cells	Potent factor in angiogenesis. Mytogenic for cells. Stimulates re-epithelisation, and matrix formation. Signals processes like inflammation, pro-inflammatory cytokines/ chemokines production in endothelial cells.	Zhang et al. 2006
TGF-β	Platelets, macrophages, keratinocytes, and fibroblasts	Chemoattractant for immune cells. Induces granulation, tissue repair and provide strength.	Wang et al. 2006
KGF	Keratinocytes	Mitogen of epithelial cells.	Traversa and Sussman 2001
GCSF		Activates bone marrow-derived stem cells.	Theiss et al. 2010
BMP	Bone, cartilage	Differentiation and migration of osteoblasts.	Fu et al. 2008
Ang-1	Heart, muscle, blood vessels	Stability and maturation of blood vessels.	Carmeliet 2005
Ang-2	Blood vessels	Disassociates endothelial cells, destabilize.	

limitation of GF is the half-life, low protein stability, safety, rapid deactivation, and cost-effectiveness. Bulk quantities of GF were directly introduced into the body via topical application, spraying, and injection. Here are some examples: FGF-2 injection for periodontal repair, GCSF for myocardial infarction, VEGF for diabetic foot ulcers, and FGF sprayed directly on burn wounds (Kiritsi and Nystrom 2018; Kitamura et al. 2011; Gainza et al. 2015; Hanft et al. 2008). The problem is that this administration does not permit enough time for reaching target tissue, rapid degradation, and fast clearance of GF. Moreover, the bioavailability of GF is very low owing to the result of diffusion. The FGF-1 treatment shows intrinsically less stability, with a poor half-life in the blood. The half-life of b-FGF was 3 min, and VEGF is only 50 min by intravenous injection (Lee and Blaber 2013; Chen et al. 2017; Waller et al. 2021). Furthermore, to increase the half-life, a high enough dose was used to reach the target site. Administration of a high dosage leads to severe side effects such as tumor formation. The clinical dose of BMP-2 used for lumbar spinal arthrodesis was high risk in new cancer development. The VEGF application causes edema and systemic hypotension in the cardiovascular and leads to serious concern. Still, GF has marginal benefits; it does not ensure the regeneration application. Additionally, combinant GF production was very expensive, which is a major obstacle to limit therapeutic application (Carragee et al. 2013; Simons and Ware 2003).

3.3   PATTERNING NANOMATERIALS FOR GF DELIVERY

Collectively, cost-effectiveness, larger size, short half-lives, and potential toxicity to the higher dose are the major drawback of GF during conventional delivery. The delivery of GF without appropriate spatiotemporal control mainly leads to burst release of GF at the non-target site and faster clearance from the damaged site. To address these difficulties, highly advanced delivery systems that provide sustained, specific, continuous, and targeted release of GF/biocomponents were used. It enables optimal doses with spatial/temporal gradients at target sites for higher tissue repair. Recently, patterned nanomaterials are capable of mimicking the ECM for cell adhesion; migration maintains the 3D network for tissue regeneration. Additionally, nanostructured delivery systems have a higher surface area, roughness, and surface energy, which offers more advantages compared to microstructure. Several factors need to be considered for patterning the nanomaterial for GF delivery.

3.4   IMMOBILIZATION OF GF

The main factor in nanomaterial-based GF delivery is the immobilization of GF into the nanosystem, and there are several advanced techniques, such as physical/chemical interaction (Mao et al. 2017). Strategies such as directive immobilization, encapsulation, adsorption, covalent conjugation, LbL self-assembly, and binding are used for the controlled delivery of GF. Table 3.2 consists of some detailed strategies of GF immobilization.

TABLE 3.2
Overview of Different Substances Used for Immobilization of Growth Factor

Substrate	GF	Immobilization Approach	Application	Reference
PLGA scaffold	VEGF	Physical encapsulation	Bone therapy	Murphy et al. 2000
Alginate scaffold	VEGF, bFGF, PDGF, TGF-β1	Physical encapsulation	Vascularization	Freeman and Cohen 2009
Chitosan film	BMP-2 or FGF-2.	Physical adsorption	Bone regeneration	Budiraharjo et al. 2013
Diblock co-polymer matrix	HGF	Physical adsorption	Vocal fold regeneration	Choi et al. 2017
Dermatan, and gum tragacanth –PLL	VEGF	Encapsulation	Tissue regeneration	Zandi et al. 2020
Porous PLA film	NGF	Encapsulation	Nerve regeneration	Uz et al. 2017
TCP-HAP	BMP-2	LbL assembly	Bone regeneration	Crouzier et al. 2011
Gelatin-based coating	NGF	LbL assembly	Alzheimer's Disease treatment	Zhang et al. 2015
PLGA scaffold	VEGF	Carbodiimide crosslinking	Angiogenesis	Sharon and Puleo 2008
Fibrin	HGF	Carbodiimide crosslinking	Skeletal muscle regeneration	Grasman et al. 2008
Titanium surface	BMP-2	Mussel-inspired crosslinking	Bone regeneration	Chien and Tsai 2013
Titanium surface	BMP-2	ECM mimic approach	Bone regeneration	Wang et al. 2015
PLGA microsphere	BMP-2	Affinity interaction	Bone regeneration	Kim et al. 2015
Hyaluronic hydrogel	BMP-2	Affinity interaction	Bone regeneration	Kisiel et al. 2013

3.4.1 PHYSICAL IMMOBILIZATION

Physical immobilization is the simplest technique to immobilize the GF into materials before attaining their matrix/scaffold/nanostructures. This delivery system has maintained their properties after incorporation of GF and also protects the bioactivity of GF from the external factors. Direct encapsulation of GF was performed by diffusion of a pre-formed delivery system in GF solution, impregnation. Advantages of this technique include low cost, accessibility, protection of the bioactivity of GF, and controlled release. The less distribution and unpredictable release attained by this process are the reason for development of different methods (Schumacher et al. 2017). As represented in Figure 3.2, the major subtypes of physical immobilization approaches are surface adsorption, encapsulation, and LbL immobilization.

Physical immobilization approaches

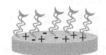
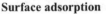

Surface adsorption

Encapsulation

Layer by layer

FIGURE 3.2 Schematic representation of various type of physical immobilization methods.

3.4.1.1 Physical Encapsulation

Physical encapsulation will also immobilize the GF into the delivery system by entrapment by hydrophobic, hydrophilic-hydrophilic, and electrostatic interactions. A diverse range of GFs were immobilized by physical encapsulation, including VEGF, BMP-2, IGF-1, CSF. GF was incorporated into the polymer matrices such as chitosan, collagen, gelatin, cellulose, alginate, PLA, PLGA, and PEG (Zhang et al. 2020; Abbah et al. 2012; Hameed et al. 2019).

3.4.1.2 Surface Adsorption

Surface adsorption is the simplest method to form an attachment between the GF and delivery system by surface adsorption. The adsorption of GF was varied based on the different types of material and their respective properties. Adsorption was controlled by the solution used to immobilizes the GF. This process used to immobilize the various GF such as FGF, FGF-2, and BMP-2. The main disadvantages of this method are the poor payload, low control over the release, and lack of space (Wang et al. 2017). Ziegler et al. prepared a synthetic bone implant with a HAP-TCP carrier for packing of BMP-2 and bFGF. The release of BMP-2 increases the activity of ALP, and it contributed to the adsorption process. It also highlighted the necessity of immobilization of GF to a delivery system for improved retention effect (Ziegler et al. 2008). Reyes et al. used a brushite and brushite-PLGA for immobilization of PDGF,TGF-β1 and VEGF. GF was directly adsorbed onto the brushite composites, whereas VEGF was pre-loaded on PLGA. Initially, a there was a 40% burst release of PDGF and TGF-β1 for 24 h and a further controlled release of 5.5% per day for the next 6 days. Ninety percent of GF was released after 3 weeks; VEGF encapsulated into PLGA and incorporated to brushite composite showed more controlled release (Reyes et al. 2012).

3.4.1.3 Layer-by-Layer (LbL)

To overcome the problem of over-controlled release and spatial distribution issue of surface adsorption technique, an alternative LbL immobilization technique was presented. In this, GF is adsorbed on the several layers of matrix and immobilization of GF mainly depends on electrostatic interaction such as hydrophobic interaction, oppositely charged electrolytes, and hydrogen bond. LbL is a simple, low-cost method, and LbL efficiency does not affect by GF size/shape, attachment of different GF improved by structural design (Gomes et al. 2015). LbL immobilization is mainly applied for wound healing, cardiac, and neural repair approaches (Liu et al. 2017; Mandapalli et al. 2017). Naves formed an LbL process with a poly(ethylene imine) combination of chitosan and heparin for acid FGF attachment. The GF release rate was inversely proportional to the number of matrix layers, and higher GF adsorption leads to increased stability and controlled the release of GF. GF immobilize on the 6-bilayer matrix shows higher stability than a 3-bilayer one. It also improves the GF release profile; a 3-bilayer substrate releases faster than a 6-bilyaer matrix due to poor stability. In other work, (FGF) FGF-2 was immobilized in a 5polyelectrolyte layer composed of PMAA, PL, and PLH. It also increases the fibroblast proliferation when compared with a single dose GF (Naves et al. 2016). Kumorek prepared a albumin/heparin bilayer for immobilization of FGF-2. It forms a covalent linkage by glutaraldehyde and FGF-2 enhances cell proliferation (Kumorek et al. 2015).

3.4.2 CHEMICAL IMMOBILIZATION OF GF

3.4.2.1 Covalent Conjugation

In covalent conjugation, functional groups of GF are usually used to immobilize them on the delivery system. The main issue in the process is the availability of functional groups near the GF active site, which affects the bioactivity of GF at the time of immobilization. Mostly the attachment is very strong and irreversible; covalent binding of GF is needed when the GF cannot be adsorbed on the substrate surface (Chiu et al. 2011).

3.4.2.2 Carbodiimide Coupling Immobilization

Carbodiimide coupling is the most commonly used method; it forms a covalent attachment between GF and substrates. Carbodiimide is a crosslinking process between the amine and carboxylic acid group to the formation of amide linkage as shown in Figure 3.3. In carbodiimide,1-ethyl3- (3- dimethyl amino propyl) carbodiimide hydrochloride (EDC) is mainly used for the bioconjugation process. The reaction provides an active o-acylisourea intermediary, which reacts with a primary amine to form an amide linkage. In some cases, hydrolyze of o-acylisourea restores the carboxylic group and fails to bind the GF. To prevent the reverse reaction, carbodiimides are combined with NHS. Carbodiimide conjugation may bind through the amine functional groups of lysine and the -COOH groups in the GF. The presence of various functional groups causes random orientation of GF on

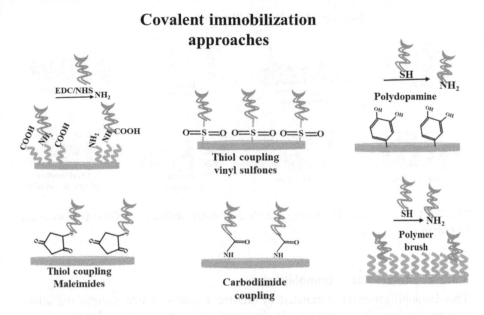

FIGURE 3.3 Overview of methods currently used in immobilization of GF via covalent immobilization.

the substrate, which affects bioactivity (Hermanson 2008). Psarra used HGF and FGF -NH2groups with the PAA for immobilization. The GF-PAA efficiency was studied with cell lines to show higher proliferation compared to free GF (Psarra et al. 2015).

3.4.2.3   Thiol Functionalized Immobilization

Another strategy of covalent attachment is thiol groups, which are able to form -SH containing GF. Mostly the conjugation follows the two reactions as shown in Figure 3.3: alkylation or di-sulfide exchange and reaction generate either -S- or -S-S. In this, the reaction of thiol groups- cysteine residues of GF form interaction with substrate thiol-reactive groups for immobilization. Zisch et al. (2003) prepared PEG divinyl sulfone-conjugated hydrogels to attached VEGF, RGD peptide, and MMP substrate peptide. The variants VEGF immobilized to promote the HUVECs, adhesion, and migration. The coupling process preserves the functionality of GF, induces angiogenesis, and vascularizes tissue formation (Zisch et al. 2003). Rahman immobilized the VEGF onto modified agarose gel to prevent hematopoietic progenitor cells. The VEGF altered with maleimide to facilitate the binding, and it was 75 times more efficient than soluble GF. Other thiol groups such as allyl ethers or norbornenes are used to immobilize the GF onto the substrate surface. The selection of the reactive group was based on the compatibility of GF during the reaction. The pH condition, organometallic catalysts, and presence of by-products are important to consider before reaction (Rahman et al. 2010).

Non covalent immobilization approaches

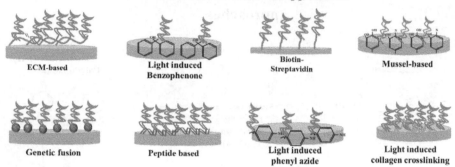

FIGURE 3.4 Overview of methods currently used in immobilization of GF via non-covalent immobilization.

3.4.2.4 Mussel-Based Immobilization

This immobilization is stimulated by marine mussels, which secrete the adhesive protein dopa. The catechol side chain and the amine group of dopa/dopamine help in immobilizing the GF to the organic/inorganic delivery system as shown in Figure 3.4. Dopamine polymerizes under an alkali condition to form a polydopamine file, which reacts with -NH2 and -SH groups. Polydopamine-mediated immobilization was performed for GF such as VEGF, NGF, bFGF, and GDNF. Mussel-based immobilization is a simple procedure without any complex modification steps (Kord Forooshani and Lee 2017).

3.4.3 OTHER COVALENT METHODS

Several other methods are available to immobilize the GF covalently to the delivery system. Plasma treatment is a simple step for the introduction of new functional groups on the surface, which form a linkage with different components such as carbodiimide. It helps for immobilization of BMP and FGF (Zhang et al. 2012). Silane and imine linkage is another process for immobilization of GF. The newly formed bond can be hydrolyzed under physiological conditions, leading to the controlled release of GF (Cabanas-Danes et al. 2018).

3.4.3.1 Light-Induced Immobilization

In light-induced immobilization, covalent immobilization of GF to the delivery system uses photoreactive groups, which convert reactive groups into strong covalent binding target material upon exposure to light. Mostly, GF is coupled to a photoreactive group, further conjugated to the delivery system, which activates upon exposure to a particular ultraviolet or visible light. In certain cases, the delivery system may be coupled with photoreactive groups as shown in Figure 3.4; then it reacts with the GF. Light-based immobilization enables high conjugation over the immobilization because the reaction is regulated by light treatment constraints. Still, light treatment is able to change the GF activity by altering the conformational, stereochemical property, aggregation, and fragmentation of protein. It can be avoided by utilizing long-wavelength UV light and reducing the time of exposure. Some photoreactive groups such as phenyl azide, benzophenone, anthraquinone, diazo compounds, and diazirine are used for coupling the GF/delivery system surface (Kawamoto et al. 2018; Pattison et al. 2012). GF can be coupled to a photoreactive group phenyl azide for immobilization to polystyrene upon UV light. It stimulates the keratinocyte migration to a higher extent than the unmodified polystyrene plate (Stefonek-Puccinelli and Masters 2008). Another photoreactive group, benzophenone, forms a carbon-carbon covalent bond with GF upon UV light exposure (Martin et al. 2011). Acrylate, a common photoreactive group, generates free radicals from photocleavable initiator molecules to form a crosslinking polyacrylate chain. This is used to immobilize GF such as SCF, FBF, VEGF, and PDGF (Lin and Anseth 2009). Another polymer crosslinking photoreactive group is riboflavin, mainly applied for ophthalmic and tissue engineering. It is mainly used with collagen for crosslinking GF such as EGF, TGF-β1, FGF. After exposure to UV, the riboflavin carboxylic group generates highly reactive oxygen species, which induce the covalent linkage formation with GF (Fernandes-Cunha et al. 2017). The main application of photoactive group-based immobilization is to allow higher conjugation and control over immobilization on both two-dimensional and three-dimensional surfaces using light.

3.4.3.2 ECM-Based GF Delivery Systems

As presented in Figure 3.4, ECM is an active microenvironment that controls several cellular processes; additionally, it serves as a source for various GFs. In particular, heparin sulfate of ECM interacts with BMP-2, BMP-7, VEGF, FGF-2. So the delivery system functionalized with heparin/heparin sulfate-mimicking molecules helps to immobilize the GF. Jha et al. loaded TGF-β1 in a heparin-functionalized hyaluronic acid-based hydrogel, which provides high loading of TGF-β1 on low molecular weight heparin (Jha et al. 2015). Interestingly, Kim et al. reported the formation of electrostatic interactions between heparin and GF, which disrupt physiological conditions to cause controlled release. Some other GF binding motifs in ECF are collagen, FN, and vitronectin, which helps to immobilize the BMP-2, PDGF, etc. In addition to the ECM bio-affinity components, ECM architecture itself plays a vital role in GF immobilization (Kim et al. 2016a).

3.4.3.3 Non-covalent Approaches

Non-covalent GF tethering is a simple process by mixing the GF with the target substrate without any functional modification of GF. Another important feature in the non-covalent process is reversible, temporal control of immobilized GF. In Figure 3.4 some other forms of non-covalent approaches are presented. Peptides/short oligomers of amino acids help in GF immobilization on a wide variety of delivery system surfaces. Some examples, such as collagen mimetic peptide, self-assemble peptide amphiphiles that were used to immobilize the VEGF and TGF-β1 (Brummelhuis et al. 2017). The coiled-coil is a protein that includes extracellular motor proteins, such as kinesin, myosin, keratin, fibrin, and transcriptional factor, etc. It consists of 2-5 helices, parallel/antiparallel, super-helical structure and characterized with seven amino acids. The high specificity and stable interaction make it advantageous for immobilizing GF. Several studies are promising in the usage of de novo coiled-coils due to their stability, degree of oligomerization, self-assembly, pH, and temperature sensitivity (Goktas et al. 2018). Another valuable technique is genetic fusion, which produced fusion protein of GF with binding tags and specific affinity peptides. Some examples of natural fusion proteins are IgG, FN collagen-binding domain, spider silk protein, β-TCP-binding peptide, and artificial fusion proteins such as hexa histidine residues and titanium-binding peptides (Worrallo et al. 2017). Next, biotin-streptavidin conjugation is one of the stable non-covalent interactions that contain the binding of biotin to avidin/streptavidin. Mostly, immobilized surfaces were functionalized with avidin/streptavidin, while the biotin was functionalized with GF. Mainly, GF immobilization via biotin-streptavidin interaction performs by tetrameric streptavidin, which makes irreversible biotin avidin/streptavidin interaction (O'Sullivan et al. 2012).

3.5 GROWTH FACTOR DELIVERY SYSTEM

Several types of delivery systems were available to provide improved stability and controlled release and to protect the bioactivity of GF. The delivery system for GF was classified into particulates, hydrogel, scaffold, and miscellaneous systems. In this section, classification, loading procedure, route of administration, dosing regimens, and therapeutic effects (Koria 2012) are described in detail.

3.5.1 PARTICULATE SYSTEMS

Particulate systems are composed of natural/synthetic polymers, protein, biomaterials, lipids, or ceramics materials, which offer great advantages in the controlled delivery of GF with enhanced therapeutic effect for various tissue regeneration as represented in Figure 3.5. The particulate delivery system is characterized by size, such as microparticles and nanoparticles (Mehnath et al. 2018a; Sumathra et al. 2020; Murugan et al. 2018). Among the several particulate systems, polymer and biomaterials are widely used for encapsulation of GF and tissue regeneration application (Wang et al. 2017).

3.5.1.1 Synthetic Polymeric Nanoparticles

The major synthetic polymers used for nanoparticle fabrication are polyesters, polyanhydrides, polyamines, polyphosphazenes, poly(alkyl cyanoacrylate). The major polymeric NPs preparation techniques are self-assembly, emulsion solvent evaporation, spray drying, and nanoprecipitation (Pradeepkumar et al. 2017; Jeyaraj et al. 2016; Mehnath et al. 2018b; Mehnath et al. 2018c; Mehnath et al. 2019). The polymeric nanoparticles are mostly biocompatible, have more GF loading efficiency, provide targeted delivery, and are able to respond to stimuli such as pH, temperature, light, magnetic field, and ultrasound (Wang et al. 2013). However, direct contact of GF with some solvents, increases in temperature, and

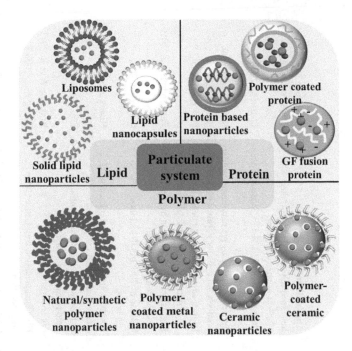

FIGURE 3.5　Schematic representation of GF loaded various kind of nanoparticles.

degradation during synthesis are the main challenges for protecting the bioactivity of GF. However, polymers are widely used because of their safety profile. In the PLGA "gold standard," synthetic polymers are approved by FDA for human clinical drug-delivery application. Additionally, different molecular sized PLGA were used for GF delivery (Degim 2008). Wei et al. prepared PLGA nanosphere via double emulsion method and loaded with rhBMP-7. PLGA nanosphere prepared with higher molecular weight exhibited controlled release of GF for 7 weeks (Wei et al. 2007).

3.5.1.2　Natural Polymeric Nanoparticles

Naturally available materials such as chitosan, cellulose, alginate, agarose, gellan gum, carrageenan, hyaluronic acid, starch, dextran, cyclodextrins, and proteins such as collagen, gelatin, albumin, elastin, fibroin, sericin also gained equal attention to synthetic polymers. These enable design of biomaterial systems promoting cross-linking with GF without affecting the bioactivity. Some physical properties are a possible problem in natural polymers, which often are regulated by chemical modi-fication (Rajam et al. 2011; Irache et al. 2005). Some examples of natural/synthetic polymeric nanoparticles most extensively used for GF delivery are given in Table 3.3.

3.5.1.3　Lipid-Based Nanoparticles

Liposomes, solid lipid nanoparticles, and lipid nanocapsules are lipid-based nanoparticles, and their main advantage is biocompatibility with mimicking cell-membrane structure. The liposomes are composed of an aqueous core surrounded

TABLE 3.3

Examples of Polymeric Nanoparticles System for GF Delivery

Polymeric Nanoparticles	Types	Form	Growth Factor	Procedure	Application	Reference
PLGA	Synthetic	Nanoparticles	IGF-I	Solvent evaporation	Sustained release IGF-I for 40 days with 70% at in vitro condition.	Chung et al. 2006
PCL-PEG-PCL	Synthetic	Nanoparticles	bFGF	Emulsion solvent evaporation	Encapsulation of 61 % GF. Sustained release for 10 days.	Gou et al. 2008
PBCA	Synthetic	Nanoparticles	NGF	Emulsion polymerization	Enhanced uptake by primary brain capillary endothelial cells for Parkinson's therapy.	Kurakhmaeva et al. 2008
Poly(metha crylic acid)	Synthetic	Nanoparticles	EGF	Dispersion copolymerization	High-loading, sustained release for 7 days, and high proliferation of A431 cells.	Park et al. 2003
Chitosan	Natural	Nanoparticles	HGF	Strong ionic interactions	Higher cell differentiation from stem cells and prolonged release.	Pulavendran et al. 2010
Chitosan	Natural	Nanoparticles	bFGF	Ionotropic gelation	Release of 70% bFGF and intact for 24 hours.	Cetin et al. 2007
Chitosan-dextran sulfate	Natural	Nanoparticles	VEGF	Coacervation	Encapsulation of 50% and release of 75% more than 10 days.	Huang et al. 2007
Alginate	Natural	Nanoparticles	BMP-2	Reverse emulsification	Enhances osteoblastic differentiation (bMSC) and release for 7 days.	Lim et al. 2010
Alginate	Natural	Nanoparticles	PLGF	Crosslinking	Enhances angiogenesis.	Binsalamah et al. 2011
Albumin	Natural	Nanoparticles	BMP-2	Glutaraldehyde crosslinking	High encapsulation and induces bone regeneration.	Zhang et al. 2008
Chitosan -BSA NPs	Natural	Nanoparticles	BMP-2	Modified desolvation	Coatings improved the stability and provide the sustained release of BMP-2.	Li et al. 2015

(Continued)

TABLE 3.3 (*Continued*)
Examples of Polymeric Nanoparticles System for GF Delivery

Polymeric Nanoparticles	Types	Form	Growth Factor	Procedure	Application	Reference
Albumin-PEI	Hybrid	Micelles	BMP-2	Conversion process.	Encapsulation of 90% and release for 10 days.	Zhang et al. 2008
Heparinconjugated Tetronic® -PCL	Synthetic	Micelles	bFGF	Bulk ring-opening polymerization.	Loading of 70% due to heparin interaction and the bFGF release for 60 days.	Lee et al. 2008
PLGA	Synthetic	Nanocapsules	BMP-2	Free-radical polymerization	Enhanced bone regeneration compared to free BMP-2.	Tan et al. 2012
Protein	Natural	Nanocapsules	VEGF	Aqueous assembly	Sustained release of VEGF and enhanced vascular formation.	Tan et al. 2011
PAMAM	Synthetic	Dendrimer	EGF	Divergent	Cell-growth stimulation higher than the free EGF.	Thomas et al. 2008
PAMAM	Synthetic	Dendrimer	VEGF	Divergent	High liver accumulation.	Backer et al. 2005

by the bilayer arrangement of amphiphilic phospholipids. The major preparation process involves high-pressure homogenization, reverse phase evaporation, detergent depletion, sonication, and freeze-dried rehydration. It has the advantage of encapsulating the hydrophobic components inside the hydrophilic moieties and trapping hydrophilic GF (Beduneau et al. 2007). The second type of particle is solid lipid nanoparticles made up of lipid core stabilized by surfactants and bilayer structure are not distinguished. High-pressure homogenization and microemulsion are common techniques for solid lipid nanoparticle synthesis. It has many advantages such as simple preparation methods, biocompatibility, and retention of the GF bioactivity; its main drawback is poor encapsulation effect. It is difficult to allot space for GF due to its dense hydrophobic lipid core in the colloidal system. Lipid nanocapsule formulations are prepared by phase the inversion temperature method and temperature recycling treatment (Simao et al. 2020; Salamanna et al. 2021). Several studies were done for delivering the GF from lipid-based nanoparticles through systemic routes such as oral and parental routes. To enhance the mucoadhesive property and improve the circulation in plasma, liposomes were coated with polymers. The coating also helps to avoid reticuloendothelial (RET). The system improves cellular internalization and further helps to immobilize targeting moieties (Lasch et al. 2003). Li et al. 2003, prepared liposomes using DPPC and PC and coated them with PEG for the delivery of recombinant EGF. Even though loading efficiency was low, PEG-coated DPPC liposomes enhance permeability and prevent enzyme degradation (Li et al. 2003). In another work, Liposome size of 91 nm exhibited 32% encapsulation efficiency and showed higher efficiency of HGF compared to control (Li et al. 2008). The PC from eggs was used for liposome preparation with magnetic nanoparticles loaded with BMP-2 (Matsuo et al. 2003), and TGF-β1 (Tanaka et al. 2005) for new bone formation in animal models. Lipid-based nanoparticles seem to be effective in penetration of the BBB and delivery of GF to the brain. Xie et al. prepared liposomes encapsulated with NGF for delivery to the brain (Xie et al. 2005).

3.5.1.4   Other Nanoparticulate Systems

A few other nanoparticles, such as ceramics, quantum dots, graphene, hybrid, inorganic nanoparticles, are used for growth factor delivery. Ceramic materials such as TCP, HAP, bioactive glass, silica, calcium sulphate, and carbonate apatite are utilized for hard-tissue regeneration applications. Park loaded PDGF into calcium sulphate nanoparticles for bone-tissue regeneration application. Calcium sulphate in nano form has more size-to-surface ratio, and a positive charge helps in protein and cell adhesion (Park et al. 2007). Pitukmanorom used HAP-PLGA microsphere for encapsulation of BMP-2 and exhibited controlled delivery for 7 weeks and collagen sponge releases BMP-2 for 3 weeks (Pitukmanorom et al. 2008). Mesoporous silica NPs get considerable attention in biomedical applications due to their high surface area, pore size, controlled particle size, easy surface modification, and biocompatibility. Mesoporous NPs grafted with BMP-2 via aminosilane linker exhibited good stability in buffer and cell media (Zhou et al. 2015). Lee used graphene oxide to transport FN and transform growth factor-β3 (TGF-β3) to enhance the cell adhesion and chondrogenic differentiation of hASCs (Lee et al. 2014). Skaat used magnetic Fe_2O_3 nanoparticles coupled with FGF with the help of gelatin for olfactory mucosa

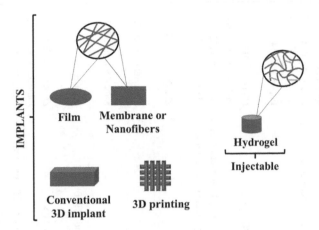

FIGURE 3.6 Illustration of different classes of scaffold such as film, membrane, conventional 3D implant, 3D printing scaffold, hydrogel.

cell proliferation. Nanoparticles exhibited higher migration and proliferation of olfactory cells compared to the control (Skaat et al. 2011). Vu used quantum dots for functionalization of β-NGF using a streptavidin-biotin immobilization method. The GF bioactivity retained efficiency due to the steric hindrance effect of bulk quantum dots and enhanced the neuronal differentiation in PC12cells (Vu et al. 2005).

3.5.2 SCAFFOLDS

Scaffolds are three-dimensional structures that assist in cell attachment and differentiation and provide a good platform for GF delivery. The scaffold delivery system is classified into the membrane, thin-film, conventional scaffold, and 3D printed scaffold types represented in Figure 3.6. Physical adsorption/encapsulation of GF was performed during scaffold preparation and the process such as lyophilization, phase separation, particulate leaching, gas foaming, electrodeposition, and solvent casting (Mehnath et al. 2020a; Sumathra et al. 2018). A wide variety of biomaterials that mimic natural ECM were used as scaffolds for stabilization of GF (Tinke et al. 2018). Currently, several types of research on the different classes of scaffold for controlled delivery of GF are presented in Table 3.4.

3.5.2.1 Nanofiber Scaffold

Nanofibers are interlinked mesh-like structures that form 3D scaffolds with more surface area to increase cell adhesion and attachment of GF. Electrospinning is the most common technique for the fabrication of nanofiber and the encapsulation of GF into the nanofiber in two ways, as represented in Figure 3.7. In the pre-fabrication method GF is immobilized in nanofiber before electrospinning process. In the post-fabrication method GF is immobilized into the nanofiber after electrospinning process via physical adsorption, affinity, and covalent-based immobilization (Mehnath et al. 2020b; Chitra et al. 2017). Several organic solvents, sonication, and a stirring process were required for nanofiber preparation, and the bioactivity of GF

TABLE 3.4

Different Types of Materials Used for Preparation of Various Type of Scaffold for GF Delivery and Its Application

Materials	Scaffold	Growth Factor	Applications	Reference
polydopamine decorated poly(l-lactide)	Nanofiber	BMP-2	Polydopamine modification helps in grafting GF, accelerate the tissue regeneration	Cho et al. 2014
Chitosan-collagen	Nanofiber	BMP-2	Bioadhesive microporous scaffold mimic the ECM	Eap et al. 2014
Silk	Nanofiber	EGF	Full-thickness dorsal skin excision in Balb/C mouse	Gil et al. 2013
PLGA	Film	IGF-1,TGF-β1	Controlled release and bone regeneration	Jaklenec et al. 2008
PLGA-poly(propylene)	Film	VEGF, BMP-2	VEGF plus BMP-2 Delivery of both factors via gelatin microspheres	Kempen et al. 2009
polycaprolactone/β-TCP	Film	BMP-2	80 % BMP-2 release for 2 days, 20% being released over 2 weeks.	Macdonald et al. 2011
Silk fibroin/ HAP	Porous	BMP-2	Continuous protein release for 7 days, Burst release of 48% on first day	Zhang et al. 2011
PDLLA	Film	BMP-2	BMP increase osteogenic differentiation at maximum rate	Kanczler et al. 2010
PDLLA	Film	VEGF	Maximum stimulation of human umbilical vascular endothelial cells	Kanczler et al. 2010
PCL/β-TCP- poly(β-aminoester)-2	Film	recombinant BMP-2	Controlled release of BMP-2 for 14 days and VEGF for 1 weeks	Shah et al. 2011
Silk	Hydrogel	rhBMP-2 and VEGF	15 % release of rhBMP-3 and VEGF for 28 days	Zhang et al. 2011
Fibrin	Hydrogel	neurotrophin-3	Treatment of spinal cord injury	Johnson et al. 2009
PEG	Hydrogel	rhBMP-2	Glycosylated rhBMP-2 exhibited 56% release for 15 days, non-glycosylated shows 35% release for 15 days	Hanseler et al. 2012
Poly-l-lactic acid- gelatin	hydrogel	FGF	Anterior cruciate ligament regeneration	Kimura et al. 2008
Alginate	Hydrogel	BMP-2	Exhibited 98% release for 7 days	Kolambkar et al. 2011
PEG heparin	Hydrogel	FGF, VEGF	Only exhibited 10 % release for 4 days	Zieris et al. 2011

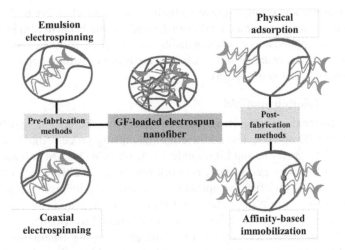

FIGURE 3.7   Different approaches for GF encapsulation inside the nanofiber using electrospinning (Hsieh et al. 2006).

was protect by using the BSA, collagen, fetal calf serum, collagen, and biomaterials (Briggs and Arinzeh 2011; Yang et al. 2011). Gil used natural silk to enhance the bioactivity of EGF and GF-loaded electrospun silk nanofibers wound dressing material, which improves collagen synthesis and re-epithelization and dermis proliferation (Gil et al. 2013). Fu et al. used a blending process for the fabrication of BMP-2/ poly-L- lactide(PLLA)/HAP scaffolds, which exhibited sustained release over two months (Fu et al. 2008). Liao used coaxial electrospinning, another pre-fabrication method for loading PDGF in core-shell nanofiber with minimum loss of GF. PEG forms the shell layer, creates the pores, and regulates the GF releases for 40 days (Liao et al. 2006). Hsieh prepared a self-assembling peptide solution to consist of PDGF that was injected into the rat myocardial infarction model, which exhibited the controlled release of PDGF for 14 days. Another method to protect GF to use the fusion protein-like cell receptor binding peptide, which covalently couples with self-assembling peptide (Liao et al. 2006). Chen prepared chemical moieties/biological epitopes to conjugate amphiphilic peptide for effective delivery of recombinant BMP (Chen et al. 2020).

3.5.2.2   Film/Membrane Scaffold

Thin-film/membrane was prepared by a solvent casting, salt leaching, and freeze-drying technique. Salt leaching uses porogens in colloidal solution, which is distributed throughout the scaffold, and the removal of porogens leads to formation of pores. In the freeze-drying process, the porous scaffolds are fabricated by sublimation for the complete removal of the solvent (Calori et al. 2020). Mizuno prepared a chitosan film by the freeze-drying method; bFGF was mixed with hydroxypropyl chitosan. The application of scaffolds into genetically diabetic mice shows increases in granulation and tissue formation (Mizuno et al. 2003). Hong performed studies on rhEGF-chitosan film for the regeneration of porcine wounds. It exhibited the controlled release and promote the re-epithelization (Hong et al. 2006). Liu used co-crosslinked -SH residues with chondroitin derivatives and heparin film encapsulated with bFGF and applied it to wounds in db/db mice. It achieved 89% of wound closure in 2 weeks after exposure of bFGF-loaded chondroitin6-sulfate-heparin films and control was 27% (Liu et al. 2007a).

3.5.2.3 3D Printing Scaffold

Three-dimensional printing is a computer-assisted technique in which material is formed into 3D objects. The additive manufacturing process like LbL arrangement to produce versatile and high-quality scaffold. CAD/CAM software permits the strategy of various geometries, network pore sizes, multilayers, and compartments. Additionally, it offers an option to translate computed tomography into 3D bio-scaffolds that mimic the tissues and organs. In this way a variety of growth factors are able to load onto different types of material to enhance the biological response. It also prefabricates patient-specific geometry for traumatic spinal cord injury/cartilage repair with more dynamic behavior (Moroni et al. 2018). Becker prepared a 3D printed HAP block loaded with BMP-2 that implanted onto the surface of the latissimus dorsi muscle. The CT and histology results indicate increases in bone density and heterotopic bone formation (Becker et al. 2012). Tarafder utilized the multi-cartridge printing poly(ε-caprolactone)/PLGA material with CTGF or TGF-β3 for TMJ disc regeneration (Tarafder et al. 2016). Vorndran suggested the degradation of rhBMP-2 bioactivity due to the damage during spraying through the nozzle (Vorndran et al. 2008).

3.5.3 Injectable Hydrogel

Hydrogels are versatile, flexible material, able to entrap bioactive GF within their hydrated matrix. They are composed of crosslinked, insoluble polymers that swell and form an insoluble 3D structure at the site of injection. Various polymers such as hyaluronic acid, chitosan, alginate, PEG, deblock, and triblock copolymer were used to prepare hydrogel that carries GF. The major common method of loading GF is simple mixing with polymer for physical entrapment of GF within the matrix (Luca et al. 2010). Zieris used amino end-functionalized four-arm star-shaped PEG to improve GF binding (Zieris et al. 2011). Luca used rhBMP-2 containing hyaluronic acid hydrogel to improve the osteo induction, and compared it with chitosan hydrogel of the same design. However, more regeneration was observed in hyaluronate hydrogel, which was described by Masson's trichrome staining and μCT imaging in a rat model (Luca et al. 2010). An additional study was performed with the same chitosan hydrogel combined with β-TCP and rhBMP-2. It exhibited less mineralization, which may lead to the high affinity of rhBMP-2 to bind on TCP leads to slower release (Luca et al. 2011). In dental applications, rhBMP-2 bound to a sandblasted, titanium implant coated by PEG, collagen/hyaluronic acid, and PEG- collagen/hyaluronic acid hydrogel combination. In this, PEG hydrogel and collagen/hyaluronic acid hydrogel control the burst release and maintain the sustained release (Wen et al. 2011). A self-assembled peptide-based hydrogel was loaded with IGF for myocardial infarction model. The GF delivery helps in cell differentiation and secretion of biochemical molecules from the cells. A topical gel made was up of carboxymethylcellulose loaded with PDGF for diabetic neuropathic ulcers (Chen et al. 2015). The adhesive, thermo-responsive Pluronic-127/chitosan hydrogels was used for delivery of rhEGF. PluronicF-127 transforms aqueous solution to hydrogel, with an increasing blend ratio hydrogel to regulate the release of rhEGF. High mucoadhesive helps improved the healing rate and epidermis regeneration of burn wounds (Kant et al. 2014). Landsman et al. used heparin and diacrylates PEG hydrogel sheet for sustained release of EGF to accelerate the wound closure process in vivo (Landsman et al. 2010).

3.5.4 MISCELLANEOUS SYSTEM

In addition to this system, there is another miscellaneous system to enhance the skin permeation delivery of GF. This burst release of GF was controlled by coacervate integration of poly(ethylene arginine aspartate diglyceride) with heparin in the particulate system (Wu et al. 2016). To increase the treatment time of GF in the repair area, conjugation of aldehyde-hyaluronic acid and -NH2 group of EGF in membrane significantly increases skin regeneration (Kim et al. 2016b). Further protein fusion such as trans activator of transcription protein or low-molecular-weight protamine, improves the penetration of a FGF and EGF without losing the biological activity (Zheng et al. 2015; Choi et al. 2012). The targeting peptide was fused with recombinant decorin, which increases the neutralizing activity of TGF-1, increases accumulation in wounds, and promotes wound regeneration (Jarvinen and Ruoslahti 2010). Nanofibrous wound dressing loaded with astragaloside IV promotes cell attachment, multiplication, inhibited scar formation closure, angiogenesis, and tissue formation (Shan et al. 2015).

3.6 STRATEGIES FOR GROWTH FACTOR DELIVERY

The application of GF for regeneration/repair forms an important armamentarium in repair therapy. It shows the degree of outcomes in ideal pre-clinical and clinical scenarios of osteoblast proliferation, wound healing, implant dentistry, and periodontal healing. Most of the methods for tissue regeneration consist of a single-time delivery of GF. It is administered through injection, direct release of GF. To avoid non-specific delivery, localized delivery at the desired site is a preferable action. A desirable nanomaterial that delivers certain molecules for a prolonged time at the targeted site and additionally providing protection to the bioactive GF molecules is needed. The delivery rates are controlled and pulsatile, and these are very important in designing a spatiotemporal delivery system. preparing To prepare a spatiotemporally controlled release it is necessary to develop a suitable formulation, determine the roles of GF in tissue repair, and identifying the biological signals. Additional considerations for regenerative strategy include the loading efficiency, protection of GF, and immobilization process, which are important for translation of clinical strategy and cost-regulatory approval barriers (Lopes et al. 2019; Pradhan et al. 2017; Mantha et al. 2019). In localized delivery, GF may be immobilized on the carrier system by covalent or non-covalent binding. The degradation and release mechanism must be considered during the fabrication process. Non-covalent internalization follows the diffusion and swelling, followed by controlled release, whereas covalent immobilization consists of a chemical/enzymatic reaction process for the controlled release mechanism. The GF encapsulated into a particulate system of a biodegradable polymer provides controlled release at a remote part of the body after implantation. It is not readily internalized into the cells; it is retained in tissue and provides controlled release. Due to their size, nanomaterials are able to penetrate the tissue, capillaries, and cells, giving several applications in GF delivery. In scaffold materials, outer structure and porosity are specifically fabricated for incorporation of GF components. A polymeric scaffold with 3D architecture serves dual purposes of cell support and GF immobilization. Scaffolds of micropores are useful for cell penetration, and micro/mesopores contribute to GF diffusion (Liu et al. 2007b; Chen et al. 2005; Chen et al. 2006). The release profile of the scaffold is altered by altering the property of the scaffold such as porosity, shape, size, tortuosity, degree of crosslinking indeed in degradation. The precise regulation of the release kinetics can be achieved by the release of GF in response to definite signals. It possible by the introduction of a stimuli-responsive component in the delivery system. The common triggering mechanism involves changes in cellular microenvironment as represented in Figure 3.8: (i) pH/temperature, (ii) enzymes/ions cleaves the crosslinker, which immobilizes the GF. Additionally, external factors such as light, electric, magnetic fields, and ultrasound alter the nanomaterial structure to regulate the GF release (Ulijn et al. 2007).

3.6.1 pH AND TEMPERATURE-TRIGGERED RELEASE

The most usual stimuli for the release is based on the varying pH of different tissues. The delivery system is composed of a crosslinked network/moiety that exhibits the transition upon pH changes for controlled release (Mehnath et al. 2017; Jeyaraj et al. 2016). The nanomaterial exhibits constancy at biological pH; the protonation at acidic pH decreases the steadiness, foremost to GF release. Popular pH-sensitive nanomaterial consists of pH-sensitive linkers, such as sulfamethazine oligomers, sulphonamide, and methacrylic acid (Kim et al. 2009; Shim et al. 2005). Recently, pH-responsive hydrogels were fabricated for sustained delivery of insulin (Huynh et al. 2008). The change in temperature was also used for the triggered release of GF from nanomaterial. A widely used polymer is PNIPAAM, which exhibits sol-to-gel transition under physiological conditions (Fundueanu et al. 2008).

3.6.2 ENZYME-TRIGGERED RELEASE

Enzyme actions were used as activating mechanism to start the GF release. The protease enzyme was susceptible to a system consisting of catalytic matrix MMP interactions. A BMP-2-loaded PEG hydrogel pendant with integrin-binding RGD peptide was amine-functionalized with MMP as a crosslinker. The protease modulates the degradability of the bifunctional matrix, which increases the BMP-2 release (Thornton et al. 2005). Similarly, VEGF coupled PEG peptide hydrogel released VEGF based upon the cellular demand (Zisch et al. 2003).

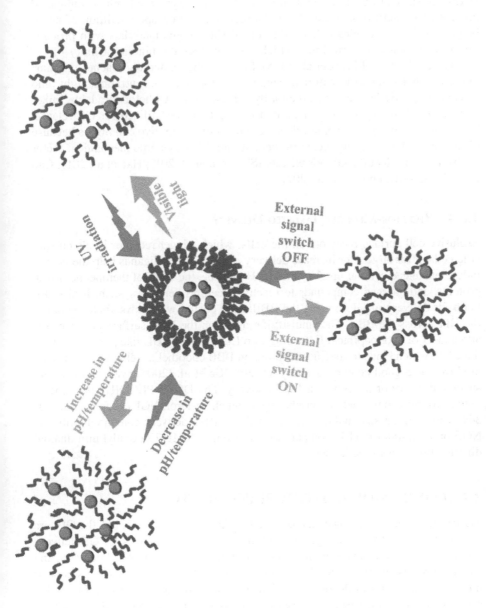

FIGURE 3.8 Different strategies of GF delivery via various triggering factors.

3.6.3 External Stimuli–Based GF Release

Stimulating progress has been made recently for GF delivery. An antibiotic-identifying hydrogel was developed for triggered and spatiotemporal release of GF. Hydrogel was fabricated by interaction with bacterial gyrase subunit B conjugated polymer. Coumermycin crosslinking changes to sol-state upon addition of novobiocin results in the release. The addition of Ca^+ to nanomaterials with proteins initiates the sol-to-gel transition, which also changes the binding affinity of GF (Ehrbar et al. 2008; Ehrick et al. 2005). Some sophisticated approaches of smart materials that respond to external triggers such as ion concentration, light, and electric/magnetic field can be potentially released GF. A photodegradable linker coupled PEG hydrogel that is degraded by light can be utilized for GF release. These smart prototype nanomaterials were not suitable in vivo conditions because of the particular wavelength/electric field signal. This dynamic mechanical factor is also able to affect the GF release rate (Sharmin et al. 2017; Han et al. 2017; Cao et al. 2018; Sarrigiannidis et al. 2021).

3.6.4 Receptor-Mediated Targeted Delivery

Exclusive cell surface receptors on the cells, which trigger receptor levels on specific cells, offer targets for increase delivery of GF. Certain ligands help the NPs to induce enhanced cellular uptake. The BBB controls the entry of therapeutic drugs, proteins, and charged compounds to reach the central nervous system. It also difficult for delivery of GF to cross the BBB; NPs coated with polysorbates enhance the NPs across the BBB. The emulsifying agent on the NPs' surface improves the attachment of apolipoprotein E, turning into LDL. These LDL-like particles mimic the LDL, which binds to specific receptors on BBB endothelial cells. Liposomes are preferred as a good cerebral delivery system. Xie et al. (2005) evaluated the site-specific delivery of liposome on NGF delivery. The DOPE-PEG-NHS was coated onto liposomes composed of phospholipids and cholesterol. NGF encapsulation was 34% with 100 nm size and delivery to evaluate BBB delivery compared with free NGF on an animal model. Compared to liposomes, RMP-7 (a bradykinin analog) directed liposomes were higher.

3.7 CONCLUSION AND FUTURE PERSPECTIVE

Tissue regeneration is an unavoidable factor in future medical care, and the GFs are vital components for tissue regeneration/repair strategy. Strategies for GF delivery related to different nanocarrier, immobilization techniques, controlled delivery, and triggered release have increased exponentially over the past 20 years. This created multiple methods for evaluation of various GF-based therapeutic effects for a wide range of disorders and tissue regeneration processes. This article provides an outline of the nanomaterial patterning for effective delivery of multiple GF, different methodology, and combination strategy for GF delivery. It is very important to study the bioactive molecules properties, complex behavior, and healing/tissue repair mechanism. The design and optimization of nanomaterials are very important to overcome the difficulty in GF delivery and allow flexible tailoring of GF to enhance its application. The controlled release system has been developed to seize and protect the GF and to release the optimal dose in a particular time based on the biological demands of target tissues. Currently, the usage of GF for clinical patients faces several challenges, such as sensitivity, inefficiency, non-specific delivery, and socioeconomic challenges. Still, several studies were continuously optimized for GF delivery for clinical therapeutic purposes. Satisfying reports of in vitro studies allow entry of in vivo and pre-clinical applications. The main role of nanomaterials is to enhance the stability of encapsulated GF protein and replicate similar results after the scaling approach. A successful, safe, and effective approach will be adapted to clinical application. To discover the latent technology for clinical application based on several scientists requires a multidisciplinary technique, a combination of biomaterials, medicine, and an engineering technique. The multiple GF delivery, recombinant protein, and miRNA-based regulation of GF will be a further advancement of tissue regeneration application. There is huge demand required from scientists and funding agencies to accelerate the availability of resources to develop clinical translation. With the co-operative action of tissue engineers, surgeons may ultimately help in filling the gap between bench and clinics. This effective GF delivery strategy will deliver a variety of therapeutic benefits in the future.

ACKNOWLEDGMENTS

We gratefully acknowledge the support from Indian Council of Medical Research, New Delhi for Senior Research Fellowship (ICMR-SRF Grant no. Fellowship/TB/32/2019/ECD-I). We thank DST-SERB for funding this project, Grant No. YSS/2015/000050.

ABBREVIATIONS

ALP	alkaline phosphatase
Ang-1	angiopoietin
BBB	blood-brain barrier
BDNF	brain-derived neurotrophic factors
BMPs	bone morphogenetic proteins
BSA	bovine serum albumin
CAD/CAM	computer-aided manufacturing/designs
CTGF	connective tissue growth factor
Dopa	3,4-dihydroxyphenylalanine
DOPE	1,2-dioleoyl-sn-glycero-3-phosphoethanolamine
DPPC	dipalmitoylphosphatidylcholine
ECM	extracellular matrix
EGF	epidermal growth factor
FGF	fibroblast growth factor
FN	fibronectin
GCSF	granulocyte colony-stimulating factor
GDNF	glial cell line-derived neurotrophic factor

GF	growth factors
HAP	hydroxyapatite
HGF	hepatocyte growth factor
HUVECs	human endothelial cells
IGF	insulin-like growth factors
KGF	keratinocyte growth factor
LbL	layer-by-layer
LDL	low-density lipoprotein
MMP	metalloproteinase
NGF	nerve growth factor
NHS	N-hydroxysuccinimide
PAA	poly(acrylic) acid
PAMAM	polyamidoamine
PBCA	poly(butyl cyanoacrylate)
PC	phosphatidylcholine
PDGF	platelet-derived growth factor
PEG	polyethylene glycol
PEI	polyethylenimine
PL	poly L-histidine
PLA	polylactic acid
PLGA	poly(lactide-co-glycolate)
PLGF	placental growth factors
PLH	poly L-histidine hydrochloride
PMAA	poly methacrylic acid
PNIPAAM	poly(N-isopropylacrylamide)
RGD	arginylglycylaspartic acid peptide
rhEGF	recombinant human epidermal growth factor
SCF	stem cell factors
TCP	tricalcium phosphate
TGF	transforming growth factor
TGF-β	transforming growth factor beta
TMJ	temporomandibular joint
VEGFs	vascular endothelial growth factors

REFERENCES

Abbah, S.A., Liu, J., Lam, R.W.M., Goh, J.C.H., Wong, H.K. (2012). *In vivo* bioactivity of rhBMP-2 delivered with novel polyelectrolyte complexation shells assembled on an alginate microbead core template. J Control Release, 162, 364–372.

Backer, M.V., Gaynutdinov, T.I., Patel, V., Bandyopadhyaya, A.K., Thirumamagal, B.T.S., Tjarks, W., Barth, R.F., Claffey, K., Backer, J.M. (2005). Vascular endothelial growth factor selectively targets boronated dendrimers to tumor vasculature. Mol Cancer Ther, 4, 1423–1429.

Becker, S.T., Bolte, H., Schunemann, K., Seitz, H., Bara, J.J., Beck-Broichsitter, B.E., Russo, P.A.J., Wiltfang, J., Warnke, P.H. (2012). Endocultivation: the influence of delayed vs. simultaneous application of BMP-2 onto individually formed hydroxyapatite matrices for heterotopic bone induction. Int J Oral Maxillofac Surg, 41, 1153–1160.

Beduneau, A., Saulnier, P., Benoit, J.P. (2007). Active targeting of brain tumors using nano-carriers. Biomaterials, 28, 4947–4967.

Binsalamah, Z.M., Paul, A., Khan, A.A., Prakash, S., Shum-Tim, D. (2011). Intramyocardial sustained delivery of placental growth factor using nanoparticles as a vehicle for delivery in the rat infarct model. Int J Nanomedicine, 6, 2667–2678.

Briggs, T., Arinzeh, T.L. (2011). Growth factor delivery from electrospun materials. J Biomed Mater Res A, 1, 129–138.

Brummelhuis, N., Wilke, P., Borner, H.G. (2017). Identification of functional peptide sequences to lead the design of precision polymers. Macromol Rapid Commun, 38, 1700632.

Budiraharjo, R., Neoh, K.G., Kang, E.T. (2013). Enhancing bioactivity of chitosan film for osteogenesis and wound healing by covalent immobilization of BMP-2 or FGF-2. J Biomater Sci Polym Ed, 24, 645–662.

Cabanas-Danes, J., Landman, E., Huskens, J., Karperien, M., Jonkheijm, P. (2018). Hydrolytically labile linkers regulate release and activity of human bone morphogenetic protein-6. Langmuir, 34, 9298–9306.

Calori, I.R., Braga, G., Jesus, P., Bic, H., Tedesco, A.C. (2020). Polymer scaffolds as drug delivery systems. Eur Polym J, 129, 109621.

Cao, L., Kong, X., Lin, S., Zhang, S., Wang, J., Liu, C., Jiang, X. (2018). Synergistic effects of dual growth factor delivery from composite hydrogels incorporating 2-N,6-O-sulphated chitosan on bone regeneration. Artif Cells Nanomed Biotechnol, 46(sup3), S1–S17.

Carmeliet, P. (2005). Angiogenesis in life, disease and medicine. Nature, 438, 932–936.

Carragee, E.J., Chu, G., Rohatgi, R., Hurwitz, E.L., Weiner, B.K., Yoon, S.T., Comer, G., Kopjar, B. (2013). Cancer risk after use of recombinant bone morphogenetic protein-2 for spinal arthrodesis. J. Bone Joint Surg Am, 95, 1537–1545.

Cetin, M., Aktas, Y., Vural, I., Capan, Y., Dogan, L.A., Duman, M., Dalkara, T. (2007). Preparation and in vitro evaluation of bFGF-loaded chitosan nanoparticles. Drug Deliv, 14, 525–529.

Chen, C.H., Hsu, E.L., Stupp, S.I. (2020). Supramolecular self-assembling peptides to deliver bone morphogenetic proteins for skeletal regeneration. Bone, 141, 115565.

Chen, F.M., Wu, Z.F., Sun, H.H., Wu, H., Xin, S.N., Wang, Q.T., et al. (2006). Release of bioactive BMP from dextran-derived microspheres: an ovel delivery concept. Int J Pharm, 307, 23–32.

Chen, F.M., Wu, Z.F., Wang, Q.T., Wu, H., Zhang, Y.J., Nie, X., et al. (2005). Preparation of recombinant human bone morphogenetic protein-2 loaded dextran-based microspheres and their characteristics. Acta Pharmacol Sin, 26, 1093–1103.

Chen, Y., Wu, Y., Gao, J., Zhang, Z., Wang, L., Chen, X., Mi, J., Yao, Y., Guan, D., Chen, B., Dai, J. (2017). Transdermal vascular endothelial growth factor delivery with surface engineered gold nanoparticles. ACS Appl Mater Interfaces, 9(6), 5173–5180.

Chen, Y.C., Ho, H.O., Liu, D.Z., Siow, W.S., Sheu, M.T. (2015). Swelling/floating capability and drug release characterizations of gastroretentive drug delivery system based on a combination of hydroxyethyl cellulose and sodium carboxymethyl cellulose. PLoS ONE, 10, e0116914.

Chien, C.Y., Tsai, W.B. (2013). Poly(dopamine)-assisted immobilization of Arg-Gly-Asp peptides, hydroxyapatite, and bone morphogenic protein-2 on titanium to improve the osteogenesis of bone marrow stem cells. ACS Appl Mater Interf, 5, 6975–6983.

Chitra, K., Mehnath, S., Ganesh Kumar, J., Rangasamy, S., Balasubramanian, S., Dhinakar Raj, G. (2017). Fabrication of Progesterone-Loaded Nanofibers for the Drug Delivery Applications in Bovine. Nanoscale Res Lett, 12, 116.

Chiu, L.L.Y., Weisel, R.D., Li, R.K., Radisic, M. (2011). Defining conditions for covalent immobilization of angiogenic growth factors onto scaffolds for tissue engineering. J Tissue Eng Regen Med, 5, 69–84.

Cho, H.J., Madhurakka Perikamana, S.K., Lee, J.H., Lee, J., Lee, K., Shin, C., Shin, H. (2014). Effective immobilization of BMP-2 mediated by polydopamine coating on biodegradable nanofibers for enhanced *in vivo* bone formation. ACS Appl Mater Interf, 6, 11225–11235.

Choi, J.K., Jang, J.H., Jang, W.H., Kim, J., Bae, I.H., Bae, J., Park, Y.H., Kim, B.J., Lim, K.M., Park, J.W. (2012). The effect of epidermal growth factor (EGF) conjugated with low-molecular-weight protamine (LMWP) on wound healing of the skin. Biomaterials, 33, 8579–8590.

Choi, J.W., Kim, Y.S., Park, J.K., Song, E.H., Park, J.H., Kim, M.S., Shin, Y.S., Kim, C.H. (2017). Controlled release of hepatocyte growth factor from MPE`G-b-(PCL-ran-PLLA) Diblock copolymer for improved vocal fold regeneration. Macromol Biosci, 17, 1600163.

Chung, Y.I., Tae, G., Yuk, S.H. (2006). A facile method to prepare heparinfunctionalized nanoparticles for controlled release of growth factors. Biomaterials, 27, 2621–2626.

Crouzier, T., Sailhan., F., Becquart, P., Guillot, R., Logeart-Avramoglou, D., Picart, C. (2011). The performance of BMP-2 loaded TCP/HAP porous ceramics with a polyelectrolyte multilayer film coating. Biomaterials, 32, 7543–7754.

Degim, Z. (2008). Use of microparticulate systems to accelerate skin wound healing. J Drug Target, 16, 437–448.

Eap, S., Ferrand, A., Schiavi, J., Keller, L., Kokten, T., Floretti, F., Mainard, D. (2014). Collagen implants equipped with 'fish scale'-like nanoreservoirs of growth factors for bone regeneration. Nanomed, 9, 1253–1261.

Ehrbar, M., Schoenmakers, R., Christen, E.H., Fussenegger, M., Weber, W. (2008). Drug-sensing hydrogels for the inducible release of biopharmaceuticals. Nat Mater, 7, 800–804.

Ehrick, J.D., Deo, S.K., Browning, T.W., Bachas, L.G., Madou, M.J., Daunert, S. (2005). Genetically engineered protein in hydrogels tailors stimuli-responsive characteristics. Nat Mater, 4, 298–302.

Fathi-Achachelouei, M., Knopf-Marques, H., Ribeiro, da Silva C.E., Barthes, J., Bat, E., Tezcaner, A., Vrana, N.E. (2019). Use of nanoparticles in tissue engineering and regenerative medicine. Front Bioeng Biotechnol, 7,113.

Fei, Y., Gronowicz, G., Hurley, M.M. (2013). Fibroblast growth factor-2, bone homeostasis and fracture repair. Curr Pharm Des, 19, 3354–3563.

Fernandes-Cunha, G.M., Lee, H.J., Kumar, A., Kreymerman, A., Heilshorn, S., Myung, D. (2017). Immobilization of growth factors to collagen surfaces using pulsed visible light. Biomacromolecules, 18, 3185–3196.

Freeman, I., Cohen, S. (2009). The influence of the sequential delivery of angiogenic factors from affinity-binding alginate scaffolds on vascularization. Biomaterials, 30, 2122–2131.

Fu, Y.C., Nie, H., Ho, M.L., Wang, C.K., Wang, C.H. (2008). Optimized bone regeneration based on sustained release from three-dimensional fi brous PLGA/Hap composite scaffolds loaded with bmp-2. Biotechnol Bioeng, 99, 996–1006.

Fundueanu, G., Constantin, M., Ascenzi, P. (2008). Preparation and characterization of pH- and temperature-sensitive pullulan microspheres for controlled release of drugs. Biomaterials, 29, 2767–2775.

Gainza G, Villullas S, Pedraz JL, Hernandez RM, Igartua M. (2015). Advances in drug delivery systems (DDSs) to release growth factors for wound healing and skin regeneration. Nanomedicine, 11, 1551–1573.

Gil, E.S., Panilaitis, B., Bellas, E., Kaplan, D.L. (2013). Functionalized silk biomaterials for wound healing. Adv Healthc Mater, 2, 206–217.

Goktas, M., Luo, C., Sullan, R.M.A., Bergues-Pupo, A.E., Lipowsky, R., Vila Verde, A., et al. (2018). Molecular mechanics of coiled coils loaded in the shear geometry. Chem Sci, 9, 4610–4621.

Gomes, A.P., Mano, J.F., Queiroz, J.A., Gouveia, I.C. (2015). Layer-by- layer assembly for biofunctionalization of cellulosic fibers with emergent antimicrobial agents. Adv Polym Sci, 271, 225–240.

Gou, M.L., Dai, M., Gu, Y.C., Li, X.Y., Wen, Y.J., Yang, L., et al. (2008). Basic fibroblast growth factor loaded biodegradable PCL-PEG-PCL copolymeric nanoparticles: preparation, in vitro release and immunogenicity study. J Nanosci Nanotechnol, 8, 2357–2361.

Grasman, J.M., Page, R.L., Pins, G.D. (2008). Design of an in vitro model of cell recruitment for skeletal muscle regeneration using hepatocyte growth factor-loaded fibrin microthreads. Tissue Eng A, 23, 773–783.

Hameed, A., Gallagher, L.B., Dolan, E., O'Sullivan, J., Ruiz-Hernandez, E., Duffy, G.P., et al. (2019). Insulin-like growth factor-1 (IGF-1) poly (lacticco- glycolic acid) (PLGA) microparticles–development, characterisation, and in vitro assessment of bioactivity for cardiac applications. J Microencapsul, 36, 267–277.

Han, T.Y., Liu, X.W., Liang, N., et al. (2017). In vitro effects of recombinant adenovirus-mediated bone morphogenetic protein 2/vascular endothelial growth factor 165 on osteogenic differentiation of bone marrow mesenchymal stem. Cells Artif Cells Nanomed Biotechnol, 45, 108–114.

Hanft, J.R., Pollak, R.A., Barbul, A., et al. (2008). Phase I trial on the safety of topical rhVEGF on chronic neuropathic diabetic foot ulcers. J Wound Care, 17(1), 30–32.

Hanseler, P., Jung, U.W., Jung, R.E., et al. (2012). Analysis of hydrolyzable polyethylene glycol hydrogels and deproteinized bone mineral as delivery systems for glycosylated and nonglycosylated bone morphogenetic protein-2. Acta Biomaterialia, 8(1), 116–123.

Hermanson, G.T. (2008). Bioconjugate techniques, 2nd Edn. London: Elsevier Academic Press.

Hong, J.P., Jung, H.D., Kim, Y.W. (2006). Recombinant human epidermal growth factor (EGF) to enhance healing for diabetic foot ulcers. Ann Plast Surg, 56, 394–400.

Hsieh, P.C.H., Davis, M.E., Gannon, J., MacGillivray, C., Lee, R.T. (2006). Controlled delivery of PDGF-BB for myocardial protection using injectable self-assembling peptide nanofibers. J Clin Invest, 116, 237–248.

Huang, M., Vitharana, S.N., Peek, L.J., Coop, T., Berkland, C. (2007). Polyelectrolyte complexes stabilize and controllably release vascular endothelial growth factor. Biomacromolecules, 8, 1607–1614.

Huynh, D.P., Nguyen, M.K., Pi, B.S., Kim, M.S., Chae, S.Y., Lee, K.C., Kim, B.S., Kim, S.W., Lee, D.S. (2008). Functionalized injectable hydrogels for controlled insulin delivery. Biomaterials, 29, 2527–2534.

Irache, J.M., Merodio, M., Arnedo, A., Camapanero, M.A., Mirshahi, M., Espuelas, S. (2005). Albumin nanoparticles for the intravitreal delivery of anticytomegaloviral drugs. Mini Rev Med Chem, 5, 293–305.

Jaklenec, A., Hinckfuss, A., Bilgen, B., Ciombor, D.M., Aaron, R., Mathiowitz, E. (2008). Sequential release of bioactive IGF-I and TGF-beta 1 from PLGA microsphere-based scaffolds. Biomaterials, 29, 1518e25.

Jarvinen, T.A., Ruoslahti, E. (2010). Target-seeking antifibrotic compound enhances wound healing and suppresses scar formation in mice. Proc Natl Acad Sci USA, 107, 21671–21676.

Jeyaraj, M., Amarnath Praphakar, R., Rajendran, C., Ponnamma, D., Sadasivuni, K.K., Munusamy, M.A., Rajan, M. (2016). Surface functionalization of natural lignin isolated from Aloe barbadensis Miller biomass by atom transfer radical polymerization for enhanced anticancer efficacy. RSC Advances, 6, 51310–51319.

Jha, A.K., Mathur, A., Svedlund, F.L., Ye, J., Yeghiazarians, Y., Healy, K.E. (2015). Molecular weight and concentration of heparin in hyaluronic acidbased matrices modulates growth factor retention kinetics and stem cell fate. J Control Release, 209, 308–316.

Johnson, P.J., Parker, S.R., Sakiyama-Elbert, S.E. (2009). Controlled release of neurotrophin-3 from fibrin-based tissue engineering scaffolds enhances neural fiber sprouting following subacute spinal cord injury. Biotechnol Bioeng, 104(6), 1207–1214.

Kanczler, J.M., Ginty, P.J., White, L., et al. (2010). The effect of the delivery of vascular endothelial growth factor and bone morphogenic protein-2 to osteoprogenitor cell populations on bone formation. Biomaterials, 31(6), 1242–1250.

Kant, V., Gopal, A., Kumar, D., Gopalkrishnan, A., Pathak, N.N., Kurade, N.P., Tandan, S.K., Kumar, D. (2014). Topical pluronic F-127 gel application enhances cutaneous wound healing in rats. Acta Histochem, 116, 5–13.

Kawamoto, M., Matsuda, M., Ito, Y. (2018). Photochemical processed materials. In: Ito Y, editor. Photochemistry for biomedical applications: from device fabrication to diagnosis and therapy. Singapore: Springer. pp. 25–50.

Kempen, D.H., Lu, L., Heijink, A., Hefferan, T.E., Creemers, L.B., Maran, A., et al. (2009). Effect of local sequential VEGF and BMP-2 delivery on ectopic and orthotopic bone regeneration. Biomaterials, 30, 2816e25.

Kim, B., Gwon, K., Lee, S., Kim, Y.H., Yoon, M.H., Tae, G. (2016a). Heparin-immobilized gold-assisted controlled release of growth factors: Via electrochemical modulation. RSC Adv, 6, 88038–88041

Kim, H., Kong, W.H., Seong, K.Y., Sung, D.K., Jeong, H., Kim, J.K., Yang, S.Y., Hahn, S.K. (2016b). Hyaluronate-epidermal growth factor conjugate for skin wound healing and regeneration. Biomacromolecules, 17, 3694–3705.

Kim, H.K., Shim, W.S., Kim, S.E., Lee, K.H., Kang, E., Kim, J.H., Kim, K., Kwon, I.C., Lee, D.S. (2009). Injectable in situ-forming pH/thermo-sensitive hydrogel for bone tissue engineering, Tissue Eng Part A, 15, 923–933.

Kim, S.E., Yun, Y.P., Shim, K.S., Park, K., Choi, S.W., Shin, D.H., Suh, D.H. (2015). Fabrication of a BMP-2-immobilized porous microsphere modified by heparin for bone tissue engineering. Colloids Surf B, 134, 453–460.

Kimura, Y., Hokugo, A., Takamoto, T., et al. (2008). Regeneration of anterior cruciate ligament by biodegradable scaffold combined with local controlled release of basic fibroblast growth factor and collagen wrapping. Tissue Eng Part C Methods, 14 (1), 47–57.

Kiritsi, D., Nystrom, A. (2018). The role of TGFbeta in wound healing pathologies. Mech Ageing Dev, 172, 51–58.

Kisiel, M., Martino, M.M., Ventura, M., Hubbell, J.A., Hiborn, J., Ossipov, D.A. (2013). Improving the osteogenic potential of BMP-2 with hyaluronic acid hydrogel modified with integrin-specific fibronectin fragment. Biomaterials, 34, 704–712.

Kitamura, M., Akamatsu, M., Machigashira, M., et al. (2011). FGF-2 stimulates periodontal regeneration: results of a multi-center randomized clinical trial. J Dent Res, 90(1), 35–40.

Kolambkar, Y.M., Dupont, K.M., Boerckel, J.D., et al. (2011). An alginate-based hybrid system for growth factor delivery in the functional repair of large bone defects. Biomaterials, 32(1), 65–74.

Kord Forooshani, P., Lee, B.P. (2017). Recent approaches in designing bioadhesive materials inspired by mussel adhesive protein. J Polym Sci A Polym Chem, 55, 9–33.

Koria, P. (2012). Delivery of growth factors for tissue regeneration and wound healing. BioDrugs, 26, 163–175.

Kumorek, M., Kubies, D., Filova, E., Houska, M., Kasoju, N., Chanova, E.M., et al. (2015). Cellular responses modulated by FGF-2 adsorbed on albumin/heparin layer-by-layer assemblies. PLoS ONE, 10, e0125484

Kurakhmaeva, K.B., Voronina, T.A., Kapica, I.G., Kreuter, J., Nerobkova, L.N., Seredenin, S.B., Balabanian, V.Y., Alyautdin, R.N. (2008). Antiparkinsonian effect of nerve growth factor adsorbed on polybutylcyanoacrylate nanoparticles coated with polysorbate-80. Bull Exp Biol Med, 145, 259–262.

Landsman, A., Agnew, P., Parish, L., Joseph, R., Galiano, R.D. (2010). Diabetic foot ulcers treated with becaplermin and TheraGauze, a moisture-controlling smart dressing: A randomized, multicenter, prospective analysis. J Am Podiatr Med Assoc, 100, 155–160.

Lasch, J., Weissig, V., Brand, M. (2003). Preparation of liposomes. In: Torchilin VP, Weissig V, editors. Liposomes: a practical approach. Oxford: Oxford University Press. pp. 3–23.

Lee, J., Blaber, M. (2013). Increased functional half-life of fibroblast growth factor-1 by recovering a vestigial disulfide bond. J Prot Proteomics, 1, 47–53.

Lee, J.S., Bae, J.W., Joung, Y.K., Lee, S.J., Han, D.K., Park, K.D. (2008). Controlled dual release of basic fibroblast growth factor and indomethacin from heparin-conjugated polymeric micelle. Int J Pharm, 346, 57–63.

Lee, T.J., Park, S., Bhang, S.H., Yoon, J.K. Jo, I., Jeong, G.J., Hong, B.H., Kim, B.S. (2014). Graphene enhances the cardiomyogenic differentiation of human embryonic stem cells. Biochem Biophys Res Commun, 452(1), 174–180.

Li, H., Song, J.H., Park, J.S., Han, K. (2003). Polyethylene glycol-coated liposomes for oral delivery of recombinant human epidermal growth factor. Int J Pharm, 258, 11–19.

Li, L., Zhou, G., Wang, Y., Yang, G., Ding, S., Zhou, S. (2015). Controlled dual delivery of BMP-2 and dexamethasone by nanoparticle-embedded electrospun nanofibers for the efficient repair of critical-sized rat calvarial defect. Biomaterials, 37, 218–229.

Li. F., Wang, J.Y., Sun, J.Y. (2008). Hepatocyte growth factor encapsulated in targeted liposomes modified with cyclic ARG-GLY-ASP peptides promotes the remission of liver cirrhosis. J Hepatol, 48, S189.

Liao, I.C., Chew, S.Y., Leong, K.W. (2006). Aligned core shell nanofibers delivering bioactive proteins. Nanomedicine, 1(4), 465–471.

Lim, H.J., Ghim, H.D., Choi, J.H. (2010). Controlled release of BMP-2 from alginate nanohydrogels enhanced osteogenic differentiation of human bone marrow stromal cells. Macromol Res, 18(8), 787–792.

Lin, C.C., Anseth, K.S. (2009). PEG hydrogels for the controlled release of biomolecules in regenerative medicine. Pharm Res, 26, 631–643.

Liu, G., Li, L., Huo, D., Li, Y., Wu, Y., Zeng, L., et al. (2017). A VEGF delivery system targeting MI improves angiogenesis and cardiac function based on the tropism of MSCs and layer-by-layer self-assembly. Biomaterials, 127, 117–131.

Liu, Y., Cai, S., Shu, X.Z., Shelby, J., Prestwich, G.D. (2007a). Release of basic fibroblast growth factor from a crosslinked glycosaminoglycan hydrogel promotes wound healing. Wound Repair Regen, 15, 245–251.

Liu, Y., Huse, R.O., DeGroot, K., Buser, D., Hunziker, E.B. (2007b). Delivery mode and efficacy of BMP-2 in association with implants. J Dent Res, 86, 84–89.

Lopes, J., Fonseca, R., Viana, T., Fernandes, C., Morouço, P., Moura, C., Biscaia, S. (2019). Characterization of biocompatible poly(Ethylene Glycol)-Dimethacrylate hydrogels for tissue engineering. Appl Mech Mater, 890, 290–300.

Losi, P., Briganti, E., Errico, C., Lisella, A., Sanguinetti, E., Chiellini, F., Soldani, G. (2013). Fibrin-based scaffold incorporating VEGF- and bFGF-loaded nanoparticles stimulates wound healing in diabetic mice. Acta Biomater, 9, 7814–7821.

Losi, P., Briganti, E., Magera, A., Spiller, D., Ristori, C., Battolla, B., et al. (2010). Tissue response to poly(ether)urethane-polydimethylsiloxane-fibrin composite scaffolds for controlled delivery of pro-angiogenic growth factors. Biomaterials, 31, 5336–5344.

Luca, L., Rougemont, A.L., Walpoth, B.H. Gurny, R., Jordan, O. (2010). The effects of carrier nature and pH on rhBMP2-induced ectopic bone formation. J Control Release, 147(1) 38–44.

Luca, L., Rougemont, A.L., Walpoth, B.H., et al. (2011). Injectable rhBMP-2-loaded chitosan hydrogel composite: Osteoinduction at ectopic site and in segmental long bone defect. J Biomed Mater Res A, 96(1) 66–74.

Macdonald, M.L., Samuel, R.E., Shah, N.J., Padera, R.F., Beben, Y.M., Hammond, P.T. (2011). Tissue integration of growth factor-eluting layer-by-layer polyelectrolyte multilayer coated implants. Biomaterials, 32(5), 1446–1453.

Mandapalli, P.K., Labala, S., Jose, A., Bhatnagar, S., Janupally, R., Sriram, D., et al. (2017). Layer-by-layer thin films for co-delivery of TGF-b siRNA and epidermal growth factor to improve excisional wound healing. AAPS Pharm Sci Tech, 18, 809–820.

Mantha, S., Pillai, S., Khayambashi, P., Upadhyay, A., Zhang, Y., Tao, O., Pham, H.M., Tran, S.D. (2019). Smart Hydrogels in Tissue Engineering and Regenerative Medicine. Materials (Basel, Switzerland), 12(20), 3323.

Mao, H., Kim, S.M., Ueki, M., Ito, Y. (2017). Serum-free culturing of human mesenchymal stem cells with immobilized growth factors. J Mater Chem B, 5, 928–934.

Martin, T.A., Caliari, S.R., Williford, P.D., Harley, B.A., Bailey, R.C. (2011). The generation of biomolecular patterns in highly porous collagen- GAG scaffolds using direct photolithography. Biomaterials, 32, 3949–3957.

Martino, M.M., Briquez, P.S. (2015). Extracellular matrix-inspired growth factor delivery systems for bone regeneration. Adv Drug Deliv Rev, 94, 41–52.

Matsuo, T., Sugita, T., Kubo, T., Yasunaga, Y., Ochi, M., Murakami, T. (2003). Injectable magnetic liposomes as a novel carrier of recombinant human BMP-2 for bone formation in a rat bone-defect model. J Biomed Mater Res A, 66, 747–754.

Mehnath, S., Arjama, M., Rajan, M., Jeyaraj, M. (2018c). Development of cholate conjugated hybrid polymeric micelles for FXR receptor mediated effective site-specific delivery of paclitaxel, New J Chem, 42, 17021–17032.

Mehnath, S., Arjama, M., Rajan, M., Premkumar, K., Karthikeyan, K., Jeyaraj, M. (2020a). Mineralization of bioactive marine sponge and electrophoretic deposition on Ti-6Al-4V implant for osteointegration. Surf Coat Technol, 392, 125727.

Mehnath, S., Arjama, M., Rajan, M., Vijayaanand, M.A., Jeyaraj, M. (2018a). Polyorganophosphazene stabilized gold nanoparticles for intracellular drug delivery in breast carcinoma cells. Process Biochem, 72, 152–161.

Mehnath, S., Ayisha Sithika, M.A., Arjama, M., Rajan, M., Praphakar, R.A., Jeyaraj, M. (2019). Sericin-chitosan doped maleate gellan gum nanocomposites for effective cell damage in mycobacterium tuberculosis. Int J Biol Macromol, 122, 174–184.

Mehnath, S., Rajan, M., Sathishkumar, G., Jeyaraj, M. (2017). Thermoresponsive and pH triggered drug release of cholate functionalized poly(organophosphazene) – polylactic acid copolymeric nanostructure integrated with ICG. Polymer, 133, 119–128.

Mehnath, S., Arjama, M., Rajan, M., Annamalai, G., Jeyaraj, M. (2018b). Co-encapsulation of dual drug loaded in MLNPs: Implication on sustained drug release and effectively inducing apoptosis in oral carcinoma cells. Biomed Pharmacother, 104, 661–671.

Mehnath, S., Chitra, K., Karthikeyan, K., Jeyaraj, M. (2020b). Localized delivery of active targeting micelles from nanofibers patch for effective breast cancer therapy. Int J Pharm, 584, 119412.

Mizuno, K., Yamamura, K., Yano, K., Osada, T., Saeki, S., Takimoto, N., Sakurai, T., Nimura, Y. (2003). Effect of chitosan film containing basic fibroblast growth factor on wound healing in genetically diabetic mice. J Biomed Mater Res A, 64, 177–181.

Moroni, L., Boland, T., Burdick, J.A., De Maria, C., Derby, B., Forgacs, G., Groll, J., Li, Q., Malda, J., Mironov, V.A. (2018). Biofabrication: a guide to technology and terminology, Trends Biotechnol, 36, 384–402.

Murphy, W.L., Peters, M.C., Kohn, D.H., Mooney, D.J. (2000). Sustained release of vascular endothelial growth factor from mineralized poly(lactide-co-glycolide) scaffolds for tissue engineering. Biomaterials, 21, 2521–2527.

Murugan, S., Rajan, M., Alyahya, S.A., Alharbi, N.S., Kadaikunnan, S., Kumar, S.S. (2018). Development of self-repair nano-rod scaffold materials for implantation of osteosarcoma affected bone tissue. New J Chem, 42(1), 725–734.

Naves, A.F., Motay, M., Mérindol, R., Davi, C.P., Felix, O., Catalani, L.H., et al. (2016). Layer-by-Layer assembled growth factor reservoirs for steering the response of 3T3-cells. Colloids Surf B Biointerfaces, 139, 79–86.

O'Sullivan, V.J., Barrette-Ng, I., Hommema, E., Hermanson, G.T., Schofield, M., Wu, S.C., et al. (2012). Development of a tetrameric streptavidin mutein with reversible biotin binding capability: engineering a mobile loop as an exit door for biotin. PLoS ONE, 7, e35203.

Okonkwo, U.A., DiPietro, L.A. (2017). Diabetes and wound angiogenesis. Int J Mol Sci, 18(7), 1419.

Park, I.K., Seo, S.J., Akashi, M., Akaike, T., Cho, C.S. (2003). Controlled release of epidermal growth factor (EGF) from EGF-loaded polymeric nanoparticles composed of polystyrene as core and poly(methacrylic acid) as corona in vitro. Arch Pharm Res, 26, 649–652.

Park, Y.B., Dziak, R., Genco, R.J., Swihart, M., Perinpanayagam, H. (2007). Calcium sulfate based nanoparticles. U.S. patent 60/887,859.

Pattison, D.I., Rahmanto, A.S., Davies, M.J. (2012). Photo-oxidation of proteins. Photochem Photobiol Sci, 11, 38–53.

Pitukmanorom, P., Yong, T.H., Ying, J.Y. (2008). Tunable release of proteins with polymer-inorganic nanocomposite microspheres. Adv Mater, 20, 3504–3509.

Pradeepkumar, P., Govindaraj, D., Jeyaraj, M., Munusamy, M.A., Rajan, M. (2017). Assembling of multifunctional latex-based hybrid nanocarriers from Calotropis gigantea for sustained (doxorubicin) DOX releases. Biomed Pharmacother, 87, 461–470.

Pradhan, S., Keller, K.A., Sperduto, J.L., Slater, J.H. (2017). Fundamentals of laser-based hydrogel degradation and applications in cell and tissue engineering. Adv Healthc Mater, 6, 1700681.

Psarra, E., Foster, E., König, U., You, J., Ueda, Y., Eichhorn, K.J., et al. (2015). Growth factor-bearing polymer brushes - Versatile bioactive substrates influencing cell response. Biomacromolecules, 16, 3530–3542.

Pulavendran, S., Rajam, M., Rose, C., Mandal, A.B. (2010). Hepatocyte growth factor incorporated chitosan nanoparticles differentiate murine bone marrow mesenchymal stem cell into hepatocytes in vitro. IET Nanobiotechnol, 4(3), 51–60.

Rahman, N., Purpura, K.A., Wylie, R.G., Zandstra, P.W., Shoichet, M.S. (2010). The use of vascular endothelial growth factor functionalized agarose to guide pluripotent stem cell aggregates toward blood progenitor cells. Biomaterials, 31, 8262–8270.

Rajam, M., Pulavendran, S., Rose, C., Mandal, A.B. (2011). Chitosan nanoparticles as a dual growth factor delivery system for tissue engineering applications. Int J Pharm, 410, 145–152.

Reyes, R., De la Riva, B., Delgado, A., Hernandez, A., Sanchez, E., Evora, C. (2012). Effect of triple growth factor controlled delivery by a brushite–PLGA system on a bone defect. Injury, 43, 334–342.

Salamanna, F., Gambardella, A., Contartese, D., Visani, A., Fini, M. (2021). Nano-based biomaterials as drug delivery systems against osteoporosis: a systematic review of preclinical and clinical evidence. Nanomaterials, 11(2), 530.

Sarrigiannidis, S.O., Rey, J.M., Dobre, O., González-García, C., Dalby, M., Salmeron-Sanchez M. (2021). A tough act to follow: collagen hydrogel modifications to improve mechanical and growth factor loading capabilities. Mater Today Bio, 10, 100098.

Schumacher, M., Reither, L., Thomas, J., Kampschulte, M., Gbureck, U., Lode, A., et al. (2017). Calcium phosphate bone cement/mesoporous bioactive glass composites for controlled growth factor delivery. Biomater Sci, 5, 578–588.

Shah, N.J., Macdonald, M.L., Beben, Y.M., Padera, R.F., Samuel, R.E., Hammond, P.T. (2011). Tunable dual growth factor delivery from polyelectrolyte multilayer films. Biomaterials, 32, 6183–6193.

Shan, Y.H., Peng, L.H., Liu, X., Chen, X., Xiong, J., Gao, J.Q. (2015). Silk fibroin/gelatin electrospun nanofibrous dressing functionalized with astragaloside IV induces healing and anti-scar effects on burn wound. Int J Pharm, 479, 291–301.

Sharmin, F., McDermott, C., Lieberman, J., et al. (2017). Dual growth factor delivery from biofunctionalized allografts: sequential VEGF and BMP-2 release to stimulate allograft remodeling. J Orthop Res, 35, 1086–1095.

Sharon, J.L., Puleo, D.A. (2008). Immobilization of glycoproteins, such as VEGF, on biodegradable substrates. Acta Biomater, 4, 1016–1023.

Shim, W.S., Yoo, J.S., Bae, Y.H., Lee, D.S. (2005). Novel injectable pH and temperature sensitive block copolymer hydrogel. Biomacromolecules, 6, 2930–2934.

Simao, P.B., Rui, M.A., Babo, P.S., Dominika, B., Margarida, S.M., Manuela, E.G., Nicholas, A.P., Rui, L.R. (2020). Epitope-imprinted nanoparticles as transforming growth factor-$\beta 3$ sequestering ligands to modulate stem cell fate. Adv Funct Mater, 31, 4.

Simons, M., Ware, J.A. (2003). Therapeutic angiogenesis in cardiovascular disease. Nat Rev Drug Discov, 2, 863–872.

Skaat, H., Ziv-Polat, O., Shahar, A., Margel, S. (2011). Enhancement of the growth and differentiation of nasal olfactory mucosa cells by the conjugation of growth factors to functional nanoparticles. Bioconjugate Chem, 22(12), 2600–2610.

Stefonek-Puccinelli, T.J., Masters, K.S. (2008). Co-immobilization of gradient-patterned growth factors for directed cell migration. Ann Biomed Eng, 36, 2121–2133.

Sumathra, M., Munusamy, M.A., Alarfaj, A.A., Rajan, M. (2018). Osteoblast response to Vitamin D_3 loaded cellulose enriched hydroxyapatite Mesoporous silica nanoparticles composite. Biomed Pharmacother, 103, 858–868.

Sumathra, M., Rajan, M., Amarnath Praphakar, R., Marraiki, N., Elgorban, A.M. (2020). In vivo assessment of a hydroxyapatite/κ-carrageenan–maleic anhydride–casein/doxorubicin composite-coated titanium bone implant. ACS Biomater Sci Eng, 6(3), 1650–1662.

Talebian, S., Mehrali, M., Taebnia, N., Pennisi, C.P., Kadumudi, F.B., Foroughi, J., Hasany, M., Nikkhah, M., Akbari, M., Orive, G., Dolatshahi-Pirouz, A. (2019). Self-healing hydrogels: The next paradigm shift in tissue engineering? Adv Sci (Weinh), 6(16), 1801664.

Tan, H., Shen, Q., Jia, X., Yuan, Z., Xiong, D. (2012). Injectable nanohybrid scaffold for biopharmaceuticals delivery and soft tissue engineering. Macromo Rapid Commun, 33, 2015–2022.

Tan, Q., Tang, H., Hu, J., Hu, Y., Zhou, X., Tan, Y., Wu, Z. (2011). Controlled release of chitosan/heparin NP-delivered VEGF enhances regeneration of decellularized tissue engineered scaffolds. Int J Nanomed, 6, 929–942.

Tanaka, H., Sugita, T., Yasunaga, Y., Shimose, S., Deie, M., Kubo, T., Murakami, T., Ochi, M. (2005). Efficiency of magnetic liposomal transforming growth factor-$\beta 1$ in the repair of articular cartilage defects in a rabbit model. J Biomed Mater Res A, 73A, 255–263.

Tarafder, S., Koch, A., Jun, Y., Chou, C., Awadallah, M.R., Lee, C.H. (2016). Micro-precise spatiotemporal delivery system embedded in 3D printing for complex tissue regeneration. Biofabrication, 8(2), 025003.

Theiss, H.D., Brenner, C., Engelmann, M.G., et al. (2010). Safety and efficacy of SITAgliptin plus GRanulocyte-colony-stimulating factor in patients suffering from acute myocardial infarction (SITAGRAMI-Trial): rationale, design and first interim analysis. Int J Cardiol, 145(2), 282–284.

Thomas, T.P., Shukla, R., Kotlyar, A., Liang, B., Ye, J.Y., Norris, T.B., Baker, J.R. (2008). Dendrimer-epidermal growth factor conjugate displays superagonist activity. Biomacromolecules, 9, 603–609.

Thornton, P.D., Mcconnell, G., Ulijn, R.V. (2005). Enzyme responsive polymer hydrogel beads. Chem Commun, 5913–5915.

Tinke, M.W., Lidy, E.F., Amir, A.Z., Nicholas, A.P. (2018). Bone tissue engineering via growth factor delivery: from scaffolds to complex matrices. Regen Biomater, 5(4), 197–211.

Traversa, B., Sussman, G. (2001). The role of growth factors, cytokines and proteases in wound management. Primary Intent, 9, 161–167.

Ulijn, R.V., Bibi, N., Jayawarna, V., Thornton, P.D., Todd, S.J., Mart, R.J., Smith, A.M., Gough, J.E. (2007). Bioresponsive hydrogels. Mater Today. 10, 40–48.

Ulubayram, K., Cakar, A.N., Korkusuz, P., Ertan, C., Hasirci, N. (2001). EGF containing gelatin-based wound dressings. Biomaterials, 22, 1345–1356.

Uz, M., Sharma, A.D., Adhikari, P., Sakaguchi, D.S., Mallapragada, S.K. (2017). Development of multifunctional films for peripheral nerve regeneration. Acta Biomater. 56, 141–152.

Vorndran, E., Klarner, M., Klammert, U., Grover, L.M., Patel, S., Barralet, J.E., Gbureck, U. (2008). 3D powder printing of β-tricalcium phosphate ceramics using different strategies. Adv Eng Mater, 10(12), B67–B71.

Vu, T.Q., Maddipati, R., Blute, T.A., Nehilla, B.J., Nusblat, L., Desai, T.A. (2005). Peptide-conjugated quantum dots activate neuronal receptors and initiate downstream signaling of neurite growth. Nano Lett, 5, 603–607.

Waller, J.P., Burke, S.P., Engel, J. et al. (2021). A dose-escalating toxicology study of the candidate biologic ELP-VEGF. Sci Rep, 11, 6216.

Wang, X.J., Han, G., Owens, P., Siddiqui, Y., Li, A.G. (2006). Role of TGF beta-mediated inflammation in cutaneous wound healing. J Investig Dermatol Symp Proc, 11, 112–117.

Wang, Y., Cooke, M.J., Sachewsky, N., Morshead, C.M., Shoichet, M.S. (2013). Bioengineered sequential growth factor delivery stimulates brain tissue regeneration after stroke. J Control Release, 172, 1–11.

Wang, Z., Li, C., Xu, J., Wang, K., Lu, X., Zhang, H., Qu, S., Zhen, G., Ren, F. (2015). Bioadhesive microporous architectures by self-assembling polydopamine microcapsules for biomedical applications. Chem Mater, 27, 848–856.

Wang, Z., Wang, Z., Lu, W.W., Zhen, W., Yang, D., and Peng, S. (2017). Novel biomaterial strategies for controlled growth factor delivery for biomedical applications. NPG Asia Mater, 9, e435.

Wei, G., Jin, Q., Giannobile, W.V., Maa, P.X. (2007). The enhancement of osteogenesis by nanofibrous scaffolds incorporating rhBMP-7 nanospheres. Biomaterials, 28, 2087–2096.

Wen, B., Karl, M., Pendrys, D., Shafer, D., Freilich, M., Kuhn, L. (2011). An evaluation of BMP-2 delivery from scaffolds with miniaturized dental implants in a novel rat mandible model. J Biomed Mater Res B, 97(2), 315–326.

Worrallo, M.J., Moore, R.L.L., Glen, K.E., Thomas, R.J. (2017). Immobilized hematopoietic growth factors onto magnetic particles offer a scalable strategy for cell therapy manufacturing in suspension cultures. Biotechnol J, 12, 1–10.

Wu, J., Ye, J., Zhu, J., Xiao, Z., He, C., Shi, H., Wang, Y., Lin, C., Zhang, H., Zhao, Y., Fu, X., et al. (2016). Heparin-based coacervate of FGF2 improves dermal regeneration by asserting a synergistic role with cell proliferation and endogenous facilitated VEGF for cutaneous wound healing. Biomacromolecules, 17, 2168–2177.

Xie, Y., Ye, L.Y., Zhang, X.B., Cui, W., Lou, J.N., Nagai, T., Hou, X.P. (2005). Transport of nerve growth factor encapsulated into liposomes across the blood-brain barrier: in vitro and in vivo studies. J Control Release, 105, 106–119.

Yamakawa, S., Kenji, H. (2019). Advances in surgical applications of growth factors for wound healing. Burns Trauma, 7, 10.

Yang, Y., Xia, T., Zhi, W., Wei, L., Weng, J., Zhang, C., Li, X. (2011). Promotion of skin regeneration in diabetic rats by electrospun core-sheath fibers loaded with basic fibroblast growth factor. Biomaterials, 32, 4243–4254.

Zandi, N., Mostafavi, E., Shokrgozar, M.A., Tamjid, E., Webster, T.J., Annabi, N., et al. (2020). Biomimetic proteoglycan nanoparticles for growth factor immobilization and delivery. Biomater Sci, 8, 1127–1136.

Zhang, S., Wang, G., Lin, X., Chatzinikolaidou, M., Jennissen, H.P., Laub, M., Uludag, H. (2008). Polyethylenimine-coated albumin nanoparticles for bmp-2 delivery. Biotechnol Prog, 24, 945–956.

Zhang, W., Wang, X., Wang, S., et al. (2011). The use of injectable sonication-induced silk hydrogel for VEGF165 and BMP-2 delivery for elevation of the maxillary sinus floor. Biomaterials, 32(35), 9415–9424.

Zhang, X., Ibrahimi, O.A., Olsen, S.K., Umemori, H., Mohammadi, M., Ornitz, D.M. (2006). Receptor specificity of the fibroblast growth factor family. The complete mammalian FGF family. J Biol Chem, 281, 15694–15700.

Zhang, X., Yao, D., Zhao, W., Zhang, R., Yu, B., Ma, G., Li, Y., Hao, D., Xu, F.J. (2020). Engineering platelet-rich plasma based dual-network hydrogel as a bioactive wound dressing with potential clinical translational value. Adv Funct Mater, 31, 8.

Zhang, Y.H., Zhu, L.J., Yao, J.M. (2011). Studies on recombinant human bone morphogenetic protein 2 loaded nano-hydroxyapatite/silk fibroin scaffolds. Adv Mater Res, 175, 253–257.

Zhang, Z., Hu, J., and Ma, P.X. (2012). Nanofiber-based delivery of bioactive agents and stem cells to bone sites. Adv Drug Deliv Rev, 64, 1129–1141.

Zhang, Z., Li, Q., Han, L., Zhong, Y. (2015). Layer-by-layer films assembled from natural polymers for sustained release of neurotrophin. Biomed Mater, 10, 55–60.

Zheng, L., Hui, Q., Tang, L., Zheng, L., Jin, Z., Yu, B., Wang, Z., Lin, P., Yu, W., Li, H., Li, X., Wang, X. (2015). TAT-mediated acidic fibroblast growth factor delivery to the dermis improves wound healing of deep skin tissue in rat. PLoS ONE, 10, e0135291.

Zhou, X., Feng, W., Qiu, K., Chen, L., Wang, W., Nie, W., Mo, X., He, C. (2015). BMP-2 derived peptide and dexamethasone incorporated mesoporous silica nanoparticles for enhanced osteogenic differentiation of bone mesenchymal stem cells. ACS Appl Mater Interf, 7, 15777–15789.

Ziegler, J., Anger, D., Krummenaner, F., Breitig, D., Fickert, S. and Guenther, K.P. (2008). Biological activity of recombinant human growth factors released from biocompatible bone implants. J Biomed Mater Res A, 86, 89–97.

Zieris, A., Chwalek, K., Prokoph, S., et al. (2011). Dual independent delivery of pro-angiogenic growth factors from starPEGheparin hydrogels. J Control Release, 156(1), 28–36.

Zisch, A. H., Lutolf, M.P., Ehrbar, M., Raeber, G.P., Rizzi, S.C., Davies, N., et al. (2003). Cell-demanded release of VEGF from synthetic, biointeractive cell ingrowth matrices for vascularized tissue growth. FASEB J, 17, 2260–2262.

4 Natural and Synthetic Tissue Regenerative Materials

Roohi Kesharwani and Dilip Kumar Patel
Sam Higginbottom University of Agriculture,
Technology and Sciences

Surendra Tripathy
Northeast Frontier Railway Hospital

Pankaj Kumar Yadav and Vikas Kumar
Sam Higginbottom University of Agriculture,
Technology and Sciences

CONTENTS

DOI: 10.1201/9781003140108-4

107

4.1 INTRODUCTION

The powerful regeneration and restoration of damaged organs and tissues relies upon prompt restoration of the bloodstream required for metabolic assistance and cell invasion. Regenerative medicine is a flourishing new zone of multidisciplinary research that can alter the treatment process of ailing and harmed tissue. The ability to create materials that can interface with tissues mechanically, biofunctionally, and structurally, is critical to the accomplishment of the methodology of regeneration (Griffith and Naughton 2002; Bonzani, George, and Stevens 2006). Currently, the ideal model of medication for regeneration the utilization of substance concerned with natural materials is the latest representation of the cross-disciplinary logical methodologies that join the latest advancement in innovation, fundamental sciences, life sciences, and materials sciences (Mano et al. 2007). The material used for implants intended to replace diseased or damaged tissues should function as scaffolds among which cells can move and build up required vascularization. Also, the polymers should be sufficiently able to withstand the biological requests put on them when embedded into a site-explicit organ framework, and after some time they should hold their mechanical properties (Hodde 2002). These days, the advancement of proficient biomaterials and scaffolds is popular for the creation of clinically usable volumes of new tissues to replace lost or failing body parts and to accomplish straightforward injury mending. Significantly, the scaffold materials can communicate with encompassing tissue to fill up the deformity yet, additionally, encourage the characteristic recovery of undifferentiated organisms (He and Lu 2016). Tissue design for the most part requires a fake extracellular matrix for tissue recovery, since cell expansion and separation, bringing about tissue recovery, would be troublesome unless that kind of lattice has capacity as a scaffold. Considering that this counterfeit extracellular matrix ought to vanish via retention into the body during recovery of new tissues, it should best and suitable from the polymers having biodegradable property (Freed, Martin, and Vunjak-Novakovic 1999; Rosso et al. 2005). With everything taken into account, regenerative planning intends to give a temporary three-dimensional atmosphere or framework, instead of the neighborhood extracellular matrix for developed cells to duplicate and recuperate tissue. Mesenchymal stem cells are prepared to isolate toward different cell lineages; they are broadly utilized because of their simplicity of detachment from various grown-up tissues and their manipulability (Frassica and Grunlan 2020).

4.2   TYPES OF TISSUE REGENERATIVE MATERIAL

There is a wide variety of biomaterials in regeneration, both synthetic and natural. They have been used for osteochondritis dissecans repair in various clinical applications. Of these materials, by and large the most utilized are reliant on proteins, for instance, silk fibroin and collagen, for their regenerative and glue-like property as discussed in the current chapter. Regardless, because of the intricate idea of cell-protein associations, we have chosen to focus on the current status of engineered-based framework techniques (Deng, Chang, and Wu 2019; Di Luca, Van Blitterswijk, and Moroni 2015). This chapter centers around the point of view of biomimicry before surveying two different categories of materials: one obtained from naturally occurring molecules and the other one prepared synthetically. These can be separated into two significant classes (Basu 2017):

1. Natural origin polymers (such as collagen, chitosan, and alginate)
2. Synthetic polymers (such as PEO, PAA, PGA, PLA)

4.3   NATURAL-ORIGIN POLYMERS

These are characterized as polymers that are delivered by the cells of a living animal, especially underlying proteins, for example, elastin, collagen, and fibronectin (Figure 4.1), which are utilized as scaffold materials in tissue engineering and as vehicles for cell transport. In this, the collagen turned out to be a scaffold and transporter

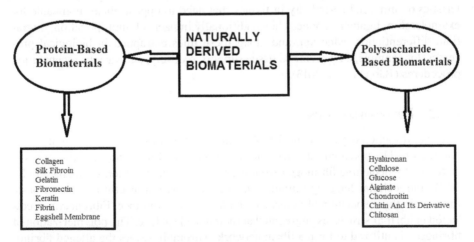

FIGURE 4.1   Classification of naturally derived biomaterials.

for cells in various tissues. Natural-occurring materials are made out of polysaccharides, polypeptides, nucleic acids, and hydroxyapatites. The natural polymer have few exceptional focal points over synthetic materials are its magnificent physiological exercises, for example, particular cell attachment, mechanical properties like normal tissues and its biodegradable behavior (Murray et al. 2003). The materials obtained naturally represent a significant subset of biodegradable materials utilized in tissue engineering due to their biocompatibility, tunable degradation bioactivity, and inherent underlying similarity to the extracellular matrix of local tissue. They are frequently handled utilizing environmentally friendly methods. These natural frameworks don't deliver cytotoxic items at the time of degradation; thus the rate might differ after adjusting the formulation conditions (Chen et al. 2016; Singh et al. 2016).

4.3.1 COLLAGEN

Collagen is a protein found abundantly in connective tissues of all animals. Collagens are pervasive proteins responsible for keeping up the underlying structural integrity of vertebrates and numerous different living organisms. More than 20 hereditarily recognizable collagens came to be distinguished mostly as types I, II and III. The structure of collagen is the triple-helical type and composed of three polypeptide chains carrying rehashed X and Y positions of Gly X-Y trios and regularly involved by 4-hydroxyproline and proline, individually. It can be promptly decontaminated from tissues of animals, e.g., skin and ligaments (Hulmes 2002; Patterson, Martino, and Hubbell 2010). It is a significant protein segment of ECM, so it is seen as a biocompatible scaffold. Various platforms (scaffolds) that are reliant on collagen protein are available for clinical use, such as those effectively applied in the field of tissue engineering (Yang et al. 2004). Any structural and physical forms created from collagen-containing tissues, such as films, gels, monofilaments, and porous matrices, can likewise be delivered utilizing it. These structures can be utilized in controlling skin recovery and tissue engineering (Huang and Fu 2010; Chen, Ushida, and Tateishi 2000). Collagen is superior in fibrils, along with the rigidity via characteristics 67 nm axial periodicity in tissues that need to oppose shear, malleable for example, skin, ligaments, bone. They additionally impact cell multiplication, migration, differentiation, adhesion, and along these lines entrapped in biological processes, for example, advancement, tissue support, recovery, and various regeneration procedures (Bao Ha et al. 2013).

4.3.2 FIBRIN/FIBRONECTIN

The multifunctional part of the ECM is fibronectin, which actively initiates cell connection. The potential for infection transmission and immunogenic responses is restricted by detaching fibrinogen from the blood plasma of patients (Huang and Fu 2010). Intracellular flagging initiated via cell bond on fibronectin assumes a basic function in the association of cytoskeleton and in cell endurance. Fibronectin is collected in fibrillar structures aggregated at their apical surface. The polymerization of fibrinogen is utilized to form a fibrin network. Thrombin severs the alleged fibrinopeptides on fibrinogen that prevent physicochemical self-assembly or polymerization of the molecule, and cross-linked, perplexing fibril structure relies on the development (Patterson, Martino, and Hubbell 2010). Fibrin assumes a significant role in unconstrained tissue repair and hemostasis. It has been a valuable cell delivery matrix for ligament tissue design. Additionally, it is utilized in skin recovery, with significant achievement, and even in the stacking and back arrival of development factors (Hubbell 2003; Mano et al. 2007). A three-dimensional fibrin gel platform can be used for vessel tissue designing. The fibrin gel structure in 3D form could fill in as a helpful framework for tissue engineering and in the advancement of tissues. The huge disadvantage of fibrin is that it is defenseless against quick corruption in vivo and encounters issues keeping up the integrity of the structure. This shortcoming can be overcome via overhauling the groupings of fibrinogen, calcium particle by bringing down cell density, or by adding specific protease inhibitors. Fibrin is additionally demonstrated as a natural platform for migration, differentiation, and proliferation of cells in tissue engineering. The three-dimensional fibrin framework in cardiovascular tissue design is created and explored by Ye and colleagues (Ye et al. 2000; Rowe, Lee, and Stegemann 2007).

4.3.3 SILK

Silk fibroin is an insoluble sinewy protein produced by silkworms (Bombyx mori), which contains about 90% amino acids, including glycine, alanine, and serine. It is generally characterized as protein polymers that are spun into filaments by lepidoptera hatchlings, for example, insects, silkworms, scorpions, bugs, etc. They are fibrous proteins combined in specific epithelial cells. These types of polymers comprise redundant protein groupings and provide primary parts in the formation of cocoons, nest building, traps, and web formation. After silk fibroin is cleaned, it is separated from degummed silk (Kundu et al. 2013; Lee and Parpura 2009; Yucel, Lovett, and Kaplan 2014). The shell is degummed in a bubbling arrangement of 0,5% sodium carbonate at 70°C for half an hour. At that point, the degummed fiber is disintegrated at 80°C in a mixture of ethanol, $CaCl_2$, and H_2O. After that, to eliminate $CaCl_2$ the silk fibroin salts, the mixture was centrifuged for 10 minutes at 5000 rpm; it was dialyzed persistently for 72 hours in running unadulterated water. Subsequently, the fluid silk fibroin was put away at 4°C and utilized in the accompanying examinations for the readiness of silk fibroin NPs. It is utilized in clinical applications as biodegradable miniature cylinders for the repair of veins and as fabricated additions for bone, ligament, and tooth recreation. The biodegradable and bioresorbable polymers can create joints and bone installations in the biomedical field to reduce pain for patients (Wang et al. 2006; Sofia et al. 2001). It is also utilized in tissue recovery for treating wound casualties and as a network in recuperating wounds. For instance, profoundly permeable silk frameworks have been joined with MSCs for in vitro ligament tissue design (Kumaresan, Sinha, and Raje Urs 2007; Wang et al. 2005; Altman et al. 2003).

4.3.4 GELATIN-ALGINATE

Gelatin is a typical regular polymer utilized in drug and clinical applications because of its biodegradability and biocompatibility in physiological conditions.

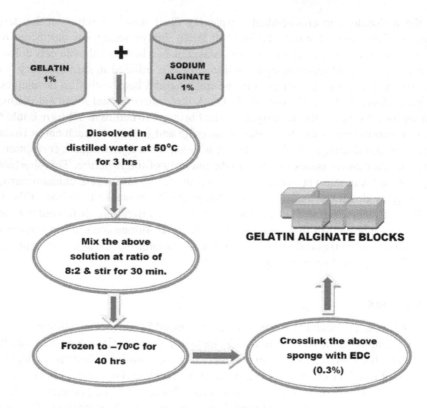

FIGURE 4.2 Manufacturing process of gelatin alginate.

It is obtained via the process of hydrolysis of collagen, and it is a significant segment of connective tissue and bone. It contains amino acids, for example, proline, hydroxyproline and glycine. The gelatin particles contain repeated groupings of glycine XY trios, where X and Y are usually proline and hydroxyproline (Kelley et al. 1989; Bao Ha et al. 2013). More explicitly, the isoelectric purpose of gelatin can be changed during the process of fabrication to obtain a contrarily charged acidic gelatin. Other than fusing growth factors, gelatin transporters can be utilized to join cells to accomplish effective design of tissue (Huang and Fu 2010). Alginate (alginic acid), made up of block copolymers of [1–4]-connected β-d-mannuronic acid (M) and α-l-guluronic acid (G) covalently connected. The polymer goes through ionotropic gelation within the sight of divalent cations, and gelling relies (Figure 4.2) upon the particle attraction (Izydorczyk, Cui, and Wang 2005). It has been utilized widely in a hydrogel structure for cell epitome and medication conveyance just as in tissue-design applications. The creation of sanitized alginates with reliably high clinical evaluation quality has been considered. Alginate has demonstrated materiality in the region of ligament recovery, as chondrocytes are accounted for to keep up their aggregate in the alginate gels (Häuselmann et al. 1994; Bhat and Kumar 2012).

4.3.5 CHITOSAN

Chitosan is a subordinate of chitin, a carbohydrate that essential underlying polymer in arthropod exoskeletons is a decidedly charged polysaccharide. Chitin is composed of (1→4)- β-N-acetyl-D-glucosamine units of polysaccharide. Chitin is effectively acquired from crab or shrimp shells and pathogenic parasites, which are framed through deacetylation. It is biocompatible, non-poisonous, and can be promptly debased by catalysts, for example, glycosyl hydrolases and lysosomes. It is insoluble in neutral pH conditions, so the materials should be added to somewhat acidic solutions to be dissolved. Its biocompatibility, just as biodegradability, makes this material reasonable as a brief framework for tissue design (Singh and Ray 2000; Dvir, Tsur-Gang, and Cohen 2005). For ligament tissue designing it observes that utilization of microsphere have principally centered concerning the utilization of chitosan-based frameworks. Kim and other researchers have planned a sort of permeable chitosan framework, containing TGF-b1, to improve chondrogenesis. It was demonstrated that the platform containing the stacked chitosan microspheres fundamentally expanded the cell expansion and creation of extracellular matrix (Kim et al. 2003; Jayakumar et al. 2010).

4.3.6 CELLULOSE

Cellulose is the most plentiful polymer, which makes it likewise the most widely recognized natural compound. Cotton contains 90% cellulose; other plants contain roughly 33% while wood contains around half. It comprises 15,000 D-glucose buildups connected by β-(1→4)- glycosidic bonds, with incredibly warm, biodegradable, mechanical properties and biocompatibility. The overall preparation of designed materials can be considered to happen in four fundamental stages: bacterial cellulose refined, pellicle the executives, water expulsion, and substance alteration (Figure 4.3). This microbial cellulose blended by acetobacter xylinum shows extensive potential as a novel injury-mending framework, coming about because of its extraordinary nanostructure (Klemm et al. 1998; Bao Ha et al. 2013). Bacterial cellulose has one of a kind properties, such as high water-holding limit, high crystallinity, a fine fiber organization and biocompatibility. Notwithstanding its cost-proficient and generally straightforward creation it has the upside of insitu moldability (Entcheva et al. 2004; Svensson et al. 2005; Singh et al. 2016).

4.4 SYNTHETIC POLYMERS

Synthetic polymers are composed of covalently bound rehashed monomer units. These rehashed units can react with one another to form high subatomic weight homopolymers, for the most part by expansion polymerization in tissue design (Vert 2005; Lee, Yoo, and Atala 2017). Engineered biodegradable polymers offer various points of interest over normal biopolymers as platform material. They can be customized to have biodegradation active profiles and mechanical strength properties as per the particular tissue application. What's more, synthetic materials don't have the complexities related to sanitization, immunogenicity, and microorganism transmission, issues that can happen with normally

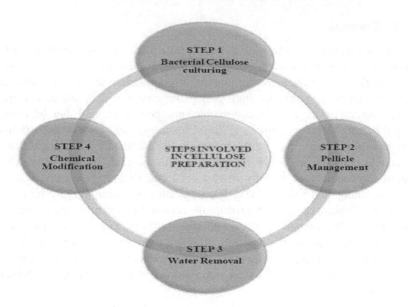

FIGURE 4.3   Steps involved in cellulose preparation.

synthesized materials. In a perfect world, a polymeric material utilized for tissue design should have the option to control cell expansion without deficiency of pluripotency and to coordinate separation into a particular cell ancestry (He and Lu 2016).

4.4.1   Polyesters of Lactic Acid and Glycolic Acid (PLGAs) and Their Copolymers

Polyesters of lactic acid and glycolic acid are the most generally utilized manufactured materials for tissue engineering. Their selection was influenced by various reasons: they are endorsed by the FDA for various clinical applications, for example, stitches, bone plates, and controlled delivered microspheres; their mechanical strength can be changed by the polymer MW; their biodegradation rate can be handily constrained by controlling the molar proportion between the constituent co-monomers; and they can be prepared into various shapes and morphologies, utilizing, for instance, pressure forming, because of their thermoplastic properties. Change of the PLGA platforms by these different strategies improved their presentation. For instance, a new investigation with a composite platform of PLGA (L/G, 50/50) blended in with dextran uncovered its potential as osteoconductive material in basic-size bone imperfections (Khabbaz et al. 2004; Kesharwani et al. 2016).

4.4.2   Poly (vinyl alcohol) (PVA)

Poly (vinyl alcohol) (PVA) has effectively controllable hydrophilicity and dissolvability that can be accomplished by changing the subatomic weight and degree of hydrolysis. Lamentably, huge numbers of the crosslinkers utilized with PVA, such as glutaraldehyde or epichlorohydrin, can be harmful and have issues with draining that can be relieved by freeze-thaw cycles. An electron beam can likewise be utilized to crosslink PVA; however, it brings about a less steady gel than the gels that have experienced the freeze-thaw cycles, which were accounted for as steady at room temperature. PVA isn't biodegradable and subsequently is helpful as a drawn-out perpetual framework (Yoshii et al. 1999; Gu, Xiao, and Zhang 1998).

4.4.3 Poly(ethylene oxide)

Poly(ethylene oxide) are another class of manufactured polymers that have been utilized as a scaffold for tissue engineering. Although they are not biodegradable and need natural explicitness, these polymers have been utilized because of their biocompatibility and endorsement by the FDA. What's more, PEOs can shape hydrogels through substance response, γ-radiation,80 or photograph polymerization81 and consequently can be made to reproduce delicate tissues in actual qualities. PEOs have low toxicity and are truly biocompatible. PEOs can be combined by anionic or cationic polymerization of ethylene oxide or through star-molded monomers or oligomers and shaped into hydrogels through UV photopolymerization. Poly(propylene oxide) (PEO PPO PEO) has a hydrophobic block that takes into account the development of reversible gels without the requirement for lasting crosslinks. This triblock (PEO, PPO, PEO) has been utilized for drug conveyance applications as it has been known to upgrade drug penetration. However, PEG-based materials are not biodegradable, conceivably restricting their utility. Poly(lactic corrosive) has been integrated with PEO and appeared to frame temperature subordinate reversible gel-sol advances at internal heat level for which the subsequent hydrogel go through a blend of hydrolytic corruption and separation (Alexandridis, Zhou, and Khan 1996).

4.4.4 Poly(acrylic acid) (PAA)

Poly(acrylic acid) (PAA) and its numerous subordinates can frame an assortment of hydrogels. Poly (2hydroxyethyl methacrylate) or poly(HEMA) has been utilized for an assortment of uses including contact lenses and in drug delivery. Macroporous gels can be shaped utilizing freeze-thaw cycling. Poly(HEMA) gels are nondegradable under ordinary physiological conditions. Dextran has been utilized to alter poly (HEMA) to take into account the subsequent hydrogels to be degradable by catalysts. Poly(N-isopropyl acrylamide) (PNIPAM) hardens at temperatures above 32°C, making it appealing for injectable applications. PNIPAM can be copolymerized with acrylic acid to adjust the gel for various applications., These gels structure non-degradable crosslinks and incorporate vinyl monomers, which can be poisonous (Lu and Anseth 1999; Meyvis et al. 2000).

4.5 BIOMATERIAL PROPERTIES

The biomaterials rely upon the class in which they are places for their properties. Yet key properties incorporate surface properties and debasement. The advantages and disadvantages of biomaterials are summarized in Table 4.1.

TABLE 4.1
Drawbacks and Advantages of Biomaterials in Tissue Regeneration

S.No.	Biomaterials	Drawbacks	Advantages
1.	Natural polymers	Transfer of pathogens possible	Biological properties
		Temperature sensitive	Hydrophilic nature
		Poor mechanical stability	Mimic natural ECM structure
		Difficult to control biodegradation rate	and composition
2.	Synthetic polymers	Hydrophobic nature	Easy to process
		Degrade to form by-products	Controlled surface characteristics
		Fewer biological properties than natural polymers	Pathogen free
			Controlled biodegradation rate
			Tunable mechanical properties

4.5.1 SURFACE

The associations between the biomaterials and have tissue is a surface marvel, so the properties of embedded materials are vital. material surface is the end of the ordinary 3D structure of a specific material. An adjustment in the polymer arrangement that builds the general development of chains thus expands the strength and diminishes the pliancy of the biomaterial.

4.5.2 DEGRADATION

Different classes of biomaterials such as polymers don't go through corrosion; however, they are vulnerable to corruption under physiological conditions. A perfect biomaterial ought to have a managed pace of debasement, which should coordinate with the neotissue arrangement. (Bhat and Kumar 2012).

4.6 EVALUATION OF BIOMATERIALS

4.6.1 IN VITRO ANALYSIS

A biomaterial of any category can be seen as "harmful" if it kills the cells either straightforwardly or by implication. So any biomaterial expected to be utilized as a clinical embed ought to be at first examined for its cytotoxicity. After the analysis of cytotoxicity, more explicit tests are performed to survey the general biocompatibility of the implanted materials. At the time of assay, the test substance might be placed directly on the cells or might be extracted in a solution. In light of how the examine is performed there are three significant techniques to examine the biocompatibility of any material: direct contact, agar diffusion, and elution. Of these techniques, direct-contact strategy is significantly utilized in the field of tissue design and regenerative therapy. For this purpose the blended monolayer of L-929 mammalian fibroblast cells was taken. For example, biomaterial was put cautiously in the way of life plates, and incubation was done for 24 hours at 37°C under damp air. The staining of the cell line was done by hematoxyline and eosin or by live fluorescent stains after incubation. The assessment of toxicity was determined by the shortfall of stained cells. Another method for assay is 3-(4,5- dimethylthiazol-2-yl)-2,5-diphenyltetrazolium bromide assay (MTT assay). In this test, cells are permitted to develop on the biomaterial for a few days. This test includes the transformation of tetrazolium salt MTT by reasonable multiplying cells to an insoluble item, purple formazan following four hours of hatching time and solubilized color complex utilized for quantitative analysis by determining its optical density spectrophotometrically.

4.6.2 IN VIVO ANALYSIS

A fundamental point of in vivo evaluation is to decide the biocompatibility of new biomaterial in the biological system physiologically. It was assessed by the accompanying strategies:

4.6.2.1 Implantation

A recently planned biomaterial is embedded precisely or is put into an embedding site in a creature model. Assessment of the obsessive impact is then done at both gross and minuscule levels.

4.6.2.2 Hemocompatibility

It is done to assess the impact of these materials on blood components. As per ISO norms, five test classes are demonstrated for hemocompatability: coagulation, thrombosis, platelets, immunology, and hematology.

4.6.2.3 Biodegradation

By this method the kinetics of degradation can be easily assayed. For this purpose biomaterial is implanted onto the experimental model. This test further gives insight regarding the type of material discharged at the time of degradation. The material belongs to ideal category if it does not form any toxic material at the time of degradation. (He and Lu 2016; Bhat and Kumar 2012).

4.7 DESIGNING OF TISSUE ENGINEERING SCAFFOLDS

Effective tissue design systems require the advancement of a satisfactory framework that upholds the process of regeneration. The platform gives a 3-D design and format whereupon the tissue-explicit cells connect, multiply, and produce extracellular matrix. In addition, the dissemination of supplements and metabolites in a 3-D climate requires exceptionally permeable scaffolds.

4.7.1 PARTICLE LEACHING

Particle leaching is quite possibly the most generally utilized handling techniques to get controlled-size scaffolds. The interaction depends on the scattering of a porogen such as sugar or salt either in a fluid, particulate, or powder-based material. The fluid might be hardened by crosslinking or solvent evaporation, and the powder might be compacted utilizing temperature and pressure. Benefits of this interaction include its effortlessness, adaptability, and effectiveness of control of the pore size and calculation. The pore geometry is achieved by the choice of the state of the porogen specialist, while the pore size is constrained by sieving the porogen particles to a particular measurement range. It is, nonetheless, troublesome by this technique to precisely plan the interconnectivity of the pores.

4.7.2 FREEZE DRYING

This process is widely utilized for the purpose of stabilization and perseverance of products having sensitivity to heat. The technique depends on the arrangement of ice crystals that actuate porosity through ice sublimation and desorption process. It is feasible to control the porosity level of froths by shifting the freezing time and the tempering stage. Advantages of porosity up to 90% with distinctive interconnectivities are basic in freeze-dried designs. The fundamental trouble related with this interaction is to guarantee primary dependability and sufficient mechanical properties of the permeable develops after resulting hydration. This restriction thwarts its utilization when the application includes conditions with mechanical pressure. The chitosan/hydroxyapatite scaffolds developed by the researcher use this strategy for this purpose.

4.7.3 FIBER MESHES AND FIBER BONDING

The researcher created a starch-based scaffolds through fiber meshes by melt-spinning a mixture of starch with ethylene vinyl alcohol copolymer, poly(3-caprolactone) (PCL) and polylactide (PLA) into fiber bundles. In this approach, fiber mesh scaffolds are produced by applying a heat treatment to bond fiber gatherings. For these scaffolds, cell survival was demonstrated to be profoundly subject to porosity of scaffolds. This could diffuse nutrients within the scaffolds more efficiently. Another method proposed by the researcher for the non-fusible materials via fiber mesh through wet spinning technique through the fibers bundles.

4.7.4 MELT PROCESSING

The non-thermoplastic conduct of regular polymers has restricted the use of dissolve-based handling techniques for the creation of Tissue engineering platforms to these materials. In any case, the researcher has proposed a few soften-based handling strategies, for example, extrusion and injection molding with blowing agents, compression molding combined with particulate leaching. Frothing during melt expulsion or infusion shaping depends on the utilization of physical or substance-blowing specialists that are liable for actuating porosity. Examination of these handling methods has primarily been centered around the utilization of synthetic blowing specialists. Up until this point, scaffolds dependent on thermoplastic mixes of starch with ethylene vinyl alcohol copolymer and cellulose acetate have been delivered by liquefying expulsion, utilizing endothermic synthetic blowing specialists dependent on combinations of citrus extract and sodium bicarbonate. It was reported more to be biocompatible and to display sufficient characteristics in terms of both geometry as well as porosity for the purpose of bone formation and cell growth. A comparative methodology has been applied for the creation of scaffolds dependent on molding through injection. Injection molding utilized the consolidated impact of shear and heat in comparison to extrusion technique to provide plasticity to the thermoplastic materials. More recently, an actual blowing substance, for example, supercritical CO_2 and water, has been utilized to deliver scaffolds via injection molding strategy.

4.7.5 BATCH FOAMING

In conventional techniques microporous materials are created on the basis of a phase separation polymer solution of homogeneous mixture via temperature extinguish or by the expansion of an anti-solvent. On the other hand, it is feasible to produce structures with porous property through the utilization of high pressure or supercritical gas for the saturation of polymer; this was done at controlled temperature conditions and submitting by rapid depressurization to pressure quenching. In this method of production of TE scaffolds, the saturation of a polymer should be done by pressurized gas, trailed by a fast pressure reduction, which is responsible for thermodynamic instability and ensuing nucleation and development of gas pores. Some researchers spearheaded the utilization of this procedure for the advancement of this scaffold dependent on PLGA, PLA, and PGA in combination with leaching of particle salt. Recently, anisotropic composites dependent on PLA and hydroxyapatite (HA) were developed by an alternate technique using immersion of the polymer over its softening temperature with supercritical CO_2 followed by quick depressurization, which brought about porosity levels up to 87.8%. Instead of the utilization of a high pressing factor or supercritical gas, other frothing techniques that depend on the utilization of synthetic frothing specialists have been researched,. Silk fibroin frameworks were created utilizing ammonium bicarbonate as a porogen specialist. For this situation, a silk fibroin arrangement containing ammonium bicarbonate was dried and settled with ethanol prior to being foamed in warm water. There is another batch-foaming strategy in which the paste of polymer and sodium bicarbonate particles is saturated with citric acid. This one is effectively utilized for the PLGA scaffolds fabrication and dexamethasone efficiently incorporated with this strategy in PLGA scaffolds.

4.7.6 RAPID PROTOTYPING

An alternative processing strategy based on solid freeform fabrication, or rapid prototyping, has been investigated due to various drawbacks and limits in the above techniques. The principle benefits of the prototyping technique is that it is rapidly involved in fabrication via computer-aided design, medical imaging for further creation of anatomically adjusted scaffolds and interior structure with customization property. Incredible emphasis has been given to the advancement of scaffolds by expulsion-based rapid prototyping. In this the strategy employed is fused deposition modeling (FDM), in which the fiber of material is warmed and softened in an expulsion spout and kept layer by layer, as indicated in a programmable way. The temperature and stream of the material are constrained by an expulsion head, while the development of scaffold in the z axis is guaranteed by the overall development of the stage to the expulsion head. Many authors detailed the development of these scaffolds by utilizing the fused deposition modeling strategy. In the synthesized 3-D deposition process, also referred to as 3-D bioplotting, the granular or powdered material is kept in a barrel and, after being melted, is ejected by the plunger, or piston. In fact, in this extrusion process the melted material is plasticized through rotating screw present in it. TE scaffolds are developed by this technique in which thermoplastic mixture of starch is utilized. For natural polymer scaffolds, the specific laser sintering strategy is utilized in which each layer present in the scaffolds is prepared through sintering, and scanning will be done by laser beam on the powdered material. The utilization of solid freeform fabrication (SFF) strategy based on melting is limited due to the non-fusible property of numerous naturally occurring polymers. An alternative approach utilized in the fabrication rapid prototyping is 3-D printing, in which starch is utilized as binding agent. This type of printing is specifically based on the bonding of the powder substrate through the binder resin deposition process. SFF methodology have likewise centered around the preparing of non-fusible natural polymers, for example, chitosan and chitosan/hydroxyapatite. In this methodology, the dispersion of a chitosan/acetic acid solution into sodium hydroxide based media is responsible for building up scaffolds layer by layer, which ultimately be the reason of neutralization of the acetic acid and the gel like chitosan strand were developed. The utilization of low temperatures in this technique enables, on a fundamental level, the epitome of cells and bioactive particles, which is excessive in melt-based measures. An illustration of this is the improvement of gelatin/alginate frameworks epitomized cells delivered by the back-to-back information of a combination of gelatin/alginate and hepatocytes cells, utilizing a microdispenser and resulting crosslinking by calcium chloride or glutaraldehyde. Different research centered on the fabrication of scaffolds by inkjet printing of fibrin hydrogen in which incorporation of the fibroblast growth factor 2 (FGF-2) and bone morphogenetic protein 2 (BMP-2) is done. Wang and other researchers developed hydroxyapatite-based scaffolds by the alleged lamination system of 3-D gel. The hydroxyapatite slurry was gelled by utilizing sodium alginate and calcium chloride. An elective technique is to utilize rapid prototyping advancements to fabricate a mold-dependent production of scaffolds.

4.7.7 Microsphere-Based Strategies

The "customary" drug conveyance approach can be applied with regard to tissue engineering when systems incorporate the embodiment of development factors or living cells inside the scaffolds. Thusly, the growth factor can be protected by designing scaffolds as a traditional system of delivery of medication that can effectively control site-specific release and time-specific release. Microsphere-based technology effectively utilized this in the application of tissue designing. Microspheres have been utilized in the field of tissue design basically to represent development components or cells. Microspheres can likewise be utilized as injectable scaffolds to help cell development and multiplication straightforwardly or can be totaled by these cells to shape living tissue-designed builds. In addition, the conglomeration of the microspheres themselves can be utilized as a preparing procedure to create scaffolds having a porous property. Another methodology that has been normally utilized is to insert stacked microspheres with growth factors in hydrogels that are then embedded as an incorporated build. Microspheres can be joined with scaffolds having a porous form by either direct consolidation inside the scaffolds, fusing together when embedded, or more infrequently, utilizing these scaffolds' covering material. Various processing techniques, such as spray drying, precipitation,, and suspension polymerization, are utilized to prepare spheres of polymer having a size of approximately 2 mm. This is a matrix-filled system in which the microcapsules and other vesicular structures are encircled through a kind of polymeric film. Cell culture procedures have become fundamental for the investigation of creature cell design, capacity, and separation and for the creation of numerous significant natural materials, such as vaccinations, chemicals, antibodies, interferons, and nucleic acids. Another procedure dependent on microsphere-based innovation is the creation of scaffolds with porous characteristics dependent on the synthetic, warm, or actual agglomeration of microspheres. (Mano et al. 2007; He and Lu 2016; Hulmes 2002; Wang et al. 2005; Kim et al. 2003).

4.8 CHALLENGES IN DESIGNING SCAFFOLDS

Each tissue normally presents a one-of-a kind course of wound-mending measures because of infection or injury as well as regular cell and subatomic occasions during ongoing tissue repair. Preferably, a cell framework, as well as being biocompatible, ought to be a biomaterial device with physical and mechanical properties that match those of the objective tissue and that contain a large number of growth factor, cytokines, and cell grip atoms that can advance a regenerative microenvironment for suitable cell populations and actuate their conduct. More often than expected, a single-part format doesn't meet the prerequisites for a regenerative biomaterial lattice because of an absence of a controlled rate of degradation; an absence of wanted mechanical properties and bioactivity; and, more critically, an absence of the ideal cell matrix collaborations to control quality articulation, cytoskeletal construction. While composite biomaterials from a similar class will create a specific level of guideline, blending biomaterials from different classes may give a more prominent degree of command over the general material properties for cell direction. For instance, crossover hydrogel scaffolds integrated from chosen biopolymers may give freedom to intently emulate the critical attributes of the local extra cellular matrix, including by showing attachment destinations and introducing growth factors, which not just instigates reparative. A developing objective in this field has been to investigate new techniques that more adequately produce multi-material and cell-loaded scaffolds with less effort. In this regard, polymer brushes with different designs and sciences, just like assorted brush-based procedures, which are both uninvolved and bioactive, might be used for biomaterial alteration. Specifically, these highlights may make the material surfaces biocompatible and non-fouling, which forestalls bothersome host reactions. Likewise, fiber-assisted molding (FAM) has been demonstrated to be a straightforward and strong technique to make biomimetic three-dimensional surfaces with a controllable curvature and helical bend. Such altered surfaces can manage cell arrangement and the get together of a helically designed extra cellular matrix, showing the capability of fiber-assisted molding for application in materials science and tissue design (Chen et al. 2016; Deng, Chang, and Wu 2019; Di Luca, Van Blitterswijk, and Moroni 2015).

4.9 CLINICAL APPLICATIONS OF DIFFERENT SCAFFOLDS

Clinical utilizations of scaffolds require the recovery of explicit sizes of surrenders, underlying trustworthiness, and adequate cell entrance, trailed by separation and multiplication. Silk fibroin has been utilized for the recovery of tendon tissue in trial on animals because of extraordinary mechanical property and suitable degradability. The US FDA has approved silk stitches for utilization in delicate tissue repair, and silk-based biomaterials are being utilized for the recovery of musculoskeletal tissue. The biomaterials that were utilized in the creation of unbending scaffolds are of incredible interest for medical procedures and are sought to control the modifying of bone and ligaments. Numerous normal polymers are popular to develop delicate frameworks. Collagen shows incredible potential in bone-tissue design. In spite of the fact that engineered or characteristic polymers are being utilized to help the development of osteoblasts and their progenitor cells to enroll their phenotypic articulation and separation. Calcium phosphate, hydroxyapatite and glass ceramics may be interesting selections of materials for the manufacture of hard tissues. Graphene-layer composites have been intended to use in bone-imperfection recovery locales to consider the penetration of delicate tissue cells into the developing cells. Graphene oxide advancement of collagen film upgrades the osteoblastic separation interaction and diminishes the irritation, filling in as a decent substitute for the conventional collagen layers.

Recently, various in vitro and a couple of in vivo methods considering use of ASCs in combination with transporter scaffolds can be found by looking on clinical preliminary sites. The utilization of refined foundational microorganisms in clinical settings is rigorously constrained by administrative guidelines across the planet, which to a great extent limits the use of ASCs in regenerative medication. One recent improvement in treating complex fistulas might be the utilization of ASCs in combination with a fibrin-stick platform depicted by a researcher. The fibrin stick utilized in this investigation contained human fibrinogen, a cow-like aprotinin, and human thrombin, and the ASCs were confined from lipoaspirated fat tissue. Two months after the last treatment, fistula repair was seen in 17 (71 percent) of 24 patients who got fibrin-stick treatment in addition to ASCs, in contrast with 4 (16 percent) of 25 patients who got fibrin stick alone. Albeit the uses of platform materials along with ASCs advances are a quickly creating field of recovery medication, they are profoundly trial so far. Thus, there is still a huge need to create effective transporter materials that may overcome any barrier and lead toward clinical applications in tissue design.

The extracellular lattice segments of the cellar film of the AM are local scaffolds for cell cultivation in tissue design. Amniotic membrane has been applied in tissue design related to eyes, skin, ligaments, and nerves, particularly malignant growth. Gelatin has been utilized in medication as plasma expander, wound dressing, cement, and permeable cushion for careful use. The silk bio-polymer is utilized in tissue recovery for treating wound casualties and as network of wound mending. In biomedical and bioengineering fields, the utilization of characteristic fiber blended with biodegradable and bio-resorbable polymers can deliver joints and bone apparatuses to mitigate torment for patients. Chitin and chitosan are known for their phenomenal organic properties, along with biocompatibility with human cells, in the arranged recovery of injured tissues. For tissue repair and recovery applications, chitosan can be functionalized by synthetic response, coupled with explicit ligands or moieties, consolidating with biomacromolecules, and crosslinking in the presence or nonattendance of crosslinkers. Articular ligament is especially powerless against injury trauma, sickness, or innate anomalies as a result of its avascular, alypmhatic, and aneural nature. A few researchers have created three-dimensional (3D) electrospun PCL/PLA mix nanofibrous frameworks and examined the in vivo bone arrangement capacity of the substrate in a clinically pertinent basic-size cranial bone-imperfection mouse model. Bone morphogenic proteins are Food and Drug Administration (FDA) endorsed for clinical use and are found generally prominent for instigating osteogenic separation. Accordingly, their consolidation with assorted autografts and allografts are in effect more popular. (Bao Ha et al. 2013; Frassica and Grunlan 2020; Di Luca, Van Blitterswijk, and Moroni 2015; He and Lu 2016).

4.10 CONCLUSION AND FUTURE PERSPECTIVE

In the new era, many disorders have been increasing in humans due to accidents, lifestyle, pollution, and stress. Mutilation in the human body leads to increased demand for replacement organs/tissue. However, the source available for organs and tissues is limited. Production of artificial organs and tissue for repairing destroyed or malfunctioning tissues and organs has become a big thrust area in material science. Naturally obtained biomaterials have been discussed and utilized in the field of regeneration of artificial tissues/organs because of their potential for biodegradability, proliferation, cell-support, and remodeling tissues. However, recent studies have not completely satisfied the clinical demand; the optimum utilization of naturally derived biomaterials is still highly considered; hence, further research on this field is now taking place all over the world. Synthetic materials can be utilized as the structural blocks of platforms for tissue design as they have the benefit of low immunogenicity. To make synthetic materials more biocompatible and bioactive, the mechanical and substance properties of a framework could epitomize these properties effectively, and it would give an ideal stage to tissue recovery. These significant advances keep on being researched for their capacity for tissue regeneration. Recent advancement recommends that tissue-designed develops may have an extended clinical pertinence later on and may speak to a suitable remedial alternative for the individuals who require tissue substitution or fix.

ABBREVIATIONS

ASCs	adipose derived stem cells
ECM	extracellular matrix
FDM	fused deposition modeling
PAA	poly acrylic acid
PCL	poly(3-caprolactone)
PEG	poly ethylene glycol
PEO	poly ethylene oxide
PLA	polylactide
PLGA	poly(lactide-co- glycolic acid)
PNIPAM	poly(N-isopropyl acrylamide)
PVA	poly vinyl alcohol
SFF	solid freeform fabrication
TE	tissue engineering

REFERENCES

Alexandridis, P., D. Zhou, and A. Khan. 1996. Lyotropic Liquid Crystallinity in Amphiphilic Block Copolymers: Temperature Effects on Phase Behavior and Structure for Poly(ethylene oxide)-b-poly(propylene oxide)-b-poly(ethylene oxide) Copolymers of Different Composition. *Langmuir.*

Altman, G.H., F. Diaz, C. Jakuba, T. Calabro, R.L. Horan, J. Chen, H. Lu, J. Richmond, and D.L. Kaplan. 2003. Silk-Based Biomaterials. *Biomaterials.*

Bao Ha, T. Le, T. Minh, D. Nguyen, and D. Minh. 2013. Naturally Derived Biomaterials: Preparation and Application. In *Regenerative Medicine and Tissue Engineering.*

Basu, B. 2017. *Biomaterials for Musculoskeletal Regeneration. Springer Nature.*

Bhat, S., and A. Kumar. 2012. Biomaterials in Regenerative Medicine. *Journal of Postgraduate Medicine, Education and Research.*

Bonzani, I.C., J.H. George, and M.M. Stevens. 2006. Novel Materials for Bone and Cartilage Regeneration. *Current Opinion in Chemical Biology.*

Chen, F.-M., X. Liu. 2016. Advancing Biomaterials of Human Origin for Tissue Engineering. *Progress in Polymer Science.*

Chen, G., T. Ushida, and T. Tateishi. 2000. Hybrid Biomaterials for Tissue Engineering: A Preparative Method for PLA or PLGA-Collagen Hybrid Sponges. *Advanced Materials.*

Deng, C., J. Chang, and C. Wu. 2019. Bioactive Scaffolds for Osteochondral Regeneration. *Journal of Orthopaedic Translation.*

Dvir, T., O. Tsur-Gang, and S. Cohen. 2005. "Designer" Scaffolds for Tissue Engineering and Regeneration. *Israel Journal of Chemistry.*

Entcheva, E., H. Bien, L. Yin, C.Y. Chung, M. Farrell, and Y. Kostov. 2004. Functional Cardiac Cell Constructs on Cellulose-Based Scaffolding. *Biomaterials.*

Frassica, M.T., and M.A. Grunlan. 2020. Perspectives on Synthetic Materials to Guide Tissue Regeneration for Osteochondral Defect Repair. *ACS Biomaterials Science and Engineering.*

Freed, L.E., I. Martin, and G. Vunjak-Novakovic. 1999. Frontiers in Tissue Engineering. *Clinical Orthopaedics and Related Research.*

Griffith, L.G., and G. Naughton. 2002. Tissue Engineering - Current Challenges and Expanding Opportunities. *Science.*

Gu, Z.Q., J.M. Xiao, and X.H. Zhang. 1998. The Development of Artificial Articular Cartilage - PVA-Hydrogel. *Bio-Medical Materials and Engineering.*

Häuselmann, H.J., R.J. Fernandas, S.S. Mok, T.M. Schmid, J.A. Block, M.B. Aydelotte, K.E. Kuettner, and E.J.M.A. Thonar. 1994. Phenotypic Stability of Bovine Articular Chondrocytes after Long-Term Culture in Alginate Beads. *Journal of Cell Science.*

He, Y., and F. Lu. 2016. Development of Synthetic and Natural Materials for Tissue Engineering Applications Using Adipose Stem Cells. *Stem Cells International.*

Hodde, J. 2002. Review: Naturally Occurring Scaffolds for Soft Tissue Repair and Regeneration. *Tissue Engineering.*

Huang, S., and X. Fu. 2010. Naturally Derived Materials-Based Cell and Drug Delivery Systems in Skin Regeneration. *Journal of Controlled Release.*

Hubbell, J.A. 2003. Materials as Morphogenetic Guides in Tissue Engineering. *Current Opinion in Biotechnology.*

Hulmes, D.J.S. 2002. Building Collagen Molecules, Fibrils, and Suprafibrillar Structures. *Journal of Structural Biology.*

Izydorczyk, M., S.W. Cui, and Q. Wang. 2005. Polysaccharide Gums: Structures, Functional Properties, and Applications. In *Food Carbohydrates.*

Jayakumar, R., M. Prabaharan, S. V. Nair, and H. Tamura. 2010. Novel Chitin and Chitosan Nanofibers in Biomedical Applications. *Biotechnology Advances.*

Kelley, S.S., T.C. Ward, T.G. Rials, and W.G. Glasser. 1989. Engineering Plastics from Lignin. XVII. Effect of Molecular Weight on Polyurethane Film Properties. *Journal of Applied Polymer Science.*

Kesharwani, S., P.K. Jaiswal, R. Kesharwani, V. Kumar, and D.K. Patel. 2016. Dendrimer: A Novel Approach for Drug Delivery. *Journal of Pharmaceutical and Scientific Innovation.*

Khabbaz, M.G., N.P. Kerezoudis, E. Aroni, and V. Tsatsas. 2004. Evaluation of Different Methods for the Root-Rnd Cavity Preparation. *Oral Surg Oral Med Oral Pathol Oral Radiol Endod. Elsevier.* 98(2):237–42.

Kim, S.E., J.H. Park, Y.W. Cho, H. Chung, S.Y. Jeong, E.B. Lee, and I.C. Kwon. 2003. Porous Chitosan Scaffold Containing Microspheres Loaded with Transforming Growth Factor-B1: Implications for Cartilage Tissue Engineering. *Journal of Controlled Release.*

Klemm, D., B. Philipp, T. Heinze, U. Heinze, and W. Wagenknecht. 1998. *Comprehensive Cellulose Chemistry: Fundamentals and Analytical Methods. Volume I.*

Kumaresan, P., R.K. Sinha, and S. Raje Urs. 2007. Sericin - A Versatile Byproduct. *Indian Silk.*

Kundu, B., R. Rajkhowa, S.C. Kundu, and X. Wang. 2013. Silk Fibroin Biomaterials for Tissue Regenerations. *Advanced Drug Delivery Reviews.*

Lee, S.J., J.J. Yoo, and A. Atala. 2017. Biomaterials and Tissue Engineering. In *Clinical Regenerative Medicine in Urology.*

Lee, W., and V. Parpura. 2009. Wiring Neurons with Carbon Nanotubes. *Frontiers in Neuroengineering.*

Lu, S., and K.S. Anseth. 1999. Photopolymerization of Multilaminated Poly(HEMA) Hydrogels for Controlled Release. *Journal of Controlled Release.*

Di Luca, A., C. Van Blitterswijk, and L. Moroni. 2015. The Osteochondral Interface as a Gradient Tissue: From Development to the Fabrication of Gradient Scaffolds for Regenerative Medicine. *Birth Defects Research Part C - Embryo Today: Reviews.*

Mano, J.F., G.A. Silva, H.S. Azevedo, P.B. Malafaya, R.A. Sousa, S.S. Silva, L.F. Boesel, et al. 2007. Natural Origin Biodegradable Systems in Tissue Engineering and Regenerative Medicine: Present Status and Some Moving Trends. *Journal of the Royal Society Interface.*

Meyvis, T.K.L., S.C. De Smedt, J. Demeester, and W.E. Hennink. 2000. Influence of the Degradation Mechanism of Hydrogels on Their Elastic and Swelling Properties during Degradation. *Macromolecules.*

Murray, M.M., K. Rice, R.J. Wright, and M. Spector. 2003. The Effect of Selected Growth Factors on Human Anterior Cruciate Ligament Cell Interactions with a Three-Dimensional Collagen-GAG Scaffold. *Journal of Orthopaedic Research.*

Patterson, J., M.M. Martino, and J.A. Hubbell. 2010. Biomimetic Materials in Tissue Engineering. *Materials Today.*

Rosso, F., G. Marino, A. Giordano, M. Barbarisi, D. Parmeggiani, and A. Barbarisi. 2005. Smart Materials as Scaffolds for Tissue Engineering. *Journal of Cellular Physiology.*

Rowe, S.L., S.Y. Lee, and J.P. Stegemann. 2007. Influence of Thrombin Concentration on the Mechanical and Morphological Properties of Cell-Seeded Fibrin Hydrogels. *Acta Biomaterialia.*

Singh, D.K., and A.R. RAY. 2000. Biomedical Applications of Chitin, Chitosan, and Their Derivatives. *Journal of Macromolecular Science - Polymer Reviews.*

Singh, N., A. Tiwari, R. Kesharwani, and D.K. Patel. 2016. Pharmaceutical Polymer in Drug Delivery: A Review. *Research Journal of Pharmacy and Technology.*

Sofia, S., M.B. McCarthy, G. Gronowicz, and D.L. Kaplan. 2001. Functionalized Silk-Based Biomaterials for Bone Formation. *Journal of Biomedical Materials Research.*

Svensson, A., E. Nicklasson, T. Harrah, B. Panilaitis, D.L. Kaplan, M. Brittberg, and P. Gatenholm. 2005. Bacterial Cellulose as a Potential Scaffold for Tissue Engineering of Cartilage. *Biomaterials.*

Vert, M. 2005. Aliphatic Polyesters: Great Degradable Polymers That Cannot Do Everything. *Biomacromolecules.*

Wang, Y., D.J. Blasioli, H.J. Kim, H.S. Kim, and D.L. Kaplan. 2006. Cartilage Tissue Engineering with Silk Scaffolds and Human Articular Chondrocytes. *Biomaterials.*

Wang, Y., U.J. Kim, D.J. Blasioli, H.J. Kim, and D.L. Kaplan. 2005. In Vitro Cartilage Tissue Engineering with 3D Porous Aqueous-Derived Silk Scaffolds and Mesenchymal Stem Cells. *Biomaterials.*

Yang, C., P.J. Hillas, J.A. Báez, M. Nokelainen, J. Balan, J. Tang, R. Spiro, and J.W. Polarek. 2004. The Application of Recombinant Human Collagen in Tissue Engineering. *BioDrugs.*

Ye, Q., G. Zünd, P. Benedikt, S. Jockenhoevel, S.P. Hoerstrup, S. Sakyama, J.A. Hubbell, and M. Turina. 2000. Fibrin Gel as a Three Dimensional Matrix in Cardiovascular Tissue Engineering. *European Journal of Cardio-Thoracic Surgery.*

Yoshii, F., Y. Zhanshan, K. Isobe, K. Shinozaki, and K. Makuuchi. 1999. Electron Beam Crosslinked PEO and PEO/PVA Hydrogels for Wound Dressing. *Radiation Physics and Chemistry.*

Yucel, T., M.L. Lovett, and D.L. Kaplan. 2014. Silk-Based Biomaterials for Sustained Drug Delivery. *Journal of Controlled Release.*

5 Peptide-Based Functional Nanomaterials for Soft-Tissue Repair

Surendra Tripathy
Northeast Frontier Railway Hospital

Dilip Kumar Patel, Roohi Kesharwani, and Vikas Kumar
Sam Higginbottom University of Agriculture, Technology and Sciences

CONTENTS

DOI: 10.1201/9781003140108-5

5.1 INTRODUCTION

Soft tissue refers to those tissues that are involved in supporting, connecting, and surrounding various internal body parts, including organs, muscles, ligaments, tendons, nerves, blood vessels, lymph vessels, and synovial membranes. These soft tissues are prone to injuries (Figure 5.1), which mostly occur in athletes and elderly people. Soft-tissue injuries commonly need surgical interventions, but many times such procedures are unable to restore the structure and function of the injured tissue and leave scars. These limitations demand some novel approaches to repair and regenerate the soft tissues [1, 2]. Tissue engineering can contribute to producing bioactive implantable structures mimicking the extracellular matrix (ECM) of the target site. These implantable structures may be a combination of scaffolds, cells, and bioactive molecules. Scaffolds usually support tissue growth, migration, and differentiation by creating a suitable microenvironment at the target site. The ideal scaffolds should be biocompatible and should have excellent mechanical properties [3, 4].

There is increasing research in incorporation of peptides within regenerative scaffolds, which is observed to enhance the cell attachment and induce the signaling pathways in the cell for tissue repairing. This leads to improved cellular infiltration and biochemical responses. Peptides naturally occur in the body; these are chains of 2 to 50 amino acids linked together. Peptides have the major role as signaling agents for various functions, including tissue repair. Synthetic peptide-based biomaterials can mimic the functions of endogenous peptides. But short peptides can be prepared

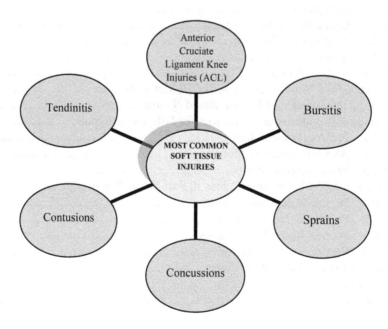

FIGURE 5.1 Most commonly occurring soft-tissue injuries.

TABLE 5.1
Natural Sources to Obtain Peptides

Plant-Derived Sources	Animal-Derived Sources
Zein	Casein
Gluten	Silk fibroin
Soy Protein	Hemoglobin
	Bovine serum albumin (BSA)
	Fibrinogen
	Elastin
	Collagen
	Gelatin
	Keratin

easily due to easy processability and modification. Therefore, short peptides are getting more attention by researchers [5, 6].

Of many self-assembly platforms, self-assembling peptides have gathered significant attention from researchers, which can be attributed to several reasons such as easy synthesis by solid-phase method, sequence specific modification, additional peptide functionalization, easy cell penetration of self-assembled structure, etc. [5–7]. The peptides have another advantage in that they can be obtained both from plant and animal protein sources and also can be synthetically obtained (Table 5.1). Self-assembled peptide nanostructures have revolutionized the research area of functional nanomaterials, which have potential for devices for repairing soft tissues.

5.2   PEPTIDE SELF-ASSEMBLING MECHANISMS AND TYPES OF PEPTIDES FOR PREPARING DIFFERENT NANOSTRUCTURES

The most common mechanisms for peptide self-assembling to form nanoscale structures are electrostatic forces, hydrophobic attraction, hydrogen bonding, and π-π stacking (Figure 5.2). Aromatic and aliphatic amino acids are non-polar and mostly involve hydrophobic interactions for self-assembly. Polar amino acids with uncharged and charged residues undergo electrostatic interactions and hydrogen bonding for self-assembly. The peptide backbone provides stability to the self-assembly through

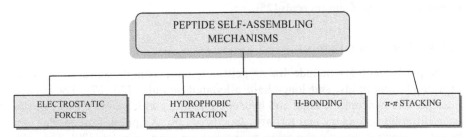

FIGURE 5.2   Self-assembly mechanisms of peptides.

hydrogen bonding [8, 9]. The aromatic amino acids with π bonds undergo π-π stacking and promote directional growth, especially in polar solvents like water. In solvents like toluene the π-π stacking mechanism may be a more prominent mechanism for self-assembly than other mechanisms [10].

Peptides can be self-assembled into different nanostructures such as nanotubes, nanofibers, monolayers, nanovesicles, etc. [11]. The self-assembled nanostructures can be formed by different types of peptides, which are as follows.

5.2.1 Dipeptides

Researchers have found that short peptides can be synthesized into multiple nanostructures with a better stability profile more easily and with lower cost of preparation [12, 13]. The most popular short-peptide–based nanostructures are prepared with dipeptides for biomedical applications. Diphenylalanine (Phe-Phe) was reported to be the first dipeptide for fabrication of different self-assembled nanostructures [14]. Different nanostructures prepared with FF dipeptide include nanoparticles, nanotubes, nanovesicles, and nanowires [15–17]. These nanostructures prepared with dipeptides reported good thermal stability [18] and higher yield [15, 16]. The diphenylalanine self-assembled nanotubes can also be synthesized by simply dissolving dipeptides in water, followed by gentle gradual heating. Similarly, nanowires can be synthesized by the same technique at a higher ionic strength of water. The dipeptide self-assembled nanotubes and nanowires are interconvertable [19, 20].

5.2.2 Cyclic Peptides

The concept of self-assembly of cyclic peptides was put forward in 1974. But the first successful self-assembly of cyclic peptide was reported in 1993, using cyclo-(LGln- D-Ala-L-Glu-D-Ala)2. The concept demonstrates that the alternating D type and L type amino acids in cyclic peptides form hydrogen bonding as the amino and carbonyl side chains lie perpendicular against the ring. This arrangement forms nanotubes. The nanotubes with these cyclic peptides as building blocks possess good stability due to the hydrogen bonding [21–24]. Major advantages of using cyclic peptides are the precise diameter control of nanostructures and functionalization with the side chains. Some cyclic peptide sequences utilized for the self-assembly include alternating D type and L type α-amino acids, alternating α- and β-amino acids, β-amino acids, and δ-amino acids [25].

5.2.3 Amphiphilic Peptides

Amphiphilic peptides include linear peptides, ionic complementary peptides, peptide phospholipids, and long-chain alkylated peptides [26, 27]. These peptides possess hydrophilic head and hydrophobic tails, which can be exploited to form different secondary and tertiary structures [28]. Amphiphilic peptides can be self-assembled into nanovesicles, nanotubes, and nanomicelles [29]. The self-assembly mechanism is based on electrostatic and hydrophobic interactions [30].

Linear peptides with hydrophilic heads and hydrophobic tails can be formed into multiple self-assembled nanostructures, whereas ionic complementary self-assembling peptides mainly form nanofibers. Ionic complementary peptides-based nanofibers have charged side chains on the outer side, and a hydrophobic side chain forms a sheet structure inside the nanofiber, which ultimately forms a stable structure with repeated positive and negative charge due to amino acids of alternating charges. These typically form β-sheet structures followed by formation of stable transparent hydrogel comprising nanofibers. Hydrogen bondings and ionic forces make the hydrogel stable in different pH and temperature levels [31]. Transparent hydrogel formation can be achieved instantaneously by exposure of amphiphilic peptides with the physiological fluids. These hydrogels have tremendous water-retention capacity, which may be above 99% water content. This water content creates a huge space for incorporation of different medications. The self-assembled nanostructures prepared with amphiphilic peptide have been used in cell growth and differentiation in soft tissues such as cartilage, heart, and neural systems [32, 33].

5.2.4   α-Helical Peptides

α- helical peptides with 25–30 amino acids are found suitable by researchers for fabrication of self-assembled nanostructures. The major advantage of these nanostructures is that they are filamentous structures, which resemble the cytoskeleton and ECM [34]. Nanofibers can be prepared from α- helical peptides with 2–5 helices, having about 30 amino acids [35, 36]. Nanofiber formation occurs due to the hydrophobic interaction. Peptides with glutamic acid and lysine located centrally can self–assembled due to ionic forces. Stimuli-responsive self-assembled hydrogel formation has also been reported using α- helical peptides with coiled-coil structure [37, 38].

5.2.5   β-Sheet Peptides

β-sheet peptides are among the most useful natural peptide motifs, having alternating hydrophilic and hydrophobic amino acid sequences providing an amphiphilic nature to the peptide structure. The amphiphilic nature is helpful for self-assembling the β-sheets [39]. The different nanostructures that can be fabricated by using these peptides are nanotubes, nanofibers, monolayers, and nanoribbons [40, 41]. Some β-sheet peptides can form hydrogels by pH-induced self-assembling at lower pH conditions.

5.3   INTERACTION OF NANOSTRUCTURES WITH CELL MATERIALS

Thermodynamically, protein/peptides in solution reduce the Gibb's free energy, which leads to formation of a distinct interface between physiological solution and the solid biomaterial [42, 43]. Proteins undergo conformational changes after biomaterials adsorb to them. These adsorptions are mostly due to hydrophobic and electrostatic interactions. These adsorbed proteins facilitate the attachment

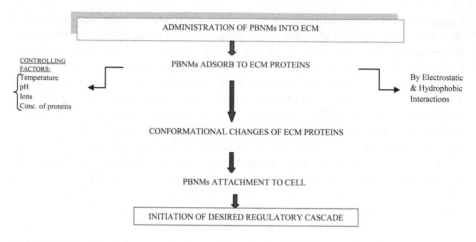

FIGURE 5.3 Illustration of attachment of PBNMs to cell.

of biomaterials to the cell through cell specific integrins. These proteins are vital constituents of the cellular matrix, which are mainly involved in transmitting biochemical signals. The versatile physicochemical features of these proteins enable them to attach to any surface in a biological system. However, the adsorption of biomaterials to proteins present in ECM is controlled by factors such as temperature, pH of solution, presence of ions, and the concentration of protein at the site [44]. The interaction of biomaterials with the cellular components can be improved by surface modification of these biomaterials with biomimetic receptor identical natural proteins derived especially from ECM. This may help in inducing the signaling pathway, followed by initiation of the desired regulatory cascade (Figure 5.3) [45, 46]. Hydrogels and nanofibers have shown promising results in such cellular interactions due to their water content and porosity respectively. Further, the surface functionalization with peptide sequences and growth factors provides biocompatibility.

Arg-Gly-Asp (RGD) functionalization helps in binding with fibronectin, which improves cell adhesion and migration of nanostructures. It has been reported that RAD16-II functionalization of nanofibers promotes their interaction with endothelial cells and helps to activate the angiogenesis cascade [47].

5.4 BIOFUNCTIONALIZATION OF PEPTIDE-BASED NANOSTRUCTURES

Biofunctionalization leads to improved biological function, retaining the bulk properties intact. The main purpose of biofunctionalization is to produce nanostructures that can achieve good cell attachment by mimicking the ECM. Here, it is notable that insoluble cell adhesive proteins are attached and processed through integrin receptors, whereas soluble molecules like cytokines and growth factors are guided via autocrine and paracrine signaling. Cell–cell contact is guided via transmembrane proteins called cadherins [48]. Biofunctionalization increases the affinity of the nanostructures to be recognized by cells [49]. It has also been reported that reduction in inflammatory responses mediated by macrophages, mast cells and T- Cells can be achieved with biofunctionalization [50].

The most common methods for biofunctionalization are adsorption, chemical crosslinking, surface attachment, and encapsulation [51]. Surface attachment is achieved by covalent bonding of the biomimicking proteins on the nanomaterial surface. In the chemical crosslinking method the protein is subjected to electrospinning with water soluble polymers, followed by crosslinking, leading to encapsulation of protein molecules within the nanomaterial. A high amount of protein molecules can be encapsulated by the crosslinking method [52].

5.5 COMMON PEPTIDE SEQUENCE MIMICS FOR SOFT-TISSUE REPAIR

Peptide sequences are used as structural mimics, which act as epitopes for binding to bioactive sites. Many short bioactive sequences have been reported, which is being exploited in tissue engineering. Some potential peptide sequences utilized by researchers have been summarized in Table 5.2.

TABLE 5.2
Some Established Potential Peptide Motifs

Extracellular Matrix Protein	Established Sequences	Major Function	Target Cells/Sites [References]
Collagen	GFOGER, DGEA	Improvement in bone growth	Fibroblasts [65, 66]
Laminin	IKVAV, LRE, PDGSR	Promotes cell adherence	Cardiomyocytes, Neural cells [67, 68]
Fibronectin	RGDS, KQAGDV	Promotes cell attachment	Endothelial cells [69]
Remodeling Enzymes			
Collagenase	GPQYILGQ, GPQGYIAGQ	Release of specific molecules after eliciting proteolytic effect	Collagen [70]
Matrix metalloproteinase	CPENYFFWGGG, APGL, LGPA	Proteolytic activity, exhibits photoresponsiveness	Fibroblasts [71, 72]
Plasmin	ELAPLRAP, YKNRD	Bone regeneration, cell attachment	Fibroblasts [73]
Target proteins/ Receptors			
VEGF	KLTWQELYQLKY-KGI	Promotes angiogenesis	Endothelial cell [74]
Glycosaminoglycan	PNDRRR	Promotes angiogenesis, Heparin binding	Endothelial cells, heparin [75]

5.5.1 Pro-Angiogenic Motifs

In angiogenesis process the endothelial cells proliferate and migrate with simultaneous remodeling of ECM to develop new blood vessels. Vascular endothelial growth factor (VEGF) acts as regulator for angiogenesis in both normal as well as diseased states. The physiological response via VEGF regulator is elicited by tyrosine kinase receptors. The VEGF peptide mimics were reported to be one of the most successful short peptide mimics in soft-tissue repair [53, 54]. An example of one successfully characterized VEGF mimic is QK peptide, which has been studied for inducing endothelial cell activation and subsequent physiological responses as self-assembled hydrogel form in a rat model [55]. Further study in this area is required to understand the binding of VEGF mimics to heparin and subsequent growth of endothelial cells and their proliferation. Hepatocyte growth factor (HGF) is a chemokine, responsible for promoting angiogenesis. HGF mimics can also be explored to find their role in angiogenesis and their feasibility to be used a short peptide mimic for repairing soft tissues [56].

5.5.2 Anti-inflammatory Motifs

Inflammation is reported to be a complex biological process that involves many sequential events that take place at the cellular level, such as angiogenesis, cell infiltration and proliferation, polarization, etc. Out of many players to bring out an inflammatory response, macrophages are the most common. Macrophages may be classified as pro-inflammatory and pro-healing. Pro-healing macrophages have receptors such as TGF-bR, IL-4R, IL-6R, IL-10R, and MCSFR, which can be modulated to repair tissue damage [57, 58]. By using short peptide mimics, which can act on immunogenic receptors of both type of macrophages, the expression of anti-inflammatory cytokines like IL6 and TNF-a can be initiated to reduce the inflammation and promote healing [59]. A short peptide of 12 Amino acids (i.e., IDR-1018) has been reported, which showed an anti-inflammatory response [60]. Matrix metalloproteinases (MMPs) are also anti-inflammatory peptides that act by regulating cytokines and chemokines. These MMPs mimicking short peptide may prove to be potential peptide sequences for combating inflammatory responses [61, 62].

5.5.3 Pro-adherence Motifs

The peptides that display a specific binding sequence can be encompassed in the nanostructures to ensure that the nanostructures are attached to the cells of interest and are supporting the growth, attachment, and proliferation of cells in that microenvironment. The most widely used binding sequences are RGD and RGDS, which are common in most of the adhesion proteins like laminin, fibronectin, fibrinogen, etc. Also, the RGDS motifs are known for their anti-platelet aggregation and anti-thrombolytic activity. Like RGD, PHSRN is also a pro-adherence sequence that acts as anchoring site for integrin binding receptors; it is derived from fibronectin [63]. Some other pro-adherence motifs are fibronectin-derived REDV, LDV and KQAGDV (helps in anchoring human umbilical vein endothelial cells) and laminin-derived IKVAV and YIGSR (helps in neurite growth) [64].

5.6 POTENTIAL PBNMS FOR APPLICATIONS IN SOFT-TISSUE REPAIR

Some PBNMs have been found to be feasible to be developed as potential devices for repairing soft-tissue injury. A handful of work has been reported for soft-tissue repair purposes despite excellent features that make them potential devices. Some of these devices have been briefly discussed below.

5.6.1 PEPTIDE-BASED NANOTUBES

Nanotubes formed by molecular self-assemblies of synthetic peptides have been reported to possess several advantages such as ease of reproducibility, affordability, large-scale production ability, and monodispersity. Smart functionalities can be attached at desired sites in the nanotubes by modulating the synthesis. Hence, the inside as well as outside wall of nanotubes can be decorated with different functionalities of interest. These features show peptide-based nanotubes as robust devices for use in biomedical applications [76].

Studies revealed that the structure and physical properties of peptide self-assembled nanotubes are dependent on the sequence of amino acids. Peptide nanotubes manage to restore the stability and properties of the smart functionalities attached on their structure, which is beneficial in molecular recognition [77, 78]. Peptide nanotubes do not aggregate in water; rather they solubilize in water, which indicates that the molecular recognition mediated self-assembly occurs readily. The nanotubes are provided with three-dimensional H-bondings that contribute to the rigid structure of peptide nanotubes, with a melting point up to 235°C; however, the nanotubes have stability issues in harsh environments. Among linear and cyclic peptide nanotubes, the cyclic peptide offers the formation of nanotubes with more precise diameters. The amino acid sequence and the number of amino acids involved in self-assembling determine the surface as well as core properties of nanotubes. Cyclic peptides with a larger ring diameter produce large-diameter peptide nanotubes. However, nanotubes with a different size range can be prepared by using linear peptide monomer units [79].

5.6.2 PEPTIDE-BASED NANOFIBERS

Peptide-based nanofibers can be prepared with different technologies (Figure 5.4), the most popular of which is electrospinning, where electrostatic forces are utilized to synthesize nanofibers. The nanofibers prepared by electrospinning possess sound features like large surface area, more porosity, tunable pore size, high permeability, etc. Peptide denaturation is a major concern for electrospinning, and the ambient condition should be set at optimum level. Parameters like

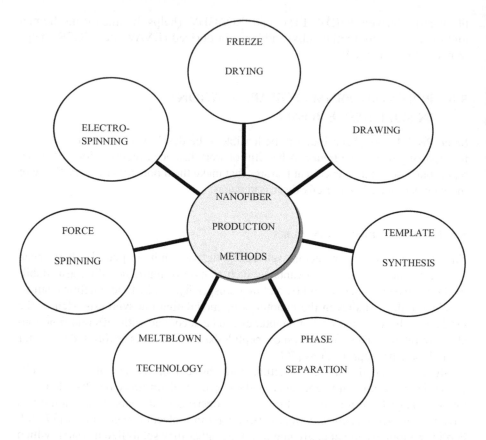

FIGURE 5.4 Schematic presentation of nanofiber production methods.

temperature, pH are optimized for preventing peptide degradation. Spinability of the peptides can be improved by mixing with organic solvents like hexafluoroisopropanol, dimethylformamide, trifluoroacetic acid, and ethanol. [80–83]. Nanofiber production using peptide/protein offers several advantages over synthetic polymers peptide nanofibers: absence of cytotoxic properties, improved cell adherence, biocompatibility, stable structure, etc. In delivering drugs to soft tissues, drug loading can also be improved by adjusting the pH, which is difficult in synthetic polymers [84].

Peptide/proteins are combined with polymers with the help of crosslinkers like glutaraldehyde, formaldehyde, genipin, etc., to improve the mechanical properties. Some widely used polymers are Eudragit®, poly-L-lactic acid (PLLA), polycaprolactone (PCL), chitosan, polylactic acid (PLA), etc. The major difficulty raised in preparing nanofibers with peptide-polymer crosslinked macromolecules is the use of organic solvents, crosslinkers, and polymers. Production and storage conditions of these nanofibers need a controlled environment [85]. A list of protein/peptide, co-polymer and crosslinker has been provided in Table 5.3.

TABLE 5.3
A List of Peptides, Co-polymers, and Solvents Used in Fabrication of Nanofibers [80]

Proteins/Peptides	Co-polymers	Crosslinkers
Soy protein	Polylactic acid	Glutaraldehyde
Silk fibroin	Chitin	Genipin
Gelatin	Alginate	Proanthocyanine
Zein	Collagen	1,6-diidohexacyanate
Gluten	Polyvinylalcohol	Glyoxal
Casein	Polyethyleneoxide	Formaldehyde
Keratin	Fibroin	Heat

5.6.3 PEPTIDE-BASED NANOVESICLES

Self-assembling peptide-based nanovesicles are promising nanoscale devices, which are potential replacement for liposomes and other lipid-based nanostructures [86, 87]. These self-assembled nanovesicles offer better stability, site specificity, and tunability over liposomes/lipid-based nanostructures [88]. Amphiphilic block copolymers are suitable macromolecules for synthesizing nanovesicles. When a polypeptide constitutes one of the segments in an amphiphilic copolymer, the resulting self-assembled vesicle-like structures are called peptide nanovesicles or peptosomes. In many instances, the polypeptide segment is linked to a hydrophobic synthetic segment [89].

Vauthey et al. [90] first reported that a simple 7–8 residue amphiphilic peptide is capable of self-assembling into nanotubes and nanovesicles. They named the peptides "surfactant-like peptides." Similar peptides with glycine and aspartic acid self-assembled to form nanotubes and nanovesicles were studied by Santos et al. (2002) [91]. Van Hell et al. (2007) [92] reported the self-assembled nanovesicles of an amphiphilic oligopeptide SA2, which had excellent biocompatibility. The nanovesicles formed were biodegradable and had a better stability profile compared to lipid- and polysaccharide-based vesicles.

5.6.4 PEPTIDE-BASED MANOLAYERS

Among the self-assembled structures, monolayers are other interesting structures as they offer advantages like easy functionalization and strictly controlled peptide backbone [93]. The self-assembly is stabilized by molecular interactions like hydrogen bonding, disulphide bridges, dipole interactions and π-π stacking [94–96].

Stable peptide monolayer on gold surfaces was reported where the peptide chain was functionalized with thiol, disulfide group, and thiol side chain of cysteine [97–99]. Lipoic acid was also functionalized on oligo- and polypeptide via disulfide functionalities at the N terminus. Synthetic linkers are nowadays replaced with peptides for surface

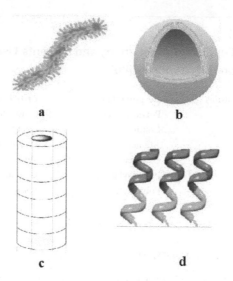

FIGURE 5.5   Diagrams of (a) nanofibers, (b) nanovesicles, (c) nanotubes, and (d) nanoscale monolayers.

attachment for synthesizing peptide-based materials. Cysteine has been used commonly to attach peptides on gold surfaces [100]. Figure 5.5 illustrates structure of a few PBNMs.

5.7   CONCLUSION AND FUTURE CHALLENGES

Peptide-based functional nanomaterials seem to be clinically translatable for tissue repair and regeneration and are promising biomaterials to improve quality of life at comparatively low cost. Advancement in solid-phase peptide synthesis and improved methods to study structure–function relationship lead the path of peptide-based nanomaterial toward clinical stages. It is becoming easier in designing target-oriented biomaterials to elicit the desired activity and provide a better biocompatibility. Short peptides are becoming the material of choice by researchers due to ease of processing, solubility, easy cross-linking with polymeric backbone, and ability to respond different stimuli.

A combinatorial approach is becoming popular as numerous peptide sequences of different structure and function can be designed. This approach will be simplified when predictive models and databases for large bioactive peptides will be available. However, compatibility with immune system, cell survival, and restoration of mechanical properties, compositional considerations, cell exhaustion and ethical regulations are the major challenges to be overcome for clinical translations of PBNMs. The diameter of PBNMs and its effect on cell orientation, cell response, and macrophage response needs a more thorough study for individual biomaterial. Although these materials are slowly approaching industrial scale, researchers should pay attention to certain concerns such as avoiding expensive techniques like chemical vapor deposition, which demands large staffing power and space for operation, and avoiding high temperature requiring methods to prevent wastage of water.

ABBREVIATIONS

ECM   extracellular matrix
HGF   hepatocyte growth factor
MMPs   matrix metalloproteinases
PBNMs   peptide-based nanomaterials
RGD   Arg-Gly-Asp
VEGF   vascular endothelial growth factor

REFERENCES

1. W. Liu, S. Thomopoulos, and Y. Xia, "Electrospun nanofibers for regenerative medicine," *Adv. Healthc. Mater.*, vol. 1, no. 1 pp. 10–25, 2012.
2. R. J. Mondschein, A. Kanitkar, C. B. Williams, S. S. Verbridge, and T. E. Long, "Polymer structure-property requirements for stereolithographic 3D printing of soft tissue engineering scaffolds," *Biomaterials*, vol. 140, pp. 170–188, 2017.
3. I. Jun, H. S. Han, J. R. Edwards, and H. Jeon, "Electrospun fibrous scaffolds for tissue engineering: viewpoints on architecture and fabrication," *Int. J. Mol. Sci.*, vol. 19, no. 3, p. 745, 2018.
4. N. Narayanan, C. Jiang, G. Uzunalli, S. K. Thankappan, C. T. Laurencin, and M. Deng, "Polymeric electrospinning for musculoskeletal regenerative engineering," *Regen. Eng. Transl. Med.*, vol. 2, no. 2, pp. 69–84, 2016.
5. R. Nayak, R. Padhye, I. L. Kyratzis, Y. B. Truong, and L. Arnold, "Recent advances in nanofiber fabrication techniques," *Text. Res. J.*, vol. 82, no. 2, pp. 129–147, 2012.
6. K. Vig, A. Chaudhari, S. Tripathi, S. Dixit, R. Sahu, S. Pillai, V. A. Dennis, and S. R. Singh, "Advances in skin regeneration using tissue engineering," *Int. J. Mol. Sci.*, vol. 18, no. 4, 789, 2017.
7. Y. M. Bello, A. F. Falabella, and W. H. Eaglstein, "Tissue-engineered skin," *Am. J. Clin. Dermatol.*, vol. 2, no. 5, pp. 305–313, 2001.
8. S. Toksoz, H. Acar, and M. O. Guler, "Self-assembled one-dimensional soft nanostructures," *Soft Matter*, vol. 6, no. 23, pp. 5839–5849, 2010.
9. D. M. Leite, E. Barbu, G. J. Pilkington, and A. Lalatsa, "Peptide self-assemblies for drug delivery," *Curr. Top. Med. Chem.*, vol. 15, no. 22, pp. 2277–2289, 2015.
10. J. Wang, K. Liu, R. Xing, and X. Yan, "Peptide self-assembly: thermodynamics and kinetics," *Chem. Soc. Rev.*, vol. 45, no. 20, pp. 5589–5604, 2016.
11. J. J. Panda and V. S. Chauhan, "Short peptide based self-assembled nanostructures: implications in drug delivery and tissue engineering," *Polym. Chem.*, vol. 5, no. 15, pp. 4418–4436, 2014.
12. C. Chen, F. Pan, and S. Zhang et al., "Antibacterial activities of short designer peptides: a link between propensity for nanostructuring and capacity for membrane destabilization," *Biomacromolecules*, vol. 11, no. 2, pp. 402–411, 2010.
13. A. S. Veiga, C. Sinthuvanich, D. Gaspar, H. G. Franquelim, M. A. R. B. Castanho, and J. P. Schneider, "Arginine-rich self-assembling peptides as potent antibacterial gels," *Biomaterials*, vol. 33, no. 35, pp. 8907–8916, 2012.
14. C. H. Görbitz, "The structure of nanotubes formed by diphenylalanine, the core recognition motif of Alzheimer's β-amyloid polypeptide," *Chem. Commun.*, no. 22, pp. 2332–2334, 2006.
15. S. Marchesan, A. V. Vargiu, and K. E. Styan, "The Phe-Phe motif for peptide self-assembly in nanomedicine," *Molecules*, vol. 20, no. 11, pp. 19775–19788, 2015.
16. L. Adler-Abramovich, D. Aronov, and P. Beker et al., "Self-assembled arrays of peptide nanotubes by vapour deposition," *Nat. Nanotechnol.*, vol. 4, no. 12, pp. 849–854, 2009.

17. M. Wang, L. Du, X. Wu, S. Xiong, and P. K. Chu, "Charged diphenylalanine nanotubes and controlled hierarchical self-assembly," *ACS Nano*, vol. 5, no. 6, pp. 4448–4454, 2011.
18. L. Adler-Abramovich, M. Reches, V. L. Sedman, S. Allen, S. J. B. Tendler, and E. Gazit, "Thermal and chemical stability of diphenylalanine peptide nanotubes: implications for nanotechnological applications," *Langmuir*, vol. 22, no. 3, pp. 1313–1320, 2006.
19. S. Scanlon and A. Aggeli, "Self-assembling peptide nanotubes," *Nano Today*, vol. 3, no. 3–4, pp. 22–30, 2008.
20. N. Hendler, N. Sidelman, M. Reches, E. Gazit, Y. Rosenberg, and S. Richter, "Formation of well-organized self-assembled films from peptide nanotubes," *Adv. Mater.*, vol. 19, no. 11, pp. 1485–1488, 2007.
21. P. De Santis, E. Forni, and R. Rizzo, "Conformational analysis of DNA–basic poly-peptide complexes: Possible models of nucleoprotamines and nucleohistones," *Biopolymers*, vol. 13, no. 2, pp. 313–326, 1974.
22. M. R. Ghadiri, J. R. Granja, R. A. Milligan, D. E. McRee, and N. Khazanovich, "Self-assembling organic nanotubes based on a cyclic peptide architecture," *Nature*, vol. 366, no. 6453, pp. 324– 327, 1993.
23. R. Chapman, M. Danial, M. L. Koh, K. A. Jolliffe, and S. Perrier, "Design and proper-ties of functional nanotubes from the self-assembly of cyclic peptide templates," *Chem. Soc. Rev.*, vol. 41, no. 18, pp. 6023–6041, 2012.
24. S. Fernandez-Lopez, H.-S. Kim, and E. C. Choi et al., "Antibacterial agents based on the cyclic D,L-α-peptide architecture," *Nature*, vol. 412, no. 6845, pp. 452–455, 2001.
25. Y. Ishihara and S. Kimura, "Nanofiber formation of amphiphilic cyclic tri-β-peptide," *J. Pept. Sci.*, vol. 16, no. 2, pp. 110–114, 2010.
26. D. W. P. M. Lowik and J. C. M. van Hest, "Peptide based amphiphiles," *Chem. Soc. Rev.*, vol. 33, no. 4, pp. 234–245, 2004.
27. R. Huang, W. Qi, R. Su, J. Zhao, and Z. He, "Solvent and surface controlled self-assembly of diphenylalanine peptide: from microtubes to nanofibers," *Soft Matter*, vol. 7, no. 14, pp. 6418–6421, 2011.
28. T. Gore, Y. Dori, Y. Talmon, M. Tirrell, and H. Bianco-Peled, "Self-assembly of model collagen peptide amphiphiles," *Langmuir*, vol. 17, no. 17, pp. 5352–5360, 2001.
29. L. Liu, K. Busuttil, and S. Zhang et al., "The role of self-assembling polypeptides in building nanomaterials," *Physical Chemistry Chemical Physics*, vol. 13, no. 39, pp. 17435–17444, 2011.
30. S. Vauthey, S. Santoso, H. Gong, N. Watson, and S. Zhang, "Molecular self-assembly of surfactant-like peptides to form nanotubes and nanovesicles," *Proceedings of the National Academy of Sciences of the United States of America*, vol. 99, no. 8, pp. 5355–5360, 2002.
31. X. Zhao, F. Pan, and H. Xu et al., "Molecular self-assembly and applications of designer peptide amphiphiles," *Chem. Soc. Rev.*, vol. 39, no. 9, pp. 3480–3498, 2010.
32. M. E. Davis, J. P. M. Motion, and D. A. Narmoneva et al., "Injectable self-assembling peptide nanofibers create intramyocardial microenvironments for endothelial cells," *Circulation*, vol. 111, no. 4, pp. 442–450, 2005.
33. Y. Wen, W. Liu, and C. Bagia et al., "Antibody-functionalized peptidic membranes for neutralization of allogeneic skin antigenpresenting cells," *Acta Biomater.*, vol. 10, no. 11, pp. 4759–4767, 2014.
34. R. Fairman and K. S. Akerfeldt, "Peptides as novel smart materials," *Curr. Opin. Struct. Biol.*, vol. 15, no. 4, pp. 453–463, 2005.
35. D. E. Wagner, C. L. Phillips, and W. M. Ali et al., "Toward the development of peptide nanofilaments and nanoropes as smart materials," *Proceedings of the National Academy of Sciences of the United States of America*, vol. 102, no. 36, pp. 12656–12661, 2005.

36. E. Moutevelis and D. N. Woolfson, "A periodic table of coiled-coil protein structures," *J. Mol. Biol.*, vol. 385, no. 3, pp. 726–732, 2009.

37. A. M. Smith, E. F. Banwell, W. R. Edwards, M. J. Pandya, and D. N. Woolfson, "Engineering increased stability into self-assembled protein fibers," *Adv. Funct. Mater.*, vol.16, no. 8, pp. 1022–1030, 2006.

38. C. Xu, V. Breedveld, and J. Kopeˇcek, "Reversible hydrogels from self-assembling genetically engineered protein block copolymers," *Biomacromolecules*, vol. 6, no. 3, pp. 1739–1749, 2005.

39. C. W. G. Fishwick, A. J. Beevers, L. M. Carrick, C. D. Whitehouse, A. Aggeli, and N. Boden, "Structures of helical β-tapes and twisted ribbons: the role of side-chain interactions on twist and bend behavior," *Nano Lett.*, vol. 3, no. 11, pp. 1475–1479, 2003.

40. A. Aggeli, M. Bell, and L. M. Carrick et al., "pH as a trigger of peptide β-sheet self-assembly and reversible switching between nematic and isotropic phases," *J. Am. Chem. Soc.*, vol. 125, no. 32, pp. 9619–9628, 2003.

41. N. Ashkenasy, W. S. Horne, and M. R. Ghadiri, "Design of self-assembling peptide nanotubes with delocalized electronic states," *Small*, vol. 2, no. 1, pp. 99–102, 2006.

42. M. C. Cross, R. G. Toomey, and N. D. Gallant, "Protein-surface interactions on stimuli-responsive polymeric biomaterials," *Biomed. Mater.*. vol. 11, p. 22002, 2016.

43. R. Klopfleisch and F. Jung, "The pathology of the foreign body reaction against biomaterials," *J. Biomed. Mater. Res. Part A*, vol. 105, pp. 927–940, 2017.

44. Y. Loo, M. Goktas, A. B. Tekinay, M. O. Guler, C. A. E. Hauser, and A. Mitraki, "Self-assembled proteins and peptides as scaffolds for tissue regeneration," *Adv. Healthc. Mater.*, vol. 4, pp. 2557–2586, 2015.

45. A. N. Moore, T. L. L. Silva, N. C. Carrejo, C. A. O. Marmolejo, I.-C. Li, and J. D. Hartgerink, "Nanofibrous peptide hydrogel elicits angiogenesis and neurogenesis without drugs, proteins, or cells, *Biomaterials*, vol. 161, pp. 154–163, 2018.

46. H. Acar, S. Srivastava, E. J. Chung, M. R. Schnorenberg, J. C. Barrett, J. L. LaBelle, and M. Tirrell," Self-assembling peptide-based building blocks in medical applications, *Adv. Drug Deliv. Rev.*, vol. 110 pp. 65–79, 2017.

47. H. Cho, S. Balaji, A. Q. Sheikh, J. R. Hurley, Y. F. Tian, J. H. Collier, T. M. Crombleholme, and D. A. Narmoneva, "Regulation of endothelial cell activation and angiogenesis by injectable peptide nanofibers," *Acta Biomater*, vol. 8, pp. 154–164, 2012.

48. M. Barbosa and M. C. L. Martins, *Peptides and proteins as biomaterials for tissue regeneration and repair*, Woodhead Publishing, Cambridge, England, 2017.

49. X. Wang, B. Ding, B. Li, "Biomimetic electrospun nanofibrous structures for tissue engineering," *Mater. Today*, vol. 16, pp. 229–241, 2013.

50. D. B. Khadka, D. T. Haynie, "Protein- and peptide-based electrospun nanofibers in medical biomaterials, nanomedicine nanotechnology," *Biol. Med.*, vol. 8, pp. 1242–1262, 2012.

51. Z.-G. Wang, L.-S. Wan, Z.-M. Liu, X.-J. Huang, Z.-K. Xu, "Enzyme immobilization on electrospun polymer nanofibers: an overview," *J. Mol. Catal. B: Enzym.*, vol. 56, pp. 189–195, 2009.

52. M. F. Canbolat, N. Gera, C. Tang, B. Monian, B. M. Rao, B. Pourdeyhimi, S. A. Khan, "Preservation of cell viability and protein conformation on immobilization within nanofibers via electrospinning functionalized yeast," *ACS Appl. Mater. Interfaces*, vol. 5, pp. 9349–9354, 2013.

53. M. Potente, H. Gerhardt, and P. Carmeliet, "Basic and therapeutic aspects of angiogenesis," *Cell*, vol. 146, pp. 873–887, 2011. doi: 10.1016/j.cell.2011.08.039

54. M. Simons, E. Gordon, and L. Claesson-Welsh, "Mechanisms and regulation of endothelial VEGF receptor signaling," *Nat. Rev. Mol. Cell Biol.*, vol. 17, pp. 611–625, 2016. doi: 10.1038/nrm.2016.87

55. V. A. Kumar, N. L. Taylor, S. Shi, B. K. Wang, A. A. Jalan, and M. K. Kang, et al., "Highly angiogenic peptide nanofibers," *ACS Nano*, vol. 9, pp. 860–868, 2015. doi: 10.1021/nn506544b

56. X. Xin, S. Yang, G. Ingle, C. Zlot, L. Rangell, and J. Kowalski, et al., "Hepatocyte growth factor enhances vascular endothelial growth factor-induced angiogenesis in vitro and in vivo," *Am. J. Pathol.*, vol. 158, pp. 1111–1120, 2001. doi: 10.1016/S0002-9440(10)64058-8

57. F. Taraballi, M. Sushnitha, C. Tsao, G. Bauza, C. Liverani, and A. Shi, et al., "Biomimetic tissue engineering: tuning the immune and inflammatory response to implantable biomaterials," *Adv. Healthc. Mater.*, vol. 7, p. 1800490, 2018. doi: 10.1002/adhm.201800490

58. F. O. Martinez and S. Gordon, "The M1 and M2 paradigm of macrophage activation: time for reassessment," *F1000Prime Rep.*, vol. 6, pp. 13–13, 2014. doi: 10.12703/P6-13

59. G. S. A. Boersema, N. Grotenhuis, Y. Bayon, J. F. Lange, and Y. M. Bastiaansen-Jenniskens, "The effect of biomaterials used for tissue regeneration purposes on polarization of macrophages," *BioResearch*, vol. 5, pp. 6–14, 2016. doi: 10.1089/biores.2015.0041

60. O. M. Pena, N. Afacan, J. Pistolic, C. Chen, L. Madera, and R. Falsafi, et al., "Synthetic cationic peptide IDR-1018 modulates human macrophage differentiation," *PLoS ONE*, vol. 8, p. e52449, 2013. doi: 10.1371/journal.pone.0052449

61. B. E. Turk, L. L. Huang, E. T. Piro, and L. C. Cantley, "Determination of protease cleavage site motifs using mixture-based oriented peptide libraries," *Nat. Biotechnol.*, vol. 19, pp. 661–667, 2001. doi: 10.1038/90273

62. J. Patterson, and J. A. Hubbell, "SPARC-derived protease substrates to enhance the plasmin sensitivity of molecularly engineered PEG hydrogels," *Biomaterials*, vol. 32, pp. 1301–1310, 2011. doi: 10.1016/j.biomaterials.2010.10.016

63. A. Mardilovich, J. A. Craig, M. Q. Mccammon, A. Garg, and E. Kokkoli, "Design of a novel fibronectin-mimetic peptide–amphiphile for functionalized biomaterials," *Langmuir*, vol. 22, pp. 3259–3264, 2006. doi: 10.1021/la052756n

64. H. Shin, S. Jo, and A. G. Mikos, "Biomimetic materials for tissue engineering," *Biomaterials*, vol. 24, pp. 4353–4364, 2003. doi: 10.1016/S0142-9612(03)0 0339-9

65. A. M. Wojtowicz, A. Shekaran, M. E. Oest, K. M. Dupont, K. L. Templeman, and D. W. Hutmacher, et al., "Coating of biomaterial scaffolds with the collagen-mimetic peptide GFOGER for bone defect repair," *Biomaterials*, vol. 31, pp. 2574–2582, 2010. doi: 10.1016/j.biomaterials.2009.12.008

66. M. Mehta, C. M. Madl, S. Lee, G. N. Duda, and D. J. Mooney, "The collagen I mimetic peptide DGEA enhances an osteogenic phenotype in mesenchymal stem cells when presented from cell-encapsulating hydrogels," *J. Biomed. Mater. Res. A.*, vol. 103, pp. 3516–3525, 2015. doi: 10.1002/jbm.a.35497

67. M. Yamada, Y. Kadoya, S. Kasai, K. Kato, M. Mochizuki, and N. Nishi, et al., "Ile-Lys-Val-Ala-Val (IKVAV)-containing laminin α1 chain peptides form amyloid-like fibrils," *FEBS Lett.*, vol. 530, pp. 48–52, 2002. doi: 10.1016/S0014-5793(02)03393-8

68. N. Huettner, T. R. Dargaville, and A. Forget, "Discovering cell-adhesion peptides in tissue engineering: beyond RGD," *Trends Biotechnol.*, vol. 36, pp. 372–383, 2018. doi: 10.1016/j.tibtech.2018.01.008

69. D. J. Leahy, I. Aukhil, and H. P. Erickson, "2.0 Å crystal structure of a four-domain segment of human fibronectin encompassing the RGD loop and synergy region," *Cell*, vol. 84, pp. 155–164, 1996. doi: 10.1016/S0092-8674(00)81002-8

70. J. A. Hubbell, S. P. Massia, N. P. Desai, and P. D. Drumheller, "Endothelial cell-selective materials for tissue engineering in the vascular graft via a new receptor," *Nat. Biotechnol.*, vol. 9, pp. 568–572, 1991. doi: 10.1038/nbt0691-568

71. C. N. Salinas, and K. S. Anseth, "The enhancement of chondrogenic differentiation of human mesenchymal stem cells by enzymatically regulated RGD functionalities," *Biomaterials*, vol. 29, pp. 2370–2377, 2008. doi: 10.1016/j.biomaterials.2008.01.035

72. P. N. Patel, A. S. Gobin, J. L. West, and C. W. Patrick, Jr., "Poly(ethylene glycol) hydrogel system supports preadipocyte viability, adhesion, and proliferation," *Tissue Eng.*, vol. 11, pp. 1498–1505, 2005. doi: 10.1089/ten.2005.11.1498

73. H. D. Singh, I. Bushnak, and L. D. Unsworth, "Engineered peptides with enzymatically cleavable domains for controlling the release of model protein drug from "soft" nanoparticles," *Acta Biomater.*, vol. 8, pp. 636–645, 2012. doi: 10.1016/j.actbio.2011.10.028

74. X. Liu, X. Wang, A. Horii, X. Wang, L. Qiao, and S. Zhang, et al., "In vivo studies on angiogenic activity of two designer self-assembling peptide scaffold hydrogels in the chicken embryo chorioallantoic membrane," *Nanoscale*, vol. 4, pp. 2720–2727, 2012. doi: 10.1039/c2nr00001f

75. L. Gilmore, S. Rimmer, S. L. Mcarthur, S. Mittar, D. Sun, and S. Macneil, "Arginine functionalization of hydrogels for heparin binding–a supramolecular approach to developing a pro-angiogenic biomaterial," *Biotechnol. Bioeng.*, vol. 110, pp. 296–317, 2013. doi: 10.1002/bit.24598

76. X. Gao and H. Matsui, "Peptide-based nanotubes and their applications in bionanotechnology," *Adv. Mater*, vol. 17, pp. 2037–2050, 2005.

77. G. J. Douberly, S. Pan, D. Walters, and H. Matsui, Fabrication of protein tubules: Immobilization of proteins on peptide tubules, *J. Phys. Chem. B.*, vol. 105, pp. 7612–7618, 2001.

78. R. Djalali, Y.-F. Chen, and H. Matsui. "Au nanowire fabrication from sequenced histidine-rich peptide," *J. Am. Chem. Soc.*, vol. 124, no. 46, 13660–13661, 2002.

79. I. A. Banerjee and H. Matsui, "Location-specific biological functionalization on nanotubes: Attachment of proteins at the ends of nanotubes using Au nanocrystal masks," *Nano Lett.*, vol. 3, no. 3, pp. 283–287, 2003.

80. A. Yildiz, A. A. Kara, and F. Acarturk, "Peptide-protein based nanofibers in pharmaceutical and biomedical application," *Int. J. Biol. Macromol.*, vol. 148, pp. 1084–1097, 2020.

81. X. Feng, J. Li, X. Zhang, T. Liu, J. Ding, and X. Chen, "Electrospun polymer micro/nanofibers as pharmaceutical repositories for healthcare," *J. Control. Release*, vol. 302, pp. 19–41, 2019. https://doi.org/10.1016/j.jconrel.2019.03.020.

82. S. Kajdič, O. Planinšek, M. Gašperlin, and P. Kocbek, "Electrospun nanofibers for customized drug-delivery systems," *J. Drug Deliv. Sci. Technol.*, vol. 51, pp. 672–681, 2019. https://doi.org/10.1016/j.jddst.2019.03.038.

83. J. Ding, J. Zhang, J. Li, D. Li, C. Xiao, H. Xiao, H. Yang, X. Zhuang, and X. Chen, "Electrospun polymer biomaterials," *Prog. Polym. Sci*, vol. 90, 1–34, 2019. https://doi.org/10.1016/j. progpolymsci.2019.01.002.

84. D. B. Khadka and D. T. Haynie, "Protein- and peptide-based electrospun nanofibers in medical biomaterials," *Nanomed.: Nanotechnol. Biol. Med.*, vol. 8 pp. 1242–1262, 2012. https://doi.org/10.1016/j.nano.2012.02.013.

85. S. Babitha, L. Rachita, K. Karthikeyan, E. Shoba, I. Janani, B. Poornima, and K. Purna Sai, "Electrospun protein nanofibers in healthcare: a review," *Int. J. Pharm.*, vol. 523, 52–90, 2017. https://doi.org/10.1016/j.ijpharm.2017.03.013.

86. S. Gudlur, P. Sukthankar, J. Gao, L. A. Avila, Y. Hiromasa, et al., "Peptide nanovesicles formed by the self-assembly of branched amphiphilic peptides," *PLoS ONE*, vol. 7, no. 9, p. e45374, 2012. doi:10.1371/journal.pone.0045374

87. D. E. Discher and F. Ahmed, "Polymersomes," *Annu. Rev. Biomed. Eng.*, vol. 8, pp. 323–341, 2006.

88. F. Meng, Z. Zhong, and J. Feijen, "Stimuli-responsive polymersomes for programmed drug delivery," *Biomacromolecules*, vol. 10, no. 2, pp. 197–209, 2009.

89. D. A. Christian, S. Cai, D. M. Bowen, Y. Kim, and J. D. Pajerowski, et al., Polymersome carriers: From self-assembly to siRNA and protein therapeutics, *Eur. J. Pharm. Biopharm.*, vol. 71, no. 3, pp. 463–474, 2009.

90. S. Vauthey, S. Santoso, H. Gong, N. Watson, and S. Zhang, "Molecular self-assembly of surfactant-like peptides to form nanotubes and nanovesicles," *Proc. Natl. Acad. Sci. U S A*, vol. 99, no. 8, pp. 5355–5360, 2002.

91. S. Santoso, W. Hwang, H. Hartman, and S. Zhang, "Self-assembly of surfactant-like peptides with variable glycine tails to form nanotubes and nanovesicles," *Nano Lett.*, vol. 2, no. 7, pp. 687–691, 2002.

92. A. J. Hell, C. I. Costa, F. M. Flesch, M. Sutter, and W. Jiskoot, et al., "Self-assembly of recombinant amphiphilic oligopeptides into vesicles," *Biomacromolecules*, vol. 8, no. 9, pp. 2753–2761, 2007.

93. E. Gatto and M. Venanzi, "Self-assembled monolayers formed by helical peptide building blocks: a new tool for bioinspired nanotechnology," *Polym. J.*, vol. 45, pp. 468–480, 2013.

94. Y. Loo, S. Zhang, and C. A. E. Hauser, "From short peptides to nanofibers to macromolecular assemblies in biomedicine," *Biotechn. Adv.*, vol. 30, pp. 593–603, 2012.

95. A. Badia, R. B. Lennox, and L. Reven, "A dynamic view of self-assembled monolayers," *Acc. Chem. Res.*, vol. 33, pp. 475–481, 2000.

96. S. Yasutomi, T. Morita, Y. Imanishi, and S. Kimura, "A molecular photodiode system that can switch photocurrent direction," *Science*, vol. 304, pp. 1944–1947, 2004.

97. K. Fujita, N. Bunjes, K. Nakajima, M. Hara, H. Sasabe, and W. Knoll, "Macrodipole interaction of helical peptides in a self-assembled monolayer on gold substrate," *Langmuir*, vol. 14, pp. 6167–6172, 1998.

98. S. Sek, A. Sepiol, A. Tolak, A. Misicka, and R. Bilewicz, "Distance dependence of the electron transfer rate through oligoglycine spacers introduced into self-assembled monolayers, "*J. Phys. Chem. B.*, vol. 108, pp. 8102–8105, 2004.

99. K. Uvdal and T. P. Vikinge, "Chemisorption of the dipeptide Arg-Cys on a gold surface and the selectivity of G-protein adsorption," *Langmuir*, vol. 17, pp. 2008–2012, 2001.

100. C. G. Worley, R. W. Linton, and E. T. Samulski, "Electric-field-enhanced self-assembly of α-helical polypeptides," *Langmuir*, vol. 11, pp. 3805–3810, 1995.

6 Scaffold Nanomaterial for Cardiac Tissue Regeneration

Narendra Maddu
Sri Krishnadevaraya University

CONTENT

6.1 INTRODUCTION

Cardiac tissue engineering includes the fields of cell biology and material sciences. Overall, scaffold materials such as collagen, alginate, gelatin or synthetic polymers, and cardiac cells are used to reconstitute tissue-like concepts in vitro, and these constructs exhibit properties of native myocardium such as coherent reductions, low diastolic tension, and syncytial propagation of action potentials (Zimmermann and Eschenhagen, 2003). Cardiovascular diseases are the foremost cause of death worldwide, and cell-based therapies represent a potential cure for patients with cardiac diseases such as heart failure, congenital heart disease, and myocardial infarction. Cardiac tissue engineering is now being examined as an approach to support cellbased treatments and enhance their effectiveness (Nunes et al., 2011). The human heart has continuously been a focus of such efforts, given its infamous inability to repair itself following damage or disease. The developing bioengineering methods are helpful for regeneration of heart muscle as a pattern for regenerative medicine (Vunjak-Novakovic et al., 2011). The bioengineering strategies that need to be followed to construct a polymeric scaffold of sufficient mechanical integrity, with superior surface morphologies, that is capable of mimicking the valve dynamics in vivo (Morsi, 2014). These biomedical engineering therapies have greatly relieved the symptoms of chronic heart failure and improved life expectancy (Hu et al., 2018). Current treatments for cardiac regeneration and tissue engineering methods have been explored for their potential to deliver mechanical support to injured cardiac tissues and improve cell-based therapeutic techniques and deliver cardio-protective molecules (Pena et al., 2018).

The growth of artificial matrices for tissue engineering is a vital area of study in the field of regenerative medicine. Positive tissue scaffolds, in comparison with the normal mammalian extracellular matrix (ECM), are multi-component, fibrous, and on the nanoscale (McCullen et al., 2009). Cardiac tissue engineering has potential to deliver functional, synchronously contractile tissue concepts for heart repair and for studies of growth and disease using in vivo–like approach yet manageable in vitro settings (Radisic et al., 2009). Tissue-engineering developments are emerging as functional substitutes for injured tissues and organs. Before replacement, cells are generally sowed on biomaterial scaffolds that review the extracellular matrix and deliver cells with data that are important for tissue development (Dvir et al., 2011a). The growth of biomaterials research in the field of cardiac tissue engineering has fixated on improving material properties by imitating the native cardiac tissue, designing materials with constant presence of incorporated cells and biomolecules, increasing vascularization within materials, and evaluating the in vivo lifetime and action of injected hydrogels or fixed scaffolds (Reis et al., 2016).

Current cardiac tissue engineering investigation has developed nanomaterial applications to combat heart failure, preserve normal heart tissue, and produce healthy myocardium around the infarcted part (Amezcua et al., 2016). Cardiac tissue engineering has developed to restore or redevelop the structure and function of native cardiac tissues. Scaffolds play a major role in construction of functional cardiac tissues, providing biodegradation, structural support, and cell affinity. However, scaffolds currently used in cardiac tissue regeneration tend to lack satisfactory electrical conductivity and favorable mechanical properties (Ahadian et al., 2017a). Different types of bioreactors are established to separately deliver electrical and mechanical stimulus to cardiomyocytes in vitro in both two- and three-dimensional tissue stages (Stoppel et al., 2016). The single presence of nanomaterials within the scaffolding matrix has additional marked influence as associated to the scaffold stiffness on the cell–cell coupling, maturation, and excitability of engineered cardiac tissues (Navaei et al., 2019). The use of nanostructured polymers and polymer nanocomposites has revolutionized the field of cardiac tissue engineering due to improved mechanical, electrical, and surface properties and promoting tissue growth (Mohammadi Nasr et al., 2020).

Original advances in stem cell separation and culture techniques in bioreactors and synthesis of bioactive materials enable the creation of cardiac tissue regeneration in vitro (Gorabi et al., 2017). Nanomedicines, as novel tool for better imaging, drug delivery, and diagnosis, have shown great potential in combating cardiovascular disease (Nakhlband et al., 2018). There is a wide range of conductive nanostructured materials for cardiac tissue engineering. These include carbon-based nanomaterials (CNFs, graphene, and CNTs), gold-based nanomaterials, and electroactive polymers (such as PPy, piezoelectric polymeric materials, and PANI) (Ashtari et al., 2019).

Molybdenum disulfide (MoS_2) and reduced graphene oxide (rGO) in nanosheets are two-dimensional nanomaterials that can be measured as great applicants for enhancing the electrical and mechanical properties of biological scaffolds for cardiac tissue engineering. Myocardial infarction is one of the main causes of mortality throughout the world. Cardiac scaffolds are tissue-engineered structures for the action of myocardial infarction and are employed for tissue provision and cell delivery to the injured area (Nazari et al., 2020). The purpose of the review chapter is the therapeutic applications of scaffold nanomaterials in the regeneration of injured cardiac tissue.

6.2 VARIOUS NANOMATERIALS AND APPLICATIONS FOR REPAIR OF CARDIAC TISSUE

6.2.1 SCAFFOLDS

A "scaffold" provides a structural platform for a new cellular microenvironment that supports new tissue formation. It allows migration, cell attachment, differentiation, and organization (Alrefai et al., 2015). Three-dimensional (3-D) cardiac muscle concepts can be engineered with cardiac-specific structural and electrophysiological properties and used for in vitro impulse propagation studies (Bursac et al., 1999). Cardiac tissue engineering has occurred as a new and determined approach that synthesizes knowledge from medicine and material chemistry with cell biology (Zammaretti and Jaconi, 2004). It is a novel strategy for cardiac repair based on magnetic nanosheets, highlighting the tremendous potential and capacities that nanoscaffolds have within the therapeutic test related to heart regeneration (Ventrelli et al., 2013). Cultivation of cardiac cells within hybrid scaffolds helped cell organization into elongated and aligned tissues, generating a durable reduction force, low excitation threshold, and high contraction rate (Sharon et al., 2014). Implanting cells into 3D biodegradable scaffolds may improve cell survival and enhance cell engraftment after transplantation, therefore improving cardiac cell therapy (Kitsara et al., 2017).

Polymer biomaterials are used in the theory of scaffolds in tissue engineering applications to assist in mechanical organization, support, and maturation of tissues (Ahadian et al., 2017b). Establishment of original conductive polymeric scaffold in the infarcted heart improves cardiac contractility and reinstates ventricular function (Saravanan et al., 2018). Cardiomyocytes fully grown on the nanofiber scaffolds developed into established and functional tissues (Ahn et al., 2018). Presently, various nanoparticles have been used alone or in combination in hydrogels or other biomimetic scaffolds to mimic the electrophysiological and morphological characteristics of native cardiac tissue for a better regenerative result (Kankala et al., 2018). Decellularized extracellular matrix (dECM) derived from myocardium has been extensively explored as a natural scaffold for cardiac tissue engineering applications (Pawan et al., 2019). Synthetic scaffolds, implantable patches, and injectable hydrogels are among the most promising solutions to restore cardiac function and foster regeneration (Solazzo et al., 2019).

Tissue engineering entails the in vitro or in vivo generation of replacement tissues from cells with the aid of secondary scaffolds and motivating biomolecules in

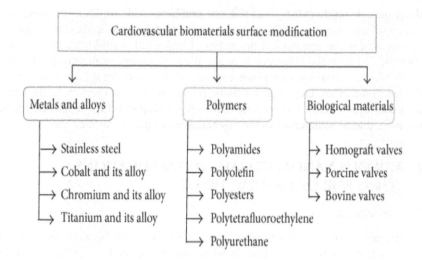

FIGURE 6.1   Classification of cardiovascular biomaterial (Jaganathan et al., 2014).

order to deliver biological replacements for restoration and maintenance of human tissue functions (Dvir and Tsur-Gang, 2005). Alginate scaffolds provide a conducive environment to facilitate the 3D culturing of cardiac cells, regeneration, and healing of the infarcted myocardium (Leor et al., 2000). Biomaterials and scaffolds fill an essential role in tissue engineering by guiding new tissue growth in vivo and in vitro (Griffith, 2002). Cardiac tissue engineering holds the potential of creating functional replacement tissues to repair heart tissue damage (Fleischer et al., 2017). Nanocarriers for cardiac regeneration-inducing biomolecules, corresponding matrices for their controlled release, injectable hydrogels for cell delivery and cardiac patches (Bar and Cohen, 2020) (Figure 6.1).

6.2.2   CARBON NANOTUBES

Carbon nanotubes (CNTs) may recover scaffold properties and improve tissue regeneration, and carbon nanotubes perform as a biomaterial for scaffold construction (Edwards et al., 2009). Carbon nanotubes can also be combined into scaffolds providing structural strengthening. In addition, imparting novel properties such as electrical conductivity into the scaffolds may aid in directing cell growth (Harrison and Atala, 2007). Carbon electrodes, exhibiting the highest charge-injection capacity and producing cardiac tissues with the best structural and contractile properties, were thus used in tissue-engineering studies (Tandon et al., 2011). Electroactive carbon nanotubes (CNTs) could be employed to direct mesenchymal stem cell (MSC) difference toward a cardiomyocyte origin (Mooney et al., 2012). Incorporation of CNTs into gelatin, and possibly other biomaterials, could be useful in creating multifunctional cardiac scaffolds for both therapeutic purposes and in vitro studies. The electrically conductive and nanofibrous networks formed by CNTs within an absorbent gelatin framework are key features of CNT-GelMA, leading to better-quality cardiac cell adhesion, cell–cell coupling, and organization, (Shin et al., 2013).

Carbon nanotubes are resonating graphitic cylinders of nanoscale dimensions and may recover scaffold properties and enhance tissue regeneration (Edwards et al., 2009). Carbon nanotubes are popular synthetic scaffolds that may revolutionize regenerative medicine. CNTs' workable properties open doors for dynamic scaffold design and provide chances for the growth of cardiac tissue constructs (Hopley et al., 2014). Carbon-based nanomaterials have generated great interest in biomedical applications such as progressive imaging, drug or gene delivery, and tissue regeneration (Zhang et al., 2014). The nanometer size and high aspect ratio of the CNTs are the two distinct structures that have contributed to varied biomedical applications. CNTs have also established great potential in diverse biomedical uses such as tissue regeneration and genetic engineering (Sharma et al., 2016).

CNTs offer a potentially harmless source for cardiac regenerative medicine (Sun et al., 2016). Carbon nanomaterials (CNMs) have outstanding mechanical and electrical properties, making them ideal candidates for refining conventional cardiac tissue scaffolds. The improved cardiac tissue concepts have the potential to advance drug discovery and allow for improving the treatment of heart disease and myocardial tissue regeneration (Dozois et al., 2017). Carbon nanotubes (CNTs) 1,8 octanedial poly (octamethylene maleate (anhydride) 1,2,4-butanetricarboxylate) (124 polymer), and developed an elastomeric scaffold for cardiac tissue engineering that delivers electrical conductivity and structural integrity to 124 polymers (Ahadian et al., 2017a). Several studies have drawn attention to the regeneration of electrically active biological tissues such as cardiac tissue and the role of heart electrophysiology and the rationale toward the use of electroconductive biomaterials for cardiac tissue engineering (Solazzo et al., 2019).

6.2.3 Gelatin, Collagen, and Fibrin Gel Scaffolds

Cardiac tissue engineering aims to develop functional tissue concepts that can re-establish the structure and function of damaged myocardium. Engineered constructs can also serve as high-fidelity models for studies of cardiac development and disease (Vunjak-Novakovic et al., 2010). The developing field of tissue engineering aims to regenerate injured tissues by combination cells from the body with highly porous scaffold biomaterials, which act as templates for tissue regeneration, to guide the growth of new tissue (O'Brien, 2011). Chitosan based hydrogel could repair the myocardial infarction (MI) microenvironment and enhance stem cell engraftment, survival, and homing in ischemic heart through ROS scavenging and chemokine recruitment, contributing to myocardial repair (Liu et al., 2012). The fibrin glue may increases/decreases infarct size, cell transplant survival, and increases blood flow to ischemic myocardium. Fibrin glue may have potential as a biomaterial scaffold to improve cellular cardiomyoplasty and treat myocardial infarction (Christman et al., 2004). GelMA hydrogels containing the aligned CNTs had superior performance in cardiac difference of stem cells upon applying electrical stimulus in contrast with control gels (Ahadian et al., 2016) (Figure 6.2).

Tissue-engineered heart muscle may be able to deliver an action modality for early-stage congestive heart failure. There is a new method to engineer functional three-dimensional heart muscle using a recyclable fibrin gel (Huang et al., 2007).

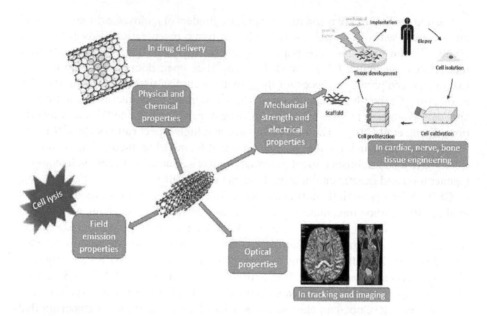

FIGURE 6.2 Applications of carbon nanotubes (CNT) in various cardiac, nerve, and bone engineering fields (Gorain et al., 2018).

Cardiac tissue engineering requires a scaffold material like hydrogel scaffold of hydroxyethyl methacrylate (HEMA) that delivers structural support and is favorable to cell growth (Cezar et al., 2007). It is possible to improve systolic heart function following myocardial infarction through establishment of differentiated muscle fibers seeded on a gel-type scaffold, despite a low rate of survival (Giraud et al., 2008). Hydrogels, due to their sole biocompatibility, flexible methods of synthesis, variety of constituents, and needed physical characteristics, have been the material of choice for many applications in regenerative medicine (Slaughter et al., 2009). Incorporating gold nanowires within alginate scaffolds can bridge the electrically resistant pore walls of alginate and recover electrical communication between together cardiac cells (Dvir et al., 2011b). Thermosensitive hydrogel can possibly be used for efficient encapsulation and defense of cell clusters during delivery, while under physiological conditions, the constructs and named cell wraps can unroll and expose the brought microtissue to the ischemic tissue (Pedron et al., 2011).

Hydrogels can serve as scaffolds that deliver structural integrity to tissue constructs, control drug and protein distribution to tissues and cultures, and serve as adhesives or fences between tissue and material surfaces (Slaughter et al., 2009). The integration of conducting nanowires within three-dimensional scaffolds may recover the therapeutic value of current cardiac patches (Dvir et al., 2011a). The unsettled elastomeric properties of natural resilin, an insect protein, are of interest in the engineering of resilin-like polypeptides (RLPs) as a potential material for cardiovascular tissue engineering (McGann et al., 2013). The incorporation of nanoscale electro-conductive gold nanoparticles (GNPs) into chitosan hydrogels improves the properties of myocardial constructs. These constructs could lead to utilization for regeneration of other electroactive tissues (Baei et al., 2016). The engineered cardiac tissue constructs using rGO incorporated hybrid hydrogels can potentially provide high-fidelity tissue models for drug studies and the investigations of cardiac tissue growth and/or disease processes in vitro (Shin et al., 2016). In cardiovascular tissue applications, creating gelatin microfiber scaffolds. Gelatin is used as a potential biomaterial for cardiac tissue repair. Collagen scaffolds, especially nanofibrous scaffolds, have been examined for cardiac tissue engineering. Fibrin was also used as a platform for inspiring cardiac angiogenesis (Mohammadi Nasr et al., 2020).

6.2.4 Bioreactors

Tissue engineering of functional cardiac patches censoriously depends on the interaction between multiple guidance cues such as topographical, adhesive, or electrical (Au et al., 2007). Bioreactors producing mechanical distortion are more appropriate with an elastomeric scaffold. Coupled electromechanical stimulation seems effective in promoting striation, elongation, and acquisition of contractile force by the stretched cells (Govoni et al., 2013). Bioreactors have been used to mimic aspects of these factors in vitro to engineer cardiac tissue, but due to design limits, previous bioreactor systems have yet to simultaneously support nutrient perfusion, electrical stimulation, and unimpeded (i.e., not isometric) tissue contraction (Maidhof et al., 2012). Cardiac tissue engineering has made considerable progress, and biomaterials are increasingly examined as potential scaffolds for cardiac tissue repair and/or regeneration (Grigore, 2017).

Cardiac patches should be able to mimic myocardium extracellular matrix for rapid addition with the host tissue, raising the need to develop cardiac constructs with complex features. In particular, cardiac patches should be electrically conductive, mechanically robust and elastic, biologically active, and pre-vascularized. A nano-reinforced hybrid cardiac patch laden with human coronary artery endothelial cells (HCAECs) has better electrical, mechanical, and biological behavior (Izadifar et al., 2018). Tissue-engineering approaches have been acknowledged for their potential to provide mechanical support to injured cardiac tissues, deliver cardio-protective molecules, and improve cell-based therapeutic techniques (Pena et al., 2018). Cardiac scaffolds are tissue-engineered structures for the treatment of myocardial infarction and are employed for tissue support and cell delivery to the injured region (Bahrami et al., 2019) (Figure 6.3).

6.2.5 Electroactive Polymers

Bio-electroactive polyurethane has potential as a platform substrate to study the effect of electrical signals on cell actions and to direct desirable cell function for tissue engineering applications (Baheiraei et al., 2014). Polypyrrole (PPy), Polyaniline (PANI), and polythiophene (PTh) are some important electroactive polymers (EAPs) that have potential applications in cardiac tissue engineering (Ashtari et al., 2019). The polypyrrole and polyaniline polymers are becoming vital materials for biosensors, neural implants, drug delivery devices, and tissue engineering scaffolds (Balint et al., 2014). The major purpose of cardiac tissue engineering is to engineer cells on scaffolds and use it as a super numeracy to infracted cardiac cells (Chaudhuri et al., 2017).

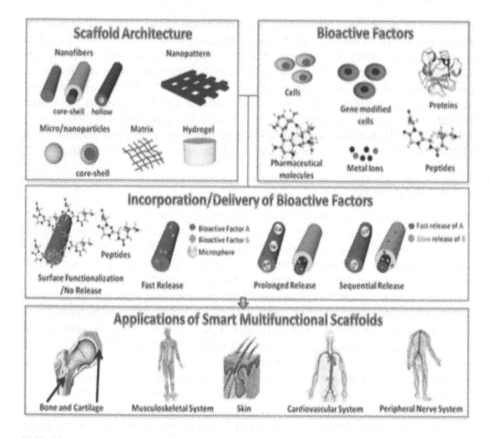

FIGURE 6.3 Applications of scaffold nanomaterials in tissue engineering (Kaliva et al., 2017).

Tissue engineering represents a forefront of current research in the treatment of heart disease. With these technologies, advancements are being made into treatments for acute ischemic myocardial damage and chronic, then non-reversible, myocardial failure (Alrefai et al., 2015). Coupling tissue-engineering technologies with patient-specific cardiac progenitor biology holds great promise for the growth of human cell models of human disease and may be the foundation for original approaches in regenerative cardiovascular medicine (Chien et al., 2008). The development of biomaterials for cardiac tissue engineering (CTE) is challenging, primarily owing to the requirement of achieving a surface with favorable features that enhances cell attachment and maturation (Tallawi et al., 2015). Strategies for cardiac tissue engineering include injection of cells, implantation of three-dimensional tissue constructs or patches, injection of acellular materials, and replacement of valves (Dunn et al., 2014).

6.2.6 STEM CELL APPROACH

The cardiomyogenic potential of hematopoietic stem cells suggests a therapeutic strategy that finally could benefit patients with myocardial infarction (Jackson et al., 2001).

Human embryonic stem cell–derived cardiomyocytes displayed structural and functional properties of early-stage cardiomyocytes. Formation of this unique differentiation system may have significant impact on the study of early human cardiac difference and tissue engineering (Kehat et al., 2001). Tissue engineering steers the principles of engineering, material science, and biology toward the development of biological substitutes that restore, maintain, or recover tissue function. Progress has been made in engineering the various components of the cardiovascular system, including blood vessels, heart valves, and cardiac muscle (Nugent and Edelman, 2003). Cardiac tissue engineering has emerged as a new and ambitious approach that combines knowledge from material chemistry with cell biology and medicine (Zammaretti and Jaconi, 2004). Cell-based cardiac repair offers the promise of rebuilding the injured heart from its component parts. Many challenges remain before the vision of healing an infarct by muscle regeneration can be realized (Laflamme and Murry, 2005).

New advances in methods of stem cell separation, culture in bioreactors, and the synthesis of bioactive materials promise to help in cardiac tissue engineering and regeneration (Leor et al., 2005). Tissue engineering approaches are designed to repair lost or damaged tissue through the use of growth factors, biomaterial scaffolds, and cellular transplantation (Christman and Lee, 2006). Stem cell–based cardiovascular regenerative medicine presents the next frontier of therapy through delivery of progenitor cells to achieve functional and structural repair of the myocardium (Bartunek et al., 2009). Cellular therapy usual cells to recover cardiac function and/or regenerate new myocardium, has been extensively examined for cardiac repair (Wang and Guan, 2010). Cardiac tissue engineering is now being acknowledged as an approach to support cell-based therapies and enhance their efficacy for cardiac disease (Wang et al., 2010). Engineering myocardial tissue is considered to be a new therapeutic method to repair infarcted myocardium and ameliorate cardiac function after MI (Sui et al., 2011). Cellular cardiomyoplasty or cellular implantation, combined with numerous tissue-engineering methods aims to regenerate functional heart tissue (Alcon et al., 2012).

Several experimental strategies to remuscularize the injured heart using adult stem cells and pluripotent stem cells, cellular reprogramming, and tissue engineering are in development (Laflamme and Murry, 2011). Cardiomyocytes for cardiac repair is emerging as an exciting treatment option for patients with postinfarction left-ventricular remodeling (Ye et al., 2013). The first clinical application of engineered cardiac tissue is a realistic option and it is predicted that cardiac tissue engineering techniques will find widespread use in the preclinical research and drug development in the near future (Hirt et al., 2014). Progress in regenerative medicine has contributed to the development of cell-based therapies as well as macro- and micro-scale tissue-engineering technologies (Mallone et al., 2016). Tissue-engineering approaches result in improved cardiomyocyte holding and sustained remuscularization but may also be explored for targeted paracrine or mechanical support (Fujita and Zimmermann, 2017). Recently, the extrinsic stimulation of cardiac regeneration has complicated the use of potential polymers to stimulate stem cells toward the differentiation of cardiomyocytes as a new therapeutic intervention in cardiac tissue engineering (Moorthi et al., 2017). New advances in tissue engineering and regenerative medicine gives hope to MI therapy and restoration of the function and structure of injured tissue by delivering exogenous cells or stimulating endogenous heart cells (Geng et al., 2018).

6.3 CONCLUSION

Cardiovascular disease persists as the foremost cause of death throughout the world, and cardiac scaffold nanomaterials are a major development in tissue engineering devices for the action of myocardial infarction. This review highlights recent applications in nanomaterials, such as scaffold nanomaterials, carbon nanotubes, gelatin hydrogel, collagen, chitosan hydrogel, and fibrin glue gel scaffolds, bioreactors, electroactive polymers, and stem cell approaches, that could provide a promising platform and advancements in cardiac tissue engineering. To recover function of heart failure following myocardial infarction and concluded imbedding of cardiac scaffolds and indicates their possibility in cardiac tissue reformative medicine.

FUNDING

No funding.

CONFLICT OF INTEREST

The authors declare that they have no conflict of interest.

REFERENCES

Ahadian S, Davenport Huyer L, Estili M, Yee B, Smith N, Xu Z, Sun Y, Radisic M. Moldable elastomeric polyester-carbon nanotube scaffolds for cardiac tissue engineering. Acta Biomater. 2017b; 52:81–91.

Ahadian S, Davenport-Huyer L, Smith N, Radisic M. Hybrid carbon nanotube-polymer scaffolds for cardiac tissue regeneration. Microfluidics, BioMEMS, and Medical Microsystems XV, 1006102, 2017a; pp. 9.

Ahadian S, Yamada S, Ramon-Azcon J, Estili M, Liang X, Nakajima K, Shiku H, Khademhosseini A, Matsue T. Hybrid hydrogel-aligned carbon nanotube scaffolds to enhance cardiac differentiation of embryoid bodies. Acta Biomater. 2016; 31:134–143.

Ahn S, Ardona HAM, Lind JU, Eweje F, Kim SL, Gonzalez GM, Liu Q, Zimmerman JF, Pyrgiotakis G, Zhang Z, Beltran-Huarac J, Carpinone P, Moudgil BM, Demokritou P, Parker KK. Mussel-inspired 3D fiber scaffolds for heart-on-a-chip toxicity studies of engineered nanomaterials. Anal Bioanal Chem. 2018; 410(24):6141–6154.

Alcon A, Cagavi Bozkulak E, Qyang Y. Regenerating functional heart tissue for myocardial repair. Cell Mol Life Sci. 2012; 69(16):2635–2656.

Alrefai MT, Murali D, Paul A, Ridwan KM, Connell JM, Shum-Tim D. Cardiac tissue engineering and regeneration using cell-based therapy. Stem Cells Cloning. 2015; 8:81–101.

Amezcua R, Shirolkar A, Fraze C, Stout DA. Nanomaterials for cardiac myocyte tissue engineering. Nanomaterials (Basel). 2016; 6(7):133.

Ashtari K, Nazari H, Ko H, Tebon P, Akhshik M, Akbari M, Alhosseini SN, Mozafari M, Mehravi B, Soleimani M, Ardehali R, Ebrahimi Warkiani M, Ahadian S, Khademhosseini A. Electrically conductive nanomaterials for cardiac tissue engineering. Adv Drug Deliv Rev. 2019; 144:162–179.

Au HT, Cheng I, Chowdhury MF, Radisic M. Interactive effects of surface topography and pulsatile electrical field stimulation on orientation and elongation of fibroblasts and cardiomyocytes. Biomaterials. 2007; 28(29):4277–4293.

Baei P, Jalili-Firoozinezhad S, Rajabi-Zeleti S, Tafazzoli-Shadpour M, Baharvand H, Aghdami N. Electrically conductive gold nanoparticle-chitosan thermosensitive hydrogels for cardiac tissue engineering. Mater Sci Eng C Mater Biol Appl. 2016; 63:131–141.

Baheiraei N, Yeganeh H, Ai J, Gharibi R, Azami M, Faghihi F. Synthesis, characterization and antioxidant activity of a novel electroactive and biodegradable polyurethane for cardiac tissue engineering application. Mater Sci Eng C Mater Biol Appl. 2014; 44:24–37.

Bahrami S, Baheiraei N, Mohseni M, Razavi M, Ghaderi A, Azizi B, Rabiee N, Karimi M. Three-dimensional graphene foam as a conductive scaffold for cardiac tissue engineering. J Biomater Appl. 2019; 34(1):74–85.

Balint R, Cassidy NJ, Cartmell SH. Conductive polymers: towards a smart biomaterial for tissue engineering. Acta Biomaterialia 2014; 10(6):2341–2353.

Bar A, Cohen S. Inducing endogenous cardiac regeneration: can biomaterials connect the dots? Front Bioeng Biotechnol. 2020; 8:126.

Bartunek J, Sherman W, Vanderheyden M, Fernandez-Aviles F, Wijns W, Terzic A. Delivery of biologics in cardiovascular regenerative medicine. Clin Pharmacol Ther. 2009; 85(5):548–552.

Bursac N, Papadaki M, Cohen RJ, Schoen FJ, Eisenberg SR, Carrier R, Vunjak-Novakovic G, Freed LE. Cardiac muscle tissue engineering: toward an *in vitro* model for electrophysiological studies. Am J Physiol. 1999; 277(2):433–444.

Cezar CA, Mortisen DJ, Ratner BD. Protein-immobilized poly (2-hydroxyethyl methacrylate-co-methacrylic acid) hydrogels for cardiac tissue engineering. J Undergraduate Res Bioeng. 2007; 7:7–12.

Chaudhuri R, Ramachandran M, Moharil P, Harumalani M, Jaiswal AK. Biomaterials and cells for cardiac tissue engineering: current choices. Mater Sci Eng C Mater Biol Appl. 2017; 79:950–957.

Chien KR, Domian IJ, Parker KK. Cardiogenesis and the complex biology of regenerative cardiovascular medicine. Science. 2008; 322(5907):1494–1497.

Christman KL, Lee RJ. Biomaterials for the treatment of myocardial infarction. J Am Coll Cardiol. 2006; 48(5):907–913.

Christman KL, Vardanian AJ, Fang Q, Sievers RE, Fok HH, Lee RJ. Injectable fibrin scaffold improves cell transplant survival, reduces infarct expansion, and induces neovasculature formation in ischemic myocardium. J Am Coll Cardiol. 2004; 44(3):654–660.

Dozois MD, Bahlmann LC, Zilberman Y, Shirley TX. Carbon nanomaterial-enhanced scaffolds for the creation of cardiac tissue constructs: a new frontier in cardiac tissue engineering. Carbon. 2017; 120:338–349.

Dunn DA, Hodge AJ, Lipke EA. Biomimetic materials design for cardiac tissue regeneration. Wiley Interdiscip Rev Nanomed Nanobiotechnol. 2014; 6(1):15–39.

Dvir T, Timko BP, Brigham MD, Naik SR, Karajanagi SS, Levy O, Jin H, Parker KK, Langer R, Kohane DS. Nanowired three-dimensional cardiac patches. Nat Nanotechnol. 2011b; 6(11):720–725.

Dvir T, Timko BP, Kohane DS, Langer R. Nanotechnological strategies for engineering complex tissues. Nature Nanotech. 2011a; 6:13–22.

Dvir T, Tsur-Gang O. "Designer" scaffolds for tissue engineering and regeneration. Special Issue: Degradable Biomaterials. Isr J Chem. 2005; 45(4):487–494.

Edwards SL, Werkmeister JA, Ramshaw JA. Carbon nanotubes in scaffolds for tissue engineering. Expert Rev Med Devices. 2009; 6(5):499–505.

Fleischer S, Feiner R, Dvir T. Cutting-edge platforms in cardiac tissue engineering. Curr Opin Biotechnol. 2017; 47:23–29.

Fujita B, Zimmermann W. Myocardial tissue engineering for regenerative Applications. Curr Cardiol Rep. 2017; 19:78.

Geng X, Liu B, Liu J, Liu D, Lu Y, Sun X, Liang K, Kong B. Interfacial tissue engineering of heart regenerative medicine based on soft cell-porous scaffolds. J Thorac Dis. 2018; 10(Suppl 20):2333–2345.

Giraud MN, Ayuni E, Cook S, Siepe M, Carrel TP, Tevaearai HT. Hydrogel-based engineered skeletal muscle grafts normalize heart function early after myocardial infarction. Artif Organs. 2008; 32(9):692–700.

Gorabi AM, Tafti SHA, Soleimani M, Panahi Y, Sahebkar A. Cells, scaffolds and their interactions in myocardial tissue regeneration. J Cell Biochem. 2017; 118(8):2454–2462.

Gorain B, Choudhury H, Pandey M, Kesharwani P, Abeer MM, Tekade RK, Hussain Z. Carbon nanotube scaffolds as emerging nanoplatform for myocardial tissue regeneration: a review of recent developments and therapeutic implications. Biomed Pharmacother. 2018; 104:496–508.

Govoni M, Muscari C, Guarnieri C, Giordano E. Mechanostimulation protocols for cardiac tissue engineering. BioMed Research International 2013; 1–10.

Griffith LG. Emerging design principles in biomaterials and scaffolds for tissue engineering. Ann N Y Acad Sci. 2002; 961:83–95.

Grigore ME. Hydrogels for cardiac tissue repair and regeneration. J Cardiovasc Med Cardiol. 2017; 4(3): 49–57.

Harrison BS, Atala A. Carbon nanotube applications for tissue engineering. Biomaterials. 2007; 28(2):344–353.

Hirt MN, Hansen A, Eschenhagen T. Cardiac tissue engineering: state of the art. Circ Res. 2014; 114(2):354–367.

Hopley EL, Salmasi S, Kalaskar DM, Seifalian AM. Carbon nanotubes leading the way forward in new generation 3D tissue engineering. Biotechnol Adv. 2014; 32(5):1000–1014.

Hu CS, Wu QH, Hu DY, Tkebuchava T. Treatment of chronic heart failure in the 21st century: A new era of biomedical engineering has come. Chronic Dis Transl Med. 2018; 5(2):75–88.

Huang YC, Khait L, Birla RK. Contractile three-dimensional bioengineered heart muscle for myocardial regeneration. J Biomed Mater Res A. 2007; 80(3):719–731.

Izadifar M, Chapman D, Babyn P, Chen X, Kelly ME. UV-Assisted 3D bioprinting of nanoreinforced hybrid cardiac patch for myocardial tissue engineering. Tissue Eng Part C Methods. 2018; 24(2):74–88.

Jackson KA, Majka SM, Wang H, Pocius J, Hartley CJ, Majesky MW, Entman ML, Michael LH, Hirschi KK, Goodell MA. Regeneration of ischemic cardiac muscle and vascular endothelium by adult stem cells. J Clin Invest. 2001; 107(11):1395–1402.

Jaganathan SK, Supriyanto E, Murugesan S, Balaji A, Asokan MK. Biomaterials in cardiovascular research: applications and clinical implications. Biomed Res Int. 2014; 2014:459465.

Kaliva M, Chatzinikolaidou M. Vamvakaki M. Applications of smart multifunctional tissue engineering scaffolds in smart materials for tissue engineering: Applications. 2017; 1–38.

Kankala RK, Zhu K, Sun XN, Liu CG, Wang SB, Chen AZ. Cardiac Tissue Engineering on the Nanoscale. ACS Biomater Sci Eng. 2018; 4(3):800–818.

Kehat I, Kenyagin-Karsenti D, Snir M, Segev H, Amit M, Gepstein A, Livne E, Binah O, Itskovitz-Eldor J, Gepstein L. Human embryonic stem cells can differentiate into myocytes with structural and functional properties of cardiomyocytes. J Clin Invest. 2001; 108(3):407–414.

Kitsara M, Agbulut O, Kontziampasis D, Chen Y, Menasche P. Fibers for hearts: a critical review on electrospinning for cardiac tissue engineering. Acta Biomater. 2017; 48:20–40.

Laflamme MA, Murry CE. Heart regeneration. Nature. 2011; 473(7347):326–335.

Laflamme MA, Murry CE. Regenerating the heart. Nat Biotechnol. 2005; 23(7):845–856.

Leor J, Aboulafia-Etzion S, Dar A, Shapiro L, Barbash IM, Battler A, Granot Y, Cohen S. Bioengineered cardiac grafts: a new approach to repair the infarcted myocardium? Circulation. 2000; 102(19 Suppl 3):56–61.

Leor J, Amsalem Y, Cohen S. Cells, scaffolds, and molecules for myocardial tissue engineering. Pharmacol Ther. 2005; 105(2):151–163.

Liu Z, Wang H, Wang Y, Lin Q, Yao A, Cao F, Li D, Zhou J, Duan C, Du Z, Wang Y, Wang C. The influence of chitosan hydrogel on stem cell engraftment, survival and homing in the ischemic myocardial microenvironment. Biomaterials. 2012; 33(11):3093–3106.

Maidhof R, Tandon N, Lee EJ, Luo J, Duan Y, Yeager K, Konofagou E, Vunjak-Novakovic G. Biomimetic perfusion and electrical stimulation applied in concert improved the assembly of engineered cardiac tissue. J Tissue Eng Regen Med. 2012; 6(10):12–23.

Mallone A, Weber B, Hoerstrup SP. Cardiovascular regenerative technologies: update and future outlook. Transfus Med Hemother. 2016; 43:291–296.

McCullen SD, Ramaswamy S, Clarke LI, Gorga RE. Nanofibrous composites for tissue engineering applications. Wiley Interdiscip Rev Nanomed Nanobiotechnol. 2009; 1(4):369–390.

McGann CL, Levenson EA, Kiick KL. Resilin-Based hybrid hydrogels for cardiovascular tissue engineering. Macromolecules. 2013; 214(2):203–213.

Mohammadi Nasr S, Rabiee N, Hajebi S, Ahmadi S, Fatahi Y, Hosseini M, Bagherzadeh M, Ghadiri AM, Rabiee M, Jajarmi V, Webster TJ. Biodegradable nanopolymers in cardiac tissue engineering: From concept towards nanomedicine. Int J Nanomedicine. 2020; 15:4205–4224.

Mooney E, Mackle JN, Blond DJ, O'Cearbhaill E, Shaw G, Blau WJ, Barry FP, Barron V, Murphy JM. The electrical stimulation of carbon nanotubes to provide a cardiomimetic cue to MSCs. Biomaterials. 2012; 33(26):6132–6139.

Moorthi A, Tyan YC, Chung TW. Surface-modified polymers for cardiac tissue engineering. Biomater Sci. 2017; 5(10):1976–1987.

Morsi YS. Bioengineering strategies for polymeric scaffold for tissue engineering an aortic heart valve: an update. Int J Artif Organs. 2014; 37(9):651–667.

Nakhlband A, Eskandani M, Omidi Y, Saeedi N, Ghaffari S, Barar J, Garjani A. Combating atherosclerosis with targeted nanomedicines: recent advances and future prospective. Bioimpacts. 2018; 8(1):59–75.

Navaei A, Rahmani Eliato K, Ros R, Migrino RQ, Willis BC, Nikkhah M. The influence of electrically conductive and non-conductive nanocomposite scaffolds on the maturation and excitability of engineered cardiac tissues. Biomater Sci. 2019; 7(2):585–595.

Nazari H, Heirani-Tabasi A, Hajiabbas M, Khalili M, Alavijeh MS, Hatamie S, Gorabi AM, Esmaeili E, Taft SHA. Incorporation of two-dimensional nanomaterials into silk fibroin nanofibers for cardiac tissue engineering. Polym Adv Technol. 2020; 31(2):248–259.

Nugent HM, Edelman ER. Tissue engineering therapy for cardiovascular disease. Circ Res. 2003; 92(10):1068–1078.

Nunes SS, Song H, Chiang CK, Radisic M. Stem cell-based cardiac tissue engineering. J Cardiovasc Transl Res. 2011; 4(5):592–602.

O'Brien FJ. Biomaterials and scaffolds for tissue engineering. Materials Today 2011; 14(3):88–95.

Pawan KC, Yi Hong, Ge Zhang. Cardiac tissue-derived extracellular matrix scaffolds for myocardial repair: advantages and challenges. Regen Biomater. 2019; 6(4):185–199.

Pedron S, van Lierop S, Horstman P, Penterman R, Broer DJ, Peeters E. Stimuli responsive delivery vehicles for cardiac microtissue transplantation. Adv Funct Mater. 2011; 21:1624–1630.

Pena B, Jett S, Rowland TJ, Taylor MRG, Mestroni L. Injectable hydrogels for cardiac tissue engineering. Macromol Biosci. 2018; 18(6):e1800079.

Radisic M, Fast VG, Sharifov OF, Iyer RK, Park H, Vunjak-Novakovic G. Optical mapping of impulse propagation in engineered cardiac tissue. Tissue Eng Part A. 2009; 15(4):851–860.

Reis LA, Chiu LL, Feric N, Fu L, Radisic M. Biomaterials in myocardial tissue engineering. J Tissue Eng Regen Med. 2016; 10(1):11–28.

Saravanan S, Sareen N, Abu-El-Rub E, Ashour H, Sequiera GL, Ammar HI, Gopinath V, Shamaa AA, Sayed SSE, Moudgil M, Vadivelu J, Dhingra S. Graphene oxide-Gold nanosheets containing chitosan scaffold improves ventricular contractility and function after implantation into infarcted heart. Sci Rep. 2018; 8(1):15069.

Sharma P, Mehra NK, Jain K, Jain NK. Biomedical applications of carbon nanotubes: a critical review. Curr Drug Deliv. 2016; 13(6):796–817.

Sharon F, Michal S, Ron F, Tal D. Coiled fiber scaffolds embedded with gold nanoparticles improve the performance of engineered cardiac tissues. Nanoscale. 2014; 6(16): 9410–9414.

Shin SR, Jung SM, Zalabany M, Kim K, Zorlutuna P, Kim SB, Nikkhah M, Khabiry M, Azize M, Kong J, Wan KT, Palacios T, Dokmeci MR, Bae H, Tang XS, Khademhosseini A. Carbon-nanotube-embedded hydrogel sheets for engineering cardiac constructs and bioactuators. ACS Nano. 2013; 7(3):2369–2380.

Shin SR, Zihlmann C, Akbari M, Assawes P, Cheung L, Zhang K, Manoharan V, Zhang YS, Yüksekkaya M, Wan KT, Nikkhah M, Dokmeci MR, Tang XS, Khademhosseini A. Reduced graphene oxide-GelMA hybrid hydrogels as scaffolds for cardiac tissue engineering. Small. 2016; 12(27):3677–3689.

Slaughter BV, Khurshid SS, Fisher OZ, Khademhosseini A, Peppas NA. Hydrogels in regenerative medicine. Adv Mater. 2009; 21(32–33):3307–3329.

Solazzo M, O'Brien FJ, Nicolosi V, Monaghan MG. The rationale and emergence of electroconductive biomaterial scaffolds in cardiac tissue engineering. APL Bioeng. 2019; 3:041501–0415015.

Stoppel WL, Kaplan DL, Black LD. Electrical and mechanical stimulation of cardiac cells and tissue constructs. Adv Drug Deliv Rev. 2016; 96:135–155.

Sui R, Liao X, Zhou X, Tan Q. The current status of engineering myocardial tissue. Stem Cell Rev Rep. 2011; 7(1):172–180.

Sun H, Mou Y, Li Y, Li X, Chen Z, Duval K, Huang Z, Dai R, Tang L, Tian F. Carbon nanotube-based substrates promote cardiogenesis in brown adipose-derived stem cells via β1-integrin-dependent TGF-β1 signaling pathway. Int J Nanomedicine. 2016; 11:4381–4395.

Tallawi M, Rosellini E, Barbani N, Cascone MG, Rai R, Saint-Pierre G, Boccaccini AR. Strategies for the chemical and biological functionalization of scaffolds for cardiac tissue engineering: a review. J R Soc Interface. 2015; 12(108):20150254.

Tandon N, Marsano A, Maidhof R, Wan L, Park H, Vunjak-Novakovic G. Optimization of electrical stimulation parameters for cardiac tissue engineering. J Tissue Eng Regen Med. 2011; 5(6):115–125.

Ventrelli L, Ricotti L, Menciassi A, Mazzolai B, Mattoli V. Nanoscaffolds for guided cardiac repair: The new therapeutic challenge of regenerative medicine. J Nanomater. 2013; 1–16.

Vunjak-Novakovic G, Lui KO, Tandon N, Chien KR. Bioengineering heart muscle: a paradigm for regenerative medicine. Annu Rev Biomed Eng. 2011; 13:245–267.

Vunjak-Novakovic G, Tandon N, Godier A, Maidhof R, Marsano A, Martens TP, Radisic M. Challenges in cardiac tissue engineering. Tissue Eng Part B Rev. 2010; 16(2):169–187.

Wang F, Guan J. Cellular cardiomyoplasty and cardiac tissue engineering for myocardial therapy. Adv Drug Deliv Rev. 2010; 62(7–8):784–797.

Wang H, Zhou J, Liu Z, Wang C. Injectable cardiac tissue engineering for the treatment of myocardial infarction. J Cell Mol Med. 2010; 14(5):1044–1055.

Ye L, Zimmermann WH, Garry DJ, Zhang J. Patching the heart: cardiac repair from within and outside. Circ Res. 2013; 113(7):922–932.

Zammaretti P, Jaconi M. Cardiac tissue engineering: regeneration of the wounded heart. Curr Opin Biotechnol. 2004; 15(5):430–434.

Zhang Y, Petibone D, Xu Y, Mahmood M, Karmakar A, Casciano D, Ali S, Biris AS. Toxicity and efficacy of carbon nanotubes and graphene: the utility of carbon-based nanoparticles in nanomedicine. Drug Metab Rev. 2014; 46(2):232–246.

Zimmermann WH, Eschenhagen T. Cardiac tissue engineering for replacement therapy. Heart Fail Rev. 2003; 8(3):259–269.

7 Nanomaterial for Kidney Disease Management

Trupti Ghatage, Srashti Goyal, Deepika Dasari, Jayant Jain, and Arti Dhar
Birla Institute of Technology and Sciences

Audesh Bhat
Central University of Jammu

CONTENTS

DOI: 10.1201/9781003140108-7

7.1 INTRODUCTION

An optimally functioning renal system is critical for survival, as it carries out vital body functions like filtration of blood, removal of waste, and maintenance of salt-water balance. Kidney diseases are one of the leading causes of mortality and morbidity worldwide, with an estimated prevalence rate of 8–16% (Jha et al. 2013). There are two main types of disorders in kidney function progression: acute kidney injury (AKI) and chronic kidney disease (CKD). AKI, also refereed as acute kidney failure, results in an acute but often reversible clinical condition linked with a rapid decrease in glomerular filtration rate (GFR). In patients with AKI, the serum creatinine increases $\geq$1.5 times from the baseline within seven days or $\geq$ 0.3 mg/dL within 48 hours, or the production of urine drops to <0.5 ml/kg/h for 6 hours. CKD is an irreversible, slow, and progressive evolving condition with a prevalence rate of 10–13% (Ammirati, 2020). In patients with CKD, there is a persistent kidney structure or function abnormality for three or more months. In most patients, CKD is diagnosed in the late stage of the disease mainly due to lack of symptoms and diagnostic resources. CKD is classified into five stages based on the GFR; with stage I and stage V having GFR of >90 ml/min/1.73 m^2 and <15 ml/min/1.73 m^2, respectively or into three stages based on the albuminuria (stage 1 <30 mg/24 hrs and stage 3 >300 mg/24 hrs) (Ammirati, 2020). The terminal stage of CKD contributes to the end-stage kidney disease (ESKD), which can be treated only by dialysis and kidney transplantation (Liu et al. 2018). CKD is mainly caused by diabetes and hypertension; however, other causes include polycystic kidney disease, a genetically inherited condition in which large cysts are formed in the kidney; glomerulonephritis, a condition caused by the inflammation of glomeruli; lupus nephritis, an autoimmune disorder; obstruction caused by tumor, kidney stone, or enlarged prostate gland; and repeated urinary tract infections (Ammirati, 2020). Unhealthy habits, older age, and genetic factors are some other contributing factors in the progression of kidney diseases. Serious secondary outcomes include increased cardiovascular risk, end-organ damage, and acute kidney injury, leading to life-threatening complications.

Treatment of kidney disease being one of the major healthcare goals has led to the development of several new promising diagnostics and therapeutic tools, including kidney replacement therapy (Breyer and Susztak, 2016; Bello et al. 2017; Kliger and Brosius, 2020; Ma et al. 2020). Besides the increasing burden of kidney diseases on healthcare, these developments were also necessitated because conventional therapeutics such as angiotensin-converting enzyme, mineralocorticoid receptor blockers, angiotensin receptor blockers, and diuretics are often not maintained at the required steady-state plasma concentration for a specific time period or the delivery system fails to deliver the drugs to the specific target organ mainly due to biological barriers in transportation. Several ongoing studies are aiming at addressing these issues by using nanomaterials for early detection and treatment of kidney diseases, including targeted drug delivery.

Expanding knowledge of nanotechnology is fast becoming an important cornerstone of modern medicine. Nanotechnology deals with the engineering of tiny atoms and biomolecules such as peptides, nucleic acids, and proteins with an ultimate aim of improving therapeutic efficacy, reducing toxicity, and achieving targeted delivery of the drugs. It also maintains the rate of drug release and minimizes off-target side effects. Nanomaterials are available in various forms, such as liposome, polymeric micelles, albumin, dendrimers, nanosized polymer-drug conjugates, hydrogels and nanocarriers (Singh et al. 2019). A variety of nanomaterials are currently undergoing clinical trial, with some already approved for clinical use in terminal complications. Use of nanomedicine is rapidly expanding in the field of nephrology, importantly for the treatment of CKDs. This chapter focuses on the major advances in nanomedicine in the preclinical and clinical study for the treatment and diagnosis of kidney diseases. It also outlines nanomaterial characteristics useful for improved targeting to renal tissue and highlights the opportunities, challenges, and future prospects of nanomaterial-based therapies for the treatment of kidney diseases.

7.2 PHYSICOCHEMICAL PROPERTIES OF NANOMATERIALS AND TARGETED DELIVERY

The primary goal of nanotechnology-based medical tools is to use them for diagnosis, prevention, and treatment of diseases, as nanomaterial provides an excellent alternative for such applications, as demonstrated by several studies (Hua et al. 2018). Nanomaterial can pass specific biological and physical barriers where conventional drugs fail to pass. Active targeting with nanomaterials involves binding of a target-specific ligand to the nanomaterial surface (Alexis, Rhee et al. 2008). These agents can be conjugated to the nanomaterial or encapsulated surface, allowing delivery of therapeutics that is more stable, soluble, or biologically activated. Solid lipid-based nanoparticles have emerged as preferred carriers for drug delivery due to multiple reasons such as biocompatibility, ease of surface modifications, encapsulation of wide varieties of drugs, feasibility to scale up, and active/passive targeting (Mohanta et al. 2019). Delivery or administration of nanoparticles is possible via several routes, such as enteral, transdermal, inhalational, and parenteral. It mainly involves mechanisms such as triggered release, solubilization, and passive or active targeting.

Physicochemical characteristics of nanomaterials, such as size, shape, density, and charge play a crucial role in improving targeted drug delivery and drug efficacy (Gatoo et al. 2014). A minor modification in physicochemical parameters contributes to the greater efficacy and stability of drugs. Nanomaterial can be either solid or have a hollow aqueous core, with a surface layer protected by inert polymers. Polyethylene glycol (PEG) is mainly used for coating the surface layer of nanomaterials. Hydrophilic or hydrophobic drugs, proteins, peptides, and nucleic acids can be incorporated within or on the surface layer of nanomaterials, facilitating the targeted delivery (Kamaly et al. 2016). The transport of nanomaterials in the systemic circulation is due to convective forces instead of Brownian motion. Nanomaterials are available in various shapes, such as rod, disc, and sphere, that can shelter cellular membrane covering processes and facilitate cellular internalization.

Likewise, size and surface area of nanomaterials can also contribute to achieving efficient therapeutic properties. Particle size and surface area can dictate the drug interaction within the biological system to distribute and eliminate materials. The particle size of nanomaterials should be <150 nm, but it should be <10 nm for kidney diseases so it can pass through a glomerular sieve (Rahman et al. 2017). The surface area increases with the decreasing size of materials; it makes the nanomaterial surface more reactive (Gatoo et al. 2014). Target delivery of nanomaterials should cross the glomerular barrier; therefore, modification in physicochemical properties can decrease nanotoxicity and increase the efficacy of therapeutic agents. Several studies were conducted to improve biological efficacy and reduce nanomaterial nephrotoxicity by changing the size and surface area of nanomaterials (Gatoo et al. 2014). As the research in nanomaterials is advancing exponentially, it is necessary to decrease the gap between physicochemical parameters and toxicity of nanomaterials in order to make them suitable for medical use.

7.3   KIDNEY ANATOMY AND FUNCTION

The bean-shaped kidneys are retroperitoneal in the lower abdominal region, protected by muscles, ribcage, and fat. The right kidney is situated slightly inferior to the left kidney because of the liver (Schott and Woodie, 2012). In the kidney, blood enters through the renal artery and leaves through the renal vein. The kidney consists of three regions: the outer part (cortex), inner part (medulla), and pelvis. The nephron is the basic structural and functional unit of a kidney. The adult healthy human kidney has approximately 1–2.5 million nephrons that maintain body homeostasis. The glomerulus is composed of glomerular basement membrane (GBM), glomerular endothelial cells (GECs), mesangial cells, parietal epithelial cells, and podocytes (Rayner, 2016). Dysfunction of these cells thus can lead to various kidney ailments.

The unique structure of a nephron contributes to the complex and vital function of the kidney. A nephron consists of glomerulus, proximal convoluted tubule (PCT), loop of Henle, distal tubule (DCT), and the collecting duct (Schott and Woodie, 2012). The glomerulus capillary bed is responsible for the filtration of blood, and Bowman's capsule collects the filtrate. Most of the water and solutes are reabsorbed in the proximal and distal convoluted tubules and the loop of Henle. The remaining filtrate is collected by the collecting ducts and the minor calyces, which combine to form major calyces, and the filtrate is finally carried toward the renal pelvis and the ureter.

7.4   TARGETED NANOMATERIAL-BASED TREATMENT

The efficiency of nanomaterial-mediated therapy and drug delivery mainly depends on the size and charge of the nanoparticles to reach the different cells of the renal system (Table 7.1).

The delicate structure of glomerulus and glomerular filtration barrier and the nanoparticles suitable to reach each cell type is illustrated in Figure 7.1.

7.4.1   GLOMERULAR ENDOTHELIAL CELL BARRIER

Endothelial cells cover the entire vascular inner surface and form a barrier between blood and renal tissue. In healthy kidneys, the glomerular barrier participates in

TABLE 7.1
Characteristics of NPs with Renal Targeting

	Characteristics	Renal Target	References
Size	80–100 nm gold core NP	Mesangium	Choi et al. 2011
	4–6 nm iron oxide core NP	Cortex, nephritis	Hauger et al. 1999
	5 nm dendrimer NPs	Renal tubular epithelial cells	Nair et al. 2015
	5 nm dextran-based NPs	Renal tubular epithelial cells	Nair et al. 2015
	~400 nm PLGA–PEG NPs	Proximal tubule epithelial cells	Williams et al. 2015
Shape	Carbon nanotubes (100–500 nm and diameter of 0.8–1.2 nm)	Proximal tubular cell	Ruggiero et al. 2010 Alidori et al. 2016
Charge	Cationic ferritin NPs	Glomerular basement membrane, podocytes	Bennett et al. 2008
	siRNA NPs	Glomerular basement membrane	Zuckerman et al. 2012
	Negatively charged quantum dots	Mesangial cells	Liang et al. 2016
	Cationic quantum dots	Tubular epithelial cells	Liang et al. 2016
Conjugation	MHC-II antibody	Medulla	Hultman et al. 2008
	Anti-CDIIb antibody	Unilateral obstruction	Shirai et al. 2012
	Integrin αvβ3 (Cyclo peptide)	Integrin αvβ3 receptor/podocytes	Pollinger et al. 2012
	Ac2-26 peptide	Collagen IV/glomerular basement membrane	Kamaly et al. 2013
	E-selectin antibody	E-selectin/glomerular endothelial cells	Ásgeirsdóttir et al. 2008
	Angiotensin I/II	Angiotensin II receptor/mesangial cells	Maslanka Figueroa et al. 2019
	Modified polymyxin	Megalin/proximal tubule epithelia cells	Oroojalian et al. 2017
Encapsulation	PLGA-coated CoQ10, superoxide scavenger	Vascular endothelium	Ankola et al. 2007
	Dendrimer	Medulla during ischemia	Kobayashi et al. 2004
	Dextran-coated iron oxide	Cortext during allograft rejection	Hauger et al. 1999
	PEG-coated nucleic acids	Cell nucleus, gene therapy	Ogris et al. 1999
	TNF-α-coated gold NPs	Tumor interstitium	Goel et al. 2009

Source: This table was adopted from Brede and Labhasetwar, 2013 and Ma et al. 2020.

blood filtration by size and charge, ensuring passage of only small-molecular-weight solutes from plasma to urine. Negatively charged and high-molecular-weight plasma components, such as albumin, are not easily filtered into the urine. Electrostatic repulsion helps filtration through the glomerular filtration barrier, which strongly favors the passage of anionic molecules. Unhealthy condition of kidneys or impairment of

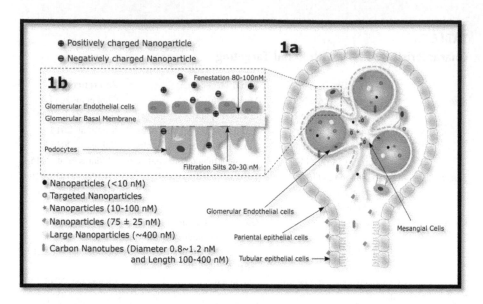

FIGURE 7.1   Targeted delivery of nanoparticles to the kidney cells. (a) Structure of the glomerulus. **(b)** Fine structure of the glomerulus filtration barrier. Depending on the size, the nanoparticles can be effectively targeted to different parts of the glomerulus for drug delivery. (Particles <10 nm size can be targeted easily to the tubular epithelial cells; particles between 10–100 nm size for the glomerular deposition; particles of ~75 ± 25 nm size to the mesangial cells; particles of ~400 nm to the proximal tubule cells and charged nanoparticles to the podocytes.) Moreover, carbon nanotubes of 0.8–1.2 nm diameter and 100–500 nm length can be targeted to the proximal tubule cells. (Recreated with permission from Ma et al. 2020. Copyright 2020: Elsevier.)

the GEC barrier leads to proteinuria and albuminuria, which causes glomerular and kidney pathology (Kamaly et al. 2016). The selective filtration process of GEC barrier, therefore, requires nanoparticles to cross this barrier for greater efficacy and targeted drug delivery. Various strategies have been attempted to restore the function of damaged GECs, such as the use of antisense oligonucleotides, short interfering RNA (siRNA), microRNA (miRNA), DNA inhibitor oligonucleotides or neutralizing antibodies. In one successful attempt, dexamethasone (DEX) liposome conjugated with an anti-E-selectin antibody was delivered to glomerular endothelium. This pharmacological activity of liposome was studied in anti-glomerular basement membrane (anti-GBM) glomerulonephritis (Ásgeirsdóttir et al. 2008). Nanoparticles conjugated to specific targeting antibodies have also been tested to increase their localization at the glomerular site (Williams et al. 2016).

7.4.2   GLOMERULAR BASEMENT MEMBRANE

Glomerular basement membrane (GBM) is the basal lamina and connective tissue barrier composed of laminin, nidogen, agrin, type IV collagen, and heparan sulfate proteoglycan proteins secreted by the glomerular endothelial cells and podocytes

(Kanwar and Farquhar, 1979; Ogawa et al. 1999; Suh and Miner, 2013). Mutation(s) in the genes expressing these proteins can lead to GBM diseases (Thorner, 2007). GBM acts as a sieve, giving entry to the negatively charged particles and bulky groups and factors that mediate communication between glomerular endothelial cells and podocytes. Nanoparticle disassembly because of electrostatic interactions is an important mechanism responsible for the rapid clearance of cyclodextrin-containing polymer-based siRNA (siRNA/CDP) nanoparticles in the GBM (Zuckerman et al. 2012).

7.4.3 Podocytes

Podocytes are specialized cells that play an essential role in maintaining the glomerular filtration barrier. They also produce growth factors for both mesangial cells and endothelial cells. Injury to the podocytes can lead to many kidney diseases, which causes proteinuria with end-stage renal disease. The types of cell surface and nanomedicine surface coatings are essential determinants in cellular response (Selc et al. 2020). Newly designed kidney-specific nano delivery of DEX with suitable size and shape successfully repaired damaged podocytes in vitro (Colombo et al. 2017). The neonatal Fc receptor (FcRn) of albumin is a novel promising therapeutic target in podocyte-associated renal diseases. Albumin-methylprednisolone nanoparticles targeting specific FcRn receptors enhanced the beneficial glucocorticosteroid effects and reduced unwanted adverse effects (Wu et al. 2017). Gold nanoparticles of 50 nm size effectively reduce renal damage by enhancing renal function and down-regulating extracellular matrix protein and inflammation markers and inhibiting renal oxidative stress and podocyte injury (Alomari et al. 2020). Renal nanoparticles cyclo-(Arg-Gly-Asp-D-Phe-Cys)-modified (Cyclo(RGDfC) quantum dots illustrate a specific and receptor-mediated binding to both podocytes and glomeruli in 2D cell culture, suggesting that these could be a promising therapeutic approach in targeted drug delivery and treatment of podocyte diseases in the future (Pollinger et al. 2012). Further, one study developed a nanocarrier with rapamycin incorporated into vascular cell adhesion molecule-1 (VCAM-1)-SAINT-O-Somes, which inhibits cellular responses in VCAM-1 expressing podocytes (Visweswaran et al. 2015).

7.4.4 Mesangial Cells

Mesangial cells sustain the glomerular capillary structure and are also responsible for glomerular matrix growth and homeostasis. Dysfunctioning in mesangial cells could contribute to the development of renal diseases. Also, diabetic-like conditions prompt excess production of reactive oxygen species, cytokines, and growth factors in mesangial cells. Hence, target-specific drug delivery to mesangial cells would be helpful in the treatment of various kidney diseases. Targeted nanoparticles ($\sim$75 $\pm$ 25 nm diameters) to the mesangial cells elicit greater biological efficacy (Choi et al. 2011). Free celastrol has severe off-target toxicity; therefore, celastrol-albumin nanoparticles offer a promising alternative in treating mesangial cell-associated glomerular diseases. It significantly alleviated inflammation, proteinuria, glomerular hypercellularity, and excessive extracellular matrix deposition in preclinical rat nephritis (Guo et al. 2017).

7.4.5　Tubular Epithelial Cells

Renal tubular epithelial cells present on the renal tubule play a vital role in absorbing amino acids, glucose, and other primary urine substances. Dysfunctioning of renal tubular epithelial cells can lead to renal fibrosis and tubule-interstitial fibrosis, which further contributes to chronic kidney diseases (Qi and Yang, 2018). Therefore, specifically designed nanoparticles to deliver drugs and nucleic acids that prevent renal fibrosis progression, inflammation, and renal tubules' regeneration could be a better alternative. Glutathione-modified fluorescent gold, a target-specific nanoparticle, significantly reduced renal fibrosis in renal fibroblast cells (Lai et al. 2020). The selective renal targeting and renal tubular localization of mesoscale nanoparticles could be the potential target in AKI and CKD (Williams et al. 2016).

7.5　APPLICATION OF NANOPARTICLES IN KIDNEY DISEASE

Chronic kidney disease poses a significant burden on the healthcare system, as current therapies have proved ineffective. Nanoparticles vary by physicochemical properties, enhancing the pharmacokinetics, target delivery, and bioavailability of drugs. Thus, the introduction of nanoparticles in medicine has provided a promising alternative to treat kidney diseases. Details of various nanoparticles undergoing clinical trial are given in Table 7.2. Nanoparticles have extended applications in the diagnosis, treatment, and prognosis of kidney diseases with high sensitivity and highly selective treatment (Figure 7.2, Table 7.3). Nanoparticles can be used as a diagnostic tool to investigate the structural and functional abnormalities in the kidney. A diagnostic tool can be extended as a therapeutic strategy for the targeted delivery of drugs and nucleic acids with improved retention and localization depending on nanoparticles' variable sizes. Also, nanotechnology can be applied as a prognostic tool to monitor the outcomes of successful intervention.

7.5.1　Nanoparticles as a Diagnostic Tool

Early detection of biomarkers is very crucial in predicting the disease progression and for selecting the proper intervention. In conventional methods, the detection of kidney diseases like acute renal failure (ARF) is not accurate and patient convenient, as the biomarkers like blood urea nitrogen (BUN) and creatinine rise over a delayed time interval of 24 hours (Waikar and Bonventre, 2009). Magnetic resonance imaging (MRI) coupled with dendrimer-encapsulated nanoparticles can detect kidney damage before it can be detected by serum biomarkers, which helps in early detection and treatment of the disease (Dear et al. 2006). Albuminuria is also a promising kidney injury biomarker, which urine albumin dipsticks or specific antibodies can detect. However, these methods are not sensitive enough as only albumin concentration >30 mg/dl can be detected. Nanoparticles coupled with surface-enhanced Raman scattering (SERS) is an emission technology; it works by inelastic scattering of incident laser light that can be measured by a Raman spectrophotometer. This technique is quite sensitive and convenient as there is no need to process the samples, and also microalbuminuria can be successfully measured at a very low level of 3µg/ml (Mosier-boss, 2017).

TABLE 7.2

Details of Clinical Trials Using Nanomaterials for Renal Disease Management

Sr. no. Drug	Clinical Trial ID	Specifications	Clinical Condition	Phase	Dates
1. Human leukocyte antigens (HLA)-coated magnetic nanoparticles	NCT04277377	Coated with donor-specific antibodies	Kidney Failure	NA	Mar 2020-Feb 2023
2. Nanoparticle albumin-bound rapamycin	NCT02646319	Albumin-bound rapamycin	Recurrent Renal Cell Carcinoma	I	Jan 2016-Apr 2018
3. NanoDoce (sterile nanoparticulate docetaxel) powder for suspension	NCT04260360	Docetaxel nanoparticles	Renal Cell Carcinoma	I	Apr 2020-Oct 2022
4. Microparticles	NCT02626663		Atypical Hemolytic Uremic Syndrome	NA	Jul 2016-Dec 2022
5. Ferumoxytol	NCT03619850	Iron oxide nanoparticle	Chronic Kidney Disease; Iron Deficiency Anemia	III IV infusion	Aug 2018-Aug 2021
6. Venofer	NCT02492672	Iron nanoparticle	Chronic Kidney Disease	IV	Sep 2014-Dec 2018
7. CRLX101	NCT01625936	Tumor-targeting nanoparticle	Renal cell carcinoma	I	June 2012-Jul 2018
8. ABI-009	NCT02587325	Albumin-bound mTOR inhibitor	Pulmonary Hypertension	I	Apr 2017-Dec 2020
9. Liposomal bupivicaine	NCT03737604		Transplant; Failure, Kidney Pain, Postoperative	IV	Oct 2018-Oct 2021
10. Mircera	NCT03552393	Methoxy polyethylene glycol-epoetin beta	Renal Insufficiency	II	May 2018-Oct 2021
11. Exosomes	NCT04053855	Tumor marker in biological fluid and urine 30 to 150 nm	Renal Cell Carcinoma	NA	Jan 2020-Sep 2021

Note: NA, Not Applicable.

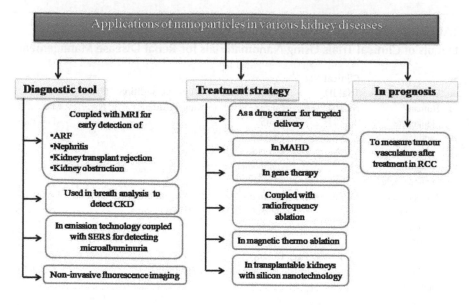

FIGURE 7.2   Applications of nanomaterials in various kidney diseases.

TABLE 7.3
Applications of Nanomaterial in Renal Disorders

Sr. No.	Nanoparticles	Application	References
1.	Polyoxometalate clusters	Ameliorates AKI and ROS associated diseases	(Ni et al. 2018)
2.	V2O5 nanowires (nanozymes)	Protects from oxidative damage in cardiac and renal diseases	(Vernekar et al. 2014)
3.	Dextran-coated iron oxide (D-IONPs) nanoparticles	Diagnostic imaging by magnetic resonance in renal diseases	(Popa et al. 2016)
4.	NIR-II gold nanoclusters	Monitors physiological behaviors in biological systems	(Song et al. 2020)
5.	Ultrasmall copper-based (Cu5.4O) nanoparticle	Protective in oxidative damage in a major organ like the kidney	(Liu et al. 2020)
6.	Gadolinium metallofullerene nanomaterials	Clinical application in the vital organ like kidney diseases	(Li and Wang, 2020)
7.	Cerium oxide nanoparticles	Prevents renal fibrosis	(Saifi et al. 2020)
8.	Black phosphorus nanosheets	Treatment of AKI and renal diseases	(Hou et al. 2020)
9.	Gold nanoparticles	5 and 200 nm AuNPs effective in tumor therapy on renal proximal tubular cells	(Zhao et al. 2020)
10.	Selenium-doped carbon quantum dots	ROS scavenger in AKI treatment	(Rosenkrans et al. 2020)

Various kidney ailments such as kidney obstruction, nephritis, and kidney transplant rejection cannot be differentiated based on kidney biopsy, which is a painful, invasive technique. In contrast, nanotechnology has massive implications for imaging the localized macrophage activity in different kidney compartments depending on disease type (Grau et al. 1998).

Using gold nanoparticle sensors to detect volatile organic compounds (VOCs) in the breath of CKD patients is another novel diagnostic tool that offers a possibility of early detection of CKD, thus increasing the chances of treating the disease at an early stage (Marom et al. 2012).

GFR is correlated with kidney functioning; however, measuring GFR is complicated and inconvenient. Hence, alternatively estimated GFR (eGFR) is measured by detecting plasma creatinine, which has limitations due to creatinine absorption and secretion by tubular cells. Fluorescent imaging, using nanoparticles has proven useful in measuring GFR more efficiently with no toxicity, as glomeruli completely filter them without being absorbed or secreted by tubules. Various fluorescent nanoparticles include fluorescent semiconductor nanocrystals, gold, and silica nanoparticles (Michalet et al. 2005).

7.5.2 Nanoparticles as Therapeutic Agents

Untreated kidney disease can lead to renal failure. However, there are limitations in the currently available treatment strategies, such as poor bioavailability, non-specificity, low aqueous solubility, and off-target side effects. When conjugated with nanoparticles, drugs show improved pharmacokinetics and targeted delivery with enhanced bioavailability (Alexis, Pridgen et al. 2008). Several studies using nanoparticles have demonstrated promising outcomes in hypertension, acute kidney injury, CKD, glomerular diseases, and kidney cancer treatment (Williams et al. 2016). Reactive oxygen species (ROS) generation during kidney ischemia caused by hypotension, renal artery stenosis, kidney transplantation, or nephrectomy leads to renal cell necrosis and release of cellular degradation products and debris, which blocks kidney tubules, causing tissue edema (Bonventre, 1993). Since the innate scavenging system is overwhelmed by ROS production during ischemic injury, potent antioxidant therapy such as superoxide dismutases (SODs) has a useful application. However, it is challenging to improve the intravascular bioavailability, short half-life, and proteolytic susceptibility of SODs (Hood et al. 2011). Interestingly, nanoparticles, as demonstrated in cultured neuronal cells and a post-injury mouse model, can successfully be used as SOD carriers (Reddy et al. 2008; Reddy and Labhasetwar, 2009).

Being a necessary intervention in managing ESRD, hemodialysis has complications and poor patient convenience. On the other hand, nanoparticle-based magnetically assisted hemodialysis (MAHD) has been proven to be a more efficient method with fewer side effects. In MAHD, ferromagnetic nanoparticles are bound with proteins, antibodies, or immunoglobulins, which act as scavengers for serum toxins. The ferromagnetic nanoparticles are infused before hemodialysis and allowed to bind with the toxins for their efficient removal. It is proven that MAHD gives eight times better clearance in one circulation of blood volume than current hemodialysis, and with improved quality of life (Stamopoulos et al. 2008).

The treatment of anemia encountered in patients with renal disorders due to decreased erythropoietin production has therapeutic limitations due to poor oral bioavailability of ferrous sulfate. However, iron oxide magnetic nanoparticles like ferumoxytol have improved bioavailability with greater efficacy to treat iron deficiency anemia in CKD patients (Pereira et al. 2014).

Although gene therapy is a promising intervention in treating renal cell carcinoma (RCC), as RCC is not sensitive to chemotherapy or radiotherapy, it has limitations since RNA and DNA have short half-lives in circulation. However, PEG-encapsulated nucleic acids have shown improved bioavailability, as PEG protects nucleic acids from enzymatic degradation and prevents kidney clearance by increasing their size (Ogris et al. 1999). Gold nanoparticles loaded with TNF-α help to sensitize the tumors before radiofrequency ablation (RFA), thereby increasing the efficiency of RFA by 23% (Pedro et al. 2010). Magnetic thermoablation is also coupled with iron oxide nanoparticles, creating an electromagnetic field in RCC ablation (Gneveckow et al. 2004). More recently it was demonstrated in both in vivo and in vitro models that modified polymyxi–PEI/DNA nanoparticles can deliver DNA efficiently to the proximal tubular epithelial cells (Figure 7.3), thus increasing the chances of effective gene therapy (Oroojalian et al. 2017).

Another emerging area of nanomaterial-enabled kidney disease management technology is the development of transplantable artificial kidneys using silicon nanotechnology. The minute slit pores of the filters used in artificial kidneys mimic the glomerular slits, thus enabling efficient blood filtration and making them suitable for kidney transplantation in the scarcity of organ donation (Brede and Labhasetwar, 2013).

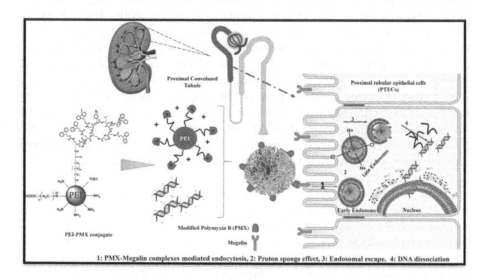

FIGURE 7.3 Schematic illustration of megalin-mediated delivery of modified-polymyxin-PEI conjugates to proximal tubular epithelial cells (PTECs). (Reprinted with permission from Oroojalian et al. 2017. Copyright 2017: Elsevier.)

7.5.3 Nanoparticles in Prognosis

Nanoparticles can also be used in monitoring successful intervention. For instance, RCC with high vasculature can be monitored with the aid of MRI coupled with magnetic nanoparticles for the extent of vascularity. This monitoring tool helps measure the efficiency of intervention and predicts the clinical outcomes and in dose adjustments and schedule (Guimaraes et al. 2011).

7.6 ASSESSMENT OF NANOMATERIALS IN KIDNEY TRANSPLANTATION

Kidney transplantation has become a standard of care for millions of kidney-failure patients due to improved surgical procedures and potent immunosuppressants (Tasciotti et al. 2016). However, due to a shortage of organ donors and a host of other issues, such as graft failures and life-long use of immunosuppressants, kidney transplantation has limited success as an effective treatment. The use of nanomaterials to address these issues is in the offing as immense progress has been made in the recent past in the field of targeted drug delivery and tissue engineering using nanotechnology (Tasciotti et al. 2016).

A significant aspect before usage and exposure of a xenobiotic nanomaterial to biological systems is to assess their toxicity, immunogenicity, and hazard capabilities of in vitro systems to predict possible risks and issues reliably. In the case of a transplantable nanomaterial, it is of extreme importance to examine its cytotoxicity effect and the immunogenic response before transplanting into animals using in vitro models. Most commonly used 2D cell culture models are not able to support complex tissue functions and are not accurate in predicting the efficacy of drugs and nanomaterials. Also, there is a high incidence of kidney toxicity reported during nanomaterial development. Hence, there is a need for new in vitro techniques to assess the efficacy of nanomaterials.

7.6.1 Microfluidics and Kidney-on-a-Chip

A microfluidic device is used to construct an in vitro model and mimic the microenvironment to investigate the molecular and cellular level activities of organs. Organs-on-chips are multiple cell types that are cultured in 2D under continuous perfusion developed by using microfluidics. These systems support the study of the molecular basis of tissue morphogenesis. Successful attempts in developing an in vitro human proximal tubule-on-a-chip might present a positive approach to studying renal physiology and diseases and toxicities (Jang et al. 2013). In recent years microfluidic devices have gained attention in the development of more relevant disease models. Several reports have supported microfluidic devices' relevance in studying gentamycin pharmacokinetics and toxicities of drugs for renal diseases (Kim et al. 2016). These microdevices mimic the renal proximal tubule cells' microenvironment and provide new insights into interactions among proximal tubular epithelial cells, tubular basement membranes, and proteinuria in in vitro studies (Zhou et al. 2014). Studies have proved that microfluidic chips are better tools for screening kidney-targeted drugs, efficacy, and toxicity than traditional cell culture systems. Some recent studies on microfluidic device systems reported potential application in various drug screening for the treatment of various disease models (Yin et al. 2020).

7.6.2   3D Culture Systems

The kidney consists of various cell types; it is difficult to portray the 2D culture renal system. In contrast, 3D structure cells grown from stem cells and organ-specific cell types, known as organoids, reflect major organs' structural and functional properties such as lung, kidney, gut, retina, and brain (Clevers, 2016). Organoids can be developed from pluripotent embryonic and organ-restricted adult stem cells. A 3D culture-based system gives improved assessment and validation of nanomaterials in kidney-related disease and gives an idea about toxicity biomarkers, drug-induced toxicity, drug interactions, and metabolism (Astashkina et al. 2012). Using a 3D kidney proximal tubule organoid model proved the model can precisely reflect nanomaterials induced toxicity biomarkers in vitro to assess kidney toxicity markers (Astashkina et al. 2014). Organoids can be used for transplantation or replace non-functional kidneys in serious kidney diseases in the future. Also, they can be a promising tool for specific target drug screening for kidney ailments. A functional 3D perfused proximal tubule model is successfully used for drug screening studies (Vormann et al. 2018).

7.6.3   Nanotoxicity Assays in Kidney Diseases

Due to a matrix of conditions and molecules that interact within a biological system, it is essential to understand nanomaterials' interaction with the system and assess its capability and toxicity. The assays are designed to contemplate the variety of possible physiological responses towards the nanomaterial using in vitro models. Cell lines (genetically altered cell lines and cancer cell lines) or primary cells (cells derived from live tissue of donor animals) are used as basal test subjects for assessment. In each specific cell line, the assays are modelled to incite response or effect, which the nanomaterial in the study is intended to perform in vivo.

7.6.4   ROS Production Assay

Stress or any foreign particle can induce production of reactive oxygen species (ROS) in a cell, which serves as a warning signal to the surrounding cells. Nanomaterial toxicity assay is often associated with material uptake by sentinel leukocytes and immune modulator cells because of their ability to uptake foreign particles and respond with cytokine release cascade and production of ROS. This assay is also performed while testing transplantable nanomaterial with specific cell lines pertaining to their intended place of use in the body and is also done to assess biocompatibility with the surroundings. The assay is performed by directly measuring ROS in cell media by reactive fluorescein probes; 2',7'-difluorescein-diacetate (DCFH-DA) and dichlorodihydrofluoresceindiacetate (H2 DCFDA) or by electron paramagnetic resonance (EPR) detection of radicals.

7.6.5   Cell Viability Assays

Nanomaterial in consideration should not cause cellular toxicity as a prerequisite. This criterion is assessed by measuring cell death by cell viability assays. Several techniques have been developed to assess the cell viability, dye-based cell viability assays being the prominent ones. They work via differential inclusion, exclusion, or conversion of the dye by cellular enzymes in living versus dead cells which is then quantified colorimetrically. Some of the routinely used dye-dependent assays include formazan-based assays (MTT, MTS, WST), lactate dehydrogenase (LDH), trypan blue, coomassie blue, mitochondrial membrane potential (MMP), and thiobarbituric (TBA) assays.

Fluorescence-activated cell sorting (FACS) is a fast and efficient way of accessing cell viability, as thousands of cells can be assessed within seconds. Other cell viability assays include enzyme-linked immunosorbent assay (ELISA), BrdU assay, Comet assay, Caspase 3 assay, Hoechst-DNA assay, and TdT-mediated dUTP-biotin nick end labeling (TUNEL) assay.

7.6.6 CELL STRESS ASSAYS

Cell stress assays are used to identify cellular behavior changes due to non-lethal injury and/or cellular stress due to nanomaterial presence. This stress/injury can disturb normal homeostasis of cells and can be detected at gene/protein expression level, change in morphology, or release of inflammatory cytokines.

Changes in gene expression can be used as markers for toxicity and the mechanism of toxicity, which can be assessed by qRT-PCR, western blotting, or ELISA. Some of the genes that are modulated under stress conditions are cell cycle arrest gene (CDKN1A), GADD45β (DNA damage-dependent), IL-6 (inflammatory response), NFκBIA (inflammatory response), NF-κB (for fibrotic/inflammatory growth factors, cytokines, and adhesion molecules), fibronectin, laminin, p-cadherin, focal adhesion kinase, and collagen IV. Some of the cytokines studied in association with nanomaterial toxicity are IL-1B, IL-6, IL-8 and TNF-A.

7.6.7 CELLULAR MORPHOLOGY AND UPTAKE

Transplantable material must possess some properties such as inertness (i.e., non-toxicity), should not entice immunological response, and should be non-degradable. Cellular uptake of transplantable material should not happen as it may be toxic and may degrade with time. Immunological cells can be used to detect nanomaterial cellular uptake, as this will also verify the degradation rate of transplantable nanomaterial. Biocompatibility of transplantable nanomaterial has to fulfil all the criteria in a cell-line–based assessment model, including toxicology and inertness parameters before switching to animal studies. The in vitro assessment thus has been judicially correlated with predictions for in vivo response analysis.

7.7 CHALLENGES IN THE CLINICAL USE OF NANOMATERIALS

Several challenges have to be addressed while moving from the development to commercialization of nanomaterial for kidney diseases. After administration, nanomaterials accumulated in various tissues due to acute and chronic exposure, leading to severe adverse effects or toxicity. These may be due to various pathological mechanisms such as endoplasmic reticulum stress, ROS generation, inflammatory mediator generation, autophagy, necrosis, and DNA damage. Furthermore, it aggravates kidney function by causing degeneration, glomerular swelling, membrane thickening and necrosis in renal tubular cells (Zhao et al. 2019). Nanomaterial toxicity also depends on the physico-chemical parameters. The small nanomaterials with a large surface area interact with the cell membrane and destroy its integrity. Physicochemical parameters are usually modified according to the severity of diseases.

Some other challenges are large-scale production, biological factors such as pathophysiological conditions, regulatory standards, costs, biocompatibility, and toxicity. Clinical application is a little costly, time-consuming, and complicated too. Scientists are working to reduce complexity, increase therapeutic potential, and reduce nanomaterials' side effects to make their use safe for medical applications (Hua et al. 2018).

7.8 FUTURE PROSPECTS AND CONCLUSION

Nanotechnology is a promising field with applications in biomedical research and clinical practice of various pathophysiological conditions. Nanomaterial efficacy and potency are mainly affected by their physicochemical properties such as size, charge, shape, and composition. Tailoring of these properties could help in potential target delivery. Nanotechnology has provided diagnosis with biomarkers such as microalbuminuria, urine creatinine, hemoglobin, and serum albumin. Conversely, noninvasive nanomaterial imaging techniques could measure GFR, kidney dysfunction, inflammation, and fibrosis. Some nanomaterial techniques proved beneficial in treating deadly renal complications such as acute kidney injury, chronic kidney diseases, hypertension, ESRD, and kidney cancer. There are several challenges while bringing nanomaterials from bench to market. However, several nanomaterials successfully reached preclinical and clinical trials. As mentioned in this chapter, few of them are marketed for the treatment of diseases. Nephrology and nanotechnology together can bring more promising and potential therapies. Expansion of this field may be able to fill the gaps in the treatment of kidney diseases.

ABBREVIATIONS

AKI	acute kidney disease
ARF	acute renal failure
BUN	blood urea nitrogen
CKD	chronic kidney disease
CoQ10	coenzyme Q10
DCFH-DA	2',7'-diflurescein-diacetate
DCT	distal convoluted tubule
DEX	dexamethasone
eGFR	estimated glomerular filtration rate
ELISA	enzyme-linked immunosorbent assay
EPR	electron paramagnetic resonance
ESKD	end stage kidney disease
FACS	fluorescence-activated cell sorting
GBM	glomerular basement membrane
GECs	glomerular endothelial cells

GFR	glomerular filtration rate
LDH	lactate dehydrogenase
MAHD	magnetically assisted hemodialysis
MHC-II	major histocompatibility complex-II
miRNA	microRNA
MMP	mitochondrial membrane potential
MRI	magnetic resonance imaging
NP	nanoparticle
PCT	proximal convoluted tubule
PEG	polyethylene glycol
PLGA	poly(lactic-co-glycolic acid)
RCC	renal cell carcinoma
RFA	radiofrequency ablation
ROS	reactive oxygen species
SERS	surface-enhanced Raman scattering
siRNA/CDP	cyclodextrin-containing polymer-based
siRNA	short interfering RNA
SODs	superoxide dismutases
TBA	thiobarbituric
TNF-α	tumor necrosis factor- α
TUNEL	TdT-mediated dUTP-biotin nick end labeling
VCAM-1	vascular cell adhesion molecule-1
VOCs	volatile organic compounds

REFERENCES

Alexis F, Pridgen E, Molnar LK, Farokhzad OC. (2008). Factors affecting the clearance and biodistribution of polymeric nanoparticles. Mol Pharm. 5(4):505–15.

Alexis F, Rhee JW, Richie JP, Radovic-Moreno AF, Langer R, Farokhzad OC. (2008). New frontiers in nanotechnology for cancer treatment. Urol Oncol. 26(1):74–85.

Alidori S, Akhavein N, Thorek DL, Behling K, Romin Y, Queen D, Beattie BJ, Manova-Todorova K, Bergkvist M, Scheinberg DA, McDevitt MR. (2016). Targeted fibrillar nanocarbon RNAi treatment of acute kidney injury. Sci Transl Med. 8(331):331ra39.

Alomari G, Al-Trad B, Hamdan S, Aljabali A, Al-Zoubi M, Bataineh N, Qar J, Tambuwala MM. (2020). Gold nanoparticles attenuate albuminuria by inhibiting podocyte injury in a rat model of diabetic nephropathy. Drug Deliv Transl Res. 10(1):216–26.

Ammirati AL. (2020). Chronic kidney disease. Rev Assoc Med Bras (1992). 66(Suppl 1):s03–s09.

Ankola DD, Viswanad B, Bhardwaj V, Ramarao P, Kumar MN. (2007). Development of potent oral nanoparticulate formulation of coenzyme Q10 for treatment of hypertension: can the simple nutritional supplements be used as first line therapeutic agents for prophylaxis/therapy? Eur J Pharm Biopharm. 67(2):361–69.

Ásgeirsdóttir SA, Zwiers PJ, Morselt HW, Moorlag HE, Bakker HI, Heeringa P, Kok JW, Kallenberg CGM, Molema G, Kamps JAAM. (2008). Inhibition of proinflammatory genes in anti-GBM glomerulonephritis by targeted dexamethasone-loaded AbEsel liposomes. Am J Physiol Renal Physiol. 294(3):554–61.

Astashkina AI, Jones CF, Thiagarajan G, Kurtzeborn K, Ghandehari H, Brooks BD, Grainger DW. (2014). Nanoparticle toxicity assessment using an in vitro 3-D kidney organoid culture model. Biomaterials. 35(24):6323–31.

Astashkina AI, Mann BK, Prestwich GD, and Grainger DW. (2012). A 3-D organoid kidney culture model engineered for high-throughput nephrotoxicity assays. Biomaterials. 33(18):4700–4711.

Bello AK, Levin A, Tonelli M, Okpechi IG, Feehally J, Harris D, Jindal K. (2017). Assessment of global kidney health care status. JAMA. 317(18):1864–81.

Bennett KM, Zhou H, Sumner JP, Dodd SJ, Bouraoud N, Doi K., Star RA, Koretsky A P. (2008). MRI of the basement membrane using charged nanoparticles as contrast agents. Magn Reson Med. 60(3):564–574.

Bonventre JV. (1993). Mechanisms of ischemic acute renal failure. Kidney Int. 43(5):1160–78.

Brede C, Labhasetwar V. (2013). Applications of nanoparticles in the detection and treatment of kidney diseases. Adv Chronic Kidney Dis. 20(6):454–65.

Breyer MD, Susztak K. (2016). Developing treatments for chronic kidney disease in the 21st century. Semin Nephrol. 36(6), 436–447.

Choi CHJ, Zuckerman JE, Webster P, Davis ME. (2011). Targeting kidney mesangium by nanoparticles of defined size. Proc Natl Acad Sci U S A. 108(16):6656–61.

Clevers H. (2016). Modeling development and disease with organoids. Cell. 165(7):1586–97.

Colombo C, Li M, Watanabe S, Messa P, Edefonti A, Montini G, Moscatelli D, Rastaldi MP, Cellesi F. (2017). Polymer nanoparticle engineering for podocyte repair: From in vitro models to new nanotherapeutics in kidney diseases. ACS Omega. 2(2):599–610.

Dear JW, Kobayashi H, Brechbiel MW, Star RA. (2006). Imaging acute renal failure with polyamine dendrimer-based MRI contrast agents. Nephron Clin Pract. 103(2):c45–9.

Gatoo MA, Naseem S, Arfat MY, Dar AM, Qasim K, Zubair S. (2014). Physicochemical properties of nanomaterials: implication in associated toxic manifestations. Biomed Res Int. 498420.

Gneveckow U, Jordan A, Scholz R, Brüss V, Waldöfner N, Ricke J, Feussner A, Hildebrandt B, Rau B, Wust P. (2004). Description and characterization of the novel hyperthermia- and thermoablation-system MFH 300F for clinical magnetic fluid hyperthermia. Med Phys. 31(6):1444–51.

Goel R, Shah N, Visaria R, Paciotti GF, Bischof JC. (2009). Biodistribution of TNF-alpha-coated gold nanoparticles in an in vivo model system. Nanomedicine (Lond). 4(4):401–10.

Grau V, Herbst B, Steiniger B. (1998). Dynamics of monocytes/macrophages and T lymphocytes in acutely rejecting rat renal allografts. Cell Tissue Res. 291(1):117–26.

Guimaraes AR, Ross R, Figuereido JL, Waterman P, Weissleder R. (2011). MRI with magnetic nanoparticles monitors downstream anti-angiogenic effects of mTOR inhibition. Mol Imaging Biol. 13(2):314–20.

Guo L, Luo S, Du Z, Zhou M, Li P, Fu Y, Sun X, Huang Y, Zhang Z. (2017). Targeted delivery of celastrol to mesangial cells is effective against mesangio proliferative glomerulonephritis. Nat Commun. 12;8(1):878.

Hauger O, Delalande C, Trillaud H, Deminiere C, Quesson B, Kahn H, Cambar J, Combe C, Grenier N. (1999). MR imaging of intrarenal macrophage infiltration in an experimental model of nephrotic syndrome. Magn Reson Med. 41(1):156–62.

Hood E, Simone E, Wattamwar P, Dziubla T, Muzykantov V. (2011). Nanocarriers for vascular delivery of antioxidants. Nanomedicine (Lond). 6(7):1257–72.

Hou J, Wang H, Ge Z, Zuo T, Chen Q, Liu X. (2020). Treating acute kidney injury with anti-oxidative black phosphorus nanosheets. Nano Lett. 20:1447–54.

Hua S, de Matos MBC, Metselaar JM, Storm G. (2018). Current trends and challenges in the clinical translation of nanoparticulate nanomedicines: pathways for translational development and commercialization. Front Pharmacol. 9:1–14.

Hultman KL, Raffo AJ, Grzenda AL, Harris PE, Brown TR, O'Brien S. (2008). Magnetic resonance imaging of major histocompatibility class II expression in the renal medulla using immunotargeted superparamagnetic iron oxide nanoparticles. ACS Nano. 2(3):477–84.

Jang KJ, Mehr AP, Hamilton GA, McPartlin LA, Chung S, Suh KY, Ingber DE. (2013). Human kidney proximal tubule-on-a-chip for drug transport and nephrotoxicity assessment. Integr Biol (Camb). 5(9):1119–29.

Jha V, Garcia-Garcia G, Iseki K, Li Z, Naicker S, Plattner B, Saran R, Wang AYM, Yang CW. (2013). Chronic kidney disease: Global dimension and perspectives. The Lancet. 382(9888):260–72.

Kamaly N, Fredman G, Subramanian M, Gadde S, Pesic A, Cheung L, Fayad ZA, Langer R, Tabas I, Farokhzad OC. (2013). Development and in vivo efficacy of targeted polymeric inflammation-resolving nanoparticles. Proc Natl Acad Sci U S A. 110(16):6506–11.

Kamaly N, He JC, Ausiello DA, Farokhzad OC. (2016). Nanomedicines for renal disease: Current status and future applications. Nat Rev Nephrol. 12(12):738–53.

Kanwar YS, Farquhar MG. (1979). Presence of heparan sulfate in the glomerular basement membrane. Proc Natl Acad Sci U S A. 76(3):1303–7.

Kim S, LesherPerez SCai, Kim BCC, Yamanishi C, Labuz JM, Leung B, Takayama S. (2016). Pharmacokinetic profile that reduces nephrotoxicity of gentamicin in a perfused kidney-on-a-chip. Biofabrication. 8(1):015021.

Kliger AS, Brosius FC. Diabetic kidney disease task force of the American Society of Nephrology (2020). Preserving kidney function instead of replacing it. Clin J Am Soc Nephrol. 15(1):129–31.

Kobayashi H, Jo SK, Kawamoto S, Yasuda H, Hu X, Knopp MV, Brechbiel MW, Choyke PL, Star RA. (2004). Polyamine dendrimer-based MRI contrast agents for functional kidney imaging to diagnose acute renal failure. J Magn Reson Imaging. 20(3):512–8.

Lai X, Geng X, Tan L, Hu J, Wang S. (2020). A pH-Responsive system based on fluorescence enhanced gold nanoparticles for renal targeting drug delivery and fibrosis therapy. Int J Nanomed. 15:5613–27.

Li X, Wang C. (2020). The potential biomedical platforms based on the functionalized Gd@C_{82} nanomaterials. View. 1:1–9.

Liang X, Wang H, Zhu Y, Zhang R, Cogger VC, Liu X, Xu ZP, Grice JE, Roberts MS. (2016). Short- and long-term tracking of anionic ultrasmall nanoparticles in kidney. ACS Nano. 10(1):387–95.

Liu C, Hu Y, Lin J, Fu H, Lim L, Yuan Z. (2018). Targeting strategies for drug delivery to the kidney: From renal glomeruli to tubules, Med Res Rev. 39(2):561–78.

Liu T, Xiao B, Xiang F, Tan J, Chen Z, Zhang X. (2020). Ultrasmall copper-based nanoparticles for reactive oxygen species scavenging and alleviation of inflammation related diseases. Nat Commun. 11:1–16.

Ma Y, Cai F, Li Y, Chen J, Han F, Lin W. (2020). A review of the application of nanoparticles in the diagnosis and treatment of chronic kidney disease. Bioact Mater. 5(3):732–43.

Marom O, Nakhoul F, Tisch U, Shiban A, Abassi Z, Haick H. (2012). Gold nanoparticle sensors for detecting chronic kidney disease and disease progression. Nanomedicine (Lond). 7(5):639–50.

Maslanka Figueroa S, Veser A, Abstiens K, Fleischmann D, Beck S, Goepferich A (2019). Influenza A virus mimetic nanoparticles trigger selective cell uptake. Proceedings of the National Academy of Sciences of the United States of America, 116(20):9831–6.

Michalet X, Pinaud FF, Bentolila LA, Tsay JM, Doose S, Li JJ, Sundaresan G, Wu AM, Gambhir SS, Weiss S. (2005). Quantum dots for live cells, in vivo imaging, and diagnostics. Science. 28;307(5709):538–44.

Mohanta BC, Dinda SC, Palei NN, Deb J. (2019). Solid lipid based nano-particulate formulations in drug targeting, role of novel drug delivery vehicles in nanobiomedicine. IntechOpen, https://www.intechopen.com/chapters/70327.

Mosier-Boss PA. (2017). Review of SERS substrates for chemical sensing. Nanomaterials (Basel). 8;7(6):142.

Nair AV, Keliher EJ, Core AB, Brown D, Weissleder R. (2015). Characterizing the interactions of organic nanoparticles with renal epithelial cells in vivo. ACS Nano, 9(4):3641–53.

Ni D, Jiang D, Kutyreff CJ, Lai J, Yan Y, Barnhart TE. (2018). Molybdenum-based nanoclusters act as antioxidants and ameliorate acute kidney injury in mice. Nat Commun. 9(1):5421.

Ogawa S, Ota Z, Shikata K, Hironaka K, Hayashi Y, Ota K, Kushiro M, Miyatake N, Kishimoto N, Makino H. (1999). High-resolution ultrastructural comparison of renal glomerular and tubular basement membranes. Am J Nephrol. 19(6):686–93.

Ogris M, Brunner S, Schüller S, Kircheis R, Wagner E. (1999). PEGylated DNA/transferrin-PEI complexes: reduced interaction with blood components, extended circulation in blood and potential for systemic gene delivery. Gene Ther. 6(4):595–605.

Oroojalian F, Rezayan AH, Mehrnejad F, Nia AH, Shier WT, Abnous K, Ramezani M. (2017) Efficient megalin targeted delivery to renal proximal tubular cells mediated by modified-polymyxin B-polyethylenimine based nano-gene-carriers. Mater Sci Eng C Mater Biol Appl. 79:770–82.

Pedro RN, Thekke-Adiyat T, Goel R, Shenoi M, Slaton J, Schmechel S, Bischof J, Anderson JK. (2010). Use of tumor necrosis factor-alpha-coated gold nanoparticles to enhance radiofrequency ablation in a translational model of renal tumors. Urology. 76(2):494–8.

Pereira DI, Bruggraber SF, Faria N, Poots LK, Tagmount MA, Aslam MF, Frazer DM, Vulpe CD, Anderson GJ, Powell JJ. (2014). Nanoparticulate iron(III) oxo-hydroxide delivers safe iron that is well absorbed and utilised in humans. Nanomedicine. 10(8):1877–86.

Pollinger K, Hennig R, Breunig M, Tessmar J, Ohlmann A, Tamm ER, Witzgall R, Goepferich A. (2012). Kidney podocytes as specific targets for cyclo(RGDfC)-modified nanoparticles. Small. 8(21):3368–75.

Popa CL, Prodan AM, Ciobanu CS, Predoi D. (2016). The tolerability of dextran-coated iron oxide nanoparticles during in vivo observation of the rats. Gen Physiol Biophys. 35:299–310.

Qi R, Yang C. (2018). Renal tubular epithelial cells: The neglected mediator of tubulointerstitial fibrosis after injury. Cell Death Dis. 9:1126.

Rahman A, Likius D, Uahengo V, Iqbaluddin S. (2017). A mini review highlights on the application of nano-materials for kidney disease: A key development in medicinal therapy. Nephrol Renal Dis. 2(2):1–6.

Rayner H. (2016). Kidney anatomy and physiology—The basis of clinical nephrology. Understanding Kidney Diseases. Springer International Publishing: Switzerland. 22:1–9.

Reddy MK, Labhasetwar V. (2009). Nanoparticle-mediated delivery of superoxide dismutase to the brain: an effective strategy to reduce ischemia-reperfusion injury. FASEB J. 23(5):1384–95.

Reddy MK, Wu L, Kou W, Ghorpade A, Labhasetwar V. (2008). Superoxide dismutase-loaded PLGA nanoparticles protect cultured human neurons under oxidative stress. Appl Biochem Biotechnol. 151(2–3):565–77.

Rosenkrans ZT, Sun T, Jiang D, Chen W, Barnhart TE, Zhang Z. (2020). Selenium-doped carbon quantum dots act as broad-spectrum antioxidants for acute kidney injury management. Adv Sci. 7:1–11.

Ruggiero A, Villa CH, Bander E, Rey DA, Bergkvist M, Batt CA, Manova-Todorova K, Deen WM, Scheinberg DA, McDevitt MR. (2010). Paradoxical glomerular filtration of carbon nanotubes. Proc Natl Acad Sci U S A. 107(27):12369–74.

Saifi MA, Peddakkulappagari CS, Ahmad A, Godugu C. (2020). Leveraging the pathophysiological alterations of obstructive nephropathy to treat renal fibrosis by cerium oxide nanoparticles. ACS Biomater Sci Eng. 6:3563–3573.

Schott H, Woodie J. (2012). Kidneys and ureters. Equine Surgery. 913–26.

Selc M, Razga F, Nemethova V, Mazancova P, Ursinyova M, Novotova M, Kopecka K, Gabelova A, Babelova A. (2020). Surface coating determines the inflammatory potential of magnetite nanoparticles in murine renal podocytes and mesangial cells. RSC Adv. 10(40):23916–29.

Shirai T, Kohara H, Tabata Y. (2012). Inflammation imaging by silica nanoparticles with antibodies orientedly immobilized. J Drug Target. 20(6):535–43.

Singh AP, Biswas A, Shukla A, Maiti P. (2019). Targeted therapy in chronic diseases using nanomaterial-based drug delivery vehicles. Sig Transduct Target Ther. 4(1):1–21.

Song X, Zhu W, Ge X, Li R Li S, Chen X, Song J, Xie J, Chen X, Yang H. (2021). A new class of NIR-II gold nanoclusters-based protein biolabels for in vivo tumor-targeted imaging. Angew Chemie Int Ed. 17:1306–12.

Stamopoulos D, Manios E, Gogola V, Benaki D, Bouziotis P, Niarchos D, Pissas M. (2008). Bare and protein-conjugated Fe_3O_4 ferromagnetic nanoparticles for utilization in magnetically assisted hemodialysis: biocompatibility with human blood cells. Nanotechnology. 17;19(50):505101.

Suh JH, Miner JH. (2013). The glomerular basement membrane as a barrier to albumin. Nat Rev Nephrol. 9(8):470–7.

Tasciotti E, Cabrera FJ, Evangelopoulos M, Martinez JO, Thekkedath U R, Kloc M, Ghobrial RM, Li XC, Grattoni A, Ferrari M. (2016). The emerging role of nanotechnology in cell and organ transplantation. Transplantation, 100(8), 1629–38.

Thorner PS. (2007). Alport syndrome and thin basement membrane nephropathy. Nephron Clin Pract. 106(2):c82–88.

Vernekar AA, Sinha D, Srivastava S, Paramasivam PU, D'Silva P, Mugesh G. (2014). An antioxidant nanozyme that uncovers the cytoprotective potential of vanadia nanowires. Nat Commun. 21(5):5301.

Visweswaran GRR, Gholizadeh S, Ruiters MHJ, Molema G, Kok RJ, Kamps JAAM. (2015). Targeting rapamycin to podocytes using a vascular cell adhesion molecule-1 (VCAM-1)-harnessed SAINT-based lipid carrier system. PLoS ONE. 10(9):1–17

Vormann MK, Gijzen L, Hutter S, Boot L, Nicolas A, van den Heuvel A, Vriend J, Ng CP, Nieskens TTG, van Duinen V, de Wagenaar B, Masereeuw R, Suter-Dick L, Trietsch SJ, Wilmer M, Joore J, Vulto P, Lanz HL. (2018). Nephrotoxicity and kidney transport assessment on 3D perfused proximal tubules. AAPS J. 20(5):90.

Waikar SS, Bonventre JV. (2009). Creatinine kinetics and the definition of acute kidney injury. J Am Soc Nephrol. 20(3):672–9.

Williams RM, Shah J, Ng BD, Minton DR, Gudas LJ, Park CY, Heller DA. (2015). Mesoscale nanoparticles selectively target the renal proximal tubule epithelium. Nano Lett. 15(4), 2358–64.

Williams RM, Jaimes EA, Heller DA. (2016). Nanomedicines for kidney diseases. Kidney Int. 90(4):740–5.

Wu L, Chen M, Mao H, Ningning W, Bo Z, Zhao X, Qian J, Xing C. (2017). Albumin-based nanoparticles as methylprednisolone carriers for targeted delivery towards the neonatal Fc receptor in glomerular podocytes. Int J Mol Med. 39(4):851–60.

Yin L, Du G, Zhang B. (2020) Efficient drug screening and nephrotoxicity assessment on co-culture microfluidic kidney chip. Sci Rep. 10:6568.

Zhao H, Li L L, Zhan H, Chu Y, Sun B. (2019). Mechanistic understanding of the engineered nanomaterial-induced toxicity on kidney. J Nanomater. 1–12.

Zhao P, Chen X, Wang Q, Zou H, Xie Y, Liu H. (2020). Differential toxicity mechanism of gold nanoparticles in HK-2 renal proximal tubular cells and 786-0 carcinoma cells. Nanomedicine. 15:1079–1096.

Zhou M, Ma H, Lin H, Qin J. (2014). Induction of epithelial-to-mesenchymal transition in proximal tubular epithelial cells on microfluidic devices. Biomaterials. 35(5):1390–1401.

Zuckerman JE, Choi CHJ, Han H, Davis ME. (2012). Polycation-SiRNA nanoparticles can disassemble at the kidney glomerular basement membrane. Proc Natl Acad Sci U S A. 109(8):3137–42.

8 Materials for Liver Regeneration, Liver-Cell Targeting, and Normal Liver Tissue Care

Ashirbad Nanda and Chinmaya Chidananda Behera
Centurion University of Technology and Management

Dilip Kumar Patel and Vikas Kumar
Sam Higginbottom University of Agriculture,
Technology and Sciences

Bhisma N Ratha and Simanchal Panda
Centurion University of Technology and Management

CONTENTS

DOI: 10.1201/9781003140108-8

8.1 INTRODUCTION

The Global Burden of Disease Study of 2017 identified chronic liver disease (CLD) as a substantial health and economic burden in most developed countries. CLD claimed 1.32 million lives in 2017 alone (GBD Cirrhosis Collaborators 2020). Not only that, there is an alarming increase in the mortality rate through the recent past. The most common aetiologies of chronic liver diseases in developed countries are ascribed to viral hepatitis and alcoholic liver disease. Moreover, the prevalence of non-alcoholic fatty liver disease (NAFLD) is rapidly increasing, and non-alcoholic steatohepatitis (NASH) has become a leading indication for liver transplantation as CLD has a long latent period, so accurate determination is difficult.

A suitable liver-to-body-weight ratio is required to maintain physiological homeostasis, and the process is termed "hepatostat" (Michalopoulos 2013; 2017). There is a correlation between liver weight and a liver-function examination such as aspartate aminotransferase (AST) or alanine aminotransferase (ALT), proving itself a milestone to detect the hepatostat (Elinav et al. 2005). However, the quest is not over yet; the availability of limited organ donors is a stumbling block with liver transplantation or CLD management (Anand et al. 2020). Either way, hepatic tissue engineering with application of nanomaterials paves a new way to overcome this problem (Vivero-Escoto et al. 2019; Giri et al. 2012). Tissue engineering utilizes various nanomaterials that mimic the hepatic cells and target them in different stages of proliferation and diseased condition (Giannitrapani et al. 2014). So briefly, tissue engineering serves as a scaffold (i.e., a three-dimensional environment for making new viable tissues with a medical purpose). For liver tissue engineering purposes, matrices of bio-compatible synthetic, bio-derived materials, surface-modified protein-coated nanofibers, and decellularized biomatrix are used to regulate cell function and activity (Sengupta and Prasad 2018; Niemczyk-Soczynska, Gradys, and Sajkiewicz 2020; Naahidi et al. 2017; Lin et al. 2004; Li et al. 2013; Arslan, Efe, and Sezgin Arslan 2019). However, these matrix-based engineered liver tissues lack a vascular system, which is highly essential to transport nutrient and oxygen. Hence, it is highly essential to develop a scaffold that will maintain the blood flow for tricky metabolic balance in the hepatic tissue fulfilling the clinical application. Recent developments in three dimensional (3D) bio-printing technology will make it possible to overcome complex issues in relation to tissue engineering (Wu et al. 2020; Egan, Shea, and Ferguson 2018). Also, it will minimize the need for organ donors. Lastly, this regenerative medicine and tissue engineering depend on two significant elements: 1) adoptable biological scaffold without any graft rejection and 2) appropriate cells—stem cells or primary cells that efficiently restore the damaged tissues without any undesirable consequences (Bracey et al. 2019; Kolios and Moodley 2013). So knowledge of hepatic cell proliferation kinetics is a must for tissue engineering.

8.2 CELL BIOLOGY OF HEPATIC CELLS

Most of the metabolic activities in our body are performed by the liver. Liver consists of precursor cells (oval cells), parenchymal cells such as Kuppfer cells, hepatocytes, fibroblasts, stellate cells, sinusoidal epithelial cells, and epithelial and biliary epithelial cells with an intricate array of vasculature cells (Begum et al. 2010). Most of the metabolic functions (i.e., 70%) such as plasma protein synthesis, glucose homeostasis, ketogenesis, urea synthesis, and xenobiotic metabolism are performed in the hepatocytes (Rui 2014). Thus, the engineered/scaffolding materials used for hepatocyte tissue regeneration must perform/support these essential functions and be non-antigenic to avoid graft rejection.

8.2.1 THE DARK SIDE OF LR: RECURRENT HEPATOCYTE PROLIFERATION

Metabolic diseases, toxic chemicals, alcohol as well as non-alcoholic steatohepatitis, and viruses are causes of hepatocyte death. Here, it's important to note that continual exposure to hepatotoxic entities, as in CLD can lead to hepatocellular carcinoma. Moreover, a clear understanding of correlation between hepatic tissue regeneration and hepatocellular carcinoma can provide a controlled hepatic cell regeneration method.

Damaged hepatocytes trigger regeneration, causing the reinstatement of hepatocyte ploidy (2n, 4n, and 8n) (Yao et al. 2012). Reactive oxygen species (ROS) and reactive electrophiles (peroxidation products) cause hepatocyte injury. These genotoxic agents are associated with genomic alterations and DNA damage (Kay et al. 2019). The genomic alteration due to the etiologies mentioned earlier triggers allelic imbalance, affecting genes for growth control such as p53, EGFR, telomerases, etc. (Liu, Chen, and St Clair 2008; Cong, Wright, and Shay 2002). It initiates clonal growth and hepatocellular carcinoma, leading to neoplastic initiation; this is the dark side of regeneration. Thus targeting of hepatic cells should be biased, avoiding the oncogene-containing cells.

8.2.2 HEPATIC CELL PROLIFERATION KINETICS

The hepatic cells (i.e. hepatocytes and cholangiocytes) are the first to proceed into mitosis. Proliferation subsides by day 5–7 (Manco et al. 2019). Accumulation of triglycerides happens at 2–3 days in the hepatocytes (Magami et al. 2002; Kawano and Cohen 2013). Activation of Cyclin D1,followed by migration to the nucleus, compels hepatocytes for DNA synthesis (Nunez et al. 2017). The proliferation of hepatocytes starts from the lobule (pericentral region) (Abu Rmilah et al. 2019). Replication of Stellate cells starts 1–2 days after the hepatocytes (Michalopoulos 2007). The incoming cells from bone marrow (endothelial cells replaced by endothelial progenitor cells) get fenestrations after the colonization of hepatic sinusoids, and they produce HGF (Wang et al. 2012). Lastly, the replication of Kupffer cells happens after monocytes migrate from blood and bone marrow (Ju and Tacke 2016).

8.3 LIVER INFLAMMATION AND FIBROSIS

Cell specificity increases the availability at the critical target cell or tissue while reducing presumed toxicity for other cell types. Researchers have proved that conventional formulations for treating liver disease containing γ (IFNγ), angiotensin II, and interleukin 10 showed significant results in the preclinical studies but lacked promising results in human trials because of low cell specificity (Zhang and Wang 2006; Lubel et al. 2008; Attallah et al. 2016). If delivered nonspecifically, IFNγ will show a proinflammatory effect on macrophages (Arango Duque and Descoteaux 2014).

Due to the advantage of cell-type specificity on binding to a specific surface structure, nanomaterial-based drugs may overcome the challenges of traditionally formulated drugs. Moreover, nanosystems may overcome biological barriers based on their sizes, protect the drug from being metabolized, facilitate the delivery of undeliverable drugs, enable a prolonged drug release, thereby enhance the pharmacological features of the drug (Bartneck, Peters, et al. 2014; Bisht et al. 2011; Dong et al. 2014; Minati et al. 2012). Since many common drugs have limited efficacy because of their low concentration at the target site. A nano-drug delivery technique may assist in overcoming the concentration based minimal efficacy because of their target specificity.

8.4 CELL TYPES OF LIVER UNDER HEALTHY AND DISEASED CONDITIONS

There are four major cell types in the liver (hepatocytes as the major parenchymal cells, and three major non-parenchymal cell types: hepatic stellate cells (HSC), macrophages, and LSEC); all of them are critically involved in liver disease progression. They could be more promising cellular targets for nanomedicine. Most of the liver volume (i.e., 80%) is occupied by hepatocytes (parenchymal cells), and the rest is made up of non-parenchymal cells. The hepatocytes have a continuous self-renewal process in the liver (i.e., 200 days in mice and 400 days in rats) (Magami et al. 2002; Macdonald 1961). Healthy hepatocytes fulfil many of the liver's key functions such as carbohydrate turnover, cholesterol synthesis, protein synthesis, bile salts and phospholipids synthesis, eliminations of exogenous substances and endogenous substances, and detoxification. Liver health is disrupted by viral infections, alcohol intake, etc., which provoke apoptosis of liver cells, ultimately causing liver fibrogenesis. For such cases, nanomedicines targeting liver cells have potential therapeutic applications.

8.5 NANOMEDICINE FOR LIVER HEALTH AND DISEASES

Various methodologies have been designed to tailor the nanomaterials based on charge, compliance, size, and synthetic construction for a significant preclinical focus for targeting specific liver cells.

8.5.1 MACROPHAGE ACTIVATION USING NANOMEDICINE

Various research groups have reported solely on the immunomodulatory activity of nanoparticles on macrophages of liver cells; mainly, the Kupffer cells are in the spotlight because of their critical role in liver inflammation and fibrogenesis. Moreover, Kupffer cells are well known for efficient and unspecific nanomaterial uptake (Bartneck, Warzecha, and Tacke 2014). Reports show the ease of polarizability of Kupffer cells macrophage by introduction of peptide-conjugated nanoparticles (van der Heide, Weiskirchen, and Bansal 2019).

Monoclonal antibody infliximab (anti-TNF antibody) is used for treating acute hepatitis. Administration of this drug in the form of conventional dosage form inhibits the proinflammatory cytokines, leading to increased bacterial infection rate. To make it target specific, the nanoparticle is a tailored mannose-modified trimethyl chitosan-cystein, which will be specifically uptaken by a macrophage-specific route of Kupffer cell through mannose receptors (He et al. 2013). This approach is more promising in lipopolysaccharide/D-galactosamine liver disease after oral administration in the mouse model (He et al. 2013). Recently, research work has focused on targeting antigen-presenting cells (APC), which are a promising target in liver cancer progression (Mossanen and Tacke 2013; Chang et al. 2020). In this way, targeting macrophages as well as APC plays a crucial role in tissue specific targeting.

8.5.2 Nanomedicine for Liver Sinusoidal Endothelial Cells (LSECs)

Liver sinusoidal endothelial cells (LSECs) have phagocytic activities similar to those of macrophages and can be a remarkable target for cell-specific drug delivery of nanoparticles. Carboxy-modified micelles, which are associated with T-cell antigens on their surface, effectively target LSES. These micelles can deliver antigens, which in turn will assist in generating regulatory T-cells to induce tolerance against autoantibodies. Taken together, the micelles with carboxy-modification will aid in overcoming autoimmune disorders, and it is a pioneering approach in the development of immunomodulatory nanoparticles with varied functions (Bartneck, Ritz, et al. 2012; Bartneck, Keul, et al. 2012; Freund et al. 2021). In another approach, researchers have demonstrated preferential in vitro uptake of viral components by LSECs, such as fluorescent viral particles and the gold nanoparticles coated with viral proteins. Such viral components masked with nanoparticles will assist specific cellular targets to deliver desired drug.

8.5.3 Role of Nanomedicine in Targeting Hepatic Cells

Liver cells lack specific receptors that can differentiate them from other cells; hence it is challenging for researchers to develop specific targeting tools for liver cells. However, developing nanocomplexes mimicking the natural macromolecules like lipoproteins have potential for development of hepatocyte targeting nanomedicines. A nano complex of lipopeptide nanoparticles (LPNPs) is used to mimic apolipoprotein, which aids in delivering siRNA to liver cells through dynamine dependent micropinocytosis. Recently peptide derived from hepatitis B virus large envelope protein (HBVpreS) was used as LPNP to specifically target the sodium-taurocholate cotransporting polypeptide, which is found the sinusoidal membrane of hepatocytes; internalization of nanoparticles was demonstrated in vitro and in vivo (Witzigmann et al. 2019). In addition, lipopeptide-based drug delivery liposomal drug delivery systems have shown promising results, such as liposomes loaded with polyphenolic compound quercetin, which have proven to reduce the hepatic fibrosis induced by arsenite poisoning (Mandal et al. 2007). Further, it was shown that glactosylation of the liposome improved the hepatic cell specificity, through interaction with the galactosyl receptor of hepatic cells (Sonoke et al. 2011; Xia et al. 2019; Mishra et al. 2013).

8.6 NANOMATERIALS FOR LIVER REGENERATION

For hepatic cell regenerative studies, mainly nanofiber materials are employed, because fiber structure can provide a scaffolding architecture for growth of the hepatic cells. Liver tissue engineering transplantation is one prominent approach for treating hepatic failure and cirrhosis. Using collagen-coated nanofibers as a supporting matrix, primary hepatic cells of rats were grown for a week, which showed certain features of hepatic cells such as albumin secretion and collagen storage activities (Bierwolf et al. 2011). Hydrogel-forming self-assembling peptide nanofibers (SAPNFs) are utilized as extracellular matrix for growing primary culture of porcine hepatic cell (Navarro-Alvarez et al. 2006). Here hepatic cells were grown on SAPNF hydrogel and collagen-coated fiber, cells grown on SAPNF hydrogel showed promising results after a week, which distinctly showed the hepatic cell morphology (Navarro-Alvarez et al. 2006). Further, the activity of the cells grown in hydrogel were maintained even after two weeks. It is worthwhile to mention that the physiochemical and biological properties of the hydrogel play crucial role in sustaining the growth and activity of the hepatic cells (Ye et al. 2019). Earlier, cells were grown as monolayer culture, but recent advancements in cell culture technology, allows 3D growth of cells under in vitro condition. (Jia et al. 2020). In 3D culture, the aggregated hepatic cell expresses connexin 32. Here, connexin 32 aids in hepatic cell communication. Such cell-to-cell communication is absent in a typical monolayer cell culture. Recently Bai et al. critically reviewed the scaffolding properties of graphene-based nanomaterials concerning hepatic cell culture. The authors argue the importance of graphene nanomaterials in tissue engineering (Bai et al. 2019). In another study, the authors have demonstrated the 60–70% increased survival of liver-cirrhosis rats by transplanting CYNK-10 human cell line, which was grown on SAPNF hydrogel scaffold (Navarro-Alvarez et al. 2010). Further advancement in 3D printing technology has enabled the use of multiple materials by the electrospinning method to produce scaffolds of desired shape and size. Using collagen, polycaprolactone, and polyethersulfone 3D-printed scaffold to grow mesenchymal stem cells isolated from human bone marrow exhibited two times higher efficiency to differentiate into hepatocytes in comparison to 2D cell culture (Kazemnejad et al. 2009). Peptides derived from natural sources have shown promising results in tissue engineering techniques, which can be further exploited for finding a suitable scaffolding material.

8.7 CONCLUSIONS AND FUTURE PERSPECTIVES

The ever-increasing global health burden of hepatic diseases requires research attention, as liver is a vital organ of the body. Though it has auto-regenerative capabilities, the fast-moving life of industrial era has hastened the regenerative ability of liver. Under such circumstances liver tissue engineering and therapeutics specifically targeting to liver cells can be of high use. It is clear from this chapter that the first generation of nanomedicine prepared with liposomes and micelles has demonstrated promising results for cell targeting. There are several approved drug products with liposomal drug formulation for targeted drug delivery. The emergence of 3D-printing technology and swelling numbers of biocompatible synthetic/natural nanomaterials together have facilitated the in vitro growth of hepatic cells. Some of the significant nanomedicine and drug combinations are listed in Table 8.1, which were tested in different disease models. Moreover, a parallel improvement in the stem cell biology has the potential to eliminate the requirement of organ donors.

TABLE 8.1
Nano Medicines and Hepatic Cell Targets

Type of Nanomedicine	Drug	Target Cell	Disease Model	Remarks	References
COOH-micelles		LSCE and T-Cell	Autoimmune disease	Improvement, restoration of tolerance	(Freund et al. 2021)
GalLip	Quercetin, galactosyl receptor	Hepatocytes	AILF	Reduction in liver fibrosis	(Mandal et al. 2007)
RGD-PM-OM	Oxymatrine, integrins	HSC	BDL-based fibrosis	Fibrosis reduction	(Yang et al. 2014)
NanoCurcTM	Integrins, curcumin	Targeting endocytic apparatus	HSC (and others), induction of HS capoptosis	Carbon tetrachloride (CCl4)-based fibrosis	(Bisht et al. 2007)
Fluorescent liposomes	Dexamethasone	Macrophages, T cells	ConA hepatitis, CCl4-based fibrosis	Prevention of hepatitis, attenuation of fibrosis	(Bisht et al. 2011)
Retinoldecorated liposomes	HSP47-siRNA, RBP	HSC	BDL, DEN, CCl4- based fibrosis	Fibrosis reversal	(Sato et al. 2008)
SSL decorated with pPB	IFNγ	HSC	TAA (chronic)- based fibrosis	Decreased fibrosis	(Li et al. 2012)
M6P-HAS liposomes	Rosiglitazone	HSC	BDL/ CCl4- based chronic liver injury	Reduction of fibrosis	(Patel, Kher, and Misra 2012; Luk et al. 2007)
MTC	TNF-siRNA, TNF	Macrophages	Acute LPS/D-GalN	Attenuation of hepatic injury, prolongation of survival	(He et al. 2013)
AuNR (gold nanorods) with RGD or GLF peptide	No drug, phagosome	Macrophages	6 weeks CCl$_4$, acute ConA	No effects on fibrosis, exacerbation of ConA hepatitis	(Bartneck, Ritz, et al. 2012)

Note: AILF(arsenic-induced liver fibrosis); AuNRs (gold nanorods); BDL (bile duct ligation); CCl4 (carbon tetrachloride); ConA(concanavalin A); COOH (carboxy group), cRGD-SSL(cyclic RGD-modified sterically stabilized liposomes); DEN (diethylnitrosamine); DMN (dimethylnitrosamine); ECM (extracellular matrix); FFA (free fatty acids); GalLip (galactosylated liposomes); GSH (glutathione); HGF (hepatocyte growth factor); HSC (hepatic stellate cells); HSP47(heat-shock protein 47); LPS/D-GalN (lipopolysaccharide/D-galactosamine); LPNP (lipopeptide nanoparticles); MTC (mannose-modified trimethyl chitosan-cysteine conjugate nanoparticles); pPB (peptide vs. PDGFβR); NanoCurc, polymeric compound; RGD-PM-OM (polymerosomes equipped with surface RGD and encapsulated oxymatrine); RGD-LP (RGD-decorated lipoprotein); RBP (retinol binding protein); SSL (sterically stabilized liposomes); TAA (thioacetamide); Treg (regulatory T cell).

ABBREVIATIONS

AILF	arsenic-induced liver fibrosis
ALT	alanine aminotransferase
APC	antigen-presenting cells
AuNRs	gold nanorods
BDL	bile duct ligation
CCl4	carbon tetrachloride
CLD	chronic liver disease
ConA	concanavalin A
cRGD-SSL	cyclic RGD-modified sterically stabilized liposomes
CYNK	natural killer cells
DEN	diethylnitrosamine
DMN	dimethylnitrosamine
ECM	extracellular matrix
EGFR	epidermal growth factor
FFA	free fatty acids
GalLip	galactosylated liposomes
GBD	Global Burden of Disease
GSH	glutathione
HBVpreS	hepatitis B virus large envelope protein
HGF	hepatocyte growth factor
LPNP	lipopeptide nanoparticle
LSEC	liver sinusoidal endothelial cell
NAFLD	non-alcoholic fatty liver disease
NASH	non-alcoholic steatohepatitis
ROS	reactive oxygen species
SAPNF	self-assembling peptide nanofiber

REFERENCES

Abu Rmilah, A., W. Zhou, E. Nelson, L. Lin, B. Amiot, and S. L. Nyberg. 2019. "Understanding the marvels behind liver regeneration." *Wiley Interdisc Rev Dev Biol* 8 (3):e340. doi: 10.1002/wdev.340.

Anand, A. C., B. Nandi, S. K. Acharya, A. Arora, S. Babu, Y. Batra, Y. K. Chawla, A. Chowdhury, A. Chaoudhuri, E. C. Eapen, H. Devarbhavi, R. Dhiman, S. Datta Gupta, A. Duseja, D. Jothimani, D. Kapoor, P. Kar, M. S. Khuroo, A. Kumar, K. Madan, B. Mallick, R. Maiwall, N. Mohan, A. Nagral, P. Nath, S. C. Panigrahi, A. Pawar, C. A. Philips, D. Prahraj, P. Puri, A. Rastogi, V. A. Saraswat, S. Saigal, Shalimar, A. Shukla, S. P. Singh, T. Verghese, M. Wadhawan, and INASL Task-Force on Acute Liver Failure. 2020. "Indian National Association for the Study of the Liver Consensus Statement on Acute Liver Failure (Part 1): Epidemiology, Pathogenesis, Presentation and Prognosis." *J Clin Exp Hepatol* 10 (4):339–76. doi: 10.1016/j.jceh.2020.04.012.

Arango Duque, G., and A. Descoteaux. 2014. "Macrophage cytokines: involvement in immunity and infectious diseases." *Front Immunol* 5:491. doi: 10.3389/fimmu.2014.00491.

Arslan, Y. E., B. Efe, and T. Sezgin Arslan. 2019. "A novel method for constructing an acellular 3D biomatrix from bovine spinal cord for neural tissue engineering applications." *Biotechnol Prog* 35 (4):e2814. doi: 10.1002/btpr.2814.

Attallah, A. M., M. El-Far, F. Zahran, G. E. Shiha, K. Farid, M. M. Omran, M. A. Abdelrazek, A. A. Attallah, A. A. El-Beh, R. M. El-Hosiny, and A. M. El-Waseef. 2016. "Interferon-gamma is associated with hepatic dysfunction in fibrosis, cirrhosis, and hepatocellular carcinoma." *J Immunoassay Immunochem* 37 (6):597–610. doi: 10.1080/15321819.2016.1179646.

Bartneck, M., H. A. Keul, M. Wambach, J. Bornemann, U. Gbureck, N. Chatain, S. Neuss, F. Tacke, J. Groll, and G. Zwadlo-Klarwasser. 2012. "Effects of nanoparticle surface-coupled peptides, functional endgroups, and charge on intracellular distribution and functionality of human primary reticuloendothelial cells." *Nanomedicine* 8 (8):1282–92. doi: 10.1016/j.nano.2012.02.012.

Bartneck, M., F. M. Peters, K. T. Warzecha, M. Bienert, L. van Bloois, C. Trautwein, T. Lammers, and F. Tacke. 2014. "Liposomal encapsulation of dexamethasone modulates cytotoxicity, inflammatory cytokine response, and migratory properties of primary human macrophages." *Nanomedicine* 10 (6):1209–20. doi: 10.1016/j.nano.2014.02.011.

Bartneck, M., T. Ritz, H. A. Keul, M. Wambach, J. Bornemann, U. Gbureck, J. Ehling, T. Lammers, F. Heymann, N. Gassler, T. Ludde, C. Trautwein, J. Groll, and F. Tacke. 2012. "Peptide-functionalized gold nanorods increase liver injury in hepatitis." *ACS Nano* 6 (10):8767–77. doi: 10.1021/nn302502u.

Bartneck, M., K. T. Warzecha, and F. Tacke. 2014. "Therapeutic targeting of liver inflammation and fibrosis by nanomedicine." *Hepatobiliary Surg Nutr* 3 (6):364–76. doi: 10.3978/j.issn.2304-3881.2014.11.02.

Begum, S., M. Joshi, M. Ek, J. Holgersson, M. I. Kleman, and S. Sumitran-Holgersson. 2010. "Characterization and engraftment of long-term serum-free human fetal liver cell cultures." *Cytotherapy* 12 (2):201–11. doi: 10.3109/14653240903398053.

Bierwolf, J., M. Lutgehetmann, K. Feng, J. Erbes, S. Deichmann, E. Toronyi, C. Stieglitz, B. Nashan, P. X. Ma, and J. M. Pollok. 2011. "Primary rat hepatocyte culture on 3D nanofibrous polymer scaffolds for toxicology and pharmaceutical research." *Biotechnol Bioeng* 108 (1):141–50. doi: 10.1002/bit.22924.

Bisht, S., G. Feldmann, S. Soni, R. Ravi, C. Karikar, A. Maitra, and A. Maitra. 2007. "Polymeric nanoparticle-encapsulated curcumin ("nanocurcumin"): a novel strategy for human cancer therapy." *J Nanobiotechnology* 5:3. doi: 10.1186/1477-3155-5-3.

Bisht, S., M. A. Khan, M. Bekhit, H. Bai, T. Cornish, M. Mizuma, M. A. Rudek, M. Zhao, A. Maitra, B. Ray, D. Lahiri, A. Maitra, and R. A. Anders. 2011. "A polymeric nanoparticle formulation of curcumin (NanoCurc) ameliorates CCl4-induced hepatic injury and fibrosis through reduction of pro-inflammatory cytokines and stellate cell activation." *Lab Invest* 91 (9):1383–95. doi: 10.1038/labinvest.2011.86.

Bracey, D. N., T. M. Seyler, A. H. Jinnah, T. L. Smith, D. A. Ornelles, R. Deora, G. D. Parks, M. E. Van Dyke, and P. W. Whitlock. 2019. "A porcine xenograft-derived bone scaffold is a biocompatible bone graft substitute: An assessment of cytocompatibility and the alpha-Gal epitope." *Xenotransplantation* 26 (5):e12534. doi: 10.1111/xen.12534.

Chang, H. C., Z. Z. Zou, Q. H. Wang, J. Li, H. Jin, Q. X. Yin, and D. Xing. 2020. "Targeting and Specific Activation of Antigen-Presenting Cells by Endogenous Antigen-Loaded Nanoparticles Elicits Tumor-Specific Immunity." *Adv Sci (Weinh)* 7 (1):1900069. doi: 10.1002/advs.201900069.

Cong, Y. S., W. E. Wright, and J. W. Shay. 2002. "Human telomerase and its regulation." *Microbiol Mol Biol Rev* 66 (3):407–25, table of contents. doi: 10.1128/mmbr.66.3. 407-425.2002.

Dong, Y., K. T. Love, J. R. Dorkin, S. Sirirungruang, Y. Zhang, D. Chen, R. L. Bogorad, H. Yin, Y. Chen, A. J. Vegas, C. A. Alabi, G. Sahay, K. T. Olejnik, W. Wang, A. Schroeder, A. K. Lytton-Jean, D. J. Siegwart, A. Akinc, C. Barnes, S. A. Barros, M. Carioto, K. Fitzgerald, J. Hettinger, V. Kumar, T. I. Novobrantseva, J. Qin,

W. Querbes, V. Koteliansky, R. Langer, and D. G. Anderson. 2014. "Lipopeptide nanoparticles for potent and selective siRNA delivery in rodents and nonhuman primates." *Proc Natl Acad Sci U S A* 111 (11):3955–60. doi: 10.1073/pnas.1322937111.

Egan, P. F., K. A. Shea, and S. J. Ferguson. 2018. "Simulated tissue growth for 3D printed scaffolds." *Biomech Model Mechanobiol* 17 (5):1481–95. doi: 10.1007/s10237-018-1040-9.

Elinav, E., I. Z. Ben-Dov, E. Ackerman, A. Kiderman, F. Glikberg, Y. Shapira, and Z. Ackerman. 2005. "Correlation between serum alanine aminotransferase activity and age: an inverted U curve pattern." *Am J Gastroenterol* 100 (10):2201–4. doi: 10.1111/j.1572-0241.2005.41822.x.

Freund, Barbara, Jörg Heeren, Peter Nielsen, Antonella Carambia, Johannes Herkel, Oliver Bruns, Ansgar Lohse, Stefan Lüth, Horst Weller, and Sunhild Salmen. 2021. *Nanoparticle compositions for generation of regulatory T cells and treatment of autoimmune diseases and other chronic inflammatory conditions.* Google Patents.

GBD Cirrhosis Collaborators. 2020. "The global, regional, and national burden of cirrhosis by cause in 195 countries and territories, 1990–2017: a systematic analysis for the Global Burden of Disease Study 2017." *Lancet Gastroenterol Hepatol* 5 (3):245–66. doi: 10.1016/S2468-1253(19)30349-8.

Geetha Bai, R., K. Muthoosamy, S. Manickam, and A. Hilal-Alnaqbi. 2019. "Graphene-based 3D scaffolds in tissue engineering: fabrication, applications, and future scope in liver tissue engineering." *Int J Nanomedicine* 14:5753–83. doi: 10.2147/IJN.S192779.

Giannitrapani, L., M. Soresi, M. L. Bondi, G. Montalto, and M. Cervello. 2014. "Nanotechnology applications for the therapy of liver fibrosis." *World J Gastroenterol* 20 (23):7242–51. doi: 10.3748/wjg.v20.i23.7242.

Giri, S., A. Acikgoz, P. Pathak, S. Gutschker, A. Kursten, K. Nieber, and A. Bader. 2012. "Three dimensional cultures of rat liver cells using a natural self-assembling nanoscaffold in a clinically relevant bioreactor for bioartificial liver construction." *J Cell Physiol* 227 (1):313–27. doi: 10.1002/jcp.22738.

He, C., L. Yin, C. Tang, and C. Yin. 2013. "Multifunctional polymeric nanoparticles for oral delivery of TNF-alpha siRNA to macrophages." *Biomaterials* 34 (11):2843–54. doi: 10.1016/j.biomaterials.2013.01.033.

Jia, Z., Y. Cheng, X. Jiang, C. Zhang, G. Wang, J. Xu, Y. Li, Q. Peng, and Y. Gao. 2020. "3D Culture System for Liver Tissue Mimicking Hepatic Plates for Improvement of Human Hepatocyte (C3A) Function and Polarity." *Biomed Res Int* 2020:6354183. doi: 10.1155/2020/6354183.

Ju, C., and F. Tacke. 2016. "Hepatic macrophages in homeostasis and liver diseases: from pathogenesis to novel therapeutic strategies." *Cell Mol Immunol* 13 (3):316–27. doi: 10.1038/cmi.2015.104.

Kawano, Y., and D. E. Cohen. 2013. "Mechanisms of hepatic triglyceride accumulation in non-alcoholic fatty liver disease." *J Gastroenterol* 48 (4):434–41. doi: 10.1007/s00535-013-0758-5.

Kay, J., E. Thadhani, L. Samson, and B. Engelward. 2019. "Inflammation-induced DNA damage, mutations and cancer." *DNA Repair (Amst)* 83:102673. doi: 10.1016/j.dnarep.2019.102673.

Kazemnejad, S., A. Allameh, M. Soleimani, A. Gharehbaghian, Y. Mohammadi, N. Amirizadeh, and M. Jazayery. 2009. "Biochemical and molecular characterization of hepatocyte-like cells derived from human bone marrow mesenchymal stem cells on a novel three-dimensional biocompatible nanofibrous scaffold." *J Gastroenterol Hepatol* 24 (2):278–87. doi: 10.1111/j.1440-1746.2008.05530.x.

Kolios, G., and Y. Moodley. 2013. "Introduction to stem cells and regenerative medicine." *Respiration* 85 (1):3–10. doi: 10.1159/000345615.

Li, F., Q. H. Li, J. Y. Wang, C. Y. Zhan, C. Xie, and W. Y. Lu. 2012. "Effects of interferon-gamma liposomes targeted to platelet-derived growth factor receptor-beta on hepatic fibrosis in rats." *J Control Release* 159 (2):261–70. doi: 10.1016/j.jconrel.2011.12.023.

Li, Y. S., H. J. Harn, D. K. Hsieh, T. C. Wen, Y. M. Subeq, L. Y. Sun, S. Z. Lin, and T. W. Chiou. 2013. "Cells and materials for liver tissue engineering." *Cell Transplant* 22 (4):685–700. doi: 10.3727/096368912X655163.

Lin, P., W. C. Chan, S. F. Badylak, and S. N. Bhatia. 2004. "Assessing porcine liver-derived biomatrix for hepatic tissue engineering." *Tissue Eng* 10 (7–8):1046–53. doi: 10.1089/ten.2004.10.1046.

Liu, B., Y. Chen, and D. K. St Clair. 2008. "ROS and p53: a versatile partnership." *Free Radic Biol Med* 44 (8):1529–35. doi: 10.1016/j.freeradbiomed.2008.01.011.

Lubel, J. S., C. B. Herath, L. M. Burrell, and P. W. Angus. 2008. "Liver disease and the renin-angiotensin system: recent discoveries and clinical implications." *J Gastroenterol Hepatol* 23 (9):1327–38. doi: 10.1111/j.1440-1746.2008.05461.x.

Luk, J. M., Q. S. Zhang, N. P. Lee, J. Y. Wo, P. P. Leung, L. X. Liu, M. Y. Hu, K. F. Cheung, C. K. Hui, G. K. Lau, and S. T. Fan. 2007. "Hepatic stellate cell-targeted delivery of M6P-HSA-glycyrrhetinic acid attenuates hepatic fibrogenesis in a bile duct ligation rat model." *Liver Int* 27 (4):548–57. doi: 10.1111/j.1478-3231.2007.01452.x.

Macdonald, R. A. 1961. ""Lifespan" of liver cells. Autoradio-graphic study using tritiated thymidine in normal, cirrhotic, and partially hepatectomized rats." *Arch Intern Med* 107:335–43. doi: 10.1001/archinte.1961.03620030023003.

Magami, Y., T. Azuma, H. Inokuchi, S. Kokuno, F. Moriyasu, K. Kawai, and T. Hattori. 2002. "Cell proliferation and renewal of normal hepatocytes and bile duct cells in adult mouse liver." *Liver* 22 (5):419–25. doi: 10.1034/j.1600-0676.2002.01702.x.

Manco, R., L. A. Clerbaux, S. Verhulst, M. Bou Nader, C. Sempoux, J. Ambroise, B. Bearzatto, J. L. Gala, Y. Horsmans, L. van Grunsven, C. Desdouets, and I. Leclercq. 2019. "Reactive cholangiocytes differentiate into proliferative hepatocytes with efficient DNA repair in mice with chronic liver injury." *J Hepatol* 70 (6):1180–91. doi: 10.1016/j.jhep.2019.02.003.

Mandal, A. K., S. Das, M. K. Basu, R. N. Chakrabarti, and N. Das. 2007. "Hepatoprotective activity of liposomal flavonoid against arsenite-induced liver fibrosis." *J Pharmacol Exp Ther* 320 (3):994–1001. doi: 10.1124/jpet.106.114215.

Michalopoulos, G. K. 2007. "Liver regeneration." *J Cell Physiol* 213 (2):286–300. doi: 10.1002/jcp.21172.

Michalopoulos, G. K. 2013. "Principles of liver regeneration and growth homeostasis." *Compr Physiol* 3 (1):485–513. doi: 10.1002/cphy.c120014.

Michalopoulos, G. K. 2017. "Hepatostat: Liver regeneration and normal liver tissue maintenance." *Hepatology* 65 (4):1384–92. doi: 10.1002/hep.28988.

Minati, L., V. Antonini, S. Torrengo, M. D. Serra, M. Boustta, X. Leclercq, C. Migliaresi, M. Vert, and G. Speranza. 2012. "Sustained in vitro release and cell uptake of doxorubicin adsorbed onto gold nanoparticles and covered by a polyelectrolyte complex layer." *Int J Pharm* 438 (1–2):45–52. doi: 10.1016/j.ijpharm.2012.08.057.

Mishra, N., N. P. Yadav, V. K. Rai, P. Sinha, K. S. Yadav, S. Jain, and S. Arora. 2013. "Efficient hepatic delivery of drugs: novel strategies and their significance." *Biomed Res Int* 2013:382184. doi: 10.1155/2013/382184.

Mossanen, J. C., and F. Tacke. 2013. "Role of lymphocytes in liver cancer." *Oncoimmunology* 2 (11):e26468. doi: 10.4161/onci.26468.

Naahidi, S., M. Jafari, M. Logan, Y. Wang, Y. Yuan, H. Bae, B. Dixon, and P. Chen. 2017. "Biocompatibility of hydrogel-based scaffolds for tissue engineering applications." *Biotechnol Adv* 35 (5):530–44. doi: 10.1016/j.biotechadv.2017.05.006.

Navarro-Alvarez, N., A. Soto-Gutierrez, Y. Chen, J. Caballero-Corbalan, W. Hassan, S. Kobayashi, Y. Kondo, M. Iwamuro, K. Yamamoto, E. Kondo, N. Tanaka, I. J. Fox, and N. Kobayashi. 2010. "Intramuscular transplantation of engineered hepatic tissue constructs corrects acute and chronic liver failure in mice." *J Hepatol* 52 (2):211–9. doi: 10.1016/j.jhep.2009.11.019.

Navarro-Alvarez, N., A. Soto-Gutierrez, J. D. Rivas-Carrillo, Y. Chen, T. Yamamoto, T. Yuasa, H. Misawa, J. Takei, N. Tanaka, and N. Kobayashi. 2006. "Self-assembling peptide nanofiber as a novel culture system for isolated porcine hepatocytes." *Cell Transplant* 15 (10):921–7. doi: 10.3727/000000006783981387.

Niemczyk-Soczynska, B., A. Gradys, and P. Sajkiewicz. 2020. "Hydrophilic Surface Functionalization of Electrospun Nanofibrous Scaffolds in Tissue Engineering." *Polymers (Basel)* 12 (11). doi: 10.3390/polym12112636.

Nunez, K. G., J. Gonzalez-Rosario, P. T. Thevenot, and A. J. Cohen. 2017. "Cyclin D1 in the Liver: Role of noncanonical signaling in liver steatosis and hormone regulation." *Ochsner J* 17 (1):56–65.

Patel, G., G. Kher, and A. Misra. 2012. "Preparation and evaluation of hepatic stellate cell selective, surface conjugated, peroxisome proliferator-activated receptor-gamma ligand loaded liposomes." *J Drug Target* 20 (2):155–65. doi: 10.3109/1061186X.2011.610800.

Rui, L. 2014. "Energy metabolism in the liver." *Compr Physiol* 4 (1):177–97. doi: 10.1002/cphy.c130024.

Sato, Y., K. Murase, J. Kato, M. Kobune, T. Sato, Y. Kawano, R. Takimoto, K. Takada, K. Miyanishi, T. Matsunaga, T. Takayama, and Y. Niitsu. 2008. "Resolution of liver cirrhosis using vitamin A-coupled liposomes to deliver siRNA against a collagen-specific chaperone." *Nat Biotechnol* 26 (4):431–42. doi: 10.1038/nbt1396.

Sengupta, P., and B. L. V. Prasad. 2018. "Surface modification of polymers for tissue engineering applications: Arginine acts as a sticky protein equivalent for viable cell accommodation." *ACS Omega* 3 (4):4242–4251. doi: 10.1021/acsomega.8b00215.

Sonoke, S., T. Ueda, K. Fujiwara, K. Kuwabara, and J. Yano. 2011. "Galactose-modified cationic liposomes as a liver-targeting delivery system for small interfering RNA." *Biol Pharm Bull* 34 (8):1338–42. doi: 10.1248/bpb.34.1338.

van der Heide, D., R. Weiskirchen, and R. Bansal. 2019. "Therapeutic targeting of hepatic macrophages for the treatment of liver diseases." *Front Immunol* 10:2852. doi: 10.3389/fimmu.2019.02852.

Vivero-Escoto, J. L., H. Vadarevu, R. Juneja, L. W. Schrum, and J. H. Benbow. 2019. "Nanoparticle mediated silencing of tenascin C in hepatic stellate cells: effect on inflammatory gene expression and cell migration." *J Mater Chem B* 7 (46):7396–7405. doi: 10.1039/c9tb01845j.

Wang, L., X. Wang, G. Xie, L. Wang, C. K. Hill, and L. D. DeLeve. 2012. "Liver sinusoidal endothelial cell progenitor cells promote liver regeneration in rats." *J Clin Invest* 122 (4):1567–73. doi: 10.1172/JCI58789.

Witzigmann, D., P. Uhl, S. Sieber, C. Kaufman, T. Einfalt, K. Schoneweis, P. Grossen, J. Buck, Y. Ni, S. H. Schenk, J. Hussner, H. E. Meyer Zu Schwabedissen, G. Quebatte, W. Mier, S. Urban, and J. Huwyler. 2019. "Optimization-by-design of hepatotropic lipid nanoparticles targeting the sodium-taurocholate cotransporting polypeptide." *Elife* 8. doi: 10.7554/eLife.42276.

Wu, L., A. Magaz, S. Huo, A. Darbyshire, M. Loizidou, M. Emberton, M. Birchall, and W. Song. 2020. "Human airway-like multilayered tissue on 3D-TIPS printed thermoresponsive elastomer/collagen hybrid scaffolds." *Acta Biomater* 113:177–195. doi: 10.1016/j.actbio.2020.07.013.

Xia, Y., J. Zhong, M. Zhao, Y. Tang, N. Han, L. Hua, T. Xu, C. Wang, and B. Zhu. 2019. "Galactose-modified selenium nanoparticles for targeted delivery of doxorubicin to hepatocellular carcinoma." *Drug Deliv* 26 (1):1–11. doi: 10.1080/10717544.2018.1556359.

Yang, J., Y. Hou, G. Ji, Z. Song, Y. Liu, G. Dai, Y. Zhang, and J. Chen. 2014. "Targeted delivery of the RGD-labeled biodegradable polymersomes loaded with the hydrophilic drug oxymatrine on cultured hepatic stellate cells and liver fibrosis in rats." *Eur J Pharm Sci* 52:180–90. doi: 10.1016/j.ejps.2013.11.017.

Yao, Q. Y., B. L. Xu, J. Y. Wang, H. C. Liu, S. C. Zhang, and C. T. Tu. 2012. "Inhibition by curcumin of multiple sites of the transforming growth factor-beta1 signalling pathway ameliorates the progression of liver fibrosis induced by carbon tetrachloride in rats." *BMC Complement Altern Med* 12:156. doi: 10.1186/1472-6882-12-156.

Ye, S., J. W. B. Boeter, L. C. Penning, B. Spee, and K. Schneeberger. 2019. "Hydrogels for Liver Tissue Engineering." *Bioengineering (Basel)* 6 (3). doi: 10.3390/bioengineering6030059.

Zhang, L. J., and X. Z. Wang. 2006. "Interleukin-10 and chronic liver disease." *World J Gastroenterol* 12 (11):1681–5. doi: 10.3748/wjg.v12.i11.1681.

9 Hydroxyapatite-Based Nanomaterials for Bone Tissue Regeneration

Sivaraj Mehnath and Murugaraj Jeyaraj
University of Madras

CONTENTS

DOI: 10.1201/9781003140108-9

9.1 INTRODUCTION

In India, bone defects and their physiological conditions are a substantial reason for the high proportion of medical expenses. In most countries, bone defects such as osteoporosis and related defective conditions account for up to 15% of the cost of healthcare services. These expenses are predicted to rise in the future with increasing case numbers of fractures, osteoporosis, obesity, and other factors (Henkel et al. 2013). Worldwide, hip fractures might reach 6.3 million per year by 2050, and several research studies have focused on cost-effective treatments for bone regeneration. More than 2.0 million people require bone grafting surgery for large-bone defects every year. For several decades, metallic bioinert implants that were accepted by the host were used for bone healing. These actively influenced the action of surrounding tissues and followed the evolution of scaffolds (Cooper et al. 1992; Javaid & Kaartinen 2013). But the failure of conventional treatment is due to the shorter life span and synthetic materials, etc. For example, bone injury needed instant postoperative repair to enhance and induce the regeneration mechanism. The treatment technique can easily compromised by post-surgical infection and reaction of metal components during repair. In larger bone defects, the use of bone autograft leads to significant donor site morbidity. In allografts/xenografts, there was risk of transfer infection from source/immunological elicitation from host (Neovius & Engstrand 2010; Mehnath et al. 2020a). So, advanced treatment techniques and novel engineering strategies are required for bone regeneration applications. Currently, biomaterial and bone tissue engineering applications lead an interdisciplinary perspective in development of a novel/better way to solve the above issues.

9.2 HYDROXYAPATITE

Hydroxyapatite (HAP)- $(Ca_{10}(PO_4)_6(OH)_2)$ is the most common mineral in natural bone. The dissolving ability of HAP is dependent on the size and chemical composition of the materials. HAP present in natural bone varies from synthetic HAP; there are variables in minor element compositions such as magnesium, zinc, and strontium. Natural HAP is brown or yellow and is available as inorganic constituents (bones, teeth, shells, fish enameloid) or pathological form such as dental enamel, urinary calculus, or stones. Synthetic HAP is highly pure, white in color, with a known Ca/P ratio of 1.67, stable, high crystalline, and less soluble (Dubok 2000). Due to its non-toxic, minimal inflammatory, biocompatible, and induction of osteoconductive properties, it was widely used in bone regeneration applications. HAP mechanical properties are based on the crystal size, density, phase composition, sintering ability, and porosity, etc. Normally, the bending, compressive, and tensile strength of HAP is in the range of 38–300 Mpa, and Young's modulus lies in the range of 35–120 GPa. The Weibull's modulus of dense HAP varies from the 5–8; Vicker's hardness is in the range of 3–7 GPa. Mostly, fine grains are harder and stronger compared to large porous grains (Hench & Thompson 2010; Dorozhkin 2012a). Recent advancement established that HAP in nanosize range exactly mimics the bone/teeth components.

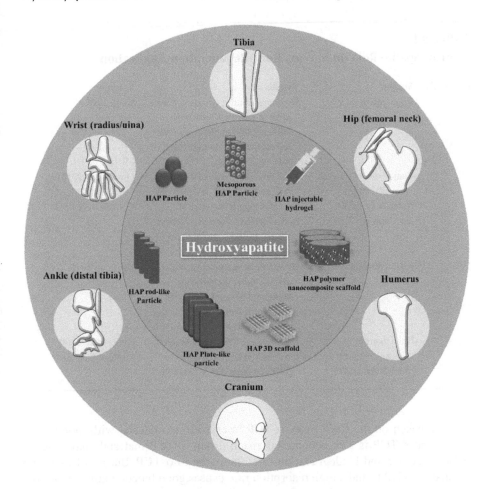

FIGURE 9.1 Hydroxyapatite-based nanomaterials, different forms and application in various bone model bone remodeling.

Hydroxyapatite-based nanomaterials and different forms and applications in various bone remodeling are presented in Figure 9.1.

HAP nanocrystalline gained better bioactivity and dissolution compared to coarser crystals. It exhibits the higher sintering effect and improved densification. It also helps in enhancing the strength and biological properties based on characteristic properties such as size, surface area, morphology, distribution, crystallinity, and agglomeration. HAP can be tailored with desired properties like bioactivity, density, thermal stability, porosity, and resorbability. It is also excellent in biological application such as cell adhesion, propagation, and maximum deposition of calcium-containing minerals on the material surface (Hing et al. 2005; Gosain et al. 2002; Mehnath et al. 2018c). Some application are briefly summarized in Table 9.1.

Different crystalline phases of calcium phosphates exhibit diverse forms of material similar to HAP. Tricalcium phosphate (TCP) was classified into α,

TABLE 9.1

Hydroxyapatite Role on Various Bone Regeneration Application

Materials	Studies	Results	Reference
	Bone tumor	Biocompatibility; porous structure helps in growth of new bone cells; suitable implant structure and mechanical strength enhances bone regeneration.	Kaito 2016
	Canine model for graft transplantation	HAP provides minimal disc height loss, good support, and strength.	Owen et al. 2018
	Anterior cervical discectomy	Provides long-term relief of radiculopathy; less risk of further operation; and superior to the autologous bone graft.	Dorozhkin & Epple 2002
HAP	Rabbit femoral condyle model	New bone development within 6 weeks; higher compression strength at 9th week; and bone marrow formation with interconnection.	Zhu et al. 2010
	Bone marrow, MSCs	Enhances the MSCs proliferation.	Predoi et al. 2008
	Osteosarcoma cell lines, MG63 and U2OS	It shows higher proliferation of U2OS compared to MG63 cells.	Matsiko et al. 2014

β-phase based on the Ca/P ratio. α-TCP is crystalline material with monoclinic space, and β-TCP is a rhombohedral space group. β-TCP materials have higher stable structure and biodegradation rate compared to α-TCP. But it is less stable compared to HAP, and a high resorption rate causes good biocompatibility. It promotes osteoprecursor cell proliferation, adhesion, and biomineralization ability (Dorozhkin et al. 201 2bKamitakahara et al. 2008). Whitlockite (WH) is another type of calcium phosphate; it contains a magnesium ion in the chemical formula $Ca_9Mg(HPO_4)(PO_4)_6$. It is crystalline material with a rhombohedral space group and is highly stable in acidic conditions. It shows higher compressive strength compared to HAP and higher solubility in physiological condition and releases more ions. The major problem is that it is difficult to synthesize WH under low-temperature conditions (Kim et al. 2017). Jang et al. reported WH in rhombohedral shape with 50 nm diameter and also showed higher osteogenic activity compared to HAP and β-TCP (Jang et al. 2015). Finally, octacalcium phosphate (OCP), shows a triclinic crystal structure; it acts as precursor of bone mineralization. Its amorphous material is used for various clinical applications by substituting different ions. Although the bioactive properties of calcium phosphate have been studied and used for bone regeneration, there are some drawbacks, such as mechanical disadvantages in clinical applications (Popp et al. 2012). Therefore, research has been carried out to utilize calcium phosphate as a composite material with other materials (Sakamoto 2010; Saiz et al. 2007).

9.3   HAP MECHANISM IN BONE REGENERATION

The involvement of nanotechnology helps to overcome the issues of bulk HAP material with enhanced integration and regeneration of bone (Sossa et al. 2018; Ryabenkova et al. 2017). Certainly, HAP in nanosize has become an alternative and effective source for bone tissue engineering. It also allows design and fabrication of nanomaterial that precisely controls bone regeneration by influencing cellular behavior. This chapter focuses on nano-HAP production methods, different forms of HAP particles, functional properties of materials, and the relevant clinical application to bone regeneration. HAP has proven to be highly bioinert, biocompatible and bioresorbable, with more osteoinductive characteristics that make it suitable for a multiple applications (Huang et al. 2011; Xiao et al. 2016). The bioactivity and porosity induces osteoinductive behavior and enhances the interaction of extracellular matrix (ECM). Different shape, dimension, architecture help trigger both osteoconduction and osteoinduction. The architecture pores of HAP increase the deposition of vital components at the surface and induce osteo cell growth and vascularization. HAP in direct contact with mesenchymal stem cells (MSCs) exhibits high osteoinductive activity to promote bone-cell differentiation and proliferation (Figure 9.2). Several studies present the effective role of HAP in signaling mechanisms. The phosphorylation of extracellular-signal-regulated kinase (ERK) initiates the stimulation of osteoblast-related genes such as OCN and Col I and initiates differentiation of MSCs to osteoblast. Material interaction with bone cells leads to activation of cytoskeletal and intracellular signaling proteins. The activation of focal adhesion kinase triggers the Ras pathway, which links with ShC proteins. The Ras stimulates the ERK signaling cascade via COL I and OCN (Ha et al. 2017; Song et al. 2008). Wang et al. cultured different concentrations of HAP onto the MC3T3-E1 cells, indicating increases in alkaline phosphatase (ALP) activity and Col expression by raising the HAP concentration. Further, there is alteration in RNA-level marker genes/proteins like ALP, BMP2, osteocalcin, RUNX2, and bone sialoprotein. The optimum HAP concentration raises the ratio of LC3II/LC3I, which confirms autophagosome formation and blocks the mTOR phosphorylation (Wang et al. 2019; Ha et al. 2015). HAP

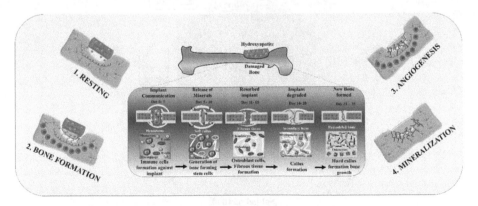

FIGURE 9.2   Hydroxyapatite mechanism on bone remodeling and steps involved in bone formation, mineralization.

alters molecular and cellular levels through surface proteins like CasR (calcium sensing receptor), PiT (Na-dependent phosphate transporters), and FGFR (fibroblast growth factor receptor) (Marie et al. 2012; Ha et al. 2017). The external stimuli from HAP induces the gene expression by activating intracellular signaling pathways like ERK1/2, p38, and Jnk pathways. The transduction of extracellular signals changes the gene expression and MAPK, which is activated by phosphorylation (Shi et al. 2009; Hauburger et al. 2009). Size, concentration, morphology, and surface topography of HAP also influence the cell signaling and gene expression. Xia et al. reported the result of HAP in various shapes, such as nanosheet, nanorod, hybrid, and spherical, on MSCs in vitro and calvarial defect animal model. Some reports indicate the HAP influence on genes was to induce the effect for longer periods, and it also implies epigenetic regulation (Xia et al. 2013). The desired HAP composition and geometry improves the formation of new blood vessels and facilitates the transport of molecular signals, which drives bone growth. Mechanically strong HAP must provide support for bone deposition and helps in bone repair and regeneration (Milovac et al. 2014).

9.4 HYDROXYAPATITE NANOPARTICLES SYNTHESIS

HAP nanomaterials are prepared in different forms such as powders, granules, porous blocks, and scaffolds. As in Figure 9.3, various methods are developed to prepare the HAP nanomaterials, which are solid and wet-state methods. These are solid-state reaction, ball milling, plasma spraying, mechanochemical methods, calcination with anti-sintering agent. Wet-state methods include, sol-gel, hydrothermal process, co-precipitation, thermal dissociation of Ca ions, and emulsion method

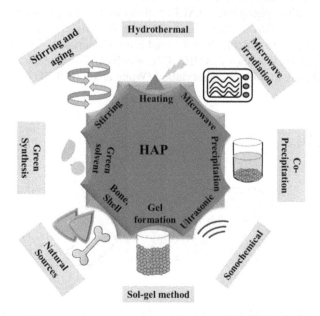

FIGURE 9.3 Representation of different techniques used for HAP preparation.

(Phatai 2019; Chen et al. 2020; Nyoo et al. 2014). In a solid-state technique, calcium and phosphor raw materials of stoichiometric levels were induced for thermal treatments of above 700°C for long treatment times. Most of the solid-state methods require the milling/grinding process to produce HAP nanomaterials. Another physical method is a plasma technique that uses a radiofrequency plasma to attain nanosize HAP (10–100 nm) in both amorphous and crystalline states. Coprecipitation is a wet-state method that starts with a combination of calcium and phosphate with a chelating agent to form a turbid solution. It forms HAP nanomaterial after a centrifugation and calcination process. In this, cysteine was used as a chelating agent to prepare HAP nanomaterial. In another method, phosphate salt was added to the Ca^{2+} solution at an alkaline pH. The mixture was mixed for 2 h and then aged to form HAP (Banerjee et al. 2018; Shen et al. 2020). In the hydrothermal method both salts were mixed and kept in a high-temperature hydrothermal treatment using an autoclave or a microwave.

Next, the sol-gel method involves the mixing of both salts to form a three-dimensional inorganic system. In this, the Ca/P ratio was maintained at ratio of 1:67, and it forms a gel that is aged and further dried in a muffle furnace (Phatai 2019). In some cases, a sample preparation was synthesized similarly with help of ultrasonic agitation to form a gel (Lett et al. 2019). This ultrasonic agitation increases the mechanical and morphological characteristics of HAP. The desired material produced depends on the stirring, sonication, Ca/P ratio, aging, and sintering process. In the sonochemical method, both salt solutions were treated with sonochemical treatment during mixing or after via ultrasonic waves. In this, alkaline pH was maintained and precursor components were slowly mixed with ultrasonic irradiation to form HAP. The nanomaterial were separated by centrifugation and dried overnight (Nyoo et al. 2014). Another technique uses an ultrasound microwave treatment during the mixing of Ca/P salt solution. The treatment condition maintains higher pH and temperature controlled by a microwave reactor. The microwave irradiation helps in controlling the size and morphology (Xiao et al. 2018).

Surfactant-based HAP synthesis, which utilizes three types of surfactants such as cationic, anionic, and non-ionic, were used (Figure 9.4). The common cationic surfactant is cetyltrimethylammonium bromide (CTAB), composed of a hydrophilic head and hydrophobic tail (Mehnath et al. 2018b). The positively charged group electrostatically interacts with the PO^{4-} and shares the tetrahedral structure (Shiba et al. 2016; Wang et al. 2015). Kolodziejczak et al. used a anionic surfactant like sodium dodecyl sulphate (SDS) for preparation of HAP nanorods. Surfactant sulphate groups electrostatically interact with calcium ions, and the addition of phosphate precursors forms a HAP nanomaterials (Kolodziejczak et al. 2014). Ethylene diamine tetracetic acid (EDTA) anionic surfactants exhibited for packing around the Ca^{2+} ions and controlling the nucleation rate (Kalita & Verma 2010). The same mechanism was exploited by adding the sodium tripolyphosphate (STPP), an effective calcium chelating agent controlling and modulating the structural morphology of HAP in plate-like shape (Zhang et al. 2009). A non-ionic surfactant such as triton X-100, pluronic F127, or polyethylene glycol (PEG) helps interaction of calcium ions to facilitate the growth of nanoparticles with the desired structural morphology.

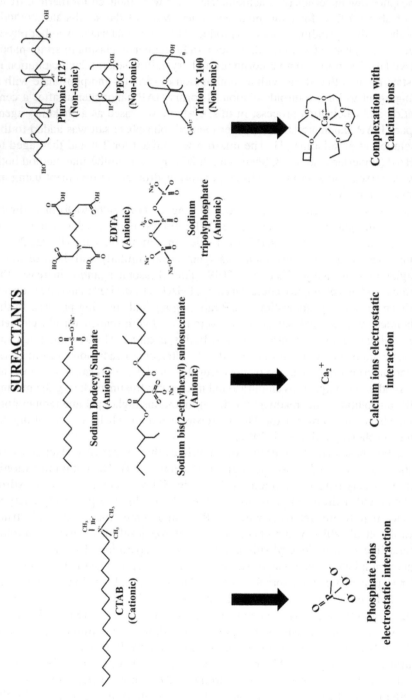

FIGURE 9.4 Various types of surfactants such as cationic, anionic, and non-ionic surfactants used for HAP preparation.

Another HAP synthesis technique is utilization of natural sources composed of calcium, which can be an alternative to conventional materials. Green sources such as eggshells, fish scales, seashells, animal bones, and algae can be utilized for synthesis of HAP. The PO^{4-} salt was slowly added to the green sources with hydrochloric acid and kept for 5–7 days. After incubation, the particles were washed and dried, and biomolecule components enhanced the properties (Vanitha et al. 2017; Nayar & Guha 2008). Some green synthesis techniques use a plant extract for HAP-nanomaterial fabrication, and this technique reduces the expense of enhancing the properties (Kumar et al. 2017). Addition of natural sources reduces the size and decreases the agglomeration (Pradeepkumar et al. 2017) (Figure 9.4). Some different methods of HAP synthesis are given in Table 9.2.

9.5 DIFFERENT FORMS OF HYDROXYAPATITE

9.5.1 PLATE-LIKE MORPHOLOGY

HAP with plate-like morphology was investigated by various research groups for mimicking natural bone and extended bone tissue–engineering applications. Synthesis methods such as hydrothermal, microwave irradiation, and emulsion were investigated to attain plate-like nanoparticles (Figure 9.5). The hydrothermal method is a common technique to alter the structure and application of surfactants to help in crystal growth. Nagata et al. used this method to prepare plate-like HAP nanoparticles with ethylamine to form a wide-plane growth. The precursor like a $CaCO_3$ and $CaHPO_4 \cdot 2H_2O$ mixture was added to the 5% of ethylamine in hydrothermal process 180°C for 5 h to prepare HAP plate like particle. (Nagata et al. 2001). Zhang et al. synthesized the plate-like HAP in different aspect ratios using hydrothermal method with STPP chelating agent. Hydrothermal treatment of $Ca(NO_3)_2$ and Na_2HPO_4 was mixed and alkaline pH maintained by ammonium hydroxide for 160°C for 4–12 h. Decreases in aspect ratio by increasing the concentration of STPP, which indicates the STPP surfactants, regulates the crystal growth of HAP particles to a form-plate like structure. Another famous technique for plate-like HAP synthesis is the emulsion method, mixing two immiscible liquids with emulsion to regulate the nucleation of HAP (Zhang et al. 2009). Sato et al. fabricated the elongated plate-like morphology via sodium bis (2-ethylhexyl) sulfosuccinate and cyclohexane as oil phase. In this precursor, components were maintained in supersaturated concentration to modulate the crystal growth (Sato et al. 2006). The formation of plate-like morphology via microwave irradiation was reported by Siddharthan et al., and desired size and shape can be synthesized by choosing the appropriate microwave power. In this, needle-shaped particles formed at 175 W, acicular at 525 W, and platelet-like particles at 660 W (Siddharthan et al. 2006).

9.5.2 ROD-LIKE MORPHOLOGY

Several research studies focus on preparation of rod-like HAP nanoparticles for their inferior biomimicry of bone components. It is obtained via hydrothermal process, microwave irradiation, emulsion, and precipitation technique with the help of

TABLE 9.2
Hydroxyapatite Synthesis Method Types, Role, and Application

Methods	Size and Morphology	Advantages	Challenges	Reference
Co-precipitation	Different size and morphology can be formed like nanorods (150:500 nm-length: width), rhombohedral (90:300 nm-length: width).	Simple technique to form stable HAP nanomaterials.	Requires several crucial dispensation parameters for synthesis.	Banerjee et al. 2018
Hydrothermal analysis	Nanorods	The approach enhances strength and morphological properties.	Mandate to maintain the ambient pressure, temperature to get desired property.	Buitrago & Patricia Ossa-Orozco 2018
Sol-gel method	Nanoparticles (50 nm), polygon morphology (20–50 nm)	Approach helps in formation of particles in advanced structure; better transparency and high surface area.	Poor crystalline compared to other method.	Amiri et al. 2017
Sonochemical method	Nanorod (18: 80 nm-length: width)	Technique improves the reaction speed with higher energy efficiency.	Maintaining the optimum conditions.	Jay et al. 2017
Ultrasound–microwave Method	Microsphere (3 to 10 µm)	Ultrasound reduces the aggregation, and microwave method improves the physical property and limits the preparation time.	Maintaining the optimum condition.	Xiao et al. 2018
Natural source: Eggshell (solid state reaction)	Spherical (10 nm)	Improves the waste management and recycling the biowaste; reduces the expense.	-	Ingole et al. 2016
Natural shells: Oyster, Seashells (wet precipitation)	Aggregated plate like structure with uneven size	Purity with high crystallinity; low cost.	Difficult in modification of material with desired property.	Hidroksiapatit & Sebagai 2017
Natural source: Fishbones (wet-impregnation method)	Aggregated particle with 33.14 nm	Easily available raw materials; enhances the properties.	-	Chakraborty & Roychowdhury 2013

(Continued)

TABLE 9.2 (*Continued*)
Hydroxyapatite Synthesis Method Types, Role, and Application

Methods	Size and Morphology	Advantages	Challenges	Reference
Natural source: Fish scale (alkaline heat treatment method)	Nanocrystals (15–20 nm)	Easily available raw materials; low energy consumption.	-	Kongsri et al. 2013
Natural source: Animal bone (heat treatment)	Crystal size	Waste recycling; improves the porosity of HAP particles	-	Ramesh et al. 2018
Natural source: Algae (ambient pressure, low temperature, basic pH)	-	Biocompatible material with good morphology; high calcite content and easily available source.	-	Walsh et al 2008
Natural source: Chicken beaks	Irregular shaped agglomerates of submicron size (300–500 nm).	Waste recycling; easily sourced; high crystalline HAP formed.	-	Alshemary et al. 2018
Green synthesis: *Azadirachta indica*	Hexagonal (10: 40 nm-length: width)	Efficient antibacterial activity against *E. coli* and *S. aureus*.	-	Kumar et al. 2017
Green synthesis: *Aloe barbadensis*	Hexagonal (43: 171 nm-length: width)	Easy altering the morphology from a sphere to a rod-like structure by raising calcination temperature.	-	Klinkaewnarong et al. 2010
Green synthesis: *Sapindus mukorossi*	Flakes (50 nm)	Altering the morphology from sphere to flake shape due to influence of source	-	Shubha et al. 2015
Green synthesis: *Daucus carota*	Capsule (45 nm)	Sugarcane sucrose as a chelating agent improved the morphology of particles without any agglomeration.	-	Gopi et al. 2013b
Green synthesis: *Musa acuminate*	Cubic (142:31 nm-length: width)	Green synthesized HAP showed effective antibacterial activity against gram positive and negative bacteria	-	Gopi et al. 2013a
Green synthesis: *Musa paradisiaca*	Spherical (35–55 nm)	HAP derived from banana peel pectin exhibited higher antibacterial activity than that of the HAP prepared in the absence of pectin.	-	Gopi et al. 2014

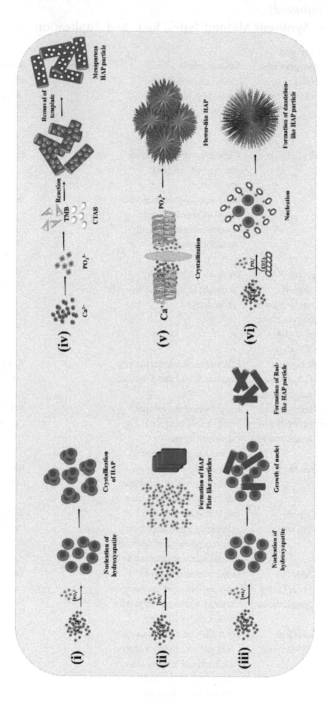

FIGURE 9.5 Different forms of HAP and synthesis techniques.

surfactants (Figure 9.5). In hydrothermal conditions, CTAB surfactant is able to direct the nucleation of PO_4^{3-} and Ca^{2+}. Wang et al. identified the importance of pH and autoclaving temperature in altering the structure of HAP. The precursors $CaCl_2$ and H_3PO_4 with CTAB form round particles at pH 13 and changed into the rod-like structure at (pH 9.0). The PO_4^{3-} and CTAB interaction changed based on the pH due to increases in hydroxyl ions concentration. This –OH group repulses the PO_4^{3-} interaction at higher pH, and decreases in pH reduce the hydroxyl group simultaneously, favoring the rod-like morphology formation. Additionally, increases in diameter and length of crystal were gained by increasing the temperature from 90°C to 150°C.

The preparation of rod-like HAP using hydrothermal technique was studied in several studies by using CTAB, SDS, SDTA, PEG, Tween-20, and trisodium citrate (Wang et al. 2006). Xin et al. evaluated the morphology of HAP by varying pH and temperature with EDTA surfactant. The HSP nanorod formed at the range of 50 to 200 nm and was obtained at pH 12 and temperature of 180°C. The major reports show that common features for nanorod formations are alkaline pH and autoclaving temperature above 100°C for 20 h. High hydrothermal temperature with longer treatment time produces advanced crystal structure with larger size. Emulsion technique was another successful technique for synthesizing the nanorod (Xin et al. 2010). Sun et al. combined a surfactant such as Triton X-100, CTAB, n-butanol or n-hexanol to form a rod-like structure with 25–50 nm length and 8–15 nm diameter. The combination of both surfactants to obtain dual stabilization results in a better control of size and growth (Sun et al. 2006). Lin et al. combined the hydrothermal and emulsion processes by heating at 180°C with W/O microemulsion containing CTAB, n-pentanol, n-heaxane, and precursor solution to form rod-like HAP particles (Lin et al. 2007). Liu et al. prepared a monodispersed single crystal HAP by the microwave irradiation method. HAP nanorods formed at pH 9.0 and 30 min microwave treatment at 700 W. Some other works focus on preparation of HAP nano-rod by reflux of precursor solution with surfactant (Liu et al. 2016). Iyyappan et al. used calcium nitrate, $(NH_4)_2HPO_4$, with surfactants refluxing for an hour and maintained in alkaline conditions to form rod-like HAP particles (Iyyappan & Wilson 2013). In another work, Shiba et al. refluxed the $K_2HPO_4 \cdot 3H_2O$, $CaCl_2$ and CTAB for 24 h at 40°C. The molar ratio of surfactant: PO_4^{3-} (2: 1) helps in formation of uniform nanorods with length of 50 nm and 20 nm diameter (Shiba et al. 2016). Wang et al. prepared the rod-like particles by a wet-chemical method along with surfactant. The mixture of $Ca(NO_3)_2$, diammonium phosphate, and ethanolamine is maintained at pH 10 for 90 min at 60°C. This is followed by aging for 24 h to help in formation of rod-like HAP particles (Wang et al. 2010). Loo et al. prepared different HAP particles by a chemical precipitation/hydrothermal method with irregular shape and morphology. But hydrothermal treatment produced highly pure single crystals, with narrow size distribution and reduced agglomeration (Loo et al. 2008). Tran and Webster prepared rod-like HAP combination with magnetic nanoparticles via a hydrothermal method. It stimulated the expression of osteoblast cell markers and exhibited higher osteogenic potential. Additionally, magnetite particles directed the nanoparticles to the osteoporotic fracture site with the help of magnetic field (Tran & Webster, 2011). Sartuqui et al. reported the hydrothermal synthesis of rod-like HAP with the help of CTAB as a templating agent. It showed increases in mechanical properties, mineralization ability, and osteoconductive potential (Sartuqui et al. 2016). Zheng et al. used hydrothermal method for preparation of HAP in rod structure using genipin as crosslinking agent. It exhibited high structural stability, compositional biomimicry, more bone cell adhesion, and maximum proliferation and differentiation rate (Zheng et al. 2017).

9.5.3 MESOPOROUS HAP

Mesoporous nanoparticles were successfully exploited in biomedical applications due to storage and release of bioactive components for bone-regeneration applications. Mainly surfactant-assisted templating approaches were used for fabrication of mesoporous HAP (Figure 9.5). In several cases, disorganized pores in the particles were reported because of the high crystallization rate of HAP. The fabrication of mesoporous HAP was sub-divided by the templating agent. Hydrothermal, microwave irradiation, and precipitation under reflux condition are common procedures for mesoporous HAP particles. Li et al. used hydrothermal treatment of temperature up to 160°C, followed by calcination at different temperature (550 to 1000°C). Increases in temperature lead to rod-like structure with an increase in crystallinity and also influence the nanopore size. At 40°C nanopores were found to be 5 nm and decreased to 2 nm at 160°C due to the tight packing of atoms (Li et al. 2008).

Wang et al. determined that CTAB affects the properties of HAP nanoparticles such as pore size, and surface area. The optimum concentration of CTAB higher surface area and pore size ranging with 2 to 7 nm. The CTAB:HA of 1:2 molar ratio shows higher surface area: $97 m^2 g^{-1}$ with pore volume-0.47 $cm^3 g^{-1}$. Increases of surfactant concentration lead to decreases in pore volume and surface area (Wang et al. 2015). Benzigar et al. utilized the same precursors, which were kept in a teflon autoclave and heated by microwave at 120°C for 8 h. HAP exhibited high crystallinity, uniform rod-like structure, width of 25 nm, and length of 100 nm. Microwave radiation favors ionic interaction with surfactant, which promotes the mesopores structure and high crystallinity (Benzigar et al. 2012). Kumar et al. prepared a mesoporous HAP particle in a rod-like structure with pores of 2 nm range. The pore formation increased after introduction of CTAB concentration above the critical micellar concentration. Different concentrations of CTAB were evaluated for optimum level to form specific pore volume and surface area. To overcome the limitations, surfactants such as pluronic F127/ P123 were used (Kumar et al. 2018).

Zhao et al. fabricated rod-like particles of diameter –50 nm, length –300 nm, using 10 wt % pluronic F127. It was refluxed for 24 h with potassium hydrogen phosphate trihydrate and calcium D-pantothenate monohydrate and maintained at pH 12 for the reaction. Further the precipitate was calcinated under 550°C for 6 h to obtain mesoporous structure (Zhao & Ma 2005). Zhang et al. obtained mesoporous rod-like HAP using same the surfactant by means of hydrothermal method (Zhang et al. 2013). Iyyappan et al. synthesized the nanoporous HAP particle via a similar hydrothermal method using surfactants. It reduces the agglomeration and improves the pore volume and percentage of pore size compared to without surfactant.

Additionally, zwitterionic surfactants' role on preparation of mesoporous HAP particles was stated by researchers (Iyyappan et al. 2016). Amer et al. used lauryl dimethylaminoacetic acid zwitterionic surfactant for preparation of HAP by microwave irradiation. A rod-like structure with diameter-19 nm, length-69 nm, and pore size-36 nm was formed (Amer et al. 2013). França et al. confirmed that high porosity is a vital factor for cell anchorage, and many studies reported that porous HAP helps in new bone formation. It also indicates that porosity is not adequate for bone formation. It helps in cell/protein adhesion, movement, differentiation, and multiplication. Interconnecting pores also affect the bone formation by preventing the diffusion of body fluids into mesoporous HAP, and they simultaneously affect the bone formation signals. Inter-pore size less than the 2–3 µm diameter is inappropriate for cell relocation. So, size of pores is vital for bone regeneration (França et al. 2014).

Tamai et al. fabricated mesoporous hydroxyapatite by foam-gel technique, forming a size of 6 mm diameter. Bone-regeneration ability was evaluated by rabbit femoral condyles. A 40-µm-size HAP was implanted in an animal model, and after 6 weeks there was formation of vessels deep in defects. The compression test of material was improved to three times after 9 weeks. So pore size and interconnection are vital factors for bone formation; it also increases the compressive strength of new bone (Tamai et al. 2002).

9.6 MODIFICATION OF HAP

9.6.1 ELEMENTS/IONS

Modified HAP has exhibited the extraordinary option of modification of its properties. Different ions can be substituted, such as Mg^{2+}, Ce^{2+}, Ni^{2+} Sr^{2+}, Zn^{2+}, Mn^{2+}, Fe^{3+}, Fe^{2+}, K^+, and Ag^+ (cations) and CO_3^{2-}, SiO_4^{3-}, and F^- (anions). The substitution of ions alters the properties of HAP, such as mechanical, biocompatibility, bone adhesion, and stimulation properties (Shepherd et al. 2012; Evis & Webster 2011). For example, conventional HAP was different from native bone minerals, whereas substitution of CO_3 into HAP shows similar physiochemical properties to bone (Cazalbou et al. 2004). For a Zn^{2+}-incorporated HAP preparation, the definite molar ratio of zinc and calcium were used. The mixture solution was heated and maintained in an alkaline pH condition to form Zn^{2+}-substituted HAP. Some studies demonstrated that the zinc substitution on the HAP improves the protein adsorption activity and increases the osteoblast cell proliferation rate (Montoyacisneros et al. 2017). Addition of strontium helps in increasing the solubility of HAP and also has a positive effect on bone regeneration by inducing ALP activity, osteocalcin level, and collage type I formation (Marie et al. 2001). Selenium is widely used in cancer inhibition and proliferation of bone cells. Manganese was also used for regulation of bone remodeling, and addition of Cl^- leads to change in environment to trigger osteoclasts. Potassium also influences bone mineralization and nucleation of apatite minerals (Supova 2015; Swetha et al. 2012). Several elements/ions are used for modification of HAP, and some of them are summarized in Table 9.3.

TABLE 9.3

Modification of Hydroxyapatites with Elements/Ions and Its Effect

Element/Ions	Effect	Reference
Strontium	It induces osteoporosis treatment; inhibits osteoclast differentiation; increases osteoblast proliferation, osteoblastic activity and stimulates the collagen synthesis.	Liu et al. 2008; Zarins et al. 2019; Conz et al. 2011
Strontium	Combination of strontium and HAP human primary osteoblast-like cells; improves the cell adhesion and faster formation of extracellular matrix.	Remya et al. 2014
Magnesium	Abundantly available in cartilage and initial phases of osteogenesis; improves the osteoconductivity and material resorption.	Wang et al. 2007; Calabrese et al. 2017
Magnesium	HAP used coating layer of magnesium which improves the corrosion resistance, reduces degradation rate, and enhances biocompatibility.	Witte et al. 2007
Silicon	Increases the differentiation, production, and collagen formation by osteoblast cells; helps in remodeling process, calcification, osteoclast growth, and resorption process.	Hao et al. 2012
Silicon	Si containing HAP raises cell growth and bone density, and enhances bone mineralization.	Balamurugan et al. 2008
Zinc	Essential trace elements plays a major role in bone growth and mineralization; stops the osteoclast differentiation, increases ALP activity, and promotes osteoblastic activity.	Anderud et al. 2016
Zinc	Zinc introduction into the HAP shows antibacterial activity.	Swetha et al. 2012
Zinc	Stimulates bone formation by initiating protein synthesis in osteoblasts and exhibits the anti-inflammatory effects.	Ashuri et al. 2012

9.6.2 TCP AND BCP COMBINATION

Tricalcium phosphates (TCP) and biphasic calcium phosphates (BCP) are ceramics similar to hydroxyapatite. These are also broadly used as grafting material and also blend with HAP to form a composite material. Cao et al. reported that HAP-TCP preparations in different ratios were used for femoral medial-epicondyle defects in rat models. The bone reorganization was begun 14 days post-operation and new bone completely replaced after 90 days. A HAP-TCP ratio of 1:3 was effective compared to the other ratio, and it also showed slow resorption. Finally, HAP-TCP exhibited the rapid mineralization and high osteogenesis compared to the control HAP group (Cao & Kuboyama 2010). In another report a different combination of biphasic calcium phosphates and HA-TCP was evaluated. In vitro and in vivo experiments on neonatal animals were performed to compare the effects of TCP and HAP. It shows that less osteoclastic resorption occurs on β-TCP, HA-TCP (Podaropoulos et al.2009). Yamada et al. studied the lower osteoclastic resorption on β-TCP compared to HA/β-TCP 25/75 group. Higher solubility increases the Ca^{2+} ions in extracellular matrix, and it also inhibits the osteoclastic activity (Yamada et al. 1997). Kurashina et al. reported the different ratio (7/3,2/8,0/10) of HAP-TCP ceramics to evaluate the intra-muscle of rabbit animal model for 6 months transplantation. Maximum degradation occurred at HAP-TCP ratios 2/8, 0/10, and morphology of composites was changed drastically. HAP-TCP 7/3 ratio exhibited less resorption/degradation and higher osteogenesis. HAP-TCP ratios 8/2 and 0/10 were degraded fast, slowly induces osteogenesis (Kurashina et al. 2002).

The alteration of organic molecules such as alcohols, carboxylic acids, and surfactant molecules leads to changes in the properties of HAP. Also a vitamin C–added HAP formation was described by using a simplified hydrothermal method (Zhou et al. 2018). The introduction of amino acids leads to modification of morphology and surface charge of HAP particles. For example, introduction of aspartic acid, glycine, glutamic acid, and serine during HAP synthesis leads to changes in morphology and increases in solubility. Introduction of amino acids such as alanine, methionine, valine, arginine, proline, and histidine does not affect the solubility, structure and crystalline behaviors (Matsumoto et al. 2002; Matsumoto et al. 2007). Uddin et al. reported that substitution of aspartic acid enhances the protein uptake due to more -COOH groups in aspartic acid (Uddin et al. 2010). HAP modification with polymers such as poly(vinyl alcohol), poly(ethylene imine), polylactic acid, polycaprolactone, poly(lactic-co-glycolic) acid, polyhydroxybutyrate, and biopolymers leads to formation of HAP/polymer composites.

9.6.3 NANOCOMPOSITES

HAP/polymer nanocomposites were developed for improved mechanical properties, bioactivity, desired morphological changes, etc. (Figure 9.6). The bioceramic/polymer composites concept was presented by Bonfield et al. They depend on the arrangement of bone tissue comprised of organic molecules reinforced by mineral compartments (Bonfield et al. 1981). For example, HAP/polyethylene combines to form like bone, and it also enhances the bioactivity and toughness of HAP. Further combination of various polymers provides desired porosity, bioactivity, biocompatibility, biodegradation, and mechanical properties (Mehnath et al. 2017; Mehnath et al. 2018a; Jeyaraj et al. 2016). Bioceramics/polymer composites are the best approach to fabricate artificial bone with the required properties (Dorozhkin 2009).

9.6.3.1 Natural Polymers

9.6.3.1.1 Chitosan

In recent years, a combination of biopolymers has been given considerable attention for fabrication of orthopedic materials. Chitosan, a natural polymer, was widely studied as a bone substitute due to its antimicrobial properties and regenerating ability. It is also excellent in binding capacity, pore-forming ability, and biodegradation property. The combination of HAP-chitosan is similar to bone and also increases the HAP strength. Among different methods, in situ is a most common method to prepare a HAP-chitosan nanocomposite. Rusu et al. used a calcium chloride and

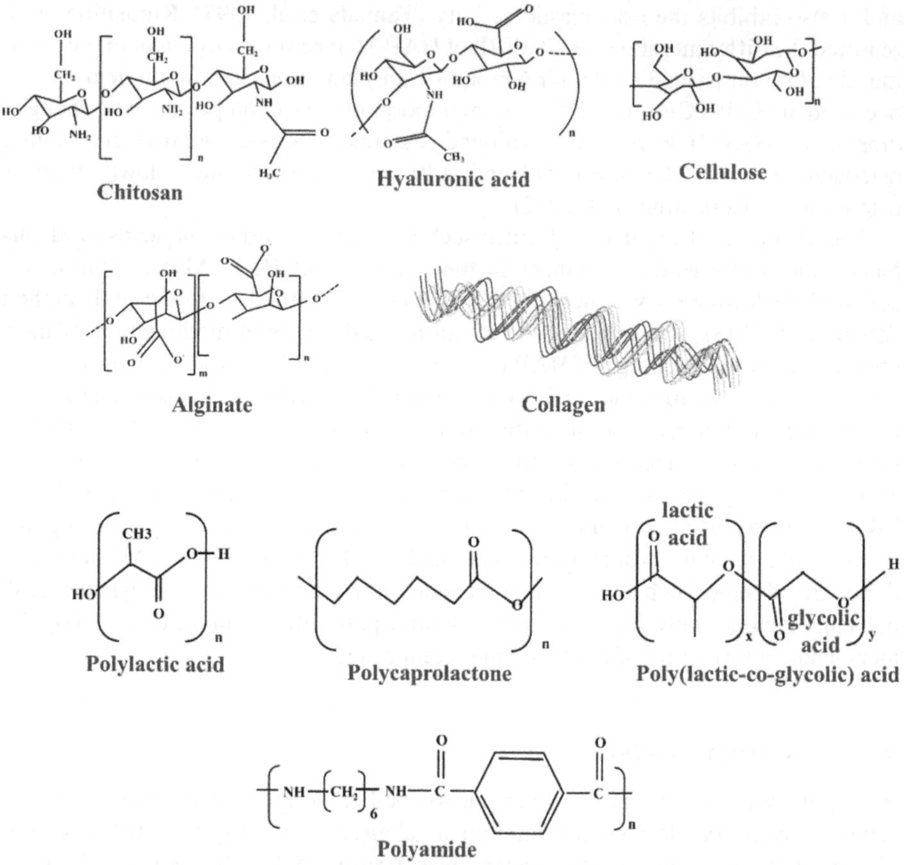

FIGURE 9.6 Different polymers used for preparation of HAP nanocomposites.

sodium dihydrogen phosphate to prepare the HA-chitosan preparation. The prepared HAP was found to be in size range of 15–50 nm, and N-carboxyethylchitosan was used for fabrication. It enhances the alkaline phosphatase activity and exhibited the compression strength around the 0.511 Mpa, which was higher than chitosan alone (Rusu et al. 2005).

Li et al. prepared a different weight ratio of HAP-chitosan (100–0, 80–20, 70–30, 60–40, 50–50, 40–60, and 30–70) using the co-precipitation method. It exhibited higher compressive strength for 70–30 ratio nanocomposites. After HAP-chitosan treatment for 7 days, proliferation rate was about 1.5 times higher compared to the pure chitosan. HAP-chitosan nanofibers induce the MSC differentiation process. It also helps in attachments and proliferation of the MSCs by upregulation of osteogenic markers. In vivo experiments indicate the maximum bone-regeneration ability of HAP-chitosan nanocomposites. In this, segmental bone defects in rabbits were a critical size; they were repaired after 12 weeks of HAP-chitosan treatments, and the defects were visible in chitosan treatment. Further bioactivity of composites was improved by inclusion of a third component such as pectin, gelatin, hyaluronic acid, tripoly phosphate, etc. (Li et al. 2007). Li et al. incorporated the gelatin via in situ chemical method. Functional groups (carboxyl and amine) play a vital role in formation of HAP on the polymer surface. HAP exhibited the crystal size of 17–19 nm and higher cell proliferation with increased ALP activity. A similar result was observed after incorporation of the collagen into the HAP-chitosan nanocomposites (Li et al. 2009).

Jiang et al. utilized HAP-chitosan mixed with carboxymethyl cellulose by freeze drying to prepare material. Carboxymethyl cellulose of 30% weight shows 100–50 nm pore size and maximum compressive strength of 3.54 MPa (Jiang et al. 2008). A further combination of montmorillonite (precipitation method) and gelatin (blending methods) shows better cell proliferation and mechanical properties (Katti et al. 2008). The combination of metal nanoparticles also improves the HAP properties. HAP-chitosan-silver particles were prepared by freeze drying techniques. The controlled amount of silver ions was reduced through chitosan functional groups (Saravanan et al. 2011). The introduction of copper into the Zn-HAP-chitosan nanocomposites leads to increases in efficiency and decreases in degradation (Tripathi et al. 2012; Lian et al. 2013). It is also non-toxic to the animal models. Li et al. prepared graphene oxide–composed HAP-chitosan nanocomposites, which show higher elastic modulus and cell proliferation in L929 and MG-63 cells (Li et al. 2013).

9.6.3.1.2 Collagen

Collagen is a major component of bone that has a fibrous morphology, and it also influences cell adhesion, proliferation, and differentiation. Several studies examined the HAP-collagen nanocomposites application for bone regeneration. It also consists of both positive and negative charges and polar and uncharged residues (Venugopal et al. 2010; Boland et al. 2004). Zhang et al. fabricated hierarchically assembled nanofibril consisting of HAP and collagen via in situ method. Collagen acted as a template for HAP formation, and it formed a collagen fibril surface layer in thicknesses of 0.75–1.45 nm. It exhibited microporous structure, able to withstand the higher compression stress compared to the control (Zhang et al. 2003). Tan et al. prepared HAP-collagen in alginate hydrogel, which showed compressive elastic modulus of 17.0–56.0 kPa and shear modulus of 24.7–55.0 kPa (Tan et al. 2009). Kim et al. fabricated HAP-collagen nanocomposites by the layer-by layer arrangement. It improved cell adhesion, proliferation, and differentiation of MSCs (Kim et al. 2010). Zhang et al. synthesized the HAP-collagen-alginate composites using calcium ions as the crosslinking agent. The strength of composites depends on the alginate ratio, and it also shows the excellent biocompatibility (Zhang et al. 2014). Li et al. used HAP-collagen nanocomposites with a goat model to evaluate bone regeneration effects. Different groups were treated with poly-l-lactic acid, HAP-collagen, and HAP-collagen chitin fibers. Both nanocomposites showed higher bone regeneration compared to the poly-l-lactic acid treated group (Li et al. 2006a). Wang et al. prepared biomimetic synthesis of HAP-collagen with polylactic acid and rhBMP-2 for improved bone formation (Wang et al. 2008). Liu et al. prepared a composite consisting of hyaluronic acid, chitosan, and collagen-HAP, which showed higher proliferation (Liu et al. 2012).

9.6.3.1.3   Gelatin

Gelatin is a solid component derivative of collagen, and in combination with HAP it was mainly studied for bone regeneration applications. Azami et al. fabricated gelatin-HAP by combination of layer solvent casting and freeze-drying techniques. Porous nanocomposites formed with interconnected structure, in size ranges from 100 nm. The nanocomposites density was around 75–93% and the compressive modulus –180 MPa. It also exhibited a good proliferation rate of L929 fibroblast cells and a higher biocompatibility effect over normal cells (Azami et al. 2010). Further studies of nanocomposites were carried out by fabrication of HAP-gelatin microsphere using water-in-oil emulsion methods. They formed needle-like HAP-gelatin crystals with a diameter range of 7.5 nm and well-defined porous structure (Teng et al. 2007). HAP-gelatin nanocomposites were prepared by a thermally assisted low-power ultrasonic irradiation method with different concentrations of gelatin. The synthesized composites were subjected to a heat treatment of 100 to 400°C to form nanosize spherical materials (Brundavanam et al. 2011). HAP-gelatin nanocomposites were prepared with minocycline, an effective antibacterial agent, and the composites were cultured with bone marrow stromal cells. The composites effectively promoted bone marrow stromal cell proliferation. TiO_2 was introduced with HAP-gelatin to form nanocomposites by the phase separation technique. The compressive strength of nanocomposites was elevated to 10.15 MPa due to the presence of titania. Nanocomposites without TiO_2 exhibited compressive strength of 4.87 Mpa, and porosity varied from 77% to 82% (Kailasanathan et al. 2012).

9.6.3.1.4   Silk Fibroin

Silk fibroin is protein isolated from silkworm cocoons, and it is in high demand in bone tissue engineering due to its biocompatibility, bioactivity, biodegradability, and low inflammatory reaction (Li et al. 2006). Nanocomposites with silk fibroin were designed by a freeze-drying technique to form needle-like HAP crystals. The nanocomposites synthesized by coprecipitation methods formed well-distributed pores (Liu et al. 2008). Wei et al. prepared a HAP-fibroin nanocomposite by calcium-phosphate alternate soaking to form electrospun nanofiber. It exhibited higher cell proliferation and functionality like alkaline phosphatase (ALP) activity (Wei et al. 2011). Another electronspun nanofiber was prepared using the polyhydroxybutyrate-co-(3-hydroxyvalerate), valerate fraction, and silk fibroin protein. It formed uniform, smooth, continuous fiber with a diameter of 10–15 μm (Pascu et al. 2013).

9.6.3.1.5   Sericin

Sericin is a protein with a globular structure composed of 18 amino acids, which exhibited hydrophobic behavior. Sericin polar side chains consist of functional groups that strongly interact with calcium and phosphate groups. It enhances critical-size nuclei formation by supersaturation, which forms HAP particles. Combinations of sericin promote good biological properties such as cell attachment and proliferation. The mechanical properties of the sericin-HAP combination are fewer compared to the fibroin-HAP because sericin is not a structural protein (Barajas-Gamboa et al. 2016; Rajput & Kumar Singh 2015). Liu et al. used various methods for preparation of HAP-sericin in a microsphere, rod-like structure using calcium carbonate and sericin as template. Rod-like structures have poor crystallinity, and microsphere exhibits the high crystallinity. Further, an increase in sericin concentration led to an increase in crystal size and agglomeration. It also stimulated the cell attachment and osteogenic differentiation of MSCs and MG-63 cells (Liu et al. 2013). Takeuchi et al. identified conditions for HAP deposition in sericin film, and it showed higher deposition only on sericin with more β-sheet content (Takeuchi et al. 2005).

9.6.3.1.6 Fibrin

Fibrin is a fibral structure and nonglobular protein that plays a vital role in hemostasis, thrombosis, and wound-healing applications. It is derived from blood by cryoprecipitation or chemical precipitation using ammonium sulphate, PEG, and ethanol. In HAP-fibrin combination, fibrin acts as a glue/sealant due to its viscoelastic nature. Mostly it is prepared by mixing HAP and fibrin glue to form a homogeneous composite. In certain cases the addition of proteins, chondrocytes, and growth factor enhance bone regeneration activity. It supports osteoblast growth, which causes bone remodeling (Noori et al. 2017). The introduction of MSCs into a HAP/fibrin composite enhances osteogenic differentiation compared to conventional MSC sheets. HAP/fibrin can also achieve a porous matrix via the sphere-templating method (Jung et al. 2014). Osathanon et al. fabricated porous scaffolds by deposition of calcium phosphate on fibrin and further cast in poly(methyl methacrylate) templates. It formed homogenous pores with interconnected structures with pore size of 200–250 μm. The biological properties of high cell adhesion and proliferation were exhibited in mineralized fibrin scaffolds (Osathanon et al. 2008). Jung et al. prepared a matrix gel made up of fibrin and HAP that was packed in a poly(L-lactic acid) polymer scaffold. It formed a porous structure with pore diameter of 100 to 300 mm and which induced osteogenic differentiation (Jung et al. 2014).

9.6.3.1.7 Keratin

Keratin is a fibrous structural protein, mostly exhibited in α-helix form and also available in β-sheet, random coil sheets. It is extracted by chemical, microbial, enzyme, and microwave irradiation methods. Incorporation of keratin improves the mechanical property and regeneration ability of material. Due to the strong mechanical property, it acts as bone-filling material, excellent in biocompatible and biodegradation properties (Shavandi et al. 2017; Wang et al. 2016). Tachibana et al. used chemically modified keratin for conjugation with HAP. It formed a microporous structure consisting of HAP and also increased osteoblast differentiation (Tachibana et al. 2005). Nakata et al. used a carboxymethylation of keratin to form a HAP/keratin hydrogel. The modified keratin increased HAP accumulation compared with keratin (Nakata et al. 2014).

9.6.3.2 Synthetic Polymers

Biodegradable polymers are widely used synthetic polymers for bone regeneration applications. Polylactic acid (PLA), polyglycolic acid (PGA), and poly(lactic-co-glycolic) acid (PLGA) are well studied for bone-tissue repair applications (Nichols et al. 2007; Pielichowska & Blazewicz 2010; Yun et al. 2014; Zhou et al. 2012).

9.6.3.2.1 Polylactic Acid (PLA)

PLA is synthetic polymer that is mainly utilized for bone regeneration applications due to its biodegradability and biocompatibility. The PLA conjugation with HAP would help in the osteoconductive, and osteoinductive process. The HAP-PLA composite was fabricated by phase separation technique and it prepared by several methods, such as mechanical stirring, ultrasound method, melt, and in situ preparation (Zhang et al. 2013; Han et al. 2013). Normally, HAP particles were dispersed in PLA polymer matrix, which forms rod-like particles in the size range of 65 nm width and 100–400 nm length (Nejati et al. 2008). The PLA combination also helps increase mechanical properties; 4% HAP content with PLA exhibited maximum tensile and bending strength. A HAP-PLA composite prepared from solid-liquid phase separation formed material with pore diameters of 64–175 nm. It also exhibited 8.46 MPa compressive strength, which was more compared with pure PLA of 1.79 MPa (Nejati et al. 2009). Zhang et al. prepared HAP-PLA nanocomposites that exhibited 155 MPa compressive strength and 3.6 GPa Young's modulus (Zhang et al. 2010). In another study, carbonated hydroxyapatite with PLA formed a nanosphere that was fabricated by selective laser sintering (Zhou et al. 2008). Nanocomposites show higher proliferation of MC3T3 osteoblast cells compared with plain PLA. Microsterolithography-based fabrication of HAP-poly(D,L-lactide) composite resin can also fabricate through liquid photointiatir diacrylate resin. The mechanical property, elastic modulus, and rigidity of material increased by raising the HAP concentration (Abdal-Hay et al. 2013). Using a blending method, ternary biocomposites were fabricated by using chitosan, PLA, and HAP. The HAP concentration of 60–67% shows higher compressive strength. A composite formed through the thermally induced phase separation method exhibited a compressive modulus of 15.4–25.5 Mpa, which was higher compared to plain PLA (1.42–1.63 MPa) (Niu et al. 2009).

9.6.3.2.2 Polycaprolactone (PCL)

Polycaprolactone is a one of the bioresorbable polymers that have huge application in bone tissue engineering. Polymer are highly stable and inexpensive, and numerous studies have focused on the HAP-PCL combination. HAP-PCL nanocomposites were prepared by the rapid-prototyping method and formed in the size range of 20–90 nm. The formation of macropores were interconnected, with pore size of 500 nm. It also indicates that MG-63 cells proliferation and attachments are higher than the control groups (Mkhabela & Sinha Ray 2014). The HAP-PCL scaffold was fabricated by the biotemplating method, with NaCl mold of cane, and further it was gas foamed by the pressure-quench method. It forms highly porous nanocomposites with larger pore size and higher compressive strength. Mechanical testing indicates an increase in Young's moduli compared to the PCL alone (Qian et al. 2013). Ternary composites were fabricated using the poly(e-caprolactone fumarate)-N-vinyl pyrrolidone142 and poly(ethylene glycol) with HAP. The solvent casting and evaporation method were used and finally formed nanofiber by electrospinning. MSCs were cultured over nanofiber, and it shows osteogenic differentiation, increase in ALP activity, mRNA expression like runx-2, and bone sialoprotein without addition of any osteogenic supplements (Polini et al. 2011; Lu et al. 2012).

9.6.3.2.3   Poly(lactic-co-glycolic) Acid (PLGA)

PLGA is an excellent biodegradable copolymer that is mainly used in drug delivery due to its controlled drug release. Some reports show the effective role of PLGA on nanocomposite preparation due to its low toxicity and its mechanical strength. HAP-PLGA nanocomposites were prepared by laser sintering, and the material exhibited a higher compressive strength. HAP and PLGA combined to form nanofibers with a diameter of 266 nm (Lao et al. 2011). Several methods, such as particulate leaching, solvent casting, and gas foaming, were used for fabrication of nanocomposites. HAP of different percentage (25%, 35%, 45% w/w) were combined with PLGA to form porous material with bioactivity and biodegradable property (Chen et al. 2011). HAP-PLGA nanocomposites containing RGD peptide and bone morphogenesis protein were prepared to evaluate the bone regeneration effect against a defective radial bone in a rabbit model. It shows the best healing effect by promoting cell adhesion and differentiation. The HAP-PLGA combination was blended with collagen, and the availability of more functional groups in collagen increases the HAP deposition. In another method, HAP-PLGA formed nanoparticles loaded with BMP-2, and it exhibited the controlled release of BMP-2 (Zhang et al. 2011).

9.6.3.2.4   Polyamides

Polyamides (PAs) have some structural and molecular similarity to the collagen that is present in human bone. They also provide good mechanical strength, biocompatibility, biodegradability, and non-toxicity effect to nanocomposites. HAP-PA nanocomposites were prepared by the co-precipitation and co-solution method to form needle-like materials. They formed a crystal size diameter of 10–20 nm and length 70–90 nm. The material exhibited porosity with a diameter of 100–300 nm, and elastic modulus material is 5.6 GPa (Jie & Yubao 2004). Another HAP-PA composite was prepared by a thermally induced phase inversion technique, and when cultured over MSCs indicates cell differentiation. A nanocomposite prepared by injection molding was implanted in the tibiae and muscle of a defective rabbit model. After 2 weeks, biocompatibility, osteogenesis, and osteoinductivity of nanocomposites were evaluated. There was an increase in osteogenesis to form new dense bone without any defects and similar to the host bone. HAP-PA composites loaded with basic fibroblast growth factor and MSCs show improvement in angiogenesis and osteogenesis on defective animal models. The introduction of growth factor and MSC-based ex vivo gene transfer accelerated the vascularization of bone (Xu et al. 2010; Qu et al. 2011).

9.6.3.2.5   Other Polymers

Polyvinyl alcohol (PVA) is a chemically stable hydrophilic polymer that has huge application in bone regeneration. The in situ development of HAP-PVA nanocomposites is carried out by freeze/thaw and spray drying methods. It showed effective results in both in vitro and in vivo studies (Sinha et al. 2008). Polyurethanes (PU) is another polymer with good thermoplasticity and elastic and durable properties. It is a porous nanocomposite composed of 30%, and 70% wt of HAP, and it has a pore size of 100–800 mm. Nanocomposites exhibited strong compressive strength of 271 kPa (Dong et al. 2009). Another nanocomposite was prepared with fluorine and formed in size range from 50–250 nm. Biocompatible-effect nanocomposites were evaluated with MSCs for viability; proliferation was 72% higher compared to control. Polyhydroxybutyrate (PHB) is a common polyester polymer like poly (hydroxyabutyrate-cohydroxyvalerate) (PHBV), and poly(3-hydroxybutyrate) was combined with HAP for bone regeneration applications. The PHBV was combined with HAP to form a nanofibrous scaffold and also combined with PLA to form a highly porous microstructure (Porter et al. 2013; Jack et al. 2009).

9.7 APPLICATION OF HYDROXYAPATITE

In several bioceramics, hydroxyapatite was widely used in clinical application due to its versatility. In bone regeneration treatment, it was fabricated into four different forms: scaffold, implant coating, injectable hydrogel, and 3D printed scaffold (Figure 9.7).

9.7.1 HAP-SCAFFOLD

Several fabrication techniques used with HAP-scaffolds have been inspired by natural bone biological features (Figure 9.8). First-generation scaffold materials bioinert scaffold; second generation materials are bioresorbable and bioactive. Currently, intensive research is being carried out in developing bio-instructive scaffolds that are able to stimulate the specific cellular response. Ren et al. prepared the HAP scaffold with microchannels and micropores on its surface. Scaffolds have a grooved structure, which increases cell adhesion and vascularization and induces bone formation. It shows high osteoinductive activity after treatment with

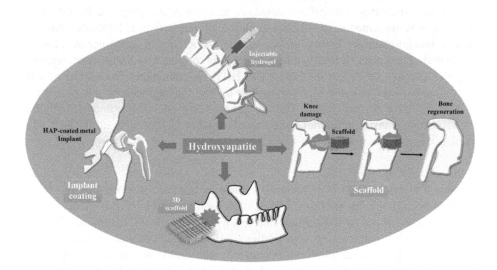

FIGURE 9.7 Application of hydroxyapatite by scaffold, injectable hydrogel, implant coating, and 3D printed scaffold.

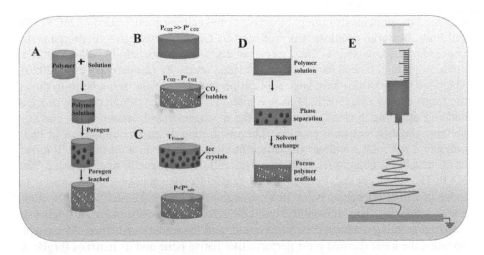

FIGURE 9.8 Scaffold preparation (A) Solvent-casting particle-leaching process, (B) Gas foaming, (C) Freeze drying, (D) Phase separation, (E) Electrospinning.

MSCs and promotes osteoblast differentiation. In in vivo studies, scaffold establishment for four weeks led to formation of a thin calcified bone layer. It also formed connective tissue and blood vessels after implantation treatment. Several techniques were available to achieve scaffolds with suitable porosity and proper surface property. It involves the introduction of organic or inorganic porogen into the mixture (Ren et al. 2018). Chen et al. utilized a chitosan and gelatin combination for fabrication of HAP scaffold for osteogenic differentiation. The scaffold exhibited high osteoconduction and osteoinduction due to the HAP and polysaccharides derived from the chitin and collagen protein. It helps in mimicking the bone matrix, which also leads to increased biocompatibility and antimicrobial and biodegradation properties (Chen et al. 2019). Addition of gelatin is due to its ability in formation of RGD (Arginyl glycyl aspartic acid)-like structure. RGD structure is very close to the structure of native bone extra cellular matrix (Mahmoudi Saber 2019). Similar components were used for preparation of electrospun nanofiber scaffolds using glutaraldehyde as a crosslinker (Chitra et al. 2017; Mehnath et al. 2020b). HAP particles were deposited by a wet-chemical process onto porous scaffold. In vitro MG-63 cells were used for evaluation of biocompatibility and proliferation. The number of cells were less in the chitosan-gelatin scaffold, and there was higher cell proliferation in the HAP-chitosan-gelatin scaffold.

Similarly migration of cells was also higher in the HAP-containing scaffold. So, the biomimetic scaffold porosity imitates the bone extracellular matrix due to availability of extensive inorganic particles. In scaffolds, HAP stimulates the cellular response such as osteoconductivity, cell growth, bioactivity, etc. (Chen et al. 2019). Januariyasa et al. prepared the fibrous scaffold structure to mimic the extra cellular matrix, and it was composed of carbonated-HAP, chitosan, and polyvinyl alcohol. Carbonated-HAP was prepared via the co-precipitation method and simultaneously added to the chitosan/PVA to form a nanofiborous scaffold. The material exhibited the protein adsorption, bioactivity, and cellular proliferation of MC3T3E1 cell lines. Bacterial cellulose was produced by *Gluconacetobacter* microorganisms via oxidative fermentation. These eco-friendly components help in cellular attachment, migration, biocompatibility, and surface reactivity (Januariyasa et al. 2020). Magnetic nanoparticles have huge application in medical field, and it helps to direct the target site by magnetic field. It was also involved in the osteoinductive process and cell signaling, such as activation of the mechano-transduction process and signalizing the differentiation pathway. The integration of magnetic material in PCL polymeric scaffolds promotes the differentiation pathway in a rat model. Torgobo et al. developed composites with bacterial cellulose, magnetic nanoparticles, and HAP. The physiochemical properties of scaffold nanocomposites were similar to those of native trabecular bone. In vitro studies using MC3T3-E1 cell lines show non-cytotoxicity, biocompatibility, and cell adhesion. Porosity plays an important role in promoting anchorage, cell migration, and biomimetic structure. Along with porosity, the ideal scaffold must perform like native bone and its matrix (Torgbo & Sukyai 2019). Some different types HAP-scaffold applications are given in Table 9.4.

9.7.2 IMPLANT COATING

The major implant materials are metal or alloys, mostly titanium alloys. Titanium is widely used for its mechanical properties, durability, low density, and higher stability. The main disadvantages of titanium are poor biocompatibility and lack of osteointegration activity. To enhance titanium implant properties, it was coated with hydroxyapatite, which exhibits good biocompatibility and osteoconductive activity (Yunan et al. 2016). The HAP coating on the implant was prepared by several methods, such as electrophoretic coating, plasma spraying, spin-coating, sol-gel, ion-beam–assisted deposition, and sputtering. The properties of implant-coating material depend on the parameters and fabrication method (Mejias et al. 2016; Levingstone et al. 2015). Narayanan et al. demonstrated good HAP-coating that exhibited high crystallinity, appropriate stoichiometry, porosity, and good adhesion to substrate. The characteristic effects of coating techniques are briefly described below (Narayanan et al. 2008). The plasma-spraying method is an easy, economically available method for coating metal implants. It exhibits various structural forms, poor bonding, non-uniform thickness. The crystalline gradient disturbs the adhesive strength of coating material because of HAP size, preheating substrate, plasma power, and post-disposition heat (Hao et al. 2011). The sol-gel method forms a chemically homogenous film with fine grains, and it is a simple method due to the low processing temperature. The pulsed-laser deposition coating process is a promising method that produces crystallinity and a high adhesive layer (Sidane et al. 2017). An electrochemical deposition technique helps for coating irregular-shaped objects at low temperature, with high control over coating thickness, phase composition, and crystallinity (He et al. 2016). Mihailescu et al. prepared an animal-derived hydroxyapatite with MgF_2 and MgO, which improves the adhesion of coating on Si-substrate by pulsed laser techniques. The addition of carbon nanotubes and graphene oxide into the HAP helps increase mechanical properties. The carbon nanotube substitution into HAP especially resulted in the formation of homogenous coating without cracking and with

TABLE 9.4
Different Types of Hydroxyapatite-Polymeric Scaffolds and Applications

Material	Application	Reference
PLA-HAP	Screw-like scaffold loaded with MSCs induces bone growth inside the bone tunnel.	Liu et al. 2016
Gelatin-Si- dopped HAP	Scaffold consisting of vancomycin release gradually inhibits bacterial growth. It also enhances the MC3T3-E1 differentiation and gene expression.	Martine-Vazquez et al. 2015
Collagen-PLGA-HAP	Scaffold encapsulated with pro-osteogenic peptide PTHrP exhibited good porosity and mechanical properties.	Lopez-Noriega et al. 2015
Collagen-HAP	Scaffold loaded with recombinant human bone morphogenetic protein 2 (rhBMP-2). It exhibited the sustained release of rhBMP-2.	Quinlan et al. 2015
HAP/β-TCP	Scaffold loaded with BMP-2 and coated with dipyridamole, which stimulates A2A receptors, enhance bone growth.	Ishack et al. 2017
Silk/calcium phosphate/PLGA	Scaffold loaded with platelet-derived growth factor (PDGF) and vascular endothelial growth factor (VEGF). The sufficient bioactivity, promote the proliferation and bone development *in vivo* studies.	Farokhi et al. 2013
Agarose-HAP	Scaffold loaded with zoledronic acid and ibuprofen.	Paris et al. 2015
HAP-icariin-vancomycin	In vivo studies shows the complete repair, improved bone formation.	Huang et al. 2013
Chitosan-Silk fibroin-polyethylene terephthalate-HAP	Introduction of silver and VEGF increases the osteocalcin, antibacterial property.	Jiang et al. 2020
Alginate-HAP	Loaded with dexamethasone and stromal cell factor 1. Stromal cell factor 1 influence cellular signaling and the release of dexamethasone directs the differentiation of cells.	Zhang et al. 2018
PCL-ZnO-HAP	Zn vital elements activates above 3000 proteins, antimicrobial activity, and osteoinductive stimulator.	Sabry et al. 2018
Carbon dots-chitosan-HAP	Carbon dots have role in decrease of bacterial growth. It also increases the osteogenesis and increases the expression of ALP.	Lu et al. 2018

high crystallinity, bonding strength, and biocompatibility (Mihailescu et al. 2016). Chitosan-graphene-oxide–containing HAP composites was coated on titanium substrate by electrophoretic deposition. The coated material forms good biocompatibility and reduces the *Staphylococcus aureus* attachment. Addition of graphene oxide-polymer increases the steadiness and enhances the HAP coating. The metal implant material needs to be free from bacteria after placement on the damaged site. Bacteria cells can easily adhere to the implant surface and initiate the formation of biofilm, leading to development of infection. So an implant surface coated with HAP needs to have antibacterial properties. An antibiotic-loaded HAP coated implant material allows delivery of antibiotics to control the infection/inflammation after surgery (Shi et al. 2016). The encapsulation of antibiotics/organic molecules with HAP was based on the physisorption, which did not allow prolonged release. So components such as silver and zinc with antibacterial property were introduced to HAP (Gautier et al. 2000; Huang et al. 2017). Guimond-Lisher et al. prepared HAP-silver nanocomposites coated on the titanium implant via vacuum plasma spray techniques. They did not exhibit any cytotoxic effect to the cells and showed antibacterial activity. The maximum silver release rate inhibited the bacteria adhering to the implant surface. HAP with zinc and HAP consisting of magnetite have higher antibacterial activity (Guimond-Lisher et al. 2016).

9.7.3 INJECTABLE HYDROGELS

Injectable hydrogels have a huge advantage for bone regeneration applications due to easy surgical procedure. A semisolid/liquid gel is introduced onto the defective sites and is hardened slowly to a gel by increases in temperature (Chatterjee et al. 2018). Thermosresponsive hydrogels are classified based on the critical solution temperature, where the polymer material undergoes a change from one phase to another at a particular temperature. In lower critical solution temperature (LCST), the polymer material poorly dissolves in water with increases in temperature. Mostly nanomaterial that exhibits phase transition near body temperature is valuable for biomedical applications (Ferreira et al. 2018). a HAP-poly(Nisopropylacrylamide) combination is used for fabrication of thermosensitive gel for bone regeneration applications. Nanocomposites undergo phase transition that changes them into compact material. Another thermosensitive material, pluronics, are combined with HAP and poly(ethylene oxide) co-polymer to form hydrogels (Li et al. 2013). In addition to temperature, environment pH alters the hydrogel behavior. The local pH changes the properties of nanocomposites and must be optimal for cell growth. Hydrogel guides cell migration by releasing chemitactic signals (Rogina et al. 2017). It also promotes bone growth by releasing signal molecules and controlling microbial growth during bone regeneration. Hydrogel properties facilitate the migration and integration of osteoblast cells. Flow properties and physical stability HAP hydrogel stimulate cell proliferation. The regenerating property of injectable hydrogels was enriched by encapsulation of MSCs (Tan et al. 2019). It differentiates into osteoblast cells, increases proliferation, and helps in regeneration of deep bone defects (Arun Kumar et al. 2015).

9.7.4   3D PRINTED SCAFFOLD

Currently additive manufacturing has gained huge attention in medical and many industrial fields. Additive manufacturing offers the possibility of getting scaffolds that perfectly fit onto the defective sites. Digital ability recreates a scaffold that mimics the damaged tissues (Zindani & Kumar 2018; Negahdari et al. 2019). Several techniques have been applied for creating tissue scaffolds in ceramics form. There are two categories for scaffold production: laser and extrusion-based techniques (Figure 9.9). Intensive research was available for the manufacture of HAP-based scaffolds able to induce osteogenesis and angiogenesis (Milazzo et al. 2019). A 3D-printed HAP scaffold with poor mechanical property was fabricated by Kim et al. To overcome this drawback, they fabricated the HAP scaffold coated with PCL loaded with BMP-2 (bone morphogenic protein). It exhibited an increase in compressive strength and BMP-2 induced-osteoinduction and accelerated bone healing. In vivo evaluation using rabbit calvarial defects exhibited the improvement of bone regeneration (Kim et al. 2018). Sun et al. integrated the BMP-2 (P28) into a HAP scaffold. It exhibited higher attachment and more proliferation of bone cells (Sun et al. 2018). Millazo et al. reported a comprehensive review of multiple HAP-based composite scaffolds prepared via 3D printing processes. They form based on a polymer matrix of different size ranges from nanometers to micrometers. A wide range of polymers, such as chitosan, hyaluronic acid, collagen, gelatin, PVA, PLA, PCL, and PGLA, were used as primary compounds along with HAP to fabricate the 3D-printed scaffolds. But the challenge is mechanical properties, which make it difficult to be processed (Milazzo et al. 2019).

9.8   CONCLUSION AND FUTURE PERSPECTIVE

The process of bone regeneration consists of numerous complexities from the starting point of design material. Hydroxyapatite has considerable promise as a candidate for bone regeneration therapy. The advanced properties, formulation, desired modification, and cost-effectiveness are the major drawbacks. In future those will be overcome by computational modelling, which will play a major role in bone regeneration application. A scaffold with anticipated geometric shape at macroscopic/microscopic level must be selected to elicit cell growth, vital fluid flow, and incorporation with surrounding tissue. Different forms of materials are used in scaffolds, and element analysis used to measure the physical properties and components (Naderi et al. 2016). In addition to modeling, finite element analysis predicts the effects of change in HAP properties. Modification of apatite composition can be due to alteration of variable in production process. In chemical synthesis, addition of Mg^{2+} or other ions in reaction will lead to incorporation into the apatite structure. Likewise, change in temperature and aging time will alter the HAP properties, which affects the resorption properties of HAP. Approaches like nonstoichiometric forms are more effective in biodegradable and bioactive properties than stoichiometric form of HAP. This preferred alteration is useful for certain clinical bone-regeneration applications (Sarkar et al. 2019).

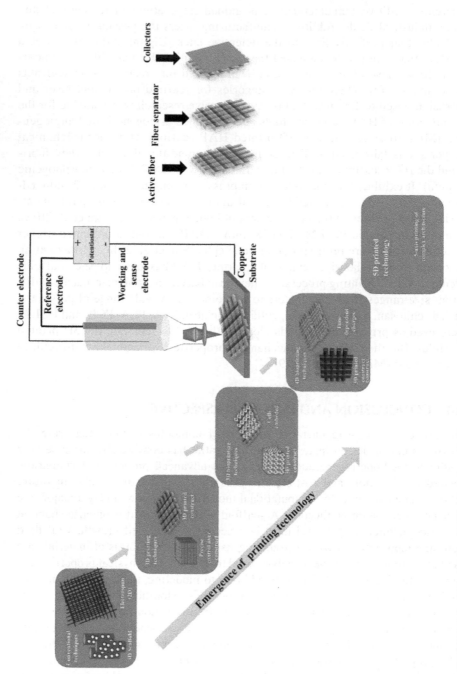

FIGURE 9.9 Fabrication of 3D printed scaffold and emergence of printing technology.

Computational modelling is the study of interactions between surface of scaffold material and proteins. It is used to design material with a higher level of relationship at the submolecular level, more specifically in the nanoscale range. Molecular dynamics simulation technique helps in evaluation of scaffold and bone protein interaction at the atomic level. (Huang et al. 2018). Some other interaction parameters, such as binding energy and desorption energy, can also be calculated (Lai et al. 2014). The new bond formation restricts the movements and generates the stick-slip motion between the two surfaces. This motion denotes the high fracture resistance of bone. Simulation studies evaluate the orientation of proteins that adsorbed on the HAP surface. The alteration in the orientation will alter the adsorption/desorption behavior of proteins. The interaction also influences the intermolecular hydrogen bonding and structural characteristics of protein (Zhou et al. 2007). It also indicates that interaction changes the conformation and orientation of the adsorbed proteins. It is based on the epitope of proteins that bond onto the HAP surface and which influence the cellular response. The high-throughput screening technique used to validate regeneration results at molecular levels. The desired pattern of cellular events was chosen before performing the physiological tests (Gu et al. 2019).

ACKNOWLEDGMENTS

We gratefully acknowledge the support from Indian Council of Medical Research, New Delhi, for a Senior Research Fellowship (ICMR-SRF Grant no. Fellowship/TB/32/2019/ECD-I). We also thank DST-SERB for funding this project, Grant No. EEQ/2020/000122.

ABBREVIATIONS

BCP   biphasic calcium phosphates
CTAB   cetyltrimethylammonium bromide
ECM   extracellular matrix
EDTA   ethylene diamine tetracetic acid
ERK   extracellular-signal-regulated kinase
HAP   hydroxyapatite
LCST   lower critical solution temperature
MSCs   mesenchymal stem cells
PCL   polycaprolactone
PEG   polyethylene glycol
PGA   polyglycolic acid
PHB   polyhydroxybutyrate
PHBV   poly (hydroxyabutyrate-cohydroxyvalerate)
PLA   polylactic acid
PLGA   poly(lactic-co-glycolic) acid
STPP   sodium tripolyphosphate
TCP   tricalcium phosphate
WH   whitlockite

REFERENCES

Abdal-Hay, A., Sheikh, F.A., Lim, J.K. (2013). Air jet spinning of hydroxyapatite/poly(lactic acid) hybrid nanocomposite membrane mats for bone tissue engineering. Colloid Surface B, 102, 635–643.

Alshemary, A.Z., Akram, M., Taha, A., Evis, Z., Hussain, R. (2018). Physico-chemical and biological properties of hydroxyapatite extracted from chicken beaks. Mater. Lett, 215, 169–172.

Amer, W., Abdelouahdi, K., Ramananarivo, H.R., Zahouily, M., Fihri, A., Coppel, Y., Varma, R.S., Solhy, A. (2013). Synthesis of mesoporous nano-hydroxyapatite by using zwitterions surfactant. Mater. Lett, 107, 189–193.

Amiri, A., Chahkandi, M., Targhoo, A. (2017). Synthesis of nano-hydroxyapatite sorbent for microextraction in packed syringe of phthalate esters in water samples. Anal. Chim. Acta, 950, 64–70.

Anderud, J., Jimbo, R., Abrahamsson, P., Adolfsson, E., Malmström, J., Wennerberg, A. (2016). The impact of surface roughness and permeability in hydroxyapatite bone regeneration membranes. Clin. Oral Implants Res, 27, 1047–1054.

Arun Kumar, R., Sivashanmugam, A., Deepthi, S., Iseki, S., Chennazhi, K., Nair, S.V., Jayakumar, R. (2015). Injectable chitin-poly (ε- caprolactone)/nanohydroxyapatite composite microgels prepared by simple regeneration technique for bone tissue engineering. ACS Appl. Mater. Interfaces, 7 (18), 9399–9409.

Ashuri, M., Moztarzadeh, F., Nezafati, N., Hamedani, A.A., Tahriri, M. (2012). Development of a composite based on hydroxyapatite and magnesium and zinc-containing sol-gel-derived bioactive glass for bone substitute applications. Mater. Sci. Eng. C, 32(8), 2330–2339.

Azami, M., Rabiee, M., Moztarzadeh, F. (2010). Glutaraldehyde crosslinked gelatin/hydroxyapatite nanocomposite scaffold, engineered via compound techniques. Polym. Compos, 31, 2112–2120.

Balamurugan, A., Rebelo, A.H.S., Lemos, A.F., Rocha, J.H.G,. Ventura, J.M.G., Ferreira, J.M.F. (2008). Suitability evaluation of sol-gel derived Si-substituted hydroxyapatite for dental and maxillofacial applications through in vitro osteoblasts response. Dent. Mater, 24(10), 1374–1380.

Banerjee, S., Bagchi, B., Bhandary, S., Kool, A. (2018). A facile vacuum assisted synthesis of nanoparticle impregnated hydroxyapatite composites having excellent antimicrobial properties and biocompatibility. Ceram. Int, 44, 1066–1077.

Barajas-Gamboa, J.A., Serpa-Guerra, A.M., Restrepo-Osorio, A., Alvarez-Lopez, C. (2016). Sericin applications: a globular silk protein. Ing. Compet, 18, 193–206.

Benzigar, M.R., Mane, G.P., Talapaneni, S.N., Varghese, S., Anand, C., Aldeyab, S.S., Balasubramanian, V.V., Vinu, A. (2012). Microwave-assisted synthesis of highly crystalline mesoporous hydroxyapatite with a rod-shaped morphology, Chem. Lett. 41, 458–460.

Boland, E.D., Matthews, J.A., Pawlowski, K.J., Simpson, D.G., Wnek, G.E., Bowlin, G.L. (2004). Electrospinning collagen and elastin: Preliminary vascular tissue engineering. Front. Biosci, 9, 1422–1432.

Bonfield, W., Grynpas, M.D., Tully, A.E., Bowman, J., Abram, J. (1981). Hydroxyapatite reinforced polyethylene – a mechanically compatible implant material for bone replacement. Biomaterials, 2, 185–186.

Brundavanam, R.K., Jiang, Z.T., Chapman, P., Le, X.T., Mondinos, N., Fawcett, D., Poinern, G.E.J. (2011). Effect of dilute gelatine on the ultrasonic thermally assisted synthesis of nano hydroxyapatite. Ultrason. Sonochem, 18(3), 697–703.

Calabrese, G., Giuffrida, R., Forte, S., Fabbi, C., Figallo, E., Salvatorelli, L., Memeo, L., Parenti, R., Gulisano, M., Gulino, R. (2017). Human adipose-derived mesenchymal stem cells seeded into a collagen-hydroxyapatite scaffold promote bone augmentation after implantation in the mouse. Sci. Rep, 7(1), 1–11.

Cao, H., Kuboyama, N. (2010). A biodegradable porous composite scaffold of PGA/β-TCP for bone tissue engineering. Bone, 46, 386–395.

Cazalbou, S., Combes, C., Eichert, D., Rey, C., Glimcher, M.J. (2004). Poorly crystalline apatites: evolution and maturation in vitro and in vivo. J. Bone Miner. Metab, 22, 310–317.

Chakraborty, R., Roychowdhury, D. (2013). Fish bone derived natural hydroxyapatitesupported copper acid catalyst: taguchi optimization of semibatch oleic acid esterification, Chem. Eng. J, 215–216, 491–499

Chatterjee, S., Hui, P.C.l., Kan, C.W. (2018). Thermoresponsive hydrogels and their biomedical applications: Special insight into their applications in textile based transdermal therapy. Polymers, 10 (5), 480.

Chen, J., Liu, J., Deng, H., Yao, S., Wang, Y. (2020). Regulatory synthesis and characterization of hydroxyapatite nanocrystals by a microwave-assisted hydrothermal method, Ceram. Int, 46, 2185–2193.

Chen, L., Tang, C.Y., Chen, D.Z., Wong, C.T., Tsui, C.P. (2011). Fabrication and characterization of poly-d-l-lactide/nano-hydroxyapatite composite scaffolds with poly(ethylene glycol) coating and dexamethasone releasing. Compos. Sci. Technol, 71(16), 1842–1849.

Chen, P., Liu, L., Pan, J., Mei, J., Li, C., Zheng, Y. (2019). Biomimetic composite scaffold of hydroxyapatite/gelatinchitosan core-shell nanofibers for bone tissue engineering. Mater. Sci. Eng. C, 97, 325–335.

Chitra, K., Mehnath, S., Ganesh Kumar, J., Rangasamy, S., Balasubramanian, S., Dhinakar Raj, G. (2017). Fabrication of progesterone-loaded nanofibers for the drug delivery applications in bovine. Nanoscale Res. Lett, 12, 116.

Conz, M.B., Granjeiro, J.M., Soares, G.A. (2011). Hydroxyapatite crystallinity does not affect the repair of critical size bone defects. J. Appl. Oral Sci, 19(4), 337–342.

Cooper, C., Campion, G., Melton, L.J. (1992). Hip fractures in the elderly: a world-wide projection. Osteoporosis Int, 1992, 2(6), 285–289.

Dong, Z., Li, Y., Zou, Q. (2009). Degradation and biocompatibility of porous nano-hydroxyapatite/polyurethane composite scaffold for bone tissue engineering. Appl. Surf. Sci, 255, 6087–6091.

Dorozhkin, S.V. (2009). Calcium orthophosphate-based biocomposites and hybrid biomaterials. J Mater Sci, 44, 2343–2387.

Dorozhkin, S.V. (2012a). Biphasic, triphasic and multiphasic calcium orthophosphates. Acta Biomater, 8, 963–977.

Dorozhkin, S.V. (2012b). Calcium Orthophosphates Applications in Nature, Biology and Medicine. Boca Raton, FL: Pan Stanford Publishing.

Dorozhkin, S.V., Epple, M. (2002). Biological and medical significance of calcium phosphates. Angew. Chem. Int. Ed, 41, 3130–3146.

Dubok, V.A. (2000). Bioceramics–yesterday, today, tomorrow. Powder Metall Met Ceram, 39, 381–394.

Evis, Z., Webster, T. (2011). Nanosize hydroxyapatite: doping with various ions. Adv. Appl. Ceram, 110, 311–321.

Farokhi, M., Mottaghitalabb, F., Ai, J., Shokrgozar, M.A. (2013). Sustained release of platelet-derived growth factor and vascular endothelial growth factor from silk/calcium delivery and bone regeneration. Acta Biomater, 15, 200–209.

Ferreira, N., Ferreira, L., Cardoso, V., Boni, F., Souza, A., Gremiaao, M. (2018). Recent advances in smart hydrogels for biomedical applications: From self-assembly to functional approaches. Eur. Polym. J, 99, 117–133.

França, R., Samani, T.D., Bayade, G., Yahia, L.H., Sacher, E. (2014). Nanoscale surface characterization of biphasic calcium phosphate, with comparisons to calcium hydroxyapatite and β-tricalcium phosphate bioceramics. J. Colloid Interface Sci, 420, 182–188.

Gautier, H., Merle, C., Auget, J.L., Daculsi, G. (2000). Isostatic compression, a new process for incorporating vancomycin into biphasic calcium phosphate: comparison with a classical method. Biomaterials, 21(3), 243–249.

Gligorijevic, B.J., Vilotijevic, M., Scepanovic, M., Vukovic, N.S., Radovic, N.A. (2016). Substrate preheating and structural properties of power plasma sprayed hydroxyapatite coatings. Ceram Int, 42, 411–420.

Gopi, D., Bhuvaneshwari, N., Indira, J., Kanimozhi, K., Kavitha, L. (2013a). A novel green template assisted synthesis of hydroxyapatite nanorods and their spectral characterization. Spectrochim. Acta: A Mol. Biomol. Spectrosc, 107, 196–202.

Gopi, D., Bhuvaneshwari, N., Indira, J., Kavitha, L. (2013b). Synthesis and spectroscopic investigations of hydroxyapatite using a green chelating agent as template. Spectrochim. Acta: A Mol. Biomol. Spectrosc, 104, 292–299.

Gopi, D., Kanimozhi, K., Bhuvaneshwari, N., Indira, J., Kavitha, L. (2014). Novel banana peel pectin mediated green route for the synthesis of hydroxyapatite nanoparticles and their spectral characterization, Spectrochim. Acta: A Mol. Biomol. Spectrosc, 118, 589–597

Gosain, A.K., Song, L., Riordan, P. (2002). A 1-year study of osteoinduction in hydroxyapatite-derived biomaterials in an adult sheep model: part I. Plast Reconstr Surg, 109, 619–630.

Gu, H., Xue, Z., Wang, M., Yang, M., Wang, K., Xu, D. (2019). Effect of Hydroxyapatite Surface on BMP-2 Biological Properties by Docking and Molecular Simulation Approaches. J. Phys. Chem. B, 123 (15), 3372–3382.

Guimond-Lisher, S., Ren, Q., Braissant, O., Gruner, P., Wampfler, B., Maniura-Weber, K. (2016). Vacuum plasma sprayed coatings using ionic silver dopped hydroxyapatite powder to prevent bacterial infection of bone implants. Biointerphases, 11, 011012.

Ha, S.W., Jang, H.L., Nam, K.T., Beck, G.R. (2015). Nano-hydroxyapatite modulates osteoblast lineage commitment by stimulation of DNA methylation and regulation of gene expression. Biomaterials, 64, 32–42.

Ha, S.W., Park, J., Habib, M.M., Beck Jr. G.R. (2017). Nanohydroxyapatite stimulation of gene expression requires Fgf receptor, phosphate transporter, and Erk1/2 signaling. ACS Appl. Mater. Interfaces, 9, 39185–39196.

Han, W., Zhao, J., Tu, M., Zeng, R., Zha, Z., Zhou, C. (2013). Preparation and characterization of nanohydroxyapatite strengthening nanofibrous poly(L-lactide) scaffold for bone tissue engineering. J. Appl. Polym. Sci, 128, 1332–1338.

Hao, J., Kuroda, S., Ohya, K., Bartakova, S., Aoki, H., Kasugai, S. (2011). Enhanced osteoblast and osteoclast responses to a thin film sputtered hydroxyapatite coating. J. Mater. Sci. Mater. Med, 22, 1489–499.

Hao, Y., Yan, H., Wang, X., Zhu, B., Ning, C., Ge, S. (2012). Evaluation of osteoinduction and proliferation on nano-Sr-HAP: a novel orthopedic biomaterial for bone tissue regeneration. J. Nanosci. Nanotechnol, 12(1), 207–212.

Hauburger, A., Von Einem, S., Schwaerzer, G.K., Buttstedt, A., Zebisch, M., Schraml, M., Hortschansky, P., Knaus, P., Schwarz, E. (2009). The pro-form of BMP-2 interferes with BMP-2 signaling by competing with BMP-2 for IA receptor binding. FEBS J, 276(21), 6386–6398.

He, D.H., Wang, P., Liu, P., Liu, X.K., Ma, F.C., Zhao, J. (2016). HA coating fabricated by electrochemical deposition on modified Ti6Al4V alloy. Surf Coat Technol, 30, 6–12.

Hench, L.L., Thompson, I. (2010). Twenty-first century challenges for biomaterials. JR Soc Interface. 7(suppl 4), S379–S391.

Henkel, J., Woodruff, M.A., Epari, D.R., Steck, R., Glatt, V., Dickinson, I.C., Choong, P.F., Schuetz, M.A., Hutmacher, D.W. (2013). Bone regeneration based on tissue engineering conceptions a 21st century perspective. Bone Res, 1(3), 216–248.

Hidroksiapatit, P., Sebagai, P. (2017). Synthesis and characterization of hydroxyapatite from bulk seashells and its potential usage as lead ions adsorbent. Malaysian J. Anal. Sci. 21, 571–584.

Hing, K., Annaz, B., Saeed, S., Revell, P., Buckland, T. (2005). Microporosity enhances bioactivity of synthetic bone graft substitutes. J. Mater. Sci. Mater. Med, 16, 467–475.

Huang, B., Lou, Y., Li, T., Lin, Z., Sun, S., Yuan, Y., Liu, C., Gu, Y. (2018). Molecular dynamics simulations of adsorption and desorption of bone morphogenetic protein-2 on textured hydroxyapatite surfaces. Acta Biomater, 80, 121–130

Huang, J.G., Pang, L., Chen, Z.R., Tan, X.P. (2013). Dual-delivery of vancomycin and icariin form an injectable calcium phosphate cement-release system for controlling infection and improving bone healing. Mol Med Rep, 8, 1221–1227.

Huang, Y., Zhang, X., Zhang, H., Qiao, H., Zhang, X., Jia, T., et al. (2017). Fabrication of silver and strontium-doped hydroxyapatite/TiO2 nanotube bilayer coatings for enhancing bactericidal effect and osteoinductivity. Ceram. Int, 43(1), 992–1007.

Huang, Y.T., Imura, M., Neheng, C.H., Yamauchi, Y. (2011). Block-copolymer-assisted synthesis of hydroxyapatite nanoparticles with high surface area and uniform size. Sci. Technol. Adv. Mater, 12, 045005.

Ingole, V.H., Hussein, K.H., Kashale, A.A., Gattu, K.P. (2016). Invitro bioactivity and osteogenic activity study of Solid state synthesized nano-hydroxyapatite using recycled eggshell bio-waste. Chemistry Select, 1, 3901–3908.

Ishack, S., Mediero, A., Wilder, T., Ricci, J.L., Cronstein, B.N. (2017). Bone regeneration in critical bone defects using three-dimensionally printed β-tricalcium phosphate/hydroxyapatite scaffolds is enhanced by coating scaffolds with either dipyridamole or BMP-2. J. Biomed. Mater. Res. B Appl Biomater, 105(2), 366–375.

Iyyappan, E., Wilson, P. (2013). Synthesis of nanoscale hydroxyapatite particles using triton X-100 as an organic modifier. Ceram. Int, 39, 771–777.

Iyyappan, E., Wilson, P., Sheela, K., Ramya, R. (2016). Role of triton X-100 and hydrothermal treatment on the morphological features of nanoporous hydroxyapatite nanorods. Mater. Sci. Eng. C, 63, 554–562.

Jack, K.S., Velayudhan, S., Luckman, P., Trau, M., Grondahl, L., Cooper White, J. (2009). The fabrication and characterization of biodegradable HA/PHBV nanoparticle-polymer composite scaffolds. Acta Biomater, 5, 2657–2667.

Jang, H.L., Lee, H.K., Jin, K., Ahn, H.Y., Lee, H.E., Nam, K.T. (2015). Phase transformation from hydroxyapatite to the secondary bone mineral, whitlockite. J. Mater. Chem. B, 3, 1342–1349.

Januariyasa, I.K., Ana, I.D., Yusuf, Y. (2020). Nanofibrous poly(vinyl alcohol)/chitosan contained carbonated hydroxyapatite nanoparticles scaffold for bone tissue engineering. Mater. Sci. Eng. C, 107, 110347.

Javaid, M.A., Kaartinen, M.T. (2013). Mesenchymal stem cell-based bone tissue engineering. Int. Dent. J. Stud. Res, 1(3), 24–35.

Jay, E., Edralin, M., Garcia, J.L., Francis, M., Punzalan, E.R. (2017). Sonochemical synthesis, characterization and photocatalytic properties of hydroxyapatite nano-rods derived from mussel shells. Mater. Lett, 196, 33–36.

Jeyaraj, M., Praphakar, R.A., Rajendran, C., Ponnamma, D., Sadasivuni, K., Munusamy, M.A., Rajan, M. (2016). Surface functionalization of natural lignin isolated from Aloe barbadensis Miller biomass by atom transfer radical polymerization for enhanced anticancer efficacy. RSC Advances, 6, 51310–51319.

Jiang, L., Li, Y., Wang, X., Zhang, L., Wen, J., Gong, M. (2008). Preparation and properties of nano-hydroxyapatite/chitosan/carboxymethyl cellulose composite scaffold. Carbohydr. Polym, 74, 680–684.

Jiang, S., Liu, X., Liu, Y., Liu, J., He,W., Dong, Y. (2020). Synthesis of silver @hydroxyapatite nanoparticles based biocomposite and their assessment for viability of Osseointegration for rabbit knee joint anterior cruciate ligament rehabilitation. J. Photochem. Photobiol. B Biol, 202, 111677.

Jie, W., Yubao, L. (2004). Tissue engineering scaffold material of nanoapatite crystals and polyamide composite. Eur. Polym. J, 40, 509–515.

Jung, O., Hanken, H., Smeets, R., Hartjen, P., Friedrich, R.E., Schwab, B., Grobe, A., Heiland, M., Al-Dam, A., Eichhorn, W., Sehner, S., Kolk, A., Woltje, M., Stein, J.M. (2014). Osteogenic differentiation of mesenchymal stem cells in fibrin-hydroxyapatite matrix in a 3-dimensional mesh scaffold. In Vivo, 28, 477–482.

Kailasanathan, C., Selvakumar, N., Naidu, V. (2012). Structure and properties of titania reinforced nano-hydroxyapatite/gelatin biocomposites for bone graft materials. Ceram. Int, 38, 571–579.

Kaito, T. (2016). Biologic enhancement of spinal fusion with bone morphogenetic proteins: current position based on clinical evidence and future perspective. J. Spine Surg, 2(4), 357–358.

Kalita, S.J., Verma, S. (2010). Nanocrystalline hydroxyapatite bioceramic using microwave radiation: synthesis and characterization. Mater. Sci. Eng. C, 30, 295–303.

Kamitakahara, M., Ohtsuki, C., Miyazaki, T. (2008). Behavior of ceramic biomaterials derived from tricalcium phosphate in physiological condition. J. Biomater. Appl, 23, 197–212.

Katti, K.S., Katti, D.R., Dash, R. (2008). Synthesis and characterization of a novel chitosan/montmorillonite/hydroxyapatite nanocomposite for bone tissue engineering. Biomed. Mater, 3, 034122.

Kim, B.S., Yang, S.S., Kim, C.S. (2018). Incorporation of BMP-2 nanoparticles on the surface of a 3D-printed hydroxyapatite scaffold using an ε-polycaprolactone polymer emulsion coating method for bone tissue engineering. Colloids Surf. B Biointerfaces, 170, 421–429.

Kim, H.D., Jang, H.L., Ahn, H.Y. Lee, H.K., Park, J., Lee, E.S., Lee, E.A., Jeong, Y.H., Kim, D.G., Nam, K.T., Hwang, N.S. (2017). Biomimetic whitlockite inorganic nanoparticles-mediated in situ remodeling and rapid bone regeneration. Biomaterials, 112, 31–43.

Kim, T.G., Park, S.H., Chung, H.J., Yang, D.Y., Park, T.G. (2010). Microstructured scaffold coated with hydroxyapatite/collagen nanocomposite multilayer for enhanced osteogenic induction of human mesenchymal stem cells. J. Mater. Chem, 20, 8927–8933.

Klinkaewnarong, J., Swatsitang, E., Masingboon, C. (2010). Synthesis and characterization of nanocrystalline HAp powders prepared by using aloe vera plant extracted solution. Curr. Appl. Phys, 10, 521–525.

Kolodziejczak, R.A., Samuel, M., Paukszta, D., Piasecki, A., Jesionowski, T. (2014). Synthesis of hydroxyapatite in the presence of anionic surfactant Physicochem. Probl. Miner. Process, 50, 225–236.

Kongsri, S., Janpradit, K., Buapa, K., Techawongstien, S., Chanthai, S. (2013). Nanocrystalline hydroxyapatite from fish scale waste: preparation, characterization and application for selenium adsorption in aqueous solution, Chem. Eng. J, 215–216, 522–532

Kumar, G.S., Karunakaran, G., Girija, E.K., Kolesnikov, E., Van, M.N., Gorshenkov, M.V., Kuznetsov, D. (2018). Size and morphology-controlled synthesis of mesoporous hydroxyapatite nanocrystals by microwave-assisted hydrothermal method. Ceram. Int, 44, 11257–11264.

Kumar, G.S., Rajendran, S., Karthi, S., Easwaradas Kreedapathy, G., Karunakaran, G., Kuznetsov, D. (2017). Green synthesis and antibacterial activity of hydroxyapatite nanorods for orthopedic applications. MRS Commu, 7, 183–188.

Kurashina, K., Kurita, H., Wu, Q., Ohtsuka, A., Kobayashi, H. (2002). Ectopic osteogenesis with biphasic ceramics of hydroxyapatite and tricalcium phosphate in rabbits. Biomaterials, 23, 407–412.

Lai, Z.B., Wang, M., Yan, C., Oloyede, A. (2014). Molecular dynamics simulation of mechanical behavior of osteopontin-hydroxyapatite interfaces. J. Mech. Behav. Biomed. Mater, 36, 12–20.

Lao, L., Wang, Y., Zhu, Y., Zhang, Y., Gao, C. (2011), Poly(lactide-coglycolide)/hydroxyapatite nanofibrous scaffolds fabricated by electrospinning for bone tissue engineering. J. Mater. Sci.: Mater. Med, 22, 1873–1884.

Lett, J.A., Sundareswari, M., Ravichandran, K., Latha, M.B. (2019). Tailoring the morphological features of sol – gel synthesized mesoporous hydroxyapatite using fatty acids as an organic modifier. R. Soc. Open Sci, 9, 6228–6240.

Levingstone, T.J., Ardhaoui, M., Benyounis, K., Loonej, L., Stokes, J.T. (2015). Plasma sprayed hydroxyapatite coatings: understanding process relationship using design of experiment analysis. Surf. Coat. Technol, 283, 29–36.

Li, C., Vepari, C., Jin, H.J., Kim, H.J., Kaplan, D.L., (2006b). Electrospun silk-BMP-2 scaffolds for bone tissue engineering. Biomaterials, 27, 3115–3124.

Li, J., Chen, Y., Yin, Y., Yao, F., Yao, K. (2007). Modulation of nanohydroxyapatite size via formation on chitosan–gelatin network film in situ. Biomaterials, 28, 781–790.

Li, J., Dou, Y., Yang, J., Yin, Y., Zhang, H., Yao, F., Wang, H., Yao, K. (2009). Surface characterization and biocompatibility of micro- and nano-hydroxyapatite/chitosan–gelatin network films. Mater. Sci. Eng. C, 29, 1207–1215.

Li, M., Wang, Y., Liu, Q., Li, Q., Cheng, Y., Zheng, Y., Xi, T., Wei, S. (2013). In situ synthesis and biocompatibility of nano hydroxyapatite on pristine and chitosan functionalized graphene oxide. J. Mater. Chem. B, 1, 475–484.

Li, X., Feng, Q., Cui, F., (2006a). In vitro degradation of porous nanohydroxyapatite/collagen/PLLA scaffold reinforced by chitin fibres. Mater. Sci. Eng. C, 26, 716–720.

Li, Y., Tjandra, W., Tam, K.C. 2008. Synthesis and characterization of nanoporous hydroxyapatite using cationic surfactants as templates. Mater. Res. Bull, 43, 2318–2326.

Li, Z., Su, Y., Xie, B., Wang, H., Wen, T., He, C., Shen, H., Wu, D., Wang, D. (2013). A tough hydrogel–hydroxyapatite bone-like composite fabricated in situ by the electrophoresis approach. J. Mater. Chem. B, 1 (12), 1755–1764.

Lian, X.J., Qiu, Z.Y. Wang, C.M., Guo, W.G., Zhang, X.J., Dong, Y.Q., Cui, F.Z. (2013). Structural and biomedical properties of zirconia-hydroxyapatite nano-crystal ceramics. J. Biomater. Tissue Eng, 3, 330–334.

Lin, K., Chang, J., Cheng, R., Ruan, M. (2007). Hydrothermal microemulsion synthesis of stoichiometric single crystal hydroxyapatite nanorods with mono-dispersion and narrowsize distribution. Mater. Lett, 61, 1683–1687.

Liu, A., Xue, G., Sun, M., Sha, H., Ma, C., Gao, Q., et al. (2016). 3D printing surgical implants at the clinic: a experimental study on anterior cruciate ligament reconstruction. Sci. Rep, 6, 21704.

Liu, J., Liu, Y., Kong, Y., Yao, J., Cai, Y. (2013). Formation of vaterite regulated by silk sericin and its transformation towards hydroxyapatite microsphere. Mater. Lett, 110, 221–224.

Liu, L., Guo, Y., Chen, X., Li, R., Li, Z., Wang, L., Wan, Z., Li, J., Hao, Q., Li, H., Zhang, X. (2012). Three-dimensional dynamic culture of pre-osteoblasts seeded in HA-CS/Col/nHAP composite scaffolds and treated with -ZAL. Acta Biochim. Biophys. Sin, 44, 669–677.

Liu, L., Liu, J., Wang, M., Min, S., Cai, Y., Zhu, L., Yao, J. (2008). Preparation and characterization of nano-hydroxyapatite/silk fibroin porous scaffolds. J. Biomater. Sci. Polym. Ed, 19, 325–338.

Loo, S.C.J., Siew, Y.E., Ho, S., Boey, F.Y.C., Ma, J. (2008). Synthesis and hydrothermal treatment of nanostructured hydroxyapatite of controllable sizes. J. Mater. Sci., Mater. Med, 19, 1389–1397.

Lopez-Noriega, A., Quinlan, E., Celikkin, N., O'Brien, F.J. (2015). Incorporation of polymeric microparticle into collagen-hydroxyapatite scaffolds for the delivery of a pro-osteogenic peptide for bone tissue engineering. Apl Materials. 3, 014910.

Lu, Y., Li, L., Li, M., Lin, Z., Wang, L., Zhang, Y., Yin, Q., Xia, H., Han, G. (2018). Zero-dimensional carbon dots enhance bone regeneration, osteosarcoma ablation, and clinical bacterial eradication. Bioconjugate Chem. 29, 2982–2993.

Lu, Z., Roohani-Esfahani, S.I., Wang, G., Zreiqat, H. (2012). Bone biomimetic microenvironment induces osteogenic differentiation of adipose tissue-derived mesenchymal stem cells. Nanomed- Nanotechnol, 8, 507–515.

Mahmoudi Saber, M. (2019). Strategies for surface modification of gelatin-based nanoparticles. Colloids Surf. B Biointerfaces, 183, 110407.

Marie, P.J., Ammann, P., Boivin, G., Rey, C. (2001). Mechanisms of action and therapeutic potential of strontium in bone. Calcif. Tissue Int, 69, 121–129.

Marie, P.J., Miraoui, H., Severe, N. (2012). FGF/FGFR signaling in bone formation: progress and perspectives. Growth Factors, 30(2), 117–123.

Martínez-Vazquez, F.J., Cabanas, M.F., Paris, J.L., Lozano, D., Vallet-Regí, M. (2015). Silk-Hydroxyapatite Nanoscale Scaffolds with Programmable Growth Factor Delivery for Bone Repair. ACS Appl. Mater. Interfaces, 8, 24463–24470

Matsiko, A., Gleeson, J.P., O'Brien, F.J. (2014). Scaffold mean pore size influences mesenchymal stem cell chondrogenic differentiation and matrix deposition. Tissue Eng. A, 21(3–4), 486–497.

Matsumoto, T., Okazaki, M., Inoue, M., Hamada, Y., Taira, M., Takahashi, J. (2002). Crystallinity and solubility characteristics of hydroxyapatite adsorbed amino acid. Biomaterials, 23, 2241–2247.

Matsumoto, T., Okazaki, M., Nakahira, A., Sasaki, J., Egusa, H., Sohmura, T. (2007). Modification of apatite materials for bone tissue engineering and drug delivery carriers. Curr. Med. Chem, 14, 2726–2733.

Mehnath, S., Arjama, M., Rajan, M., Jeyaraj, M. (2018a). Development of cholate conjugated hybrid polymeric micelles for FXR receptor mediated effective site-specific delivery of paclitaxel, New J. Chem, 42, 17021–17032.

Mehnath, S., Arjama, M., Rajan, M., Premkumar, K., Karthikeyan, K., Jeyaraj, M. (2020a). Mineralization of bioactive marine sponge and electrophoretic deposition on Ti-6Al-4V implant for osteointegration. Surf. Coat. Technol, 392, 125727.

Mehnath, S., Arjama, M., Rajan, M., Vijayaanand, M.A., Jeyaraj, M. (2018b). Polyorganophosphazene stabilized gold nanoparticles for intracellular drug delivery in breast carcinoma cells. Process Biochem, 72, 152–161.

Mehnath,S., Arjama, M., Rajan, M., Annamalai, G., Jeyaraj, M. (2018c). Co-encapsulation of dual drug loaded in MLNPs: Implication on sustained drug release and effectively inducing apoptosis in oral carcinoma cells. Biomed. Pharmacother, 104, 661–671.

Mehnath,S., Chitra, K., Karthikeyan, K., Jeyaraj, M. (2020b). Localized delivery of active targeting micelles from nanofibers patch for effective breast cancer therapy. Int. J. Pharm, 584, 119412.

Mehnath, S., Rajan, M., Sathishkumar, G., Jeyaraj, M. (2017). Thermoresponsive and pH triggered drug release of cholate functionalized poly(organophosphazene) polylactic acid copolymeric nanostructure integrated with ICG. Polymer, 133, 119–128.

Mejias, A., Candidato Jr, R.T., Pawłowski, L., Chicot, D. (2016). Mechanical properties by instrumented indentation of solution precursor plasma sprayed hydroxyapatite coatings: analysis of microstructural effect. Surf Coat Technol, 298, 93–102.

Mihailescu, N., Stan, G.E., Duta, L., Chifiriuc, M.C., Bleotu, C., Sopronyi, M., et al. (2016). Structural, compositional, mechanical characterization and biological assessment of bovine-derived hydroxyapatite coatings reinforced with MgF2 or MgO for implants functionalization. Mater. Sci. Eng. C, 59, 853–874.

Milazzo, M., Contessi Negrini, N., Scialla, S., Marelli, B., Fare, S., Danti, S., Buehler, M.J. (2019). Additive manufacturing approaches for hydroxyapatite-reinforced composites. Adv. Funct. Mater, 29, 1903055.

Milovac, D., Gallego, G., Ivankovic, M., Ivankovic, H. (2014). PCL-coated hydroxyapatite scaffold derived from cuttle fish bone: morphology, mechanical properties and bioactivity, Mater. Sci. Eng. C, 34, 437–445.

Mkhabela, V.J., Sinha Ray, S. (2014). Poly(-caprolactone) nanocomposite scaffolds for tissue engineering: A brief overview. J. Nanosci. Nanotechnol, 14, 535–545.

Montoya-cisneros, K.L., Rendon-angeles, J.C., Matamoros-veloza, Z., Yanagisawa, K. (2017). Rapid synthesis and characterization of Zn substituted hydroxyapatite nanoparticles via a microwave-assisted hydrothermal method. Mater. Lett, 195, 5–9.

Naderi, S., Dabbagh, A., Hassan, M.A., Razak, B.A., Abdullah, H., Kasim, N.H.A. (2016). Modeling of porosity in hydroxyapatite for finite element simulation of nanoindentation test. Ceram. Int, 42 (6), 7543–7550.

Nagata, F., Toriyama, M., Teraoka, K., Yokogawa, Y. (2001). Influence of ethylamine on the crystal growth of hydroxyapatite crystals. Chem. Lett, 30, 780–781.

Nakata, R., Tachibana, A., Tanabe, T. (2014). Preparation of keratin hydrogel/hydroxyapatite composite and its evaluation as a controlled drug release carrier. Mater. Sci. Eng. C, 41, 59–64.

Narayanan, R., Seshadri, S.K., Kwon, T.Y., Kim, K.H. (2008). Calcium phosphate-based coatings on titanium and its alloys. J. Biomed. Mater. Res. Part B, 85(1), 279–299.

Nayar, S., Guha, A. (2008). Waste utilization for the controlled synthesis of nanosized hydroxyapatite. Mater. Sci. Eng. C, 29(4), 1326–1329.

Negahdari, R., Pakdel, S.M.V., Ghavimi, M.A., Daryakenari, N., Bohlouli, S., Dizaj, S.M. (2019). Comparison of reconstruction of cement space in resin copings fabricated with the use of a 3D printer in single-and three-unit restorations. Biointerface Res. Appl. Chem, 9, 3919–3925.

Nejati, E., Firouzdor, V., Eslaminejad, M.B., Bagheri, F. (2009). Needle like nano hydroxy-apatite/poly(l-lactide acid) composite scaffold for bone tissue engineering application. Mater. Sci. Eng. C, 29, 942–949.

Nejati, E., Mirzadeh, H., Zandi, M. (2008). Synthesis and characterization of nano-hydroxyapatite rods/poly(l-lactide acid) composite scaffolds for bone tissue engineering. Compos. Part A Appl. S, 39, 1589–1596.

Neovius, E., Engstrand, T. (2010). Craniofacial reconstruction with bone and biomaterials: review over the last 11 years. J Plast Reconstr Aesthet Surg, 63(10), 1615–1623.

Nichols, H.L., Zhang, N., Zhang, J., Shi, D., Bhaduri, S., Wen, X. (2007). Coating nanothick-ness degradable films on nanocrystalline hydroxyapatite particles to improve the bonding strength between nanohydroxyapatite and degradable polymer matrix. J. Biomed. Mater. Res. A, 82, 373–382.

Niu, X., Feng, Q., Wang, M., Guo, X., Zheng, Q. (2009). Porous nano-HA/collagen/PLLA scaffold containing chitosan microspheres for controlled delivery of synthetic peptide derived from BMP-2. J. Control. Release, 134, 111–7.

Noori, A.; Ashrafi, S.J.; Vaez-Ghaemi, R.; Hatamian-Zaremi, A.; Webster, T.J. (2017). A review of fibrin and fibrin composites for bone tissue engineering. Int. J. Nanomed, 12, 4937–4961.

Nyoo, J., Handoyo, N., Kristiani, V., Adi, S. (2014). Pomacea sp shell to hydroxyapatiteusing the ultrasound – microwave method (U – m), Ceram. Int. 40, 11453–11456.

Osathanon, T., Linnes, M.L., Rajachar, R.M., Ratner, B.D., Somerman, M.J., Giachelli, C.M. (2008). Microporous nanofibrous fibrinbased scaffolds for bone tissue engineering. Biomaterials, 29, 4091–4099.

Owen, G.R., Dard, M., Larjava, H. (2018). Hydroxyapatite/beta-tricalcium phosphate bipha-sic ceramics as regenerativematerial for the repair of complex bone defects. J. Biomed Mater. Res. B Appl. Biomater, 106(6), 2493–2512.

Paris, J.L., Roman, J., Manzano, M., Cabanas, M.V., Vallet-Regi, M. (2015). Tuning dual-drug release from composite scaffolds for bone regeneration. Int. J. Pharm, 486(1–2), 30–37.

Pascu, E.I., Stokes, J., McGuinness, G.B. (2013). Electrospun composites of PHBV, silk fibroin and nano-hydroxyapatite for bone tissue engineering. Mater. Sci. Eng. C, 33, 4905–4916.

Phatai, P. (2019). Structural characterization and antibacterial activity of hydroxyapatite synthesized via sol-gel method using glutinous rice as a template. J. Solgel Sci. Technol, 89, 764–775

Pielichowska, K., Blazewicz, S. (2010). Biopolymers, edited by A. Abe, K. Dusek, and S. Kobayashi, Advances in Polymer Science, Springer, New york, 232, 97–207.

Podaropoulos, L., Veis, A.A., Papadimitriou, S., Alexandridis, C., Kalyvas, D. (2009). Bone Regeneration Using B-Tricalcium Phosphate in a Calcium Sulfate Matrix. J. Oral Implantol, 35(1), 28–36.

Polini, A., Pisignano, D., Parodi, M., Quarto, R., Scaglione, S. (2011). Osteoinduction of human mesenchymal stem cells by bioactive composite scaffolds without supplemental osteogenic growth factors. PLoS One, 6, e26211.

Popp, J.R., Laflin, K.E., Love, B.J., Goldstein, A.S. (2012). Fabrication and characterization of poly (lactic-co-glycolic acid) microsphere/amorphous calcium phosphate scaffolds. J Tissue Eng Regen Med, 6, 12–20.

Porter, M.M., Lee, S., Tanadchangsaeng, N., Jaremko, M.J., Yu, J., Meyers, M., McKittrick, J. (2013). Mechanics of Biological Systems and Materials, Springer, New York, Vol. 5, pp. 63–71.

Pradeepkumar, P., Govindaraj, D., Jeyaraj, M., Munusamy, M.A., Rajan, M. (2017). Assembling of multifunctional latex-based hybrid nanocarriers from Calotropis gigantea for sustained (doxorubicin) DOX releases. Biomed. Pharmacother, 87, 461–470.

Predoi, D., Vatasescu-Balcan, R.A., Pasuk, I., Trusca, R., Costache, M. (2008). Calcium phosphate ceramics for biomedical applications. J. Optoelectron. Adv. Mater, 10(8), 2151–2155.

Qian, J., Xu, M., Suo, A., Yang, T., Yong, X. (2013). An innovative method to fabricate honeycomb-like poly(-caprolactone)/nanohydroxyapatite scaffolds. Mater. Lett, 93, 72–76.

Qu, D., Li, J., Li, Y., Gao, Y., Zuo, Y., Hsu, Y., Hu, J. (2011). Angiogenesis and osteogenesis enhanced by bFGF ex vivo gene therapy for bone tissue engineering in reconstruction of calvarial defects. J. Biomed. Mater. Res. A, 96A, 543–551.

Quinlan, E., Thompson, E.M., Matsiko, A., O'Brien, F.J., Lopez-Noriega, A. (2015). Long term controlled delivery of rhBMP-2 from collagen–hydroxyapatite scaffolds for superior bone tissue regeneration. J Control Release, 207, 112–119.

Rajput, S.K., Kumar Singh, M. (2015). Sericin - A unique biomaterial. IOSR J. Polym. Text. Eng, 2, 2348–181.

Ramesh, S., Loo, Z.Z., Tan, C.Y., Chew, W.J.K., Ching, Y.C., Tarlochan, F., Chandran, H., Krishnasamy, S., Bang, L.T., Sarhan, A.A.D. (2018). Characterization of biogenic hydroxyapatite derived from animal bones for biomedical applications. Ceram. Int, 44, 10525–10530.

Remya, N.S., Syama, S., Gayathri, V., Varma, H.K., Mohanan, P.V. (2014). An in vitro study on the interaction of hydroxyapatite nanoparticles and bone marrow mesenchymal stem cells for assessing the toxicological behavior. Colloids Surf. B: Biointerfaces, 117, 389–397.

Ren, X., Tuo, Q., Tian, K., Huang, G., Li, J., Xu, T., Lv, X., Wu, J., Chen, Z., Weng, J., et al. (2018). Enhancement of osteogenesis using a novel porous hydroxyapatite scaffold in vivo and vitro. Ceram. Int, 44, 21656–21665.

Rogina, A., Ressler, A., Maticc, I., Ferrer, G.G., Marijanovicc, I., Ivankovic, M.; Ivankovic, H. (2017). Cellular hydrogels based on pHresponsive chitosan-hydroxyapatite system. Carbohydr. Polym, 166, 173–182.

Rusu, V.M., Ng, C.H., Wilke, M., Tiersch, B., Fratzl, P., Peter, M.G. (2005). Size-controlled hydroxyapatite nanoparticles as selforganized organic–inorganic composite materials. Biomaterials, 26, 5414–5426.

Ryabenkova, Y., Pinnock, A., Quadros, P., Goodchild, R., Moobus, G., Crawford, A., Hatton, P., Miller, C. (2017). The relationship between particle morphology and rheological properties in injectable nano-hydroxyapatite bone graft substitutes. Mater. Sci. Eng. C, 75, 1083–1090.

Sabry, N.M., Tolba, S.T.M., Abdel-Gawad, F.K., Bassem, S.M., Nassar, H., El-Taweel, G.E., Ibrahim, M.A. (2018). On the molecular modeling analyses of the interaction between nano zinc oxide and bacteria. Biointerface Res. Appl. Chem, 8, 3294–3297.

Saiz, E., Gremillard, L., Menendez, G., Miranda, P., Gryn, K., Tomsia, A.P. (2007). Preparation of porous hydroxyapatite scaffolds. Mater. Sci. Eng. C, 27, 546–550.

Sakamoto, M. (2010). Development and evaluation of superporous hydroxyapatite ceramics with triple pore structure as bone tissue scaffold. J Ceram Soc Jpn, 118, 753–757.

Saravanan, S., Nethala, S., Pattnaik, S., Tripathi, A., Moorthi, A., Selvamurugan, N. (2011). Preparation, characterization and antimicrobial activity of a bio-composite scaffold containing chitosan/nanohydroxyapatite/nano-silver for bone tissue engineering. Int. J. Biol. Macromol, 49, 188–193.

Sarkar, K., Kumar, V., Devi, K.B., Ghosh, D., Nandi, S.K., Roy, M. (2019). Effects of Sr doping on biodegradation and bone regeneration of magnesium phosphate bioceramics. Materialia, 5, 100211.

Sartuqui, J., Gravina, A.N., Rial, R., Benedini, L.A., Yahia, L., Ruso, J.M., Messina, P.V. (2016). Biomimetic fiber mesh scaffolds based on gelatin and hydroxyapatite nanorods: designing intrinsic skills to attain bone reparation abilities. Colloids Surfaces B, 145, 382–391.

Sato, K., Hotta, Y., Nagaoka, T., Yasuoka, M., Watari, K. (2006). Agglomeration control of hydroxyapatite nano-crystals grown in phase-separated microenvironments. Mater Sci, 41, 5424–5428.

Shavandi, A., Silva, T.H., Bekhit, A.A., Bekhit, A.E. (2017). Keratin: dissolution, extraction and biomedical application. Biomater. Sci, 5, 1699–1735.

Shen, H.Z., Guo, N., Zhao, L., Shen, P. (2020). Role of ion substitution and lattice water in the densification of cold-sintered hydroxyapatite. Scr. Mater, 177, 141–145.

Shepherd, J.H., Shepherd, D.V., Best, S.M. (2012). Substituted hydroxyapatites for bone repair. J Mater. Sci. Mater. Med, 23, 2335–2347.

Shi, Y., Li, M., Liu, Q., Jian, Z.J., Xu, X.C., Cheng, Y., et al. (2016). Electrophoretic deposition of graphene oxide reinforced chitosan–hydroxyapatite nanocomposite coatings on Ti substrate. J. Mater. Sci. Mater. Med, 27, 48, 13.

Shi, Z., Huang, X., Liu, B., Tao, H., Cai, Y., Tang, R. (2009). Biological response of osteosarcoma cells to size controlled nanostructured hydroxyapatite. J. Biomater. Appl, 25(1), 19–37.

Shiba, K., Motozuka, S., Yamaguchi, T., Ogawa, N., Otsuka, Y., Ohnuma, K., Kataoka, T., Tagaya, M. (2016). Effect of cationic surfactant micelles on hydroxyapatite nanocrystal formation: an investigation into the inorganic-organic interfacial interactions. Cryst. Growth Des, 16, 1463–1471.

Shubha, P., Varun Prashanth, B., Rajendran, A., Kavita, R., Kulandaivelu, R. (2015). Synthesis and characterization of nano-hydroxyapatite using Sapindus Mukorossi extract. AIP Conf. Proceedings, 1665(1), 050127.

Sidane, D., Rammal, H., Beljebbar, A., Gangloff, S.C., Chicot, D., Velard, F., et al. (2017). Biocompatibility of sol-gel hydroxyapatite-titania composite and bilayer coatings. Mater. Sci. Eng. C, 72, 650–658.

Siddharthan, A., Seshadri, S.K., Kumar, T.S.S. (2006). Influence of microwave power on nanosized hydroxyapatite particles. Scr. Mater, 55, 175–178.

Silk-Hydroxyapatite Nanoscale Scaffolds with Programmable Growth Factor Delivery for Bone Repair. ACS Appl. Mater. Interfaces, 8, 24463–24470.

Sinha, A., Mishra, T., Ravishankar, N. (2008). Polymer assisted hydroxyapatite microspheres suitable for biomedical application. J. Mater. Sci.: Mater. Med, 19, 2009–2013.

Song, J.H., Kim, J.H., Park, S., Kang, W., Kim, H.W., Kim, H.E., Jang, J.H. (2008). Signaling responses of osteoblast cells to hydroxyapatite: the activation of ERK and SOX9. J. Bone Miner. Metab, 26(2), 138–142.

Sossa, P.A.F., Giraldo, B.S., Garcia, B.C.G., Parra, E.R., Arango, P.J.A. (2018). Comparative study between natural and synthetic Hydroxyapatite: structural, morphological and bioactivity properties. Rev. Mater, 23(4), 12217.

Sun, T., Zhou, K., Liu, M., Guo, X., Qu, Y., Cui, W., Shao, Z., Zhang, X., Xu, S. (2018). Loading of BMP-2-related peptide onto three-dimensional nano-hydroxyapatite scaffold accelerates mineralization in critical-sized cranial bone defects. J. Tissue Eng. Regen. Med, 12, 864–877.

Sun, Y., Guo, G., Wang, Z., Guo,H. (2006). Synthesis of single crystal HAP nanorods. Ceram. Int, 32, 951–954.

Supova, M. (2015). Substituted hydroxyapatites for biomedical applications: a review. Ceram. Int, 41(8), 9203–9231.

Swetha, M., Sahithi, K., Moorthi, A., Saranya, N., Saravanan, S., Ramasamy, K., Srinivasan, N. Selvamurugan, N. (2012). Synthesis, characterization, and antimicrobial activity of nano-hydroxyapatite-zinc for bone tissue engineering applications. J. Nanosci. Nanotechnol, 12(1), 167–172.

Tachibana, A., Kaneko, S., Tanabe, T., Yamauchi, K. (2005). Rapid fabrication of keratin-hydroxyapatite hybrid sponges toward osteoblast cultivation and differentiation. Biomaterials, 26, 297–302.

Takeuchi, A., Ohtsuki, C., Miyazaki, T., Kamitakahara, M., Ogata, S., Yamazaki, M., Furutani, Y., Kinoshita, H., Tanihara, M. (2005). Heterogeneous nucleation of hydroxyapatite on protein: structural effect of silk sericin. J. R. Soc. Interface, 2, 373–378.

Tamai, N., Myoui, A., Tomita, T., Nakase, T., Tanaka, J., Ochi, T., Yoshikawa, H. (2002). Novel hyd roxyapatite ce ramics with an interconnective porous structure exhibit superior osteoconduction in vivo. J. Biomed. Mater. Res, 59A, 110–117.

Tan, J., Zhang, M., Hai, Z., Wu, C., Lin, J., Kuang, W., Tang, H., Huang, Y., Chen, X., Liang, G. (2019). Sustained release of two bioactive factors from supramolecular hydrogel promotes periodontal bone regeneration. ACS Nano, 13 (5), 5616–5622.

Tan, R., Niu, X., Gan, S., Feng, Q. (2009). Preparation and characterization of an injectable composite. J. Mater. Sci.: Mater. Med, 20, 1245–1253.

Teng, S., Chen, L., Guo, Y., Shi, J., (2007). Formation of nanohydroxyapatite in gelatin droplets and the resulting porous composite microspheres. J. Inorg. Biochem, 101, 686–691.

Torgbo, S., Sukyai, P. (2019). Fabrication of microporous bacterial cellulose embedded with magnetite and hydroxyapatite nanocomposite scaffold for bone tissue engineering. Mater. Chem. Phys, 237, 121868.

Tran, N., Webster, T.J. (2011). Increased osteoblast functions in the presence of hydroxyapatite-coated iron oxide nanoparticles, Acta Biomater, 7, 1298–1306.

Tripathi, A., Saravanan, S., Pattnaik, S., Moorthi, A., Partridge, N.C., Selvamurugan, N. (2012). Bio-composite scaffolds containing chitosan/nano-hydroxyapatite/nano-copper-zinc for bone tissue engineering. Int. J. Biol. Macromol, 50, 294–299.

Uddin, M.H., Matsumoto, T., Ishihara, S., Nakahira, A., Okazaki, M., Sohmura, T. (2010). Apatite containing aspartic acid for selective protein loading. J Dent Res, 89, 488–492.

Vanitha, C., Kuppusamy, M.R., Sridhar, T.M., Sureshkumar, R., Mahalakshmi, N. (2017). Synthesis, characterization of Nano - Hydroxyapatite from white snail shells and removal of Methylene blue. Int. J. Innov. Res. Adv. Eng, 4, 82–86.

Buitrago, V.M., Patricia Ossa-Orozco, C. (2018). Hydrothermal synthesis of hydroxyapatite nanorods using a fruit extract template. Dyna, 85, 283–288.

Venugopal, J., Prabhakaran, M.P., Zhang, Y., Low, S., Choon, A.T., Ramakrishna, S. (2010). Biomimetic hydroxyapatite-containing composite nanofibrous substrates for bone tissue engineering. Philos. T. Roy. Soc. A, 368, 2065–2081.

Walsh, P.J., Buchanan, F.J., Dring, M., Maggs, C., Bell, S., Walker, G.M. (2008). Low-pressure synthesis and characterisation of hydroxyapatite derived from mineralise red algae. Chem. Eng. J, 137, 173–179.

Wang, B., Yang, W., McKittrick, J., Meyers, M.A. (2016). Keratin: Structure, mechanical properties, occurrence in biological organisms, and efforts at bioinspiration. Prog. Mater. Sci, 76, 229–318.

Wang, H., Li, Y., Zuo, Y., Li, J., Ma, S., Cheng, L. (2007). Biocompatibility and osteogenesis of biomimetic nano-hydroxyapatite/polyamide composite scaffolds for bone tissue engineering. Biomaterials, 28, 3338–3348.

Wang, J., Huang, S.P., Hu, K., Zhou, K.C., Sun, H. (2015). Effect of cetyltrimethylammonium bromide on morphology and porous structure of mesoporous hydroxyapatite. Trans. Nonferrous Met. Soc. China (English Ed.), 25, 483–489.

Wang, P., Li, C., Gong, H., Jiang, X., Wang, H., Li, K. (2010). Effects of synthesis conditions on the morphology of hydroxyapatite nanoparticles produced by wet chemical process. Powder Technol, 203, 315–321.

Wang, R., Hu, H., Guo, J., Wang, Q., Cao, J., Wang, H., Li, G., Mao, J., Zou, X., Chen, D., Tian, W. (2019). Nano-hydroxyapatite modulates osteoblast differentiation through autophagy induction via mTOR signaling pathway. J. Biomed. Nanotechnol, 15(2), 405–415.

Wang, Y., Chen, J., Wei, K., Zhang, S., Wang, X. (2006). Surfactant assisted synthesis of hydroxyapatite particles. Mater. Lett, 60, 3227–3231.

Wang, Y., Cui, F.Z., Hu, K., Zhu, X.D., Fan, D.D. (2008). Bone regeneration by using scaffold based on mineralized recombinant collagen. J. Biomed. Mater. Res. B, 86, 29–35.

Wei, K., Kim, B.S., Kim, I.S. (2011). Fabrication and biocompatibility of electrospun silk biocomposites. Membranes, 1, 275–298.

Witte, F., Feyerabend, F., Maier, P., Fischer, J., Stormer, M., Blawert, C., Dietzel, W., Hort, N. (2007). Biodegradable magnesiumhydroxyapatite metal matrix composites. Biomaterials, 28(13), 2163–2174.

Xia, L., Lin, K., Jiang, X., Xu, Y., Zhang, M., Chang, J., Zhang, Z. (2013). Enhanced osteogenesis through nano-structured surface design of macroporous hydroxyapatite bioceramic scaffolds viaactivation of ERK and p38 MAPK signaling pathways. J. Mater. Chem. B, 1, 5403–5416.

Xiao, W., Gao, H., Qu, H., Liu, X., Zhang, J., Li, H. (2018). Rapid microwave synthesis of hydroxyapatite phosphate microspheres with hierarchical porous structure. Ceram. Int, 44, 6144–6151.

Xiao, W., Sonny Bal, B., Rahaman, M.N. (2016). Preparation of resorable carbonate-substituted hollow hydroxyapatite microspheres and their evaluation in osseous defects in vivo. Mater. Sci. Eng. C, 60, 324–332.

Xin, R., Ren, F., Leng, Y. (2010). Synthesis and characterization of nano-crystalline calcium phosphates with EDTA-assisted hydrothermal method. Mater. Des, 31, 1691–1694.

Xu, Q., Lu, H., Zhang, J., Lu, G., Deng, Z., Mo, A. (2010). Tissue engineering scaffold material of porous nanohydroxyapatite/polyamide. Int. J. Nanomed, 5, 331–335.

Yamada, S., Heymann, D., Bouler, J.M., Daculsi, G. (1997). Osteoclastic resportion of calcium phosphate ceramics with different hydroxyapatite/β-tricalcium phosphate ratios. Biomaterials, 18, 1037–1041.

Yun, Y.P., Kim, S.J., Lim, Y.M., Park, K., Kim, H.J., Jeong, S.I., Kim, S.E., Song, H.R. (2014). The effect of alendronate-loaded polycarprolactone nanofibrous scaffolds on osteogenic differentiation ofadipose-derived stem cells in bone tissue regeneration. J. Biomed. Nanotechnol, 10, 1080–1090.

Yunan, Q., Qin, C., Wu, J., Xu, A., Zhang, Z., Liao, J., et al. (2016). Synthesis and characterization of cerium-doped hydroxyapatite/polylactic acid composite coatings on metal substrate. Mater. Chem. Phys, 182, 324–32.

Zarins, J., Pilmane, M., Sidhoma, E., Salma, I., Locs, J. (2019). The role of strontium enriched hydroxyapatite and tricalcium phosphate biomaterials in osteoporotic bone regeneration. Symmetry, 11(2), 1–18.

Zhang, B., Li, H., He, L., Han, Z., Zhou, T., Zhi, W., Lu, X., Lu, X., Weng, J. (2018). Surface-decorated hydroxyapatite scaffold with on-demand delivery of dexamethasone and stromal cell derived factor-1 for enhanced osteogenesis. Mater. Sci. Eng. C, 89, 355–370.

Zhang, C.Y., Zhang, C.L., Wang, J.F., Lu, C.H., Zhuang, Z., Wang, X.P., Fang, Q.F. (2013). Fabrication and in vitro investigation of nanohydroxyapatite, chitosan, poly(L -lactic acid) ternary biocomposite. J. Appl. Polym. Sci, 127, 2152–2159.

Zhang, C., Lu, H., Zhuang, Z., Wang, X., Fang, Q. (2010). Nanohydroxyapatite/poly(l-lactic acid) composite synthesized by a modified in situ precipitation: Preparation and properties. J. Mater. Sci.: Mater. Med, 21, 3077–3083.

Zhang, H., Zhou, K., Li, Z.Y., Huang, S. (2009). Plate-like hydroxyapatite nanoparticles synthesized by the hydrothermal method. J. Phys. Chem. Solids, 70, 243–248.

Zhang, H., Zhou, K., Li, Z.Y., Huang, S. (2009). Plate-like hydroxyapatite nanoparticles synthesized by the hydrothermal method. J. Phys. Chem. Solids, 70, 243–248.

Zhang, P., Wu, H., Wu, H., Lu, Z., Deng, C., Hong, Z., Jing, X., Chen, X. (2011). RGD-conjugated copolymer incorporated into composite of poly(lactide-co-glycotide) and poly(l-lactide)-grafted nanohydroxyapatite for bone tissue engineering. Biomacromolecules, 12, 2667–2680.

Zhang, W., Chai, Y., Xu, X., Wang, Y., Cao, N. (2014). Rod-shaped hydroxyapatite with mesoporous structure as drug carriers for proteins. Appl. Surf. Sci, 322, 71–77.

Zhang, W., Liao, S., Cui, F. (2003). Hierarchical self-assembly of nanofibrils in mineralized collagen. Chem. Mater, 15, 3221–3226.

Zhao, Y.F., Ma, J. (2005). Triblock co-polymer templating synthesis of mesostructured hydroxyapatite. Micropor. Mesopor. Mat, 87, 110–117.

Zheng, X., Hui, J., Li, H., Zhu, C., Hua, X., Ma, H., Fan, D. (2017). Fabrication of novel biodegradable porous bone scaffolds based on amphiphilic hydroxyapatite nanorods. Mater. Sci. Eng. C, 75, 699–705.

Zhou, H., Lawrence, J.G., Bhaduri, S.B. (2012). Fabrication aspects of PLA-CaP/PLGA-CaP composites for orthopedic applications: A review. Acta Biomater, 8, 1999–2016.

Zhou, H., Wu, T., Dong, X., Wang, Q., Shen, J. (2007). Adsorption mechanism of BMP-7 on hydroxyapatite (001) surfaces. Biochem. Biophys. Res. Commun, 361 (1), 91–96.

Zhou, H., Yang, Y., Yang, M., Wang, W., Bi, Y. (2018). Synthesis of mesoporous hydroxyapatite via a vitamin C templating hydrothermal route. Mater. Lett, 218, 52–55.

Zhou, W.Y., Lee, S.H., Wang, M., Cheung, W.L., Ip, W.Y. (2008). Selective laser sintering of porous tissue engineering scaffolds from poly(L-lactide)/carbonated hydroxyapatite nanocomposite microspheres. J. Mater. Sci. Mater. Med, 19, 2535–2540.

Zhu, X.D., Zhang, H.J., Fan, H.S., Li, W., Zhang, X.D. (2010). Effect of phase composition and microstructure of calcium phosphate ceramic particles on protein adsorption. Acta Biomater, 6(4), 1536–1541.

Zindani, D., Kumar, K. (2018). 3D printing of biomaterials: A review. Biointerface Res. Appl. Chem, 8, 3023–3033.

10 Polymeric Biomaterials for Bone Tissue Repair and Regeneration

Sesha Subramanian Murugan
Yenepoya (Deemed to be University)

Sukumaran Anil
Qatar University

Jayachandran Venkatesan
Yenepoya (Deemed to be University)

Gi Hun Seong
Hanyang University

CONTENTS

DOI: 10.1201/9781003140108-10

10.1   INTRODUCTION

From ancient times, bone tissue has been the most needed material to restore essential functions by repairing bone defects caused by infection, illness, and trauma. In recent days, the management of bone defects has been transferred to artificial tissue transplants, instead of traditional autograft or allograft transplants, to overcome problems such as pathogen transfer and immune rejection (Tamura, Uragami, and Sugihara 1981). Since 1950, many biomaterials, including metals, alloys, etc., have been invented and used as implant biomaterials, but that has not overcome the challenge of degradation, as it requires a second surgery to remove (Arthanareeswaran, Devi, and Raajenthiren 2008). Therefore, researchers find that scaffolding material is an alternative source in bone tissue engineering for further development in clinical application. In the past century, many biomaterials have been widely used in surgical implants. Biomaterials had the characteristics of being biocompatible, biodegradable, non-toxic, non-immunogenic, and durable and facilitating tissue healing, integration, and regeneration. Biomaterials may have biophysical and biochemical cues to instruct the cells to activate specific signaling pathways and control cell response. Scientists and researchers believe that biomaterials originated from polymer sources. The source might be natural or synthetic (Table 10.1). Natural sources are collagen, chitosan, gelatin, silk fibroin, alginate, albumin, hyaluronate, and cellulose. Those naturally sourced polymers are studied in bone tissue engineering applications as they have low toxicities, non-immunogenic, enhanced cell growth, and better biocompatibility behavior. Due to the low mechanical properties, these natural polymers can be mixed with synthetic polymers or bioceramics to improve composite biomaterials (Zarif 2018). Synthetic biopolymers are prepared by using the familiar structure of fundamental building blocks. These polymers include polycaprolactone (PCL), poly (lactic acid) (PLA), poly (glycolic acid) (PGA), poly (ethylene glycol) (PEG), poly (vinyl alcohol) (PVA), polyether ether ketone (PEEK), polyurethanes (PU), and poly (p-dioxanone) (PDO).

10.2   TISSUE ENGINEERING

Tissue engineering (TE) is the primary area of regenerative medicine for tissue repair (such as for injury due to illness or trauma). TE has been a key focus over the past few years because of its innovative approaches to healing damaged tissue. It is an area of biomedical engineering that integrates biology and engineering to develop tissues or external cell products (ex vivo) or to make use of advanced knowledge to better handle the repaired tissues inside the body (in vivo). It aims to regenerate damaged tissues and to stimulate endogenous regeneration. It covers a wide range of biology, including cell-molecular biology, stem cell biology and cell lineage, systems

TABLE 10.1

A Comparative Study on Natural and Synthetic Polymers for Potential Use in Bone Tissue Repair and Regenerations

Scaffold Type	Advantages	Disadvantages	Reference
Natural	Bioactivity Biocompatibility Bioavailability Natural Remodeling	Microbial contamination Low mechanical strength Low tunability rate Uncontrolled degradation rate	(Chocholata, Kulda, and Babuska 2019)
Collagen	Mimics the extracellular matrix FDA approved Biocompatibility Biodegradability	Low mechanical strength	(Zhang et al. 2018)
Chitosan	Cytocompatibility High proliferation and differentiation rate Biodegradability	Rapid *in-vivo* degradation rate Low mechanical strength	(Saravanan, Leena, and Selvamurugan 2016)
Gelatin	Osteo conductivity Enhanced proliferation Biodegradability	Low stability and mechanical strength	(C Echave et al. 2017)
Silk fibroin	Easy modification Cytocompatibility Immune activity High thermal stability	Production of spider silk is low	(Garg et al. 2011)
Alginate	Possesses easily tunable properties Cytocompatibility Bioavailability	Low mechanical strength	(Venkatesan et al. 2015)
Hyaluronic acid	Enzymatic biodegradability Biocompatibility Viscoelasticity	Rapid degradation Low mechanical strength	(Zhu et al. 2017)
Synthetic Polymer	Water Solubility High mechanical strength Reproducibility Crystalline nature Flexible physical and mechanical properties	Poor cell adhesion Poor osteoconductivity Low bioactivity	(Chocholata, Kulda, and Babuska 2019)
PCL	Biodegradability Cytocompatibility Slow degradation	Poor bioactivity Hydrophobicity	(Dwivedi et al. 2020)
PLA	Thermal stability	Less osteo conductivity	(Gregor et al. 2017)
PLGA	Tunable and degradation properties Degradation	Less osteo conductivity Optimal mechanical strength	(Gentile et al. 2014)

biology, chemistry, and endocrine science (endocrinology). These combined sciences have led to regenerative medicine, which currently serves two clinical purposes. 1. A cellular therapy for restoring damaged tissue through injection or transplantation of cells or cell suspensions/cells combined with scaffold material. 2. Validation of tissue ex vivo for transplantation. To make tissue engineering successful, stem cells (embryonic stem cells, adult stem cells, and induced pluripotent stem cells) are the practical tools because they can differentiate themselves in a large number of cells based on the stimuli supplied. The stem cells need suitable media (selective differential media) with a supplementing factor for desired differentiation. The media should provide the desired stimulators with optimum temperature and pH for adequate cell growth, proliferation, and cell specialization. The proper choice of bio-compatible and bio-active materials is essential for repairing or regenerating the desired tissue. The prepared materials should comprise the mechanical properties for both soft and hard tissue. Materials should have interatomic and intermolecular bonding to obtain hydrolytic degradation to degrade the materials. The choice of materials should be tuned according to the desired site of the regeneration. The tuning includes stiffness, structure, and topography. It should achieve a suitable surface area, porosity, and pore size for maximum mechanical strength. The fundamental challenges faced by the tissue engineer in the implantation of cellular therapies or fabrication designs are as follows.

- In bio-engineered structures, tissue compartments must be adjusted to mimic the nutrient transport present in natural capillary beds found in the structured physical body.
- Identify the methods used to build a suitable scaffold design and arrangements for proper cell adhesion, growth, and migration include gas foaming, porogen leaching, fiber bonding, and solid free-form fabrication freeze-drying, electrospinning, 3D printing, and microsphere sintering.
- Identify the angiogenic gene within individual tissues.
- Utilize the angiogenic genes to stimulate the secretion of angiogenic factors in the desired tissue.
- Moreover, there is a need to address technical and economic barriers before technology-based therapies reach millions of potential patients (Bhattacharyya, McCarthy, and Grives 1974; Furth and Atala 2014; Sabir, Xu, and Li 2009; Tonelli et al. 2017).

10.3 BONE TISSUE ENGINEERING

Bone possesses a hierarchically porous structure ranging from 20 to 400 μm. It is a complex and intense connective tissue that keeps the body organized and safe, and it is used for locomotion. Bone is unique from a structural and chemical perspective to withstand loads and shocks. The structure of bone comprises two types of layers with different densities. The outside is compact bone with a spongy interior bone. Osteoblasts and osteoclasts are two types of cells involved in bone remodeling. In recent days the need for a bone graft is high due to the increasing number of common bone defects. The anatomical and physiological mimicking of bone through scaffold fabrication is an alternative method to remodel bone defects. Many new manufacturing techniques have been developed to prepare scaffolds. Each technique has a specific drawback and cannot meet all requirements of the native tissue. The development of a scaffold with unique properties in the native tissue is the first essential parameter. There is an exciting synergy between biomaterials and cell therapy. Mesenchymal stem cells (MSCs) are a potential source for bone regeneration. Biomaterial success rates are very high in in vitro and in vivo conditions; however, they are low in clinical practice. This is due to the clinical practice of using biomaterials with desired seeded cells as an implant for more significant human defects, and the scarcity of blood supply (vascularization) leads to cell death immediately (Sabir, Xu, and Li 2009; Zarif 2018).

10.4 BIOMATERIALS

The biomaterials field is an emerging and interdisciplinary area of research aiming to develop artificial tissue or organs. The interdisciplinary area includes material science, biology, and medicine. The developed biomaterials should be bioresorbable, bioactive, biocompatible, bioavailable, and bio-inert. The materials can apply for an extended period and are used to interact with the human tissues for the regeneration of the damaged tissues. Natural sources of biomaterials include collagen, chitosan, gelatin, silk fibroin, and alginate. Polycaprolactone, polylactic acid, poly (Lactic – co – glycolic acid), and polyether ether ketone are sources of synthetic materials (Ambrogi et al. 2003). Each biomaterial has its own specific functions in the healing and regeneration of the tissues. Natural biopolymers are well suited for biocompatibility and bioavailability but have a disadvantage in mechanical strength. Since synthetic materials provide excellent mechanical strength, semi-synthetic materials may overcome the challenge of both natural and synthetic materials disadvantage (Rubežić et al. 2020).

10.5 NATURAL BIOPOLYMERS

10.5.1 Collagen

Collagen (Figure 10.1) is a naturally occurring protein extensively present in mammals at about 30% of body weight (Ricard-Blum 2011). It is present in skin, bone, cartilage, corneal tissue, tendons, and ligaments and is an abundant source of natural

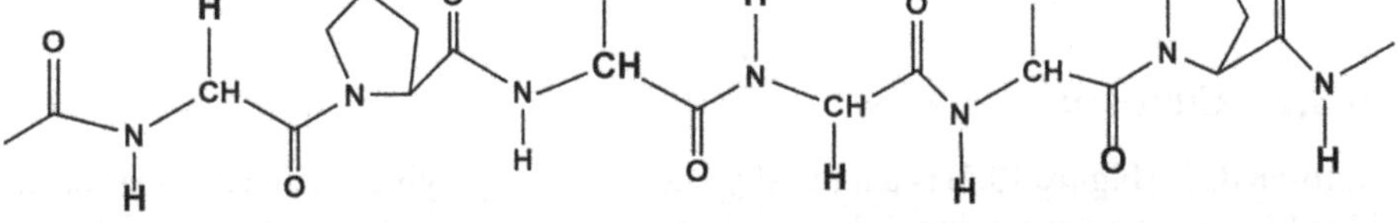

FIGURE 10.1 Chemical structure of collagen. Figure is redrawn from the reference research article (Naomi, Ratanavaraporn, and Fauzi 2020).

hydrocolloids (Caliari and Burdick 2016). It is reported that 28 different types of collagen proteins were identified and classified as type I, II, III, and IV. Collagen I is mainly found in the tissues of higher animals. It has two $\alpha 1$ chains and one $\alpha 2$ chain. Collagen II has three $\alpha 1$(II) chain forms. Collagen III attains three $\alpha 1$(III) chains (Dong and Lv 2016). Collagen is the main protein component of the extracellular matrix (ECM) of most tissue types and plays a vital part in cellular adhesion, proliferation, survival, and differentiation (Appukuttan 1987). Animal collagen has been applied in medicine and TE for many years, but it is threatened by the possible spread of multiple cattle diseases. The most significant portion of the bone matrix was 35% collagen based. In particular, type I collagen is known for forming and making bones as well as a bone-mineral deposition. However, collagen on its own is not as effective for bone formation. It has the characteristics of a bone conductive material when combined with a ceramic component. Once growth factors are blended with bone marrow components, they act like a bone-stimulating material. Oh et al. have developed a 3D PCL scaffolds with fish collagen (Col) and the osteogenic abalone intestine gastrointestinal digests (AIGIDs) (PCL/AIGIDs/Col). This scaffold combination showed higher calcium content and induced ALP expression than PCL, PCL/Collagen, and PCL/AIGIDS in MSCs. The 3-(4,5-dimethylthiazol-2-yl)-2,5-diphenyl-2H-tetrazolium bromide (MTT) assay showed adverse cytotoxicity effects and better proliferation results. An *in vivo* experiment with a rabbit tibia was carried out to examine the PCL and PCL/AIGIDs/Col scaffolds. The μ-CT and histological analysis showed that the PCL/AIGIDs/Col has excellent bone formation. These PCL/AIGIDs/Col scaffolds may be considered as possible material for bone repairing. Their results showed that the proliferation and differentiation of the cells are possible by growth factors, cytokines, and cell signaling from the dynamic bio-environment of the extracellular matrix (Oh et al. 2020). De Melo Pereira et al. attempted the composition and arrangement of the extracellular matrix by using the biomineralized collagen. It exposes a positive effect on RUNX2, SPP1, ENPP1, OCN, and COL1A1 osteo genes studies of hMSCs (de Melo Pereira et al. 2020). Laiva et al. developed a scaffold to influence angiogenesis using pro-angiogenesis through paracrine signaling. They combined the stromal-derived factor-1 alpha (SDF-1α) gene with polyethyleneimine and collagen-chondroitin sulfate for scaffold preparation. Growth of MSCs with an expression of SDF-1α mRNA and activation of vegetative endothelial growth factor (VEGF) and C-X-C chemokine receptor type - 4 (CXCR4) were identified. The MSCs on the scaffold showed SDF-1α mRNA over-expression associated with VEGF and CXCR4 activation, which are angiogenic factors. They concluded that combination of the SDF-1α gene with collagen-based scaffolds can provide a suitable niche condition for an angiogenic response during wound closure (Laiva et al. 2018)

10.5.2 CHITOSAN

Chitosan (CS) (Figure 10.2) is a naturally occurring biopolymer, a linear polysaccharide of N-acetyl glucosamine. It has (1–4) d-glucosamine and N-acetyl glucosamine subunits (Venkatesan et al. 2014). The source of CS is chitin, which is found abundantly in fungi, bacteria, crabs, prawns, and crustacean exoskeletons. It is reported

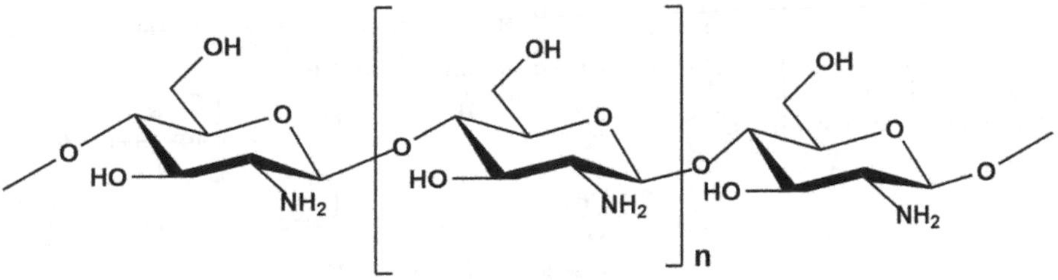

FIGURE 10.2   Chemical structure of chitosan. Figure is redrawn from the reference research article (Sami El-banna et al. 2019).

that the shells of crabs and shrimps have 30–40% protein, 30–50% calcium carbonate, and 20–30% chitin. It is produced by the deacetylation process and contains 60% glucose amine residue (Ibrahim and El-Zairy 2015). CS is a non-toxic, biocompatible, adsorbing biopolymer widely used for wound healing (Zarif 2018). It has been approved by the Food and Drug Administration (FDA) for the application of bone tissue engineering and wound dressing. In bone tissue engineering, many forms were used as fibers, films, and sponges (LogithKumar et al. 2016; Preethi Soundarya et al. 2018). Due to the low osteoinductive and mechanical properties, researchers have reinforced the nanomaterials of hydroxyapatite, bioactive glass ceramics, zirconia, and other polymers to improve the disadvantageous properties (LogithKumar et al. 2016; Balagangadharan, Dhivya, and Selvamurugan 2017). CS had an excellent antibacterial effect to overcome the use of specific antibiotics, reduced the viability of the osteoblast, and slowed down the proliferation rate of human mesenchymal (stromal) cells. Hydroxypropyl trimethylammonium chitosan chloride was added with bone cement and showed better antibacterial activity, better cell fixation, differentiation, and hydroxyapatite formation (Balagangadharan, Dhivya, and Selvamurugan 2017; LogithKumar et al. 2016). The carboxymethylic chitosan (CMC) is a chitosan derivative that includes N-CMC, O-CMC, or N, O-CMC. The depositing CMC on titanium implants inhibits the bacterial activity of *S aureus and S epidermidis*. The N-CMC induces biomineralization, O-CMC promotes the fibroblastic self-renewing capacity of bone cells, and N, O-CMC-n-β-tricalcium phosphate (β-TCP) was capable of producing hydroxyapatite at their surface (Balagangadharan, Dhivya, and Selvamurugan 2017). Several natural and synthetic polymers, including collagen, poly(lactic-co-glycolic acid), polycaprolactone, alginate, hydroxyapatite, polyethylene terephthalate, and polyvinyl alcohol, were added to chitosan to improve the cellular growth, cellular adhesion, and mechanical toughness (Balagangadharan, Dhivya, and Selvamurugan 2017; LogithKumar et al. 2016). Also, chemical modifications on the chitosan could be made to achieve superior results. Chitosan modified with enzymes, dendrimers, cyclodextrin, and crown ethers is reported for biomedical applications. Besides this, several research reports have proven that chemically modified chitosan surfaces can enhance cell biomaterials interactions. However, chemically modified chitosan blended with ceramics, alloys, and metals can enhance mechanical and osteogenic properties (Khor and Whey 1995; Wang, Kao, and Hsieh 2003; Sashiwa and Aiba 2004; Zima 2018).

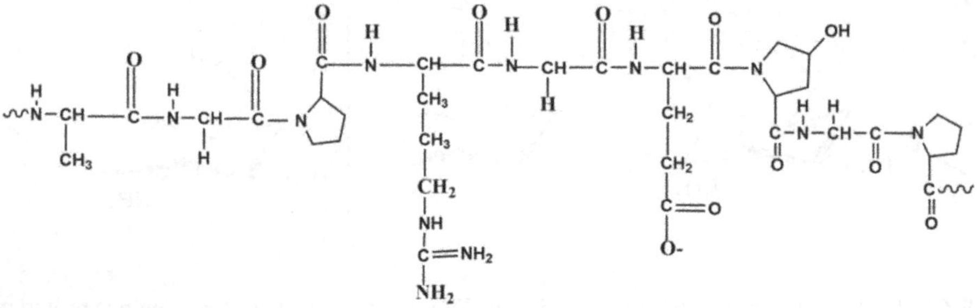

FIGURE 10.3 Chemical structure of gelatin. Figure is redrawn from the reference research article (Elzoghby 2013).

10.5.3 GELATIN

Gelatin (Figure 10.3) is a natural denatured polymer, and it is a breakdown product of insoluble collagen by disintegration and denaturation. Gelatin has a very similar molecular structure to collagen. Like collagen, gelatin crosslinked with supplementary biomaterials has promising applications in bone tissue engineering (BTE) (Van Vlierberghe et al. 2011; Feng et al. 2016; Liu et al. 2019; Bello et al. 2020). Gelatin is obtained from type 1 collagen using alkaline or acid hydrolysis. Type A is derived from the acid pre-treatment, and type B is derived from the alkali process. The integrin proteins present in the gelatin enhance cellular adhesion, migration, and proliferation. Gelatin extends its broad areas into many medical applications such as interactive cell coatings, drug delivery vehicles, and tissue-based scaffolds. Due to poor stability, gelatin was mixed with several other compounds to obtain a gelatin-based biomaterial. The gelatin-containing biocomposite materials showed increased mechanical strength and boosted bioactivity for bone regeneration applications (Bello et al. 2020). Gelatin is used in orthopedic applications because of its biodegradation and biocompatible behavior. It is typically blended with other polymer composites in a crosslinking process to improve the scaffolding system in a better tissue compatible and mechanically. It has a broad spectrum of uses (Bose, Koski, and Vu 2020; Azizian, Hadjizadeh, and Niknejad 2018). Gelatin is considered an appropriate biomaterial to imitate the extracellular matrix due to its functional groups and the development of 3D scaffolds. New approaches of hybrid scaffolds were carried out between polycaprolactone-58S bioactive glass sodium/ and alginate-gelatin by melt molding method. The prepared microspheres were used as the scaffold as they had excellent mechanical strength and degradation (Mao et al. 2018). A scaffold was developed in combination with gelatin-carboxymethyl-chitosan (CMC)-hydroxyapatite. It was then subjected to crosslinking with glutaraldehyde and lyophilized. The results show that the CMC-hydroxyapatite has good mechanical strength and shows a high degradation rate (Zarif 2018). A combination of vitamin D3, gelatin, and double hydroxides-hydroxyapatite nanolayered composite was used as scaffold structure to compensate for osteoporosis vitamin deficiency. Glutaraldehyde was used as a crosslinker. In vitro studies showed that G-292 cells grown on the scaffold have good proliferative ability, cell viability, and

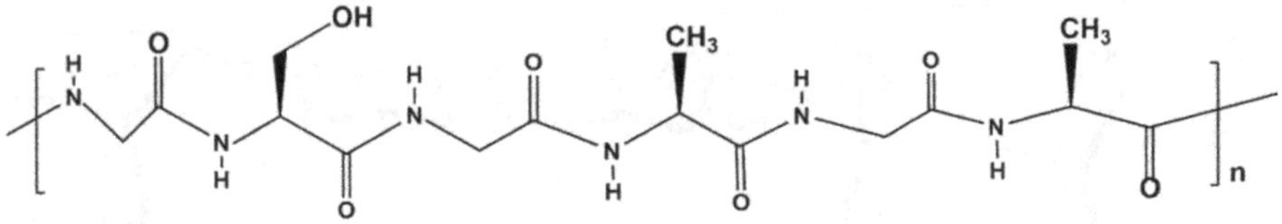

FIGURE 10.4 Chemical structure of silk fibroin. Figure is redrawn from the reference research article (Naomi, Ratanavaraporn, and Fauzi 2020).

less cytotoxicity. This scaffold system can be helpful in the future to treat osteoporosis as well as bone diseases (Fayyazbakhsh et al. 2017). A new scaffold containing bovine serum albumin chitosan nanoparticles with chitosan gelatin scaffolds was synthesized. As a result of chitosan nanoparticles, the porosity has increased. For the in vitro test, the scaffolds show an enhanced proliferation rate of human dermal fibroblasts (Azizian, Hadjizadeh, and Niknejad 2018).

10.5.4 Silk Fibroin

Globular protein (sericin) and fibrous protein (silk fibroin) (Figure 10.4) are the two significant silk proteins. Globular protein is primarily produced from silkworms and spiders. Serine, arginine, glycine, and aspartic acid are the molecular composition of the silk fibroin (SF); which stimulate cell attachment, cell growth, and proliferation (Mhuka, Dube, and Nindi 2013). Due to a highly compatible nature, the US Food and Drug Administration (FDA) approved the silk fibroin as a biomaterial for the suture implant. Seri scaffold and seri ACL are the FDA-certified silk fibrin surgical mesh. It has been proven that the degeneration rate of silk fibroin and regeneration rate of bone formation occurs in a controlled way (Wharram et al. 2010; Horan et al. 2005). To check the toxicity effect of degradation byproduct of silk fibroin, the SF was subjected to a cytotoxicity test. It showed no significant toxicity. Then SF was mixed with cryogel scaffolds which shows the 50 MPa compression modules (Ak et al. 2013). SF hydrogel was incorporated with bone morphogenic protein 2 (BMP-2) and vascular endothelial growth factor (VEGF) to enhance angiogenesis and new bone formation. Animal studies showed that the combination of the VEGF and BMP-2 induced vascularization and exposed slower degradation and the sustainable release of growth factor and platelet-derived growth factor (Correia et al. 2012). The silk fibroin was exposed to hexafluoro-2-propanol treatment and pre-seeded with adipose-derived stem cells (ADSCs). This study showed increased levels of type 1 collagen, bone sialoprotein, calcium deposits, and mineralization (Melke et al. 2016). The globular protein silk sericin contains a high volume of sericin, which has 10 to 400 kDa protein. Sericin is the compound of both mulberry and non- mulberry silkworms. It is the hot-water–soluble glue protein that makes up 20–30% of the cocoon. Four types of sericin genes secrete it. Sericin is partially unfolded, with a -sheet content in 35% and a random coil content of 63%, with no helical content. Silk sericin has been widely used in wound dressing, drug delivery, bone regeneration, and cosmetic applications (Kundu et al. 2008).

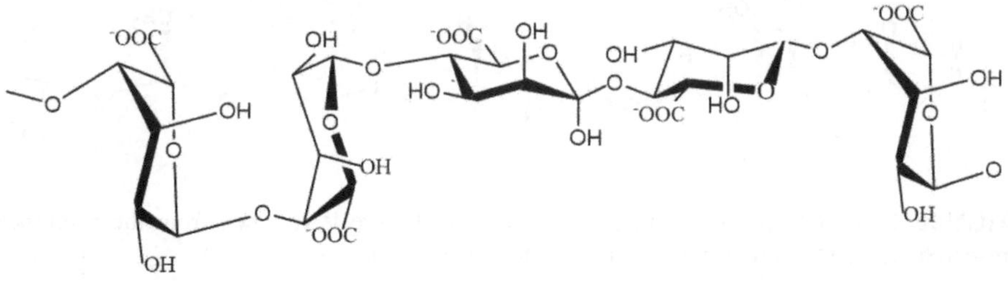

FIGURE 10.5 Chemical structure of alginate. The figure is redrawn from the reference research article (Szekalska et al. 2016).

10.5.5 ALGINATE

Alginate (Figure 10.5) is a natural organic polysaccharide derived from brown algae. It is recognized for its biocompatible, biodegradable, and hydrophilic properties. In physiological conditions, alginate may form porosity, which allows cells to fill the network. In addition, nutrients and oxygen could readily enter into the biomaterials and offer a secure environment for tissue regeneration. Alginate is a non-branched polysaccharide made of β-D-mannuronic acid and α-L-guluronic acid. In addition to the biocompatibility and biodegradability properties, gelation with divalent cations is the main characteristic. Alginate has a negatively charged carboxylic acidic group on its surface, facilitating chemical interaction with other opposite charge biomaterials. It has the properties to increase the viscosity of polymeric solutions (Gupta and Edwards 2019). A blend of gelatin, alginate, and hydroxyapatite was a novel hydrogel compound for bone regeneration (Wust et al. 2014). A study by Abouzeid et al. concentrated on the preparation of TEMPO-oxidized Cellulose nanofibrils (T-CNF)/Sodium alginate (SA) hydrogel scaffolds by using 3D extrusion printing to replace damaged hard tissue and repair the bone defects. The T-CNF/SA scaffolds show excellent mechanical strength in the range of 419~455 MPa at compressive strain 50% and modulus 1078~1233 MPa. The biomimetic mineralized study on T-CNF/SA shows 20.1% hydroxyapatite formed confirmed by FTIR, XRD, TGA, and FEG-SEM. This 3D printed combination of alginate/oxidized TEMPO cellulose nanofibril hydrogel may be a promising material for bone replacement (Abouzeid et al. 2018). The reinforced silicocarnotite of chitosan and alginate composite enhances cell proliferation, differentiation, and mechanical strength (Karimi, Mesgar, and Mohammadi 2020). Fu et al. fabricated the mesoporous bioactive glass/sodium alginate scaffolds using 3D printing. To raise the mechanical strength, crosslinking was carried out by $CaCl_2$. Due to the large pore size and excellent surface area, the target drug is released in a controlled manner (Fu et al. 2019). The new alginate composite was prepared using a mixture of three materials of chitosan, alginate, and cellulose nanocrystals at different concentrations of (0.5%, 1%, and 2%). Individual samples of concentrated cellulose nanocrystals were subjected to a cytotoxicity test. Samples of 1% cellulose nanocrystals show the best results of cytotoxicity measurement and 100% cell viability

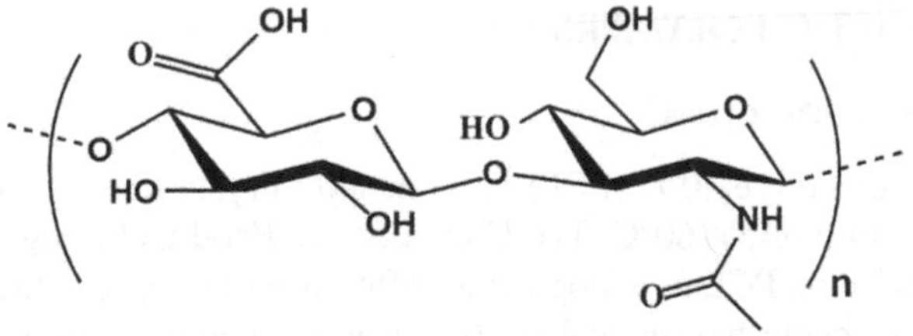

FIGURE 10.6 Chemical structure of hyaluronic acid. The figure is redrawn from the reference research article (Gupta et al. 2019).

was up to 3 days (Shaheen, Montaser, and Li 2019). An alginate composition with 17β-estradiol, BMP2, and plasma has been prepared as a composite for bone regeneration. Alginate in the prepared scaffolds enhances the stability. Subsequently, a composite scaffold was implanted on female Sprague Dawley rats. In vivo results showed that BMP-2 improved 17β-estradiol response and increased bone mineral formation (Segredo-Morales et al. 2018). Moraes et al. fabricated sodium alginate and silk fibroin containing miscible bend. It was observed that amino groups present in the silk fibroin form chemical interaction with functional groups of sodium alginate. Wang et al., have reported that hydrogen bonding between sodium alginate and silk fibroin affects crystallinity, morphology, and thermal stability (de Moraes et al. 2014; Venkatesan, Bhatnagar, and Kim 2014; Wang, Yang, and Zhu 2019; Eivazzadeh-Keihan et al. 2020). Therefore, alginate or alginate with other biomaterials containing bio composites would be developed quickly in the desired shape and size for tissue regeneration applications.

10.5.6 Hyaluronic Acid

Hyaluronic acid (Figure 10.6) is a non-sulfated and simple glycosaminoglycan anionic compound. It contains D-glucuronic acid and N-acetyl glucosamine. The average molecular weight is about 4 million daltons. Generally, hyaluronic acid presents in all body fluids and tissues extracellular matrix. The primary important function is to maintain the hydration of the body fluids such as synovial fluid. Also, it promotes cellular adhesion and proliferation differentiation and induces the angiogenesis of the tissues (Xing et al. 2020). It has the bacteriostatic and anti-adhesive ability. The literature reported that hyaluronic acid has better anti-microbial effects on *Staphylococcus aureus, Pseudomonas aeruginosa, and Aggregatibacter actinomycetemcomitans* (Drago et al. 2014). The hyaluronic acid in bone tissue engineering regulates the osteoprogenitor cells and promotes cell proliferation and differentiation (Zhai et al. 2020). Besides, it is reported that the low molecular weight of the hyaluronic acid showed the enhanced proliferation of bone marrow mesenchymal stem cells. In comparison, the high molecular weight of the hyaluronic acid has a high expression osteogenic genes of RUNX-2, ALP, and OCN. Also, the literature reported that the use of hyaluronic acid enhances the expression of the vegetative endothelial growth factor (Ciccone, Zazzetta, and Morbidelli 2019).

10.6 SYNTHETIC POLYMERS

10.6.1 POLYCAPROLACTONE

Polycaprolactone (Figure 10.7) (PCL) is a partially crystalline polymer with a low melting temperature of 55–60°C. The United States Food and Drug Administration (FDA) recognized the PCL as a biopolymer often used to improve the implants with characteristics of being biodegradable (2–4 years), biocompatible, tissue adaptable, and having cell-penetrating capacity. Physiochemical properties of PCL depend on the molecular weight and degree of crystallinity of the PCL. PCL is soluble at room temperature and viscoelastic, and can quickly fabricate PCL-containing blends with other bioactive polymers. Because it is hydrophobic, PCL lacks the osteoconductive character and integrin-binding sites required for cell adhesion. Therefore, PCL needs additional materials to improve the usage in bone tissue engineering. Blending is a widely used method to modify the surface of the hydrophobic PCL (Gandhimathi et al. 2019; Cipitria et al. 2011; Nair and Laurencin 2007). In the work of Kong et al., BMP-2/MPEG-PCL microspheres fabricated by the double emulsion method. These scaffolds have controlled drug release, stability, biocompatibility, improved proliferation, and differentiation of MSCs from myoblast in vitro. Their work showed that such microspheres have 4.30 ± 0.19 μm in size, which is suitable for cell adhesion, spread, and cell growth (Kong et al. 2020). An effort was made to reinforce PCL by the addition of silk fibroin and silica nanoparticles. This scaffold attains suitable fiber architecture in the range of 164 ± 18.65 nm to 215 ± 32.12 nm. Porosity was achieved in the range of 90 ± 7.5%. Added to this, the pore size distribution attained was around 1.45–2.35 μm. The structural space might give an appropriate place for oxygen, minerals, and nutrients exchange of niche factors into the scaffolds for essential proliferation, adhesion, differentiation, spreading, and infiltration of cells. The in vitro study on hMSCs results in the expression of a high level of alkaline phosphatase (ALP) and osteocalcin (OCN) (Gandhimathi et al. 2019). Huang, et al., proposed to combine the use of 3D printed PCL/HA/MWCNTs (CNT) as a mimic of nanostructured natural bone component. The CNT walls covalently bind with hydroxyapatite (HA) which might change the surface and may influence the activation of the focal adhesion kinase signaling pathway. PCL/HA/MWCNTs composites have significant mechanical strength. Further studies are needed to optimize the concentration of both MWCNTs and HA, which is essential to strengthening the physiochemical properties and cellular response (Huang et al. 2020). Martins et al. have proven that surface modification on the PCL nanofiber meshes can enhance the physical performance of the PCL (Martins et al. 2009). Sarasam and his co-workers have fabricated a PCL-chitosan blend for BTE. Finding results reveals that the developed blend has higher

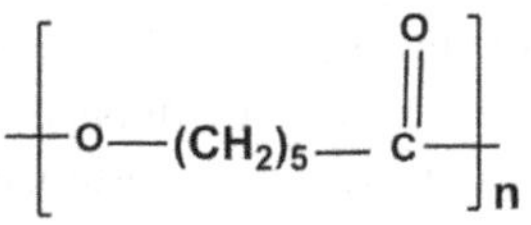

FIGURE 10.7 Chemical structure of polycaprolactone. The figure is redrawn from the reference research article (Ramanujam et al. 2018).

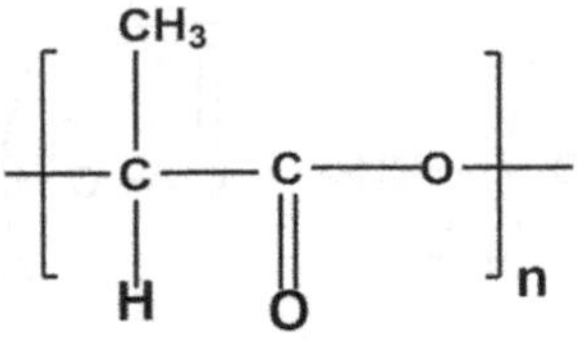

$$CH_3$$

FIGURE 10.8 Chemical structure of polylactic acid. The figure is redrawn from the reference research article (Galindo and Ureña-Núñez 2018).

mechanical strength and showing higher biological properties than individual materials (Sarasam and Madihally 2005; Guarino et al. 2002)

10.6.2 POLYLACTIC ACID

Polylactic acid (PLA) (Figure 10.8) is a monomer of lactic acid and has been a vital part of the glycolytic energy cycle for maintaining the growth and development of an organism. It is the most studied polymer and is used in pharmaceutical, medical, food, and packaging applications. Due to the semi-crystalline nature with disordered amorphous phases, it can form a nanotopography unique structure with dense lamellae (Wang et al. 2021). It has good biocompatibility, stretchability, and degradability behavior, but the mechanical properties are not perfect and still need improvement. The hydrophobic behavior of this polymer, which is inappropriate for the cell adhesion and drug-delivering system, is the main drawback. The impact toughness is extremely low, unsuited for medical implants. The above deficiency might be improved with specific innovative methods by blending with other polymers/copolymer or engineered additives during the synthesis process. Most biopolymers can biodegrade within one year, but polycaprolactone (PCL), PLA, L-PLA, and DL-PLA required a long year. The highly impaired bone conditions of an aged person need prolonged time for fracture treatment. At most, L-PLA provides the suitable tensile strength of 150MPa, to secure bone graft substitute material (Seitz et al. 2015). Wang et al. performed the experiments on 3D printed nanotopography scaffolds with the chemical cue of PDA coating via self-polymerization. They did an in-vitro study using autologous bone marrow stromal cells (BMSCs), and the results show excellent osteoblast adhesion and proliferation. Also, they did a critical-sized (4 mm × 4 mm) femoral condylar defect to a Sprague Dawley (SD) rat and implanted the PDA-coated 3D printed scaffolds on the defect site. New bone tissues developed between the pores of the scaffold were observed after surgery through micro-CT. Histological analysis gave the perfect result of cytoplasmic and nuclei gene expression (OCN, OPN, and RUNX2) (Wang et al. 2021). A PLA/CA nanofiber composite scaffold was analyzed by Ye et al. Initially, the PLA/SA fibers were obtained by an electrospinning process then subjected to $CaCl_2$ crosslinking to get PLA/CA at different ratios. The CA (calcium alginate) in the composite promotes the cell mineralization levels of calcium. The stable fibrous structures of the scaffolds promote the cell adhesion of periodontal ligament cells (PDLCs) and bone marrow stromal cells. The PLA/CA nanofiber composite enhanced the expression of

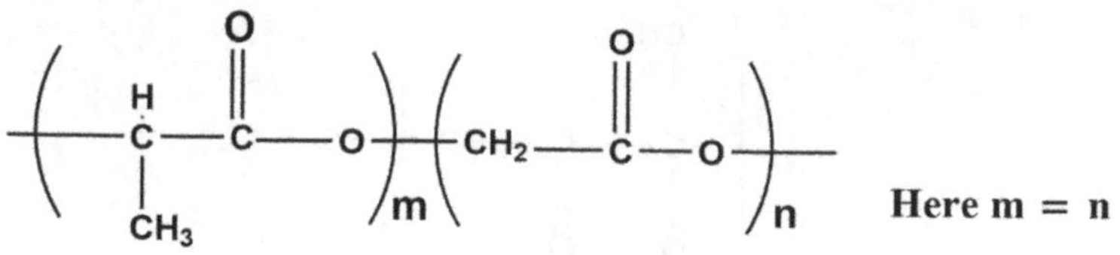

Here m = n

FIGURE 10.9 Chemical structure of poly (lactic-co-glycolic acid). The figure is redrawn from the reference research article (Bubb et al. 2002).

the inflammatory regulatory genes of Toll-like receptor 4 (TLR4), IL-6, IL-8, and IL-1b needed for fracture healing (Ye et al. 2020). Vascularity plays a significant role at the time of the healing process at the injury site. According to Guduric et al., the blood vessels (Vasculature) were developed through the 3D form of layer-by-layer bio-assembly (LBL) of PLA (assembly of the preformed cell containing fabrication units). The experiment was achieved with the coculture of human bone marrow stem cells (HBMCs) and endothelial progenitor cells (EPCs). In-vivo studies were carried on NOG SCID immunodeficient 8-week-old male mice. The LBL composite produced the vascularized blood vessels that might be provided with oxygen diffusion, nutrients, and waste product elimination (Guduric et al. 2019).

10.6.3 Poly (Lactic-co-Glycolic Acid)

Poly (a- hydroxy esters), such as poly (L-lactic acid) (PLLA) and poly (DL-lactic-co-glycolic acid) (PLGA) (Figure 10.9), are special synthetic polymers accepted for clinical use. These polymers are biocompatible, biodegradable, and easy to treat. PLGA was used as a suturing material as a medical implant. The physical, chemical, and degrading properties of PLGA served best for bone regeneration. Also, it requires mixing with other materials, including ceramics, bioactive glass, and hydroxyapatite materials that encourage bone conductivity and mechanical strength (Ferrone and Raut 2012). The Food and Drug Administration (FDA) approved PLGA for human therapy. It can be formulated as hydrogels, sponges, microparticles, and membranes. Kim et al. outline a new approach to constructing the polymeric/nano-HA composite scaffold. The method includes gas foaming and particulate leaching (GF/PL) instead of conventional solvent/particulate leaching (SC/LP). The nano- HA was well exposed on the surface of the scaffold GF/PL method and has high porous structures, good mechanical strength, and better cell growth (Kim et al. 2006). The BMP-2/Polyethyleneimine nanoparticles were entrapped with PLGA microsphere by the double emulsion method. These nanoparticles with BMP-2 lasted for 35 days, promoting osteoblast differentiation (Qiao et al. 2013). PLGA nanospheres have allowed targeted administration of cell-specific drugs to improve proteins or nucleic acid within or near mesenchymal stem cells (Vo, Kasper, and Mikos 2012).

Silk hydroxyapatite and PLGA nanoparticles hybrid scaffolds were investigated in F.A. Sheikh et al. studies. In vivo studies found that composite scaffolds exhibited complete bone formation and superior mechanical properties (Sheikh et al. 2016). J.Y. Kim et al. developed the PCL/PLGA composite through solid free-form fabrication

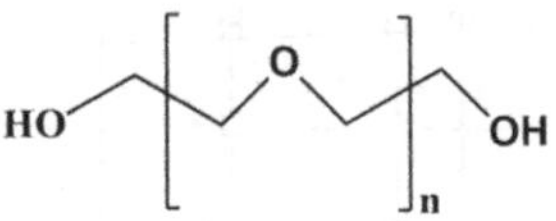

FIGURE 10.10 Chemical structure of polyethylene glycol. The figure is redrawn from the reference research article (Bitounis et al. 2012).

technology. The in vitro studies were carried out using MC3T3-E1 cells, and the results show that the scaffold has better biocompatibility and proper cell growth (Kim and Cho 2009). Chemical synthetic modifications of PLGA with biomaterials and surface modifications on PLGA significantly affect the biological properties of the PLGA. Kay et al. have developed nanostructured PLGA through surface modifications by using an optimized concentration of sodium hydroxide (Kay et al. 2002). Further study on the PLGA reveals that nano PLGA enhances osteoblast and chondrocytes cell adhesion. Also, several research reports have proven that synthetic modifications can tune the biodegradability and mechanical strength of the composite materials containing PLGA. However, PLGA crosslinked with polymers, ceramics, and alloys can enhance osteogenic properties (Katti, Vasita, and Shanmugam 2008; Bhuiyan et al. 2016)

10.6.4 POLY (ETHYLENE GLYCOL)

Poly (ethylene glycol) (PEG) (Figure 10.10) has unique physiochemical and biological properties. It has non-toxic effects on the cells. The hydrophilic nature of these polymers favors cellular attachments, proliferation, and differentiation. It is widely used in biomedical applications in the absence of antigenicity and immunogenicity. PEG was extensively used in the pharmaceutical industry for drug formulations and studies. Yang et al. blended the PEG with silk fibroin and hydroxyapatite. These composites mimic the natural extracellular matrix of the bone and sufficiently support the bone marrow mesenchymal stem cell adhesion, proliferation, and differentiation. Also, the osteogenic markers of the Runx2 showed regulatory function (Yang et al. 2020). Pazarceviren et al. developed highly porous CLN/PCL-PEG-PCL (CLN-Clinoptilolite) composites for bone tissue engineering applications. The scaffolds have high mechanical strength, better alkaline phosphatase activity, and cellular adhesion (Pazarceviren et al. 2020). The research of PEG and PLA composite scaffolds showed improved biomineralization (Bhaskar et al. 2018). Ni et al. developed the hybrid fibrous scaffolds of PEG with PLA. The hybrid scaffolds have shown better growth of the mesenchymal stem cell and are favored for expressing the osetogenes of OCN and OPN. The alizarin red S staining results showed excellent growth of the osteoblast cells (Ni et al. 2011). The hydroxyapatite composites of PEG with PCL were developed by Han-Tsung Liao for bone tissue engineering applications. The porcine bone marrow stem cells were used to test the osteogenesis activity for bone regeneration. The composite scaffolds have a suitable pore size, pore volume, and hydrophilic nature for better cellular attachments and proliferation. The vegetative endothelial growth factor gene expression was well recorded in this study (Liao et al. 2014).

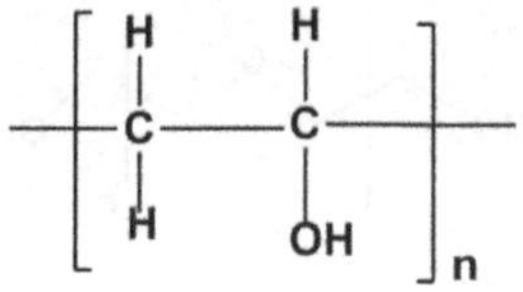

FIGURE 10.11 Chemical structure of polyvinyl alcohol. The figure is redrawn from the reference research article (Salman, Bakr, and Homad 2018).

10.6.5 POLY (VINYL ALCOHOL)

Poly (vinyl alcohol) (Figure 10.11) is a colloidal water-soluble synthetic compound with C-C bonds and acetate groups. Better biocompatibility, bioavailability, thermostability, and biodegradability made the PVA usable in biomedical applications. Instant dissolution and excessive swelling rate are the main limitations in the PVA. Crosslinkers of glutaraldehyde were used to overcome this disadvantage. Glutaraldehyde was used as an effective stabilizer as it is easily accessible and low cost. In recent days, physical crosslinking of the PVA was processed through freeze-thawing of ultraviolet radiation to increase the non-toxicity effects and efficacy to deliver the proteins, drugs, and cells (Teixeira, Amorim, and Felgueiras 2020). Enayati et al. developed the poly (vinyl alcohol)-based-nanohydroxyapatite-cellulose nanofibers bio nanocomposite for bone regeneration applications. Cell viability, adhesion, and osteoblast activity of MG-63 hold a more significant activity (Enayati et al. 2018). Also, the literature reported that the PVA and the bioactive glass were currently used as nanofibers for bone tissue engineering applications (Mansur and Costa 2008).

10.6.6 POLYETHER ETHER KETONE

Polyether ether ketone (PEEK) (Figure 10.12) is a polycyclic aromatic polymer. It is a stiff material with high thermal stability. The non-allergic and radiolucent properties of the PEEK made the clinician and the scientist believe it is an alternative for metallic implants, which overcomes the problems of stress shielding and inflammation response at the surgical site. Its mechanical and chemical strength is very high relative to human bone. The hydrophobic nature of PEEK makes it unsuitable for cell

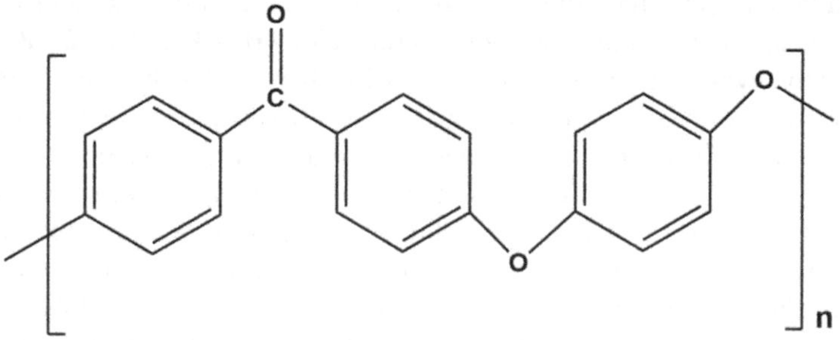

FIGURE 10.12 Chemical structure of polyether ether ketone. The figure is redrawn from the reference research article (Najeeb et al. 2015).

adhesion. Surface modifications were carried out to overcome this challenge, and results showed better cell adhesion (Almasi et al. 2016). Early studies were carried out to combine the PEEK materials with electrical glass (E-Glass) as a bone replacement implant (Chan and Leong 2008). The bone regeneration study was carried out by C. Von Wilmonsky et al. They prepared the composite according to 3D laser-sintered PEEK with βTCP. The in vivo studies were carried out on porcine animals. The results showed that the composite scaffolds had better bone regeneration (Von Wilmonsky et al. 2009). The nanocomposite of titanium dioxide and PEEK incorporated as composite were studied by Wu et al. The PEEK bioactivity was improved on its rough composite surface by n-TiO$_2$. The MG-63 cells were used for the in vitro studies and revealed better cell proliferation. The cytotoxicity assessment was confirmed by MTT assay. The in vivo studies on beagle dogs show that the n-TiO$_2$ enhances osteoblast differentiation and proliferation (Wu et al. 2012).

10.7 CONCLUSION

We discussed the role, selection, and tuning of polymeric biomaterials for bone tissue engineering applications. In particular, fabrication methods for preparing the composite materials, including technologies of 3D printing, electrospinning, and microsphere sintering, were widely observed. In particular, composite materials such as polymer matrix composites and ceramic matrix composites were elaborately discussed. From the records, the importance of materials selection and tuning method is clearly understood. The biomaterials of natural sources provide excellent biocompatibility, bioavailability, and biodegradable properties, but they fail to provide the mechanical property, whereas synthetic biomaterials provide mechanical strength. However, the composition of both natural and synthetic (semi-synthetic) compensates for the limitations. A wide variety of biocomposites were reported in the literature for bone tissue engineering applications but failed to provide the vascularization effect. In the future, vascularization effects need much attention. It is also essential to fabricate the scaffolds to mimic the exact natural bone and make it more suitable for the technology process in bone tissue regeneration.

ACKNOWLEDGMENTS

This research was supported by the Basic Science Research Program through the National Research Foundation (NRF) of Korea (2018R1A6A1A03024231 and 2021R1A2C1003566). The book chapter is also supported by a seed grant of Yenepoya (Deemed to be University), Mangalore.

ABBREVIATIONS

ADSCs adipose-derived stem cells
AIGIDs abalone intestine gastro-intestinal digests
BMP-2 bone morphogenetic protein 2
BMSCs bone marrow stromal cells
BTE bone tissue engineering

CMC	carboxymethylic chitosan
CNF	cellulose nanofibrils
Col	collagen
CS	chitosan
CXCR4	C-X-C chemokine receptor type 4
ECM	extracellular matrix
E-Glass	electrical glass
FDA	Food and Drug Administration
hMSCs	human mesenchymal stem cells
IL	interleukin
LBL	layer-by-layer bio-assembly
MSCs	mesenchymal stem cells
MWCNTs	multi-walled carbon nanotubes
nHA	nano-hydroxyapatite
PCL	polycaprolactone
PDLCs	periodontal ligament cells
PDO	poly (p-dioxanone)
PEEK	polyether ether ketone
PEG	poly (ethylene glycol)
PGA	poly (glycolic acid)
PLA	poly (lactic acid)
PLGA	poly (DL-lactic-co-glycolic acid)
PLLA	poly (L-lactic acid)
PU	polyurethanes
PVA	poly (vinyl alcohol)
rhBMP-2	recombinant human bone morphogenetic protein-2
SA	sodium alginate
SBF	simulated body fluid
SD	Sprague Dawley
SDF-1α	stromal derived factor-1 alpha
SF	silk fibroin
T-CNF	TEMPO-oxidized cellulose nanofibrils
TCP	tricalcium phosphate
TE	tissue engineering
TLR4	toll-like receptor 4
VEGF	vegetative endothelial growth factor
β-TCP	β-tricalcium phosphate

REFERENCES

Abouzeid, R. E., R. Khiari, D. Beneventi, and A. Dufresne. 2018. Biomimetic Mineralization of Three-Dimensional Printed Alginate/TEMPO-Oxidized Cellulose Nanofibril Scaffolds for Bone Tissue Engineering. *Biomacromolecules* 19 (11):4442–4452.

Ak, F., Z. Oztoprak, I. Karakutuk, and O. Okay. 2013. Macroporous Silk Fibroin Cryogels. *Biomacromolecules* 14 (3):719–727.

Almasi, D., N. Iqbal, M. Sadeghi, I. Sudin, M. R. Abdul Kadir, and T. Kamarul. 2016. Preparation Methods for Improving PEEK's Bioactivity for Orthopedic and Dental Application: A Review. *Int J Biomater* 2016:8202653.

Ambrogi, Valeria, Giuseppe Fardella, Giuliano Grandolini, Morena Nocchetti, and Luana Perioli. 2003. Effect of Hydrotalcite-Like Compounds on the Aqueous Solubility of Some Poorly Water-Soluble Drugs. *J Pharm Sci* 92 (7):1407–1418.

Appukuttan, K. K. 1987. Pearl Oyster Culture in Vizhinjam Bay. *CMFRI Bull* 39:54–61.

Arthanareeswaran, G., T. K. Sriyamuna Devi, and M. Raajenthiren. 2008. Effect of Silica Particles on Cellulose Acetate Blend Ultrafiltration Membranes: Part I. *Sep Purif Technol* 64 (1):38–47.

Azizian, S., A. Hadjizadeh, and H. Niknejad. 2018. Chitosan-gelatin porous scaffold incorporated with Chitosan nanoparticles for growth factor delivery in tissue engineering. *Carbohydr Polym* 202:315–322.

Balagangadharan, K., S. Dhivya, and N. Selvamurugan. 2017. Chitosan Based Nanofibers in Bone Tissue Engineering. *Int J Biol Macromol* 104 (Pt B):1372–1382.

Bello, A. B., D. Kim, D. Kim, H. Park, and S.-H. Lee. 2020. Engineering and Functionalization of Gelatin Biomaterials: From Cell Culture to Medical Applications. *Tissue Eng Part B Rev* 26 (2):164–180.

Bhaskar, B., R. Owen, H. Bahmaee, Z. Wally, P. Sreenivasa Rao, and G. C. Reilly. 2018. Composite Porous Scaffold of PEG/PLA Support Improved Bone Matrix Deposition in vitro Compared to PLA-Only Scaffolds. *J Biomed Mater Res A* 106 (5):1334–1340.

Bhattacharyya, D., J. M. McCarthy, and R. B. Grives. 1974. Charged membrabe ultrafiltration of inorganic ions in single annd multi-salt systems. *AIChE J* 20 (6):1206–1212.

Bhuiyan, D. B, J. C. Middleton, R. Tannenbaum, and T. M. Wick. 2016. Mechanical Properties and Osteogenic Potential of Hydroxyapatite-PLGA-Collagen Biomaterial for Bone Regeneration. *J Biomater Sci Polym Ed* 27 (11):1139–1154.

Bitounis, D., R. Fanciullino, A. Iliadis, and J. Ciccolini. 2012. Optimizing Druggability Through Liposomal Formulations: New Approaches to an Old Concept. *ISRN Pharm* 2012 (1):1–12.

Bose, S., C. Koski, and A. A. Vu. 2020. Additive Manufacturing of Natural Biopolymers and Composites for Bone Tissue Engineering. *Mater Hori* 7 (8):2011–2027.

Bubb, D. M., B. Toftmann, R. F. Haglund Jr, et al. 2002. Resonant Infrared Pulsed Laser Deposition of Thin Biodegradable Polymer Films. *Appl Phy A* 74 (1):123–125.

C Echave, M., L. S. Burgo, J. L Pedraz, and G. Orive. 2017. Gelatin as Biomaterial for Tissue Engineering. *Curr Pharm Des* 23 (24):3567–3584.

Caliari, S. R., and J. A. Burdick. 2016. A Practical Guide to Hydrogels for Cell Culture. *Nat Methods* 13 (5):405–14.

Chan, B. P., and K.W. Leong. 2008. Scaffolding in Tissue Engineering: General Approaches and Tissue-Specific Considerations. *Eur Spine J* 17 (4):467–479.

Chocholata, P., V. Kulda, and V. Babuska. 2019. Fabrication of Scaffolds for Bone-Tissue Regeneration. *Materials* 12 (4):568.

Ciccone, V., M. Zazzetta, and L. Morbidelli. 2019. Comparison of the Effect of Two Hyaluronic Acid Preparations on Fibroblast and Endothelial Cell Functions Related to Angiogenesis. *Cells* 8 (12):1479.

Cipitria, A., A. Skelton, T. R. Dargaville, P. D. Dalton, and D. W. Hutmacher. 2011. Design, Fabrication and Characterization of PCL Electrospun Scaffolds—A Review. *J Mater Chem* 21 (26):9419–9453.

Correia, C., S. Bhumiratana, L. P. Yan, et al. 2012. Development of Silk-Based Scaffolds for Tissue Engineering of Bone from Human Adipose-Derived Stem Cells. *Acta Biomater* 8 (7):2483–92.

de Melo Pereira, D., M. Eischen-Loges, Z. T. Birgani, and P. Habibovic. 2020. Proliferation and Osteogenic Differentiation of hMSCs on Biomineralized Collagen. *Front Bioeng Biotech* 8:554565.

de Moraes, M. A., M. F. Silva, R. F. Weska, and M. M. Beppu. 2014. Silk Fibroin and Sodium Alginate Blend: Miscibility and Physical Characteristics. *Mater Sci Eng C Mater Biol Appl* 40 (1):85–91.

Dong, C., and Y. Lv. 2016. Application of Collagen Scaffold in Tissue Engineering: Recent Advances and New Perspectives. *Polymers* 8 (2):42.

Drago, L., L. Cappelletti, E. De Vecchi, L. Pignataro, S. Torretta, and R. Mattina. 2014. Antiadhesive and Antibiofilm Activity of Hyaluronic Acid Against Bacteria Responsible for Respiratory Tract Infections. *APMIS* 122 (10):1013–1019.

Dwivedi, R., S. Kumar, R. Pandey, et al. 2020. Polycaprolactone as Biomaterial for Bone Scaffolds: Review of Literature. *J Oral Biol Craniof Res* 10 (1):381–388.

Eivazzadeh-Keihan, R., F. Radinekiyan, H. Madanchi, H. A. M. Aliabadi, and A. Maleki. 2020. Graphene Oxide/Alginate/Silk Fibroin Composite as a Novel Bionanostructure with Improved Blood Compatibility, Less Toxicity and Enhanced Mechanical Properties. *Carbohydr Polym* 248 (1):116802.

Elzoghby, A. O. 2013. Gelatin-Based Nanoparticles as Drug and Gene Delivery Systems: Reviewing Three Decades of Research. *J Control Release* 172 (3):1075–1091.

Enayati, M. S., T. Behzad, P. Sajkiewicz, et al. 2018. Development of Electrospun Poly (vinyl alcohol)- Based Bionanocomposite Scaffolds for Bone Tissue Engineering. *J Biomed Mater Res A* 106 (4):1111–1120.

Fayyazbakhsh, F., M. Solati-Hashjin, A. Keshtkar, M. A. Shokrgozar, M. M. Dehghan, and B. Larijani. 2017. Release Behavior and Signaling Effect of Vitamin D3 in Layered Double Hydroxides-Hydroxyapatite/Gelatin Bone Tissue Engineering Scaffold: An in Vitro Evaluation. *Colloids Surf B Biointerfaces* 158:697–708.

Feng, Q., K. Wei, S. Lin, et al. 2016. Mechanically Resilient, Injectable, and Bioadhesive Supramolecular Gelatin Hydrogels Crosslinked by Weak Host-Guest Interactions Assist Cell Infiltration and In Situ Tissue Regeneration. *Biomaterials* 101 (1):217–228.

Ferrone, M. L., and C. P. Raut. 2012. Modern Surgical Therapy: Limb Salvage and the Role of Amputation for Extremity Soft-Tissue Sarcomas. *Surg Oncol Clin N Am* 21 (2):201–13.

Fu, S., X. Du, M. Zhu, Z. Tian, D. Wei, and Y. Zhu. 2019. 3D Printing of Layered Mesoporous Bioactive Glass/Sodium Alginate-Sodium Alginate Scaffolds with Controllable Dual-Drug Release Behaviors. *Biomed Mater* 14 (6):065011.

Furth, M. E., and A. Atala. 2014. Tissue Engineering: Future Perspectives. In *Principles of Tissue Engineering*. Academic Press. 83–12.

Galindo, S, and F Ureña-Núñez. 2018. Enhanced Surface Hydrophobicity of Poly (Lactic Acid) by Co60 Gamma Ray Irradiation. *Revista Mexicana De Física* 64 (1):1–7.

Gandhimathi, C., Y. J. Quek, H. Ezhilarasu, S. Ramakrishna, B. H. Bay, and D. K. Srinivasan. 2019. Osteogenic Differentiation of Mesenchymal Stem Cells with Silica-Coated Gold Nanoparticles for Bone Tissue Engineering. *Int J Mol Sci* 20 (20).

Garg, T, A. Bilandi, B. Kapoor, S. Kumar, and R. Joshi. 2011. Scaffold: Tissue Engineering and Regenerative Medicine. *Int Res J Pharm* 2 (12):37–42.

Gentile, P., V. Chiono, I. Carmagnola, and P. V. Hatton. 2014. An Overview of Poly (lactic-co-glycolic) Acid (PLGA)-Based Biomaterials for Bone Tissue Engineering. *Int J Mol Sci* 15 (3):3640–3659.

Gregor, A., E. Filová, and M. Novák, et al. 2017. Designing of PLA Scaffolds for Bone Tissue Replacement Fabricated by Ordinary Commercial 3D Printer. *J Biol Eng* 11 (1):1–21.

Guarino, V., G. Gentile, L. Sorrentino, and L. Ambrosio. 2002. Polycaprolactone: Synthesis, Properties, and Applications. *Encyclopedia of Polymer Science and Technology* 1 (1):1–36.

Guduric, V., R. Siadous, J. Babilotte, et al. 2019. Layer-by-Layer Bioassembly of Poly(lactic) Acid Membranes Loaded with Coculture of HBMSCs and EPCs Improves Vascularization In Vivo. *J Biomed Mater Res A* 107 (12):2629–2642.

Gupta, B. S., and J. V. Edwards. 2019. Textile materials and structures for topical management of wounds. In *Advanced Textiles for Wound Care*. Woodhead Publishing. 55–104.

Gupta, R. C, R. Lall, A. Srivastava, and A. Sinha. 2019. Hyaluronic Acid: Molecular Mechanisms and Therapeutic Trajectory. *Front Vet Sci* 6 (1):192.

Horan, R. L., K. Antle, A. L. Collette, et al. 2005. In Vitro Degradation of Silk Fibroin. *Biomaterials* 26 (17):3385–93.

Huang, B., C. Vyas, J. J. Byun, M. El-Newehy, Z. Huang, and P. Bartolo. 2020. Aligned Multi-Walled Carbon Nanotubes with Nanohydroxyapatite in a 3D Printed Polycaprolactone Scaffold Stimulates Osteogenic Differentiation. *Mater Sci Eng C Mater Biol Appl* 108:110374.

Ibrahim, H. M., and E. M. R. El-Zairy. 2015. Chitosan as a Biomaterial—Structure, Properties, and Electrospun Nanofibers. *Concepts, Compounds and the Alternatives of Antibacterials* 1 (1):81–101.

Karimi, M., A. S. Mesgar, and Z. Mohammadi. 2020. Development of Osteogenic Chitosan/Alginate Scaffolds Reinforced with Silicocarnotite Containing Apatitic Fibers. *Biomed Mater* 15 (5):055020.

Katti, D. S., R. Vasita, and K. Shanmugam. 2008. Improved Biomaterials for Tissue Engineering Applications: Surface Modification of Polymers. *Curr Top Med Chem* 8 (4):341–353.

Kay, S., A. Thapa, K. M. Haberstroh, and T. J. Webster. 2002. Nanostructured Polymer/Nanophase Ceramic Composites Enhance Osteoblast and Chondrocyte Adhesion. *Tissue Eng* 8 (5):753–761.

Khor, E, and J L. H. Whey. 1995. Interaction of Chitosan with Polypyrrole in the Formation of Hybrid Biomaterials. *Carbohydr Polym* 26 (3):183–187.

Kim, J. Y., and D.-W. Cho. 2009. Blended PCL/PLGA Scaffold Fabrication Using Multi-Head Deposition System. *Microelectronic Engineering* 86 (4–6):1447–1450.

Kim, S. S., M. S. Park, O. Jeon, C. Y. Choi, and B. S. Kim. 2006. Poly(lactide-co-glycolide)/Hydroxyapatite Composite Scaffolds for Bone Tissue Engineering. *Biomaterials* 27 (8):1399–409.

Kong, D., Y. Shi, Y. Gao, M. Fu, S. Kong, and G. Lin. 2020. Preparation of BMP-2 loaded MPEG-PCL Microspheres and Evaluation of Their Bone Repair Properties. *Biomed Pharmacother* 130:110516.

Kundu, S. C., B. C. Dash, R. Dash, and D. L. Kaplan. 2008. Natural Protective Glue Protein, Sericin Bioengineered by Silkworms: Potential for Biomedical and Biotechnological Applications. *Prog Polym Sci* 33 (10):998–1012.

Laiva, A. L., R. M. Raftery, M. B. Keogh, and F. J. O'Brien. 2018. Pro-Angiogenic Impact of SDF-1α Gene-Activated Collagen-Based Scaffolds in Stem Cell Driven Angiogenesis. *Int J Pharm* 544 (2):372–379.

Liao, H.-T., Y.-Y. Chen, Y.-T. Lai, M.-F. Hsieh, and C.-P. Jiang. 2014. The Osteogenesis of Bone Marrow Stem Cells on mPEG-PCL-mPEG/Hydroxyapatite Composite Scaffold Via Solid Freeform Fabrication. *BioMed Research International* 2014 (1):1–14.

Liu, Yi, S. C. Ng, J. Yu, and W.-B. Tsai. 2019. Modification and Crosslinking of Gelatin-Based Biomaterials as Tissue Adhesives. *Colloids Surf B Biointerfaces* 174 (1):316–323.

LogithKumar, R., A. KeshavNarayan, S. Dhivya, A. Chawla, S. Saravanan, and N. Selvamurugan. 2016. A Review of Chitosan and its Derivatives in Bone Tissue Engineering. *Carbohydr Polym* 151:172–188.

Mansur, H. S., and H. S. Costa. 2008. Nanostructured Poly (vinyl alcohol)/Bioactive Glass and Poly (Vinyl Alcohol)/Chitosan/Bioactive Glass Hybrid Scaffolds for Biomedical Applications. *Chem Eng J* 137 (1):72–83.

Mao, D., Q. Li, D. Li, Y. Tan, and Q. Che. 2018. 3D Porous Poly(ε-Caprolactone)/58S Bioactive Glass–Sodium Alginate/Gelatin Hybrid Scaffolds Prepared by a Modified Melt Molding Method for Bone Tissue Engineering. *Mater Des* 160:1–8.

Martins, A., E. D. Pinho, S. Faria, et al. 2009. Surface Modification of Electrospun Polycaprolactone Nanofiber Meshes by Plasma Treatment to Enhance Biological Performance. *Small* 5 (10):1195–1206.

Melke, J., S. Midha, S. Ghosh, K. Ito, and S. Hofmann. 2016. Silk Fibroin as Biomaterial for Bone Tissue Engineering. *Acta Biomater* 31:1–16.

Mhuka, V., S. Dube, and M. M. Nindi. 2013. Chemical, Structural and Thermal Properties of GONOMETA POSTICA SILK FIBROIN, A Potential Biomaterial. *Int J Biol Macromol* 52:305–11.

Nair, L. S., and C. T. Laurencin. 2007. Biodegradable Polymers as Biomaterials. *Prog Polym Sci* 32 (8–9):762–798.

Najeeb, S., Z. Khurshid, J. P. Matinlinna, F. Siddiqui, M. Z. Nassani, and K. Baroudi. 2015. Nanomodified Peek Dental Implants: Bioactive Composites and Surface Modification—A Review. *Int J Dent* 2015 (1):1–8.

Naomi, R., J. Ratanavaraporn, and M. B. Fauzi. 2020. Comprehensive Review of Hybrid Collagen and Silk Fibroin for Cutaneous Wound Healing. *Materials* 13 (14):3097.

Ni, P., S. Fu, M. Fan, et al. 2011. Preparation of Poly (Ethylene Glycol)/Polylactide Hybrid Fibrous Scaffolds for Bone Tissue Engineering. *Int J Nanomed* 6 (1):3065.

Oh, G. W., V. T. Nguyen, S. Y. Heo, et al. 2020. 3D PCL/Fish Collagen Composite Scaffolds Incorporating Osteogenic Abalone Protein Hydrolysates for Bone Regeneration Application: In vitro and in vivo Studies. *J Biomater Sci Polym Ed* 1–17.

Pazarceviren, A. E., T. Dikmen, K. Altunbaş, et al. 2020. Composite Clinoptilolite/PCL-PEG-PCL Scaffolds for Bone Regeneration: In vitro and in vivo Evaluation. *J Tissue Eng Regen Med* 14 (1):3–15.

Preethi Soundarya, S., A. Haritha Menon, S. Viji Chandran, and N. Selvamurugan. 2018. Bone Tissue Engineering: Scaffold Preparation Using Chitosan and Other Biomaterials with Different Design and Fabrication Techniques. *Int J Biol Macromol* 119:1228–1239.

Qiao, C., K. Zhang, H. Jin, et al. 2013. Using Poly(lactic-co-glycolic acid) Microspheres to Encapsulate Plasmid of Bone Morphogenetic Protein 2/Polyethylenimine Nanoparticles to Promote Bone Formation in vitro and in vivo. *Int J Nanomedicine* 8:2985–95.

Ramanujam, R., B. Sundaram, G. Janarthanan, E. Devendran, M. Venkadasalam, and M. C. John Milton. 2018. Biodegradable Polycaprolactone Nanoparticles Based Drug Delivery Systems: A Short Review. *Biosci Biotechnol Res Asia* 15 (3):679–685.

Ricard-Blum, S. 2011. The Collagen Family. *Cold Spring Harb Perspect Biol* 3 (1):a004978.

Rubežić, M. Z, A. B. Krstić, H. Z. Stanković, R. B. Ljupković, M. S. Ranđelović, and A. R. Zarubica. 2020. Different Types of Biomaterials: Structure and Application: A Short Review. *Advanced Technologies* 9 (1):69–79.

Sabir, M. I., X. Xu, and L. Li. 2009. A Review on Biodegradable Polymeric Materials for Bone Tissue Engineering Applications. *J Mater Sci* 44 (21):5713–5724.

Salman, S. A., N. A. Bakr, and H. T. Homad. 2018. Section C: Physical Sciences DSC and TGA Properties of PVA Films Filled with $Na_2S_2O_3 \cdot 5H_2O$ Salt. *J Chem Biol Phys Sci* 8 (1):001–011.

Sami El-banna, F., M. E. Mahfouz, S. Leporatti, M. El-Kemary, and N. A. N. Hanafy. 2019. Chitosan as a Natural Copolymer with Unique Properties for the Development of Hydrogels. *Appl Sci* 9 (11):2193.

Sarasam, A., and S. V. Madihally. 2005. Characterization of Chitosan–Polycaprolactone Blends for Tissue Engineering Applications. *Biomaterials* 26 (27):5500–5508.

Saravanan, S., R. S. Leena, and N. Selvamurugan. 2016. Chitosan Based Biocomposite Scaffolds for Bone Tissue Engineering. *Int J Biological Macromol* 93 (1):1354–1365.

Sashiwa, H., and S.-i. Aiba. 2004. Chemically Modified Chitin and Chitosan as Biomaterials. *Prog Polym Sci* 29 (9):887–908.

Segredo-Morales, E., P. Garcia-Garcia, R. Reyes, E. Perez-Herrero, A. Delgado, and C. Evora. 2018. Bone Regeneration in Osteoporosis by Delivery BMP-2 and PRGF from Tetronic-Alginate Composite Thermogel. *Int J Pharm* 543 (1–2):160–168.

Seitz, J. M., M. Durisin, J. Goldman, and J. W. Drelich. 2015. Recent Advances in Biodegradable Metals for Medical Sutures: A Critical Review. *Adv Healthc Mater* 4 (13):1915–36.

Shaheen, T. I., A. S. Montaser, and S. Li. 2019. Effect of Cellulose Nanocrystals on Scaffolds Comprising Chitosan, Alginate and Hydroxyapatite for Bone Tissue Engineering. *Int J Biol Macromol* 121:814–821.

Sheikh, F. A., H. Woo Ju, B. Mi Moon, et al. 2016. Hybrid Scaffolds Based on PLGA and Silk for Bone Tissue Engineering. *J Tissue Eng Regen Med* 10 (3):209–221.

Szekalska, M., A. Puciłowska, E. Szymańska, P. Ciosek, and K. Winnicka. 2016. Alginate: Current Use and Future Perspectives in Pharmaceutical and Biomedical Applications. *Int J Polym Sci* 2016 (1):1.

Tamura, M., T. Uragami, and M. Sugihara. 1981. Studies on Syntheses and Permeabilities of Special Polymer Membranes: 30. Ultrafiltration and Dialysis Characteristics of Cellulose Nitrate-Poly(Vinyl Pyrrolidone) Polymer Blend Membranes. *Polymer* 22 (6):829–835.

Teixeira, M. A., M. T. P. Amorim, and H. P. Felgueiras. 2020. Poly (Vinyl Alcohol)-Based Nanofibrous Electrospun Scaffolds for Tissue Engineering Applications. *Polymers* 12 (1):7.

Tonelli, F. M. P., N. de Cássia Oliveira Paiva, R. V. B. de Medeiros, M. C. X. Pinto, F. C. P. Tonelli, and R. R. Resende. 2017. Tissue engineering: the use of stem cells in regenerative medicine. In *Current Developments in Biotechnology and Bioengineering: Human and Animal Health Applications.* 315–324

Van Vlierberghe, S., E. Vanderleyden, V. Boterberg, and P. Dubruel. 2011. Gelatin Functionalization of Biomaterial Surfaces: Strategies for Immobilization and Visualization. *Polymers* 3 (1):114–130.

Venkatesan, J., I. Bhatnagar, and S.-K. Kim. 2014. Chitosan-Alginate Biocomposite Containing Fucoidan for Bone Tissue Engineering. *Mar Drugs* 12 (1):300–316.

Venkatesan, J., I. Bhatnagar, P. Manivasagan, K.-H. Kang, and S.-K. Kim. 2015. Alginate Composites for Bone Tissue Engineering: A Review. *Int J Biol Macromol* 72 (1):269–281.

Venkatesan, J., B. Lowe, R. Pallela, and S.-K. Kim. 2014. Chitosan-Based Polysaccharide Biomaterials. *Polysaccharides: Bioactivity and Biotechnology.* Springer 1 (1): 1837–1850.

Vo, T. N., F. K. Kasper, and A. G. Mikos. 2012. Strategies for Controlled Delivery of Growth Factors and Cells for Bone Regeneration. *Adv Drug Deliv Rev* 64 (12):1292–309.

Von Wilmonsky, C., R. Lutz, U. Meisel, et al. 2009. In Vivo Evaluation of ß-TCP Containing 3D Laser Sintered Poly(ether ether ketone) Composites in Pigs. *J Bioact Compat Polym* 24 (2):169–184.

Wang, P., H. M. Yin, X. Li, et al. 2021. Simultaneously Constructing Nanotopographical and Chemical Cues in 3D-Printed Polylactic Acid Scaffolds to Promote Bone Regeneration. *Mater Sci Eng C Mater Biol Appl* 118:111457.

Wang, Y.-C., S.-H. Kao, and H.-J. Hsieh. 2003. A Chemical Surface Modification of Chitosan by Glycoconjugates To Enhance the Cell– Biomaterial Interaction. *Biomacromolecules* 4 (2):224–231.

Wang, Z., H. Yang, and Z. Zhu. 2019. Study on the Blends of Silk Fibroin and Sodium Alginate: Hydrogen Bond Formation, Structure and Properties. *Polymer* 163:144–153.

Wharram, S. E., X. Zhang, D. L. Kaplan, and S. P. McCarthy. 2010. Electrospun Silk Material Systems for Wound Healing. *Macromol Biosci* 10 (3):246–57.

Wu, X., X. Liu, J. Wei, J. Ma, F. Deng, and S. Wei. 2012. Nano-TiO2/PEEK Bioactive Composite as a Bone Substitute Material: In vitro and in vivo Studies. *Int J Nanomedicine* 7:1215–25.

Wust, S., M. E. Godla, R. Muller, and S. Hofmann. 2014. Tunable Hydrogel Composite With Two-Step Processing in Combination with Innovative Hardware Upgrade for Cell-Based Three-Dimensional Bioprinting. *Acta Biomater* 10 (2):630–40.

Xing, Fei, C. Zhou, D. Hui, et al. 2020. Hyaluronic Acid as a Bioactive Component for Bone Tissue Regeneration: Fabrication, Modification, Properties, and Biological Functions. *Nanotechnol Rev* 9 (1):1059–1079.

Yang, Y., Y. Feng, R. Qu, et al. 2020. Synthesis of Aligned Porous Polyethylene Glycol/Silk Fibroin/Hydroxyapatite Scaffolds for Osteoinduction in Bone Tissue Engineering. *Stem Cell Res Ther* 11 (1):1–17.

Ye, Z., W. Xu, R. Shen, and Y. Yan. 2020. Emulsion Electrospun PLA/Calcium Alginate Nanofibers for Periodontal Tissue Engineering. *J Biomater Appl* 34 (6):763–777.

Zarif, M.-E. 2018. A Review of Chitosan-, Alginate-, and Gelatin-Based Biocomposites for Bone Tissue Engineering. *Biomater Tissue Eng Bull* 5:97–109.

Zhai, P., X. Peng, B. Li, Y. Liu, H. Sun, and X. Li. 2020. The Application of Hyaluronic Acid in Bone Regeneration. *Int J Biol Macromol* 151:1224–1239.

Zhang, D., X. Wu, J. Chen, and K. Lin. 2018. The Development of Collagen Based Composite Scaffolds for Bone Regeneration. *Bioact Mater* 3 (1):129–138.

Zhu, Z., Y.-M. Wang, J. Yang, and X.-S. Luo. 2017. Hyaluronic Acid: A Versatile Biomaterial in Tissue Engineering. *Plast Aesthet Res* 4 (1):219–227.

Zima, A. 2018. Hydroxyapatite-Chitosan Based Bioactive Hybrid Biomaterials with Improved Mechanical Strength. *Spectrochim Acta A Mol Biomol Spectrosc* 193 (1):175–184.

11 Nanotherapeutics for Enhancing Burn Wound Healing

Zahid Hussain
University of Sharjah

Hnin Ei Thu
Lincoln University College

Shahzeb Khan
University of Malakand

Mohammad Sohail
COMSATS University Islamabad

Ohnmar Htwe
Universiti Kebangsaan Malaysia

Nor Amlizan Ramli
Universiti Teknologi MARA

Rai Muhammad Sarfraz
University of Sargodha

CONTENTS

DOI: 10.1201/9781003140108-11

11.1 INTRODUCTION: BURN WOUNDS (BWs)

11.1.1 PREVALENCE AND CAUSES OF BWs

Skin injuries are considered among the most common injuries encountered in all age groups. Unlike acute injuries (which can easily heal), chronic injuries (e.g., burn wounds) present substantial challenges to patients and the healthcare system [1, 2]. Among these challenges, a prolonged healing time is one of the key hurdles in the chronic wound healing, particularly second- and third-degree burns due to involvement of a large surface area and devitalization of deep skin substructures (dermis, hypodermis, and muscles). The prolonged healing time may result in greater risks of development of microbial infections that can further impede healing speed and eventually may lead to amputation [1, 2]. If remaining unnoticed, chronic injuries may progress to mortality or various other local or systemic morbidities [3]. It has been estimated that the mortality rate among burn victims is approximately 15% across the globe [3].

Burns, which cause damage to skin substructures at various levels (i.e., epidermis, dermis, hypodermis, tendon, bone, muscles, nerves, etc.), can be caused as a result of exposure to radiation, such as microwave or ionizing radiations such as X-ray or ultraviolet light (radiation burns); exposure to certain chemicals, such as strong acids or bases (chemical burns); exposure to high- or low-voltage electricity (electrical burns); prolonged or excessive sun exposure (sun burns); or exposure to wet heat, such as boiling liquids, or dry heat, such as fires (thermal burns). Among the aforementioned types, heat-induced burns are the most prevalent types of burn injuries. According to the World Health Organization (WHO) and the American Burn Association, it has been estimated that approximately 80% of the yearly reported burn cases (i.e., 6.6 million injuries and 300,000 deaths) are thermal burns, either due to dry heat (fire or flame) or wet heat (scalding). Unfortunately, the mortality rate due to burn injuries is very high in low- and middle-income countries such as South East Asia [4]. Furthermore, thermal injuries are among the most commonly encountered household injuries in children, with a high mortality rate in children between 1 and 9 years. On the other hand, patients with underlying medical conditions, such as diabetic neuropathy, vasculopathy, or mental illness, are more susceptible to burn injuries [5].

Besides causing severe damage to the skin (a highly immunocompetent organ), burn injuries may also lead to serious impairment of vascular supply and immunosuppression (suppression of both non-specific and specific immune system) [6]. In extensive burn injuries, increased blood capillary permeability causes great plasma loss, which could lead to hypovolemic shock. Apart from a high loss of plasma, down-regulation of cell-mediated immunity and cytokine release has been found compromised in extensive burn injuries. A compromised immune response that usually occurs after a burn injury is a prominent complaint that predisposes patients to develop microbial infections on local tissues (burned area) or systemically. Microbial infection causes significant delay in healing rate and may result in sepsis, which could further reduce the tissue regeneration ability of the body [6]. The maximum occurrence of microbial infection in burn victims happens in the first ten days after the injury because during this span the titer of the immunoglobulins (a chief defense against infections) is strikingly low [7]. Hence, the microbial infection (particularly septicemia) is a key reason of mortality and morbidity in burn victims, particularly when involving a larger body surface area. Souto et al. [6] reported that, although a burn area is initially sterile, at later stages it may get colonized with microorganisms, which habituate in the epithelial appendages of hair follicles and sebaceous glands and start growing, multiplying, and eventually inhabit the surface of the burned skin. It has been estimated that a 75% mortality rate has been observed in burn victims having bacteremia or septicemia, particularly when 40% of the total body surface area (TBSA) is involved. Therefore, one way to estimate the degree of burn in a patient is the assessment of TBSA involved. Another approach for determination of the severity of burn is by evaluating the depth of the skin damage. Therefore, burn cases, particularly thermal injuries involving a large TBSA, require intensive care and therapies to prevent/eradicate microbial infection [8]. Fortunately, the survival rate in burn victims has been markedly improved during the past few decades due to improvement in modern medical care and burn therapies, including burn wound care, nutritional support, and pulmonary management [9].

11.1.2 Types of BWs

Generally, BWs can be classified into four types: first-, second-, third-, and fourth-degree burns based on the degree and extent of involvement of skin tissues [1, 2]. In first-degree burns (also called as epithelial burns), only the uppermost layer of the skin (epidermis) is affected, and it typically displays signs such as erythema, pain, and dryness at the site of burn with no blister formation (Figure 11.1). Due to the involvement of epidermis only, these burns are also called superficial burns or epidermal loss. Epithelial burns cause minimal skin damage and are considered mild burns in which symptoms usually disappear within 7 to 10 days with no signs of vesication and scarring.

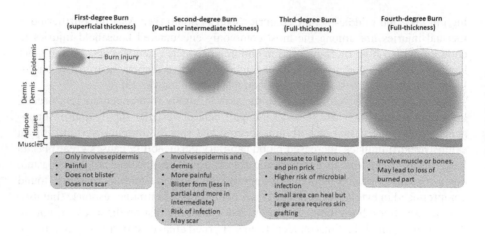

FIGURE 11.1   The pathophysiologic representation of different types of BWs.

On the other hand, second-degree burns (also called partial thickness burns) involve both papillary and reticular layers of the dermis in addition to the epidermis. Based on the dermal layers affected, second degree burns are sub-classified into superficial and deep-loss burns [1, 2]. For example, if only the papillary layer is affected, it is known as superficial loss with obvious signs of inflammation and vesication, while if deep dermal layer (reticular layer) is involved, it is known as deep loss with scar/eschar formation on the burned area [1, 2]. Typical symptoms of second-degree burns include discoloration (white or yellow) of the burned skin, blistering and thickening, and moist and shiny appearance of the burned skin. Blister formation promotes local and systemic microbial infections in burn patients via the blister fluid. Owing to its protein rich nature, blister fluid is a good growth media for microorganisms; therefore, it is strongly suggested not to leave the blister fluid on the burned skin for long (wipe it off) [10, 11]. Owing to involvement of microbial infection, second-degree burns require more intensive care and treatment compared to first-degree burns. Depending upon the dermal skin layers involved, some second-degree burns take 2 to 3 weeks to heal, but others may take more than 3 weeks to completely heal. However, as with the first-degree burns, second-degree burns rarely leave scars upon completing healing; however, discoloration of the burned skin is common in both sub-types of second-degree burns.

Contrary to the first- and second-degree burns, third-degree burns are characterized by fully destroyed epidermis and dermis and also involve hypodermal layers of the skin; therefore, they are also called full-thickness burns. Due to the high intensity of burns and great susceptibility of microbial infection, third-degree burns take longer to heal and require very intensive care and treatment [10, 11]. Typical symptoms of third-degree burns include waxy, white color appearance with raised and leathery texture. Moreover, similar to second-degree burns (particularly deep-loss), eschar formation is a typical symptom of third-degree burns [12, 13].

Having all the signs and symptoms of third-degree burns, fourth-degree burns (also known as full-thickness burns) are usually associated with severe damage to underlying tissues, muscles, bones, tendons, and ligaments [14]. Management of BWs presents a great challenge to the healthcare system; however, certain measures undertaken during the wound management can improve the therapeutic outcomes and patient compliance as well as shorten the hospital stay. These include prevention or eradication of microbial infection (local and systemic), timely support to vital organs (i.e., lungs), promotion of healing rate, decrease in scar formation, and minimization of permanent damage to the skin and bone tissues, [5]. The pathophysiologic and symptomatic representation of different types of BWs is presented in Figure 11.1.

Microbial infection is one of the most common complications of burn injuries; it mainly occurs due to immunosuppression. Exogenous and endogenous microbes may colonize into skin tissues (superficially or deeply) or may enter into systemic circulation (sepsis or septicemia) as a result of damaged/compromised skin barriers (stratum corneum) [15]. The risk of local and systemic microbial infections (sepsis and tetanus) is greater in third- and fourth-degree burns compared to the first- and second-degree burns. If remained untreated, microbial infection can involve the nervous system, which can lead to muscle contractions (tetanus). Besides bacterial infections, hypothermia (critically low body temperature) and hypovolemia (low intravascular volume due to a low blood volume) are other possible complications that can be encountered with severe burns. The risks of mortality associated with these complications (i.e., hypovolemia and hypothermia) are relatively high in third- and fourth-degree burns compared to first- and second-degree burns [7].

11.1.3 PATHOPHYSIOLOGY OF BWs

For effective management of burn injuries, it is essential to understand the pathophysiology. Apparently only one organ (i.e., skin) is involved in a burn injury; however, it actually involves various organs/tissues of the body, making it a generalized disorder. Since heat can exert both local (skin) and generalized effects on the body, the pathophysiology of burn can be classified into two responses: local or systemic. Besides causing severe local damage to the skin tissues at different levels (i.e., epidermis, dermis, hypodermis, tendon, ligaments, and bones), heat can induce systemic destruction to various organs and tissues of the body. One generalized response is an increase in permeability of the blood vasculature, which leads to leakage of plasma from the blood vessels into extracellular spaces (usually lasting for 48 hours). This loss of plasma from the blood vasculature depends upon the degree and extent of the burn and may lead to hypovolemic shock; hence, it requires immediate fluid resuscitation (administration of isotonic intravenous (IV) infusion) [16, 17]. Other generalized responses encountered in thermal injuries may include coagulation disorders, thrombosis, ischemia, hypoxia, tissue necrosis and apoptosis, and systemic edema [16, 17].

Generally, upon exposure of the skin to massive heat, a burn radiates outward from the point of initial contact and forms a local response with three zones in all directions [18]. Jackson and colleagues introduced three different zones of burn (i.e., zone of coagulation, zone of stasis and zone of hyperemia). All these zones were classified based on modulation of blood flow and severity of tissue damage [19–21].

The maximum damage occurs when a higher amount of heat is exposed to the zone of coagulation (also known as central part of BWs). Direct exposure of skin tissue to an extensive amount of heat causes denaturation of proteins (at >41°C or 106°F), which undergo complete or partial coagulation and vasculature tissue necrosis. This coagulation causes thrombosis in the vasculature of tissues around the central zone of coagulation (zone of stasis or ischemia), which is characterized by salvageable tissues with reduced blood/oxygen perfusion [22]. The severity of tissue necrosis in the zone of stasis could be prevented by restoring/improving the blood/oxygen perfusion to the burned area. The zone of stasis is also known as zone of ischemia due to its poor blood perfusion, which can lead to ischemia/hypoxia followed by tissue necrosis and apoptosis. Within 48 h post-trauma, tissue necrosis (occurring within the first 24 h) and apoptosis (occurring around 24 to 48 h) can be seen in the zone of ischemic; these are ultimate outcomes of prolonged hypoxia and ischemia [23]. Both of these tissue-destructive mechanisms (necrosis and apoptosis) involve a series of morphologic and biochemical changes in the cells/tissues that could lead to cell death in the ischemic zone [24]. One of the emergency approaches to restore the blood perfusion and to prevent irreversible tissue damage in the burned area is fluid resuscitation and proper wound management [16, 17]. In the periphery of zone of stasis, the zone of hyperemia (increased blood supply) is located. This zone represents the body response in the form of inflammation (protective inflammatory response) to burn injury and is characterized by synthesis and chemotaxis of inflammatory mediators, causing vasodilation resulting in enhanced blood supply (erythema). The zone of hyperemia lasts for at least 24 to 48 h in severe burns post-trauma [25].

Apart from damage to the skin tissues, burn trauma may cause epithelial cells apoptosis and decreased cell proliferation in other organs, which may ultimately lead to reduced functionality of those organs, including the gastrointestinal system (GI), liver, heart, lung, kidney, etc. [26–28]. Cumming and co-workers [28] carried out a human clinical study in which 85 burn victims with more than 20% of TBSA involved were admitted in a center for more than one year. Based on the type and intensity of the burn trauma, multiple organs (i.e., liver, lungs, kidney, and heart) were affected, with noticeable dysfunctioning post-burn trauma. The study findings revealed that organ dysfunction was observed in 28% of burn victims, which was associated with patient age, gender, and TBSA. However, among burn victims with organ dysfunction, 71% survived [29]. To improve the survival rate in burn victims by protecting the functionality of vital organs, Jeschke and co-researchers [27] conducted an in vivo study on rats and demonstrated that an oral administration of hepatocyte growth factor (HGF) can significantly improve mucosal cell proliferation by increasing the mucosal epithelial cells' proliferative mediators such as Bcl-2. Thus, HGF can improve small-bowel homeostasis and morphology after severe burn trauma [27]. Likewise, another vital organ that is highly susceptible to generalized effect of burn injuries is the lung, causing inhalational trauma (IHT) (breathing difficulty), which is among the primary causes of high mortality rate in burn victims. Colohan [3] studied the prognosis factors in burn patients and reported that the mortality rate among burn victims with IHT was 27.6%. They suggested that apart from TBSA and age, the presence of IHT is also a strong predictor of mortality [3]. If left untreated, IHT may lead to severe pneumonia in burn victims, which significantly increase the mortality rate [30]. Respiratory dysfunction (and other organs dysfunction) could be further aggravated if the burn victims acquire systemic microbial infection (sepsis or septicemia) [31].

Other generalized responses (i.e., burn shock) observed in burn victims include increased permeability of vasculature [32]. The increased permeability of vasculature is thought to be due to excessive outbreak of inflammatory mediators (i.e., prostaglandins, cytokines, chemokines, and white blood cells). The increased permeability of vasculature may lead to leakage of plasma fluid and proteins to extravascular tissues (i.e., interstitial space) [33]. Other symptoms of burn shock include reduced cardiac output, enhanced vascular resistance, increased hydrostatic pressure across the microvasculature, and hypovolemia, which further increase the workload on the heart [34]. Furthermore, extravasation of plasma fluid in the interstitial spaces can result in development of local and/or generalized edema, which occurs within the first 8 hours after the burn injury and may continue to worsen for next 18 hours [35]. The development of edema can further delay burn wound healing by limiting the exchange of vital nutrients [36, 37].

An altered immune status is another generalized response of burn injuries. The lowered immune response can aggravate susceptibility to microbial infection, either local or systemic (sepsis or septicemia) [38, 39]. BWs are sterile initially; however, if not taken care properly, BWs may get heavily contaminated with internal or external microbes within few days (72 hours onwards). The microbial contamination may lead to significant delay in BW healing, prolongation of hospitalization, increased healthcare costs, and significantly enhanced mortality rate (particularly in case of septicemia) [7]. Therefore, it is recommended to perform surgical excision in extensive burns within 72 hours; however, surgical excision should be performed after complete resuscitation or stabilization of the patient [40].

11.1.4 BWs Healing Process

To comprehend the healing mechanism of BWs, it is imperative to understand the healing process in normal/acute wounds. The cycle of skin injuries and tissue repair is repeatedly experienced by the body. The wound healing process of acute wounds consists of four distinct stages, where each stage plays an important role in accomplishing the healing process in a timely manner.

The first stage is called "hemostasis," which starts immediately after the body gets injured [41]. In this stage, body activates its emergency repair system, the blood clotting system to stop bleeding via forming a blood clot. Moreover, during this stage, the blood vessels start constricting around the injury/wounds to help stop the bleeding. Once the bleeding stops, the wound healing process enters into the second stage "inflammation stage," which involves cleaning of wounds by removing the debris (to prepare the wound bed for healing) and fighting against microbes to avoid wound infection (which can slow down the healing process) [42]. Further, in order to promote wound healing, the fresh blood brings essential nutrients and oxygen to the injured site and white blood cells (i.e., macrophages) facilitate this process. Macrophages play two important roles at this stage: 1) fight with microbes in the surrounding tissues to avoid infection and 2) secrete growth factors, which attract immune cells to facilitate wound repair [43]. Once the wound bed is clean, the healing process enters into the third stage called "rebuilding or proliferative stage." During the proliferative stage (which lasts for 2 days to 3 weeks), the wound undergoes filling with new tissues made up of collagen and extracellular matrix (ECM), contraction at margins, and neovascularization [44]. Moreover, re-epithelization (arising of epithelial cells from the margins or wound bed) occurs, which results in complete coverage of wound.

Finally, the healing mechanism enters the last stage of wound healing (maturation or the remodeling stage). During this stage (which lasts from 21 days to 2 years), the synthesis of collagen fibers continues to strengthen the newly formed tissues, which also increase tensile strength of the wound site, followed by remodeling of collagen from type III to type I. The aim of this stage is to achieve maximum tensile strength through organization, degradation, and re-synthesis of the ECM and to remodel collagen from type III to type I. Furthermore, apoptosis process takes place during maturation stage. During the apoptosis process, the inflammatory cells and the fibroblasts disappear from the wound area (emigration process) [45–49]. The healing process of acute wounds is presented in Figure 11.2.

The pathophysiology of BWs is different from that of acute wounds, but they share the same wound healing process. The main difference between the wound healing process in different types of wounds is the duration of each wound-healing stage [7]. For burns, the healing duration also depends on the depth of the burns and the intensity of deeper tissue involvement. Generally, the first two stages of wound healing are similar in all traumatic injuries, particularly the inflammatory stage. The proliferative stage in partial thickness burns usually take 5–7 days, in which re-epithelialization begins within a few hours after the burn injury. Similarly, the duration of the remodeling stage, particularly in the third- and fourth-degree burns (full-thickness burns), might extend to years depending upon the degree and extent of burns [50]. The duration of wound healing is further hindered if microbial infection involves fungus (*Candida species*), gram-positive (*S. aureus*), or gram-negative (*P. aeruginosa*) bacteria [31, 51] because microbial contamination is one of the main reasons which delay BW healing due to immunosuppression. Microbial containments

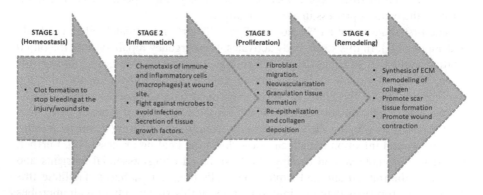

FIGURE 11.2 Healing process of acute wounds.

protect themselves from antimicrobial therapies by forming biofilms in the ECM and delay the wound healing process [31].

11.2 MANAGEMENT OF SKIN BWs

11.2.1 CONVENTIONAL APPROACHES FOR BW MANAGEMENT

The management of BWs largely depends upon severity of burns (i.e., minor, major, and clinical burns). Minor burns are burns involving less than 10% of TBSA in children and less than 15% in adults. Major burns are burns that involve up to 30% TBSA in children and 35% in adults;, if more than 30% TBSA is involved in children and more than 35% in adults, they are called critical burns (also known as life-threatening burns). Both major and critical burns require hospitalization and intensive care due to hypovolemic shock. Furthermore, long-term rehabilitation and recovery are required in patients with major or critical burns to reduce the mortality rate and to impede development of secondary morbidities.

As with other types of wounds, skin damage is the main symptom of BWs; however, due to their systemic responses such as hypothermia, hypovolemia, compromised immunity, microbial infection, blistering, and scarring, the management of burn injuries requires a separate medical superspeciality [52]. Scarring and blistering disposed causing local (beneath or at the surface of the skin) or systemic microbial infection; hence, special treatment protocols such as burn wound excision and skin grafting are the main focused following the fluid resuscitation of the patients. Further, it has been observed that conventional wound healing agents such as topical antimicrobial agents (i.e., povidone iodine and neomycin) remain ineffective on BWs as they fail to penetrate into the eschar to control sub-eschar bacterial invasion in deep burns. Thus, for managing the BWs, it is essential to use antibiotics that have greater ability to penetrate into eschars to kill the habituating and proliferating microorganisms [52]. Furthermore, owing to severe tissue damage encountered in the burn injuries, a larger amount of antimicrobial agent(s) is usually required to manage the extensive BWs; thus, it is essential to use antibiotics that are non-toxic and have minimal side effects because the applied antimicrobial agents can absorb into the general circulation. In addition, the antimicrobial agents employed to manage the burn injuries should face minimal resistance from growing microbes [7]. Among various conventionally available anti-microbial formulations, 1% silver sulfadiazine is considered a mainstay topical therapy for the management of major and clinical burns.

Besides topical antimicrobial therapy, a systemic antibiotics regimen also plays a crucial role in alleviating systemic microbial infection. It has been estimated that more than 60% of burn patients receive local or systemic anti-microbial therapies for a prolonged duration [53, 54]. The systemic administration of anti-microbial agents is beneficial to prophylactically minimize potential systemic infection; however, it has also been associated with development of bacterial resistance [55, 56]. Moreover, the limitation of systemically administered antimicrobial agents in reaching the sub-eschar level (habitat of microbes) also reduces its clinical significance. Due to these limitations associated with systemic antibiotic regimen, local antimicrobial treatments are largely replacing systemic therapies and have become the first choice for management of burn injuries [57, 58]. Other benefits of local antimicrobial therapies include low cost; need for low doses of antimicrobial agents, which can avoid/minimize systemic toxicity; diversity of novel antimicrobial agents for which systemic formulations are not available; better care of wounds due to direct application of drugs to burned areas; self-administration of medication; and reduction of need for institutional care [59]. Therefore, topical antimicrobial agents, including silver sulfadiazine, topical antibiotics, povidone-iodine, mafenide acetate, and chlorhexidine, are being widely employed as conventional topical treatments for the management of infected BWs [60]. Topical agents offer tremendous benefits, but therapeutic outcomes obtained with these therapies is still suboptimal [61, 62].

To optimize the therapeutic outcomes of the topical anti-infective agents, several innovative delivery devices have been designed to maximize permeation and retention of antimicrobial agents into various skin layers to effectively manage burn injuries with greater improvement in tissue regeneration, wound healing rate, and antimicrobial efficacy [55, 58, 63]. These management strategies include biological antimicrobial macromolecules (i.e., polypeptides like defensins, nitric oxide generators, and therapeutic microbes such as probiotics and bacteriophages) [4]. Moreover, excellent outcomes with improved healing rate have also been reported with other state-of-the-art strategies such as light therapies (i.e., visible light— blue or green— NIR, combination of light with photosensitizing dyes and ultraviolet light), stem cells, and other types of cell therapy [63].

11.2.2 MANAGEMENT OF PATHOPHYSIOLOGICAL COMPLICATIONS ENCOUNTERED IN BURN INJURIES

Unlike with acute injuries, hypovolemic shock associated with plasma loss due to leaky vasculature (increased permeability of capillaries) is one of the most common pathophysiologic complications encountered in burn victims [7]. Hence, burn patients require blood/plasma transfusion, which usually should begin after 48 hours. On the other hand, accumulation of plasma fluid in the interstitial spaces may develop systemic edema, which can delay wound healing and may even develop lung edema (which significantly enhances the mortality rate in burn victims) and thus requires immediate management. Excessive local wound inflammation can further stimulate systemic inflammation, which can further cause activation of an inflammatory cascade in distant organs, including the lungs. Edgar and co-researchers [33] conducted a study and reported that administration of vitamin C as a continuous infusion in patients with major burn significantly decreased local and lung edema and hence reduce the mortality rate. Moreover, electrical stimulation with usual physiotherapy following a burn injury can also reduce local edema and increase the functionality of organs [33]. Since edema promotes requirement of fluid therapy in combating the hypovolemia, fluid resuscitation is usually conducted by using the isotonic sodium chloride fluids (normal saline) or lactated Ringer's solution.

Another pathologic complication associated with burn injury is eschar formation (also known as black wound formation), which requires surgical removal (escharectomy) to prevent infection in the immunocompromised burn patient. Complications associated with eschar formation depend on the regions of its development. For example, eschar formation on the lower extremities may reduce blood supply proximally; however, eschar development at the chest area may compromise breathing. Hence, the escharotomy (surgical removal of eschar) is recommended in certain situations to avert such co-morbidities.

Coagulation and tissue necrosis at the burned area is another critical systemic complication that contributes to enhancing the mortality rate in burn victims. An excessive burn can cause extensive coagulation and tissue necrosis with completely thrombosed blood vessels as a result of degradation and denaturation of constituent proteins (as proteins denature above 41°C or 106°F) caused by direct exposure to excessive amount of heat or thermal energy at the trauma site. The coagulation and thrombosis of vasculature results in significant reduction or sluggishness of tissue perfusion (ischemic insult) [63], leading to hypoxia followed by tissue necrosis [64–67]. Within 48 h post trauma, tissue necrosis (occurring within first 24 h) and apoptosis (occurring around 24 to 48 h) can be seen in the burn tissues of the patients [22]. To combat these systemic complications, fluid resuscitation is one of the immediate approaches to restore tissue perfusion and prevent any form of irreversible damage [23, 63]. Furthermore, to combat hypo-perfusion, which is associated with blockage of vasculature due to thrombosis and hyper-coagulation, a variety of drugs such as anticoagulants, antioxidants, and anti-thrombotic and anti-inflammatory agents have shown satisfactory results; however, none of these drugs has earned clinical recognition. A study was performed using one of the safe and well tolerated physiologic anticoagulants such as activated protein C (APC), which was administered at a dose of 100 µg/kg to the experimental rat burn model. APC was approved by the Food and Drug Administration (FDA) for management of severe sepsis in burn victims. Results showed a significant improvement, which was attributed to the anticoagulant and anti-inflammatory effect of APC. The clinical significance of APC in managing systemic complications in burn patients has also been validated by Nisanci et al. [63]. They demonstrated that APC decreases the area of necrosis by improving the perfusion in the ischemic zone due to exhibiting the dual effect such as anti-inflammatory (via downregulating the pro-inflammatory cytokines such as IL-6, IL-8, IL-1β and TNF-Alpha from cells as well as leucocytes activation) and anti-thrombotic (via inhibition of activated factor V and VIII) [63].

11.3 NANOTHERAPEUTICS FOR MANAGEMENT OF BWs AND ASSOCIATED COMPLICATIONS

Owing to its complex pathophysiology and associated local and generalized complications, the management of BWs is far more challenging than that of the acute wounds [68]. The systemic administration of antimicrobial agents showed good efficacy; however, the prolonged systemic use of antibiotics may result in increased risks of developing bacterial resistance [56]. Thus, local antibiotic therapy has remained the most favorable approach because it overcomes risks associated with bacterial resistance encountered with systemic antibiotic therapy [57]. Local application of drugs has shown better tolerance compared to systemically administered antimicrobial agents; however, the local application of therapeutic agents also faces substantial challenges, such as low or sub-optimal penetration to deeper skin tissues particularly in case of third- or fourth-degree burns where tissue destruction occurs in hypodermis and underlying tissues (i.e., tendon, bones, ligaments, etc.). Hence, to augment the local delivery of drugs to deeper tissues and to eradicate the risks of systemic microbial infection, various newer therapeutic modalities have been adapted [57]. These therapeutic options include stem cell therapy, antimicrobial agents, light or ultrasound therapy (such as phototherapy, shockwave, or ultrasound), biological therapies (i.e., antimicrobial peptides, interferons, reactive oxygen species (ROS), NO generators, and microbiome therapy) as well as various types of nanomaterials [4]. Surgical excision, wound dressing, skin grafting, (i.e., autograft, allograft, etc.), negative pressure therapy, tissue engineering, and various other biomedical methods are being employed as alternative therapeutic options for the management of BWs with or without associated microbial infections [24, 69, 70].

Among the various newer therapeutic approaches available to manage skin BWs, nanotechnology-based wound healing approaches have shown exceptional efficacy in enhancing the burn wound healing rate as well as precluding various obstacles (i.e., sepsis, delayed wound healing, sub-optimal penetration to deeper tissues, etc.) that are encountered with conventional burn wound healing modalities [4, 71]. The versatility of nanomedicines has been significantly established due to their physiochemical properties and efficiency to deliver a wide range of therapeutic and diagnostic moieties (i.e., growth factors, gene therapy, cell therapies, antibiotics, and numerous other therapeutic moieties) for superior BW healing and skin regeneration [72–76].

The biomedical viability of nanotherapeutics is attributed to their physicochemical and biopharmaceutical properties, including 1) ultra-small size (ranging from 10–100 nm) [77, 78], 2) high encapsulation efficiency [79, 80], 3) ability to create moist environment at wound site, which promotes wound healing, 4) better transmembrane permeability and penetrability to deeper tissues, 5) protection of labile drugs from biodegradation by proteases in wound microenvironment [81], 6) sustained/controlled release of encapsulated drugs in the necrotic area via bio-responsive features [82], 7) reduced frequency of administration due to prolonged localization and maintenance of effective drug concentration into the local skin tissues [77] 8) targeted delivery of drugs to target organs/tissues [83], 9) improved pharmacokinetic profile [84], and 10) reduced cost of health and improved patient compliance.

Nanomaterials used to manage burn injuries can be classified into two major categories: 1) organic (i.e., polymeric nanoparticles, micelles, nanoemulsion, liposomes, ethosomes, nanogels, and solid-lipid NPs) and 2) inorganic nanoparticles (NPs) (i.e., metal nanoparticles, carbon nanotubes, magnetic NPs, and quantum dots) [85]. These two classes of nanomaterials display distinct properties and exhibit promising efficacy in BW healing [71, 76, 86, 87]. A pictorial image of different types of nanomaterials that have been employed for management of BWs is presented in Figure 11.3, and these are critically discussed in the following sections.

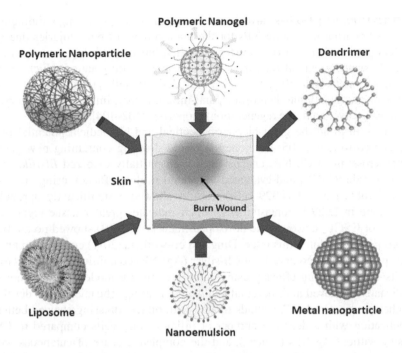

FIGURE 11.3 A pictorial image of organic and inorganic NPs that have been employed for the management of BWs.

11.3.1 ORGANIC NPs

11.3.1.1 Polymeric NPs

Polymeric NPs have extensively been employed in different applications owing to their remarkable features, including the colloidal-range size (1–500 nm) [86], biodegradability, biocompatibility, controlled release [88], high encapsulation efficiency, prevention of premature degradation of labile drugs via encapsulation into polymeric matrix, efficient permeability across biological barriers [89–91], and flexibility of functionalization of surfaces with targeting moieties for active targeting to specific tissues/cells [82, 92]. The characteristic features of polymeric NPs depend on the nature/type of the polymer (i.e., natural or synthetic and biodegradable or non-biodegradable) used for engineering of the polymeric NPs [93, 94]. The use of natural polymers (i.e., chitosan (CS), poly(lactic-co-glycolic acid) (PLGA), polyethylene glycol (PEG), and hyaluronic acid (HA)) is more prevalent due to their abundance in nature, biodegradability, and biocompatibility; however, certain risks (i.e., immunogenicity and batch variability) associated with their use limit their pharmaceutical viability [95].

Owing to their remarkable features [96, 97], a variety of polymeric nanomedicines (i.e., polymeric NPs, dendrimers, hydrogel NPs) have been synthesized and screened for treatment of BWs [93]. Among various naturally originating polymers used for design of polymeric NPs, chitosan (CS) has been one of the most tunable polymers [98, 99]. CS has been expansively investigated for application in various fields, including the food industry, pharmaceuticals, cosmetic, and agricultural industries [100, 101]. CS has earned great recognition as a promising building material for fabricating polymeric NPs for the management of burn injuries due to its excellent physicochemical (i.e., biodegradability, biocompatibility, low immunogenicity), biopharmaceutical (i.e., mucoadhesive and in situ gelation which promote transmembrane permeability, controlled drug delivery ability), and biomedical (i.e., antimicrobial, antioxidant, hemostatic, anti-inflammatory, immunomodulatory, low immunogenicity, and tissue regeneration) properties [102–104].

Keeping in mind the great biopharmaceutical and biomedical potential of CS, Ding and co-workers [105] developed a wound dressing containing new genipin-assisted crosslinked CS-NPs encapsulated with partially oxidized *Bletilla striata* polysaccharide (CSGB) and evaluated its wound healing efficacy using an in vitro mouse fibroblast model (L929 cells). Results showed a significantly upregulated proliferation in L929 fibroblasts cells, which indicates greater tissue regeneration potential of CSGB; however, the developed material (CSGB) showed no antibacterial action. To overcome this issue, Ding and co-workers (2017) constructed another novel spongy bilayer composite of CS-silver (Ag) NPs containing CSGB and evaluated its wound healing efficacy using an in vivo mouse model. Results showed a significantly improved antimicrobial and wound healing efficacies of the developed nanotherapeutic. On day 7, wounds treated with bilayer dressing showed better re-epithelization with a decrease number of inflammatory cells compared to CSGB dressing without Ag-NPs (control), and the complete closure of cutaneous wound was observed on day 14 of treatment (Figure 11.4) [105]. It was concluded that a combination of CS with Ag in the form of polymeric NPs can significantly improve tissue regeneration efficacy of CSGB [105].

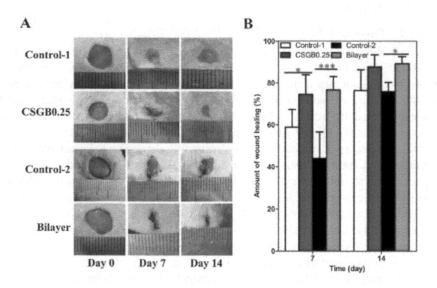

FIGURE 11.4 Time-mannered (0–14th days) wound closure of full-thickness wounds treated with bilayer composites of CS-Ag NPs containing CSGB compared to controls and CSGB0.25 groups; photomicrographs (A) and quantitative analysis of wound closure data) [105]. Permission to reprint has been granted by Elsevier Ltd. (Copyright © 2017).

Similarly, El-Feky and co-workers [106] developed CS-Ag NPs for delivery of sulfadiazine (SSD) as a promising wound dressing for management of BWs. The resulting data revealed that the fabricated NPs released SSD at the burned areas in a controlled manner. The developed polymeric NPs showed greater potential in suppressing the proliferation and differentiation of gram+ve, gram-ve and *C. albicans* in the infected BWs [106]. To further establish the capability of polymeric NPs in promoting the wound healing in BWs, Blažević and co-investigators [107] designed CS/lecithin NPs for the delivery of melatonin. Melatonin has been extensively used for tissue regeneration due to its good anti-inflammatory, scar forming via maturation and orientation of collagen fibers, and antioxidant efficacy. The fabricated melatonin-impregnated CS/lecithin NPs were evaluated for tissue regeneration ability in vitro, using human keratinocyte (HaCaT cells). The developed NPs exhibit good biocompatibility, biphasic release of melatonin, and improved wound healing rate. Interpretation of the resulting data predicted that the higher wound healing rate observed in the experimental group treated with melatonin impregnated CS/lecithin NPs was due to enhanced re-epithelialization by promoting the migration, proliferation, and differentiation of keratinocytes in the wound microenvironment. Researchers also reported that the wound healing efficacy of CS is intendent of its molecular weight [107].

Another feature of CS NPs in promoting the wound healing are their hemostatic ability, which facilitate wound healing and tissue regeneration by enhancing the mechanical strength of newly formed tissues at wound site [108]. Furthermore, CS-NPs promote healing of various types of wounds including the BWs by enabling the immune cells (inflammatory cells) to promote migration of fibroblasts at the wound area [4, 29, 108]. Excellent antimicrobial efficacy of CS-NPs against a wide variety of microbes (which can delay wound healing) also contributes to its exceptional wound healing efficacy [108]. CS-NPs display their antimicrobial efficacy by modifying the permeability of microbial cells that cause leakage of bacterial cell contents and eventual death [109–111]. The interference of CS-NPs (cationic) with the cell wall (anionic) of microbes for permeabilization is attributed to a strong ionic interaction between them. Other mechanisms that contribute to antimicrobial efficacy of CS-NPs include 1) chelation with essential metals and nutrients which are key components of bacterial growth, 2) mRNA expression and protein synthesis inhibition, and 3) alleviation of oxygenation and respiration of bacterial cells (particularly aerobic bacteria) due to shielding of bacterial cell with polymer membrane.

Bacterial infection (local and systemic) is one of the major challenges in the management of BWs, which is principally due to the suppressed immune status of a burned patient. Therefore, the wound healing potential of polymeric NPs for highly infected (with *P. aeruginosa and P. mirabilis*) full-thickness excisional wounds [112] and third-degree BWs [113] has been investigated. Results of these studies revealed that CS not only promoted wound healing but also remained adhered to the burned area for up to 21 days and killed all the microbes and saved the animals from developing fatal systemic infections (septicemia). For wounds infected with both of the pathogenic bacterial species, the survival rate of mice exposed to CS-based bandages was significantly increased (73.3% and 66.7%, respectively) compared to nanocrystalline Ag dressing (27.3% and 62.5%) and untreated mice (13.3% and 23.1%) [112,

113]. Similar results were also evidenced by Yagci et al. [114] that CS-based wound dressings eradicate microbial growth more efficiently (faster) compared to clinically approved nanocrystalline bandages. Similarly, Burkatovskaya et al. [115] reported that CS-based wound dressings applied to heavily infected BWs resulted in a promising control over the growth of microbes and prevented the systemic infection [115]. Similar results have also been validated in other animal models (i.e., rat, mice, swine, etc.) [116, 117].

The possible mechanisms by which CS-based wound dressings enhance wound healing include a decreased inflammatory outbreak, enhanced collagen expression and deposition, ECM formation, formation of granulation tissue, and antimicrobial potential [113, 117]. Moreover, an increased re-epithelialization along with improved tensile strength of wounds and accelerated dermoepidermal junction formation have also been evident in different types of wounds treated with CS-based dressings [118].

To further reduce the number of fatalities associated with BWs (particularly third- and fourth-degree burns), CS-based hybrid nanodelivery systems have also been developed by some researchers [119]. They developed CS-based composites impregnated with Ag NPs and evaluated the wound healing efficacy against infected BWs. Results showed that Ag NPs-impregnated CS composites showed excellent antimicrobial efficacy against both gram-positive (methicillin resistant *S. aureus*, MRSA) and gram-negative (*P. aeruginosa, A. baumannii, and P. mirabilis*) microbes compared to the control groups treated with CS dressing alone [119]. The antimicrobial efficacy of developed hybrid Ag NPs-impregnated CS composites was also validated in another in vivo burn wound model infected with *P. aeruginosa,* and results showed a promising control of the hybrid NPs over septicemia (by estimating the number of microbes in the blood specimen) compared to the CS dressing and CS NPs.

The proposed mechanism by which CS-based hybrid Ag NPs impregnated composites exhibited antimicrobial efficacy was disruption of cell membrane via electrostatic interaction between the cationic functional group ($-NH_3^+$) groups on the backbone of CS and anionic phospholipid components of bacterial cell membranes [120]. Likewise, Vimala and co-workers [121] developed a hybrid nanosystem composed of porous CS film impregnated with Ag NPs (nanocomposite) and examined its antibacterial activities. The resulting data showed superior antimicrobial efficacy with chitosan-silver nanocomposite (CSSNC) films [121]. Similar resulting trends were reported by other researchers in which Ag NPs-impregnated CS microporous films exhibited excellent antimicrobial efficacy against *Bacillus* and *E. coli* [122].

Natural bioactive compounds have shown greater efficacy in various skin diseases with minimal side effects [123, 124]. Curcumin (CUR), a natural biomolecule sourced from roots of *Curcuma longa,* has been widely applied due to its wide range of biomedical efficacy, including anti-inflammatory, antioxidant, antimicrobial [125], bone regeneration [126], anti-proliferative, immunomodulatory, and anticancer efficacy [127]. Being a multifunctional compound, it had been previously reported as having excellent wound healing efficacy of CUR by another research group [92, 128]. Although, CUR has been exploited in several biomedical applications, its applicability is inadequate owing to its low aqueous solubility and erratic oral bioavailability. Moreover, the phenolic functional groups present in the chemical structure of CUR make it highly liable to photo-degradation and may provoke serious adverse effects after a prolong dermal exposure. Therefore, various attempts have been made to miti-gate the aforementioned challenges associated with CUR and to improve its biomedi-cal properties. Mirnejad et al. [129] fabricated CS-based polymeric NPs using an ionic gelation method and evaluated their bactericidal activity against *S. aureus* and *P. aeru-ginosa*. The CUR-loaded CS NPs showed a momentous decline in the growth of both microbes [129]. Other studies have also reported that encapsulation of CUR into the polymeric NPs not only improved its anti-inflammatory and antibacterial effects but also facilitated its internalization into damaged body tissues for repairmen [130, 131].

Similarly, poly(lactic-co-glycolic acid) (PLGA) which is also a natural polymer has gained remarkable recognition for being used as a building material for BW dressings due to its exceptional physicochemical and pharmaceutical properties. Keeping in mind its intrinsic features, Chereddy et al. [132] developed a PLGA-based nanodelivery system impregnated with LL-37 (endogenous human catheli-cidin host defense peptide that regulates angiogenesis and exhibits antimicrobial efficacy). The application of PLGA-LL37 NPs in an in vivo full-thickness excisional wound model showed remarkable wound healing efficacy, which was evidenced by improved collagen deposition, formation of granulation tissues, neo-vascularization, re-epithelization, and excellent antimicrobial efficiency (Figure 11.5). Greater wound healing efficacy of PLGA-LL37 NPs was attributed to synergistic tissue regenerating and antimicrobial effects of LL37, lactate, and PLGA [132].

11.3.1.2 Nanoemulsions (NEs)

Nanoemulsions (NEs) are highly stable colloidal-size emulsions that constitute a kinetically stabilized heterogeneous system containing two non-miscible liquids (i.e., oil droplets dispersed in an aqueous phase and aqueous droplets dispersed in an oil phase) stabilized using suitable emulsifying agent(s) [133]. The emulsifying agent (surfactant) plays a key role in stabilizing this heterogeneous system by lowering the interfacial tension between the two immiscible phases via forming an interfacial film at the oil/water interface [134]. One of the key features of NEs is their nanoscale size ranges between 20 and 400 nm (must be below 500 nm) [135]. Due to hav-ing greater surface area, NEs provide greater absorption and higher bioavailability. Moreover, being a heterogeneous (dispersion of oil/water) system, NEs can be used for the delivery of hydrophobic, hydrophilic, or both types of therapeutic agents. Furthermore, due to their improved functional properties, NEs possess superior fea-tures over the conventional emulsions such as non-toxicity, non-irritancy, flexibility of compounding in the form of different types of pharmaceutical dosage forms (i.e., sprays, foams, creams, and liquids), and improved thermodynamic stability [134, 136]. NEs have been broadly used as efficient carriers for different types of therapeu-tic and diagnostic agents through different routes of administration (i.e., parenteral and non-parenteral, transdermal, topical, ophthalmic, etc.) [134, 135].

Owing to their remarkable physicochemical, biopharmaceutical, and biomedical features, NEs have been used as nanotherapeutics for management of various dis-eases including BWs. NEs have been extensively employed to carry different types of therapeutic agents, such as antimicrobial agents (to reduce microbial bioburden), anti-inflammatory agents (to reduce inflammation at the wound site), and tissue-regenerating moieties to enhance wound healing and regeneration potential [136]. To

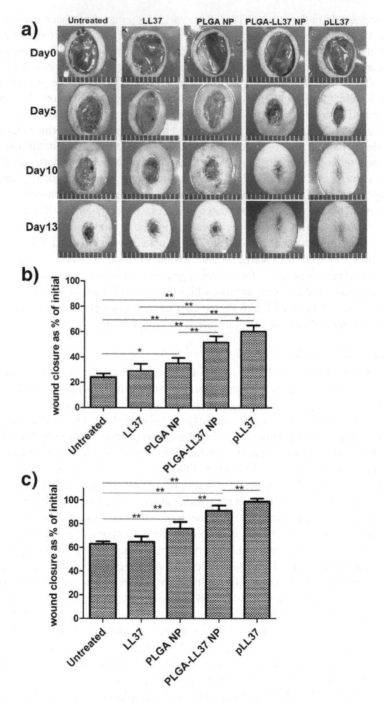

FIGURE 11.5 Wound healing proficiency of PLGA-LL37 NPs; a) photomicrographs of wounds treated with PLGA-LL37 NPs compared to other treatment and control groups, b) wound closure rate at day 5, and c) wound closure rate at day 10 [132]. Permission to reprint has been granted by Elsevier B.V. (Copyright © 2014).

validate the antimicrobial, anti-inflammatory and wound healing potential of NEs, Dolgachev et al. [137] developed an NE formulation for efficient management of BWs and alleviation of advancement BWs from partial-thickness to full-thickness. They evaluated the wound healing potential of NEs against partial-thickness BWs infected with *S. aureus* and *P. aeruginosa* in male Sprague Dawley rats. The results showed excellent wound healing efficacy along with a decreased microbial biobur-den, inflammatory cascades, and improved tissue rejuvenation (re-epithelization and formation of granulation tissues) in experimental animals treated with NEs [137].

Similarly, Song and co-researchers [138] investigated anti-biofilm activity of novel NEs encapsulated with chlorhexidine acetate (CANE) against skin BWs infected with MRSA. MRSA is a global health threat for patients with burn trauma because it significantly prolongs hospitalization. Notably, colonization with MRSA is reported to have increased risks of severe local and systemic co-morbidities [139] and hence has become one of the major causative factors for morbidities and mortalities, espe-cially in older people [140]. Moreover, an extracellular adherence protein secreted by MRSA may significantly contribute to impairing the wound healing process by inhibiting the migration, proliferation, and differentiation of keratinocytes due to its ability to alter the morphology and adhesion properties of keratinocytes [141, 142]. Results obtained from their study revealed that CANE formulations exhibited better and faster action against MRSA-infected BWs. They further demonstrated the mech-anism of antibacterial efficacy of CANE and suggested that CANE tends to disrupt the cell walls and cell membranes of MRSA, leading to increased electrical conduc-tivity and seepage of cell contents, DNA, and cell proteins, resulting in the death of MRSA. Moreover, the formulations exerted an efficient anti-biofilm activity by inhibition of new biofilm formation and clearance of pre-developed biofilms [138].

Thakur et al. [143] also validated the clinical significance of NEs in eradiating MRSA infections from BWs. They developed a cationic-charged bilayer NE loaded with fusidic acid (a potent antibacterial agent) used to treat gram+ve infections and evaluated its wound healing efficacy against MRSA infected BWs [143]. The developed NEs were characterized for physicochemical characteristics and evaluated in vitro using human keratinocyte cells (HaCat cells) and in vivo using full-thickness murine second-degree burn infected with MRSA 33591. The resulting data revealed that the NE formula-tion facilitated the permeation of loaded drug into the burned tissues, reduced bacte-rial bioburden onto burned tissues, upregulated the wound contraction, and enhanced re-epithelialization in BWs. Re-epithelialization plays an essential role in restoring the major barrier function of the skin for body protection against the invading pathogens. In burn injuries the barrier function of the skin is severely damaged, and hence microbes can invade the body. In an attempt to counter the invading pathogens, the immune system strongly reacts via excessive production of cytokines [143]. The excessive production of cytokines (known as a cytokine storm) can result in over-inflammation, further leads to organ failure and ultimately high rate of mortality. The risks of cytokine storm (over-inflammation) can be reduced by stimulating the wound healing process, particularly the re-epithelialization in order to close the wound as well as to restore the barrier function of the skin. Furthermore, the fusidic-acid–loaded NEs showed sustained release of the loaded drug for a longer time, which resulted in reduced frequency of administration, diminished scar formation, and enhanced angiogenesis and collagen formation [143].

Simultaneous delivery of multiple therapeutics usually shows better therapeutic outcomes compared to a single therapeutic [144]. Keeping mind the therapeutic advantages of combined therapy, Bonferoni et al. [145] fabricated CS-oleate based NEs for the co-delivery of Ag sulfadiazine and α-tocopherol (aTph) for skin wounds treatment. A significant increase in the differentiation and proliferation of keratinocytes and fibroblasts has been observed. Moreover, the in vivo data demonstrated an excellent wound healing efficacy of aTph/Ag sulfadiazine co-loaded NEs by promoting the tissue regeneration, fibroblast recruitment, and granulation tissue formation [145].

11.3.1.3 Nanogels

Nanogels are 3-dimensional crosslinked, swellable hydrogels having the size in the nanoscale range (10–200 nm). They are formed as a result of physical or chemical crosslinking of natural and/or synthetic polymers. They have numerous characteristic features, such as capacity to uptake a larger amount of fluid (even 100 times more than their weight), ideal hydration environment on wound bed without dissolving in the aqueous medium, preservation of gaseous permeability, controlled-release characteristics, and tissue-regenerative effects [146–148]. The water-holding capacity of nanogels makes them an ideal nanodelivery system for wound healing because it helps in maintaining the moist environment at the wound bed (which is highly favorable for tissue regeneration) as well as absorbing wound exudate, which assists in removal of enzymatic and tissue debris (for facilitating the tissue regeneration) [148–150]. Other advantages of nanogels include high encapsulation efficiency, protection of entrapped drugs from enzymatic degradation, hydrophilicity (made up of hydrophilic polymers), biocompatibility, non-immunogenicity, and non-toxicity [146, 151]. Owing to their great water-holding capacity and maintenance of moist environment at BW bed, nanogels exhibit promising wound healing efficacy [146].

BWs present a great challenge to the healthcare system; however, many studies have demonstrated the efficacy nanogels as promising wound healing nanotherapeutics [147, 151]. Loo et al. [152] developed novel ultrashort aliphatic peptides-enriched hydrogel nanofibers to meet all criteria of ideal wound healing for the treatment of second-degree BWs. The inclusion of smart peptides (which stimulate tissue regeneration) into the nanogels (having non-toxic and non-immunogenic nature) make this novel hydrogel scaffold biomimetic. Furthermore, these biomimetic nanogels were able to hold up to a maximum (i.e., 99.9%) amount of water and biological fluid (wound exudate). The peptide-based nanogels were targeted for management of second- and third-degree BWs, which usually take a prolonged period (2 to 10 weeks) to heal and leave residual amounts of viable cells for regeneration due to higher destruction of the top (epidermis) and underlying (dermis) skin layers [152]. The nanofibrous networks acted as barriers against infection and abrasion. The in vivo data showed that the nanofibrous hydrogels enhanced wound closure in partial thickness BWs in rat models. Within 14 days of the treatment, the developed hydrogels demonstrated earlier onset with completion of autolytic debridement (achieved by day 12), facilitated epithelial and dermal regeneration, and achieved highest wound closure (i.e., 92.9%) compared to a marketed product (i.e., Mepitel®, a flexible silicone-coated polyamide dressing), which showed a

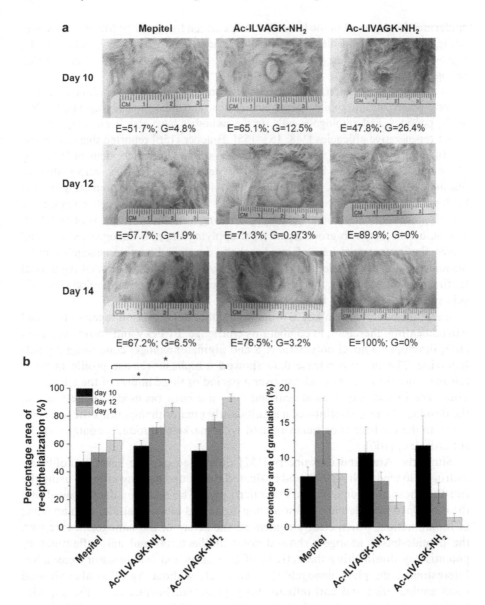

FIGURE 11.6 Wound healing efficacy of ultrashort peptide incorporated nanogels; a) photomicrographs of BWs treated with different treatments at different points and b) percentage of re-epithelization and granulation tissue formation [152]. Permission to reprint has been granted by Elsevier B.V. (Copyright © 2014).

wound closure rate of only 62.8% (Figure 11.6). Furthermore, a digital planimetry was used to measure the area of granulation, and the result indicated that wounds exposed to peptide hydrogels showed higher extent of granulation, which began to decline as the wound re-epithelialized. The histological analysis depicted significant alterations (such as disorganized ECM along with the loss of hair follicles and epidermal detachment) in the burned skin specimen treated with Mepitel-dressing, while complete wound closure with substantial signs of recovery including the regrowth of hair follicles was observed in BWs treated with peptide-incorporated nanogels [152].

Likewise, the inclusion of other bioactive moieties, such as cytokines, growth factors, potent antimicrobial agents, analgesics, anti-inflammatory agents, nucleic acids, peptides, and autologous cells, in the nanogels have also been suggested for better regenerative efficacies [148, 153–155]. Butcher [156] reported that one of the key functions of nanogels, when applied on BWs, is autolytic debridement (cleaning of wounds by removal of hyperkeratotic, viable/non-viable tissues, germs, dirt, or residual stuff of dressing), which plays a very important role in promoting wound healing. The researchers have also highlighted that the new nanogels enhance the overall process of burn wound healing by creating a structural framework on which new skin cells begin to grow. Apart from applying the new nanogels as a wound healer, the investigators have claimed that the developed peptide nanogels can be manufactured in dry powder form that could be activated with water, making it ideal for first aid kits. Moreover, the formulated nanogels can be used to develop synthetic skin substitutes for deeper burns [156].

Bacterial infection is a key BW hallmark that delays tissue regeneration and wound healing; therefore, to combat this challenge, El-Feky and co-investigators [106] developed a novel polymeric (CS and alginate) nanogel containing Ag sulfadiazine. The in vitro release data showed a biphasic release profile (a burst release followed by a slow release over a period of three hours) of the entrapped drug. The in vivo experiments carried out on a burn rat model suggested that the developed nanogel exhibited a significantly greater therapeutic efficacy compared to the controls (i.e., burns treated with marketed products containing Ag sulfadiazine) [106].

Similarly, Arab and co-workers [157] developed peptide-based nanofibrous hydrogels loaded with Ag NPs and evaluated the wound healing efficacy using the full-thickness excisional wounds on micro pigs. The resulting data showed that the developed peptide nanogels were non-toxic and biocompatible, with no signs of inflammation, which clearly evidenced the safety of the nanogels. Moreover, the peptide-based nanogels showed good antibacterial and anti-inflammatory potential by diminishing the activity of proteases and inflammatory cascades. Interestingly, the plain nanogels (i.e., nanogels without Ag NPs) also showed good antibacterial and anti-inflammatory potential. Furthermore, the peptide-loaded nanogels showed excellent wound healing efficacy against full-thickness excisional wounds [157].

Another novel hybrid nanogel system was recently developed by Soriano and co-workers [158]. This nanogel system was composed of poloxamer 407, CS, and hyaluronic acid (HA) for the delivery of melatonin. HA has been widely used as a biological macromolecule for improving therapeutic outcomes against various diseases due to its wide spectrum of biomedical activities, such as wound healing [159], tissue regeneration [160], dermal penetration [161, 162], inflammatory skin and joint diseases [163], and targeted delivery of therapeutic payloads [81, 126]. The aim of this nanogel system was to bring all the pharmaceutical and biomedical advantages of CS, HA, and hydrogel together for the stimulation of burn wound injuries [158]. The resultant nanogels were tested for various physicochemical properties, in vitro release profile, biocompatibility with human keratinocytes, in vitro antibacterial efficiency against different microbes as well as wound healing efficacy using the rat model. The resulting data showed that the developed formulation showed optimal physicochemical properties along with the release of melatonin following the first order kinetics. Compared to the commercial reference materials, the antimicrobial and wound healing efficacies of melatonin loaded nanogels were significantly high, which was evidence in terms of eradication of microbes from the culture as well as efficient re-epithelization and granulation tissue formation [158].

11.3.1.4 Liposomes

Liposomes are spherical-shaped vesicles having at least one lipid bilayer. Among various nanocarriers employed for topical drug delivery, liposomes have shown great potential due to their structural resemblance to biological membranes [164]. Liposomal nanoformulations engineered with natural polymers have been extensively investigated for biomedical implications (i.e., cancer, skin diseases, burns injuries, etc.) due to various intrinsic features such as high encapsulation efficiency, greater permeation efficiency across biological membranes, biodegradability, protection of encapsulated payload, biocompatibility, sustained release characteristics, flexibility of functionalization for active drug delivery [165] and targeted delivery [166, 167]. Being an important component of body tissue as well as ability to release the encapsulated drugs in a controlled manner, a novel collagen-based liposomal formulation has been recently proposed by Cheng et al. [168]. Moreover, the implication of liposome as a drug-carrier has shown remarkable efficiency in achieving the targeted delivery of drugs to specific tissues, such as various skin layers, as well as in lowering the systemic toxicity of various drugs in comparison with traditional dosage forms [169, 170].

One of the key reasons for therapeutic recognition of liposomes for the treatment of skin diseases, particularly BWs, is that these spherical-shaped vesicles not only cover the wound area efficiently but also create an ideal microenvironment (moist) at the wound area, which significantly promotes wound healing and tissue regeneration [171]. Thus, various research studies have concentrated on the applications of liposomes as one of the promising drug delivery vehicles for different types of agents. Madecassoside (MA) is a highly potent drug for managing different types of skin diseases, including burn traumas, owing to its proficiency to stimulate cell proliferation and differentiation, accelerate wound healing, and exert various pharmacological effects such as antibacterial, antioxidant, and anti-inflammatory [172]. However, being a polar molecule with a large molecular weight, MA faces substantial hurdles for its permeation (absorption) across the stratum corneum (a major barrier for topical absorption of drugs). Due to its poor membrane permeability, the topical wound healing effect of such a drug is hampered [173]. In order to overcome this issue, MA was encapsulated into liposomes via a double emulsion method [174] and was tested for its ability to permeate across the stratum corneum, retention into skin layers, and wound healing efficacy. The results showed a significant improvement in permeation of MA across the stratum corneum when administered in the form of liposomes and good wound healing efficacy. These results validate that the liposomal delivery system is a promising nanosystem for topical delivery of MA for better wound healing and tissue regeneration efficacy [174].

Growth factors (GFs) are polypeptide macromolecules that are present throughout our body in a miniscule quantity; yet they play very important and powerful roles in maintaining the hemostasis by modulating different activities in the body. GFs play a critical role during different stages of wound healing in terms of migration, proliferation, differentiation, and maturation of various cells involved in the wound repair mechanism [175, 176]. GFs interact with different cells and chemokines, attract various cells at wounded site, and facilitate clearing out the wound debris and promoting the wound healing processes. Many liposomal formulations have been established for targeted delivery of a wide range of GFs and evaluated for ability to promote healing in various acute and chronic wounds. Xu and co-workers [177] successfully developed a novel liposome (LP) with hydrogel core of silk fibrin containing basic fibroblast growth factor (bFGF). Their resulting findings revealed that the developed formulation (bFGF-LP) effectively improved the stability of encapsulated bFGF in wound exudates (where usually drugs encounter enzymatic degradation). Moreover, in vivo data revealed that the developed liposomal formulation significantly accelerated wound closure in a mouse model with second-degree BWs. The enhanced wound closure efficacy of bFGF-LPs was attributed to its promising permeation efficiency, which promotes tissue regeneration, re-epithelization, and angiogenesis at the wound area. Therefore, the authors of this study proposed that bFGF-loaded liposomal formulation could be a potential nanotherapeutic for management of BWs [177].

Another liposomal formulation was developed by Değim and co-investigators [178]. They developed a CS gel formulation containing liposomes loaded with epidermal growth factor (EGF) and evaluated the wound healing efficiency in second-degree BWs in the female Sprague Dawley rats. For better comparison they also prepared two control groups (EGF-loaded liposomes, EGF-loaded gel). Results showed that EGF-loaded liposomes containing chitosan gel (ELJ) exhibited a significantly higher proliferation, differentiation, and migration of keratinocytes, re-epithelization, formation of granulation tissues, and higher wound closure efficiency at different time points (3rd, 7th and 14th days) compared to both control groups [178]. Similarly, Lu et al. [179] developed a highly deformable liposomal formulation (ointment) comprising retinoic acid and EGF to improve deep partial thickness burn wound healing therapy. The results confirmed a higher entrapment efficiency and sustained-release behavior characteristics of developed liposomal formulation. Moreover, improved skin permeation, along with enhanced deposition of the encapsulated drugs, has been observed. In vitro cell culture results also indicated that application of liposomes as a dual combination therapy produced a synergistic effect, with remarkable enhanced cell proliferation and migration. In vivo animal data also highlighted that BWs treated with developed liposomal formulation showed faster closure, better debridement, higher tensile strength due to pronounced deposition and maturation of collagen from type III to type I, and development of skin appendages, all of which indicate restoration of skin structure and functionality [179]. They further demonstrated that retinoic acid enhanced the therapeutic effect of EGF by upregulating the expression of EGFR and HB-EGF. These results suggested that dual liposomal ointment can be used as a promising topical application for management of burn injuries [179]. A similar trend had been noticed in a study conducted in 1991 in which the wound healing efficacy of EGF on second-degree BWs was evaluated in a rat model [180]. In this study, the effect of a protease inhibitor (nafamostat mesilate (NM)) on the wound healing efficiency of EGF had been investigated on burn wound model. A significant improvement in BWs healing efficacy of EGF was noticed when co-administered with NM. These results illustrate that co-administration of EGF and NM (protease inhibitor) in the form of a liposomal formulation can produce a synergistic effect and further accelerate the burn wound healing rate. Moreover, a noticeable increase in the dry weight of granulation tissues was observed on the wounded area of BWs exposed to EGF/NM co-loaded liposomal formulation compared to controls (EGF alone or NM alone). Interestingly, the findings of this study also demonstrated that co-administration of EGF and NM also protect from burn shock, which was observed in the control groups [180]. Apart from the EGF, granulocyte colony-stimulating factor (G-CSF) and granulocyte-macrophage colony-stimulating factor (GM-CSF) also play essential roles in the management of various skin injuries including the BWs [181].

The wound healing efficiency of liposomal formulations has also been validated by Nunes et al. [182]. They developed a gelatin-based membrane containing liposomes loaded with usnic acid (a potent bioactive molecules used for wound healing) [183] and evaluated for BW healing. Authors of this study observed that encapsulation of usnic acid into liposomal formulation improved its solubility, membrane permeability, and stability from enzymatic degradation on the wound bed. To evaluate BW healing efficacy, second-degree BWs (5 cm^2) were created on the dorsal region of the porcine model and results were compared with wounds treated with Ag sulfadiazine ointment and a commercial well-recognized wound dressing (duoDerme®). A time-mannered increase in BWs healing was observed in the experimental animals treated with liposomal formulation. The enhanced wound healing observed in liposomal formulation was attributed to improved migration, proliferation, and differentiation of keratinocytes, higher collagen maturation, and enhanced granulation tissue formation and re-epithelization compared to the control groups (Figure 11.7) [182]. The same research group had conducted a similar study in 2011 in which they developed a collagen membrane embedded with usnic acid loaded liposomes and evaluated its BWs healing efficacy in Wistar rats [184]. They observed superior BW healing efficacy of collagen membrane embedded with usnic acid-loaded liposomes compared to the control groups. On days 14 and 21, a significant reduction in inflammatory reaction with remarkable infiltration of plasma cells was observed in the wounds exposed to usnic acid-loaded liposomal formulation. Moreover, enhanced collagen deposition, granulation tissue formation and maturation, re-epithelization, and fibroblast proliferation were evident on day 21. Thus, the resulting data obtained from both studies revealed that both gelatin [182] and collagen [184] membranes embedded with usnic acid-loaded liposomes are promising therapeutic platforms for efficient management of BWs.

Deformable liposomes, also known as transfersomes, are a new generation of liposomal drug carrier systems, mainly composed of phospholipids and an edge activator

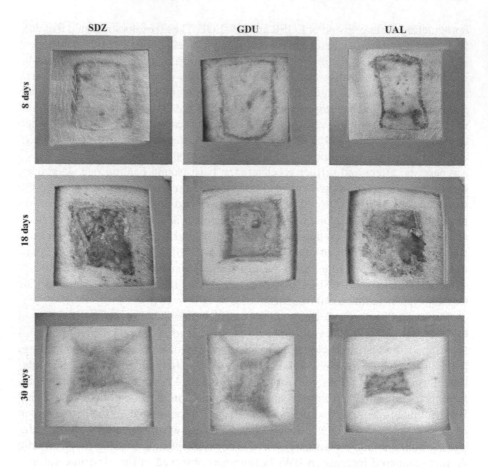

FIGURE 11.7 Time-mannered BWs healing efficacy of usnic acid-loaded liposomes embedded in gelatin membrane (UAL) compared to controls (SDZ, Ag sulfadiazine and GDU, DuoDerme®) [182]. Permission to reprint has been granted by Elsevier B.V. (Copyright © 2016).

(i.e., Tween-80, sodium cholate, and/or sodium deoxycholate) [185]. Deformable liposomes have revolutionized topical drug delivery due to their outstanding features compared to the traditional liposomes. The presence of edge activator makes deformable liposomes highly flexible to cross the stratum corneum and reach to different layers of the skin [186]. Keeping in mind the physiochemical and biopharmaceutical features of deformable liposomes, Choi et al. [187] developed a novel cationic deformable liposomal system composed of hyaluronic acid and a growth factor having good skin permeability (GF-HA) and evaluated its wound healing potential against diabetic wounds. The resulting data showed that that the GF-HA-based deformable liposomes remarkably enhanced wound closure in the tested animals (mouse model with induced diabetes mellitus) compared to those of other experimental groups (i.e., wounds treated with native growth factor complex) [187].

Similarly, Manconi et al. [188] designed a novel liposomal formulation by incorporating baicalin (a potential antioxidant and anti-inflammatory agent used for wound healing) into the self-assembled core-shell gellan-transferosome. The baicalin-loaded gellan-transferosomes showed the highest propensity of drug deposition into the skin (11% baicalin retained into whole skin in which about 8% was deposited only into the dermis). Furthermore, the wound repair experiments revealed that the developed gellan-transferosomes exhibited promising anti-inflammatory and skin repair capability in restoring the skin architecture and inhibition of excessive inflammation by downregulation of various inflammatory mediators (i.e., tumor necrosis factor-α (TNF-α) and interleukin-1β (IL-1β)) on the wounded skin [188].

As mentioned earlier, CUR and its analogs have been extensively used in various applications due to their remarkable biomedical potential; however, their therapeutic viability is hampered due to various issues (i.e., poor aqueous solubility, photo-degradation, low bioavailability, and low transmembrane permeability, which resists its topical application). To combat the aforementioned issues and to improve biopharmaceutical properties (i.e., BWs wound healing efficacy), various liposome-based nanotherapeutics have been designed and evaluated. One such study was carried out by Kianvash and co-authors [189] in which they successfully developed CUR-loaded propylene glycol (PEG)based liposomal formulations and investigated their wound healing potential for BWs. One reason for incorporating PEG into these liposomal nanosystems was to confer hydrophilic behavior onto the nanosystem to improve the plasma elimination half-life [85, 190]. Besides, PEG can also be used in formulation as a penetration enhancer and emulsifier for improving the transmembrane permeability and thermodynamic stability of the topical formulations [85, 190]. Results obtained from their study revealed that the PEG-based liposomal formulations provided good stability to curcumin, sustained release from the liposomal matrix, and prolonged plasma circulation time. Furthermore, the in vivo data showed that within 18 days of treatment wounds treated with PEG-based CUR-encapsulated liposomal formulation showed complete wound closure with no signs of bacterial growth on the wound bed [189]. The wounds treated with liposomal formulation showed better wound healing efficacy for management of BWs, compared to wounds treated with silver sulfadiazine cream 1%, ethosomes and conventional liposomes. It was anticipated that better penetration of PEG liposomes through the skin could have played an important role in improving the wound healing efficacy of PEG-based liposomal formulation [189]. In a similar attempt to improve the physicochemical and biopharmaceutical properties of CUR, Zhao and co-workers [85] encapsulated CUR into various liposomal formulations such as PEG liposomes (PEGL), conventional liposomes, and ethosomes and evaluated their BW healing efficacy. They demonstrated that PEGL showed the smallest particle size, highest encapsulation efficacy, and better protection of CUR against photo-degradation compared to other types of nanosystems (liposomes and ethosomes). Further, the resulting data showed that CUR-loaded PEGL showed significantly higher anti-inflammatory and anti-edema efficacy against paw edema in experimental animals [85]. The biopharmaceutical and therapeutic feasibility of liposomal formulation for an effective delivery of different types of bioactive molecules was also reported by El Maghraby et al. [191]. They performed a critical literature survey and demonstrated the superiority of liposomal nanosystems in enhancing the topical and transdermal delivery of drugs and improving their therapeutic potential for management of different types of damage, including BW [191].

Besides in vitro and in vivo studies, the wound healing potential of liposomal nanocarriers has also been validated through clinical studies. Luo et al. [192] conducted a clinical study involving 42 patients with second-degree BWs for screening the wound healing efficacy of Suyuping (a potent wound healer) after encapsulating it into a liposomal formulation. Results showed that the wounds treated with suyuping-loaded liposomal dressings showed merely mild wound pain along with less bleeding at the wounded sites, minimal allergy, and other side effects, compared to control (suyuping and plain liposomes). Thus, it was concluded that liposomal formulation can be used satisfactorily as a potential topical wound healer for managing second-degree BWs [192].

Liposomal formulations have also shown a greater potential in targeted delivery of other agents, including antimicrobial agents (i.e., mupirocin) [193]. The clinical applicability of mupirocin (a potent antibacterial that is being used for treatment of various skin diseases particularly skin wounds infected with MRSA) is hampered due to its intrinsic physicochemical properties. To combat these issues and to improve its wound healing effects, Hurler et al. [193] developed a liposomal formulation and evaluated its wound healing efficacy against BWs colonized with MRSA, one of the most virulent bacteria. Results showed a significant increase in wound healing rate with complete wound closure observed in 28 days. Further, a complete eradication of MRSA had been observed on wounds treated with liposomal formulations, which indicates a great potential of mupirocin-loaded liposomal formulations in eradicating local as well as systemic bacterial infection [193].

Despite the great potential of liposomal formulations for the delivery of a wide range of bioactive molecules and their tremendous wound healing and tissue regeneration potential, a significant improvement in the design and characteristics of liposomal formulations is still needful due to various shortfalls associated with them. These deficits, which include 1) premature seepage of encapsulated bioactive moieties and 2) poor thermodynamic stability and reproducibility, are the major hindrances for the clinical translation of liposomal formulations [194, 195].

11.3.2 INORGANIC NPS

11.3.2.1 Metal NPs

Metallic NPs have also been expansively applied for various purposes, including environmental sensors, diagnostic agents, antimicrobial coatings, medical imaging, and drug delivery [196, 197]. Owing to their exceptional antimicrobial efficacy, metallic NPs (i.e., Ag NPs, TiO_2 NPs, etc.) have been expansively used alone or embedded into composites, films, or other dressings for the management of various types of infections [198]. A plentiful use of metal NPs in various applications is due to many reasons, including but not limited to 1) versatility and broad spectrum antimicrobial activity, which make them capable of killing more than 650 types of micro-organisms, 2) strong potency, which makes them able to kill multiple types of microbes within an ultra-short period (i.e., within a few minutes) [199], and 3) least possibility of development of bacterial resistance against them compared to other antibiotics [200–202]. Though the exact pathway underlying the antimicrobial activity of metal NPs has not been fully understood yet, various studies have suggested different mechanisms by which metal NPs (Ag NPs) can kill microbes. For example, some studies suggested that electrostatic interference of metal NPs with microbial cell membrane causes damage to membrane proteins, resulting in compromising the cell membrane integrity and enhancing the permeability. Due to enhanced permeability of the cell membrane, bacterial cell cytoplasmic contents can leak out of the cell, which eventually causes the death of microbes [202–207]. Other researchers demonstrated that metal NPs (Ag NPs) damage bacterial cell membrane by generating the ROS and silver ions, which react with bacterial functional proteins and DNA, leading to disturbance in the metabolism and DNA replication [208–210]. Besides their outstanding antimicrobial activity, meta NPs demonstrate excellent anti-inflammatory activity in various skin injuries [211–213] and in intestines and bladder [214, 215].

Owing to their remarkable antimicrobial and anti-inflammatory activities, metal NPs have been extensively used in various treatments for the management of different types of wounds (i.e., acute, chronic, and BWs) [216, 217]. It has been reported that the anti-inflammatory, bactericidal, and wound healing efficacy of metal NPs is very much dependent on their physicochemical properties (i.e., particle size, shape, and surface charge) [218, 219]. Generally, the nanoscale metal particles exert stronger antimicrobial, anti-inflammatory, and wound healing efficacy compared to micron-scale metal particles. This is attributed to the larger surface area of nanoscale metal particles compared to micron-scale metal particles, their easy transmembrane permeability to reach intracellularly, and super-reactivity with nuclear components of bacterial cells [218–220]. Xiu and co-workers [221] have also reported that metallic NPs larger than 10 nm exhibit poor permeability and may remain on cell surfaces; however, metallic NPs smaller than 10 nm can efficiently penetrate across the bacterial cell membrane and enter bacteria cells to interact with bacterial sub-cellular structures (i.e., DNA, nuclear enzymes, and ribosomes) [221]. Therefore, the incorporation of Ag NPs (having diameter less than 10 nm) into wound dressing provides controlled and slow release of Ag clusters and Ag+ ions to exert strong antibacterial and anti-inflammatory effects [221, 222].

One of the serious challenges in the BWs healing is bacterial infection; therefore, for efficient control over microbial infection, wound dressings with strong antimicrobial agents are highly recommended. The *E. coli*, *S. aureus*, and *P. aeruginosa* are the most commonly encountered microbes that develop local or systemic microbial infections. Hence, the antibacterial efficacy of metallic NPs (Ag NPs) has been investigated against these most commonly encountered microorganisms [223, 224]. Interestingly, metallic NPs (Ag NPs) have shown a promising antibacterial efficacy against all these different types of microbes [225, 226]. Keeping in mind their exceptional antibacterial and anti-inflammatory properties, Zhang and co-workers [227] recently engineered Ag NPs and investigated their pro-healing effect on BWs using a mouse model (wild-type and Smad 3-/- mice). They observed and reported interesting findings that Ag NPs showed promising wound healing efficacy in BWs, but they delay wound closure time. They explained that early inflammation after getting a burn injury plays crucial role in clearing out the invaded microbes and preparing the wound bed for wound healing; therefore, early inflammation should not be prevented by application of Ag NPs. A slight delay in the application of Ag NP-based dressing facilitates BWs healing [227]. Results of this study were similar to those of a previous study [211]. In that study, it was demonstrated that the application of Ag NP-based dressings could significantly reduce inflammation and microbial burden on the wound bed, which plays a very important role in improving the wound healing mechanism; however, a slight delay in applying the Ag NP-embedded wound dressing will allow the occurrence of early episodes of inflammation (regulated by IL-10 and IL-6) post-burn injury, which play a key role in clearing out the microbes and tissue debris from the wound bed and hence improve wound healing in BWs [211].

Recently, Wasef et al. [212] also examined the wound healing viability of Ag NPs on BWs using the murine mouse model. In this study, deep second-degree BWs were created on the back of the experimental animals and were treated with Ag NPs for 28 days. The wound healing efficacy of Ag NPs was compared with an Ag-sulfadiazine–treated group. Furthermore, safety evaluation of the Ag NP treatment was performed by measuring the deposition rate of silver in the liver, brain, and kidney of treated mice. A significantly improved wound healing and antibacterial efficacy was observed in animals treated with Ag NPs compared to those of the silver sulfadiazine treated group. The superior wound healing efficiency of Ag NPs was attributed to excellent antibacterial effects by reducing the bioburden of aerobic microorganism i.e., S. aureus and E. coli on the wound beds. Moreover, burns exposed to Ag NPs displayed a lower degree of inflammation (in terms of redness and swelling) compared to those exposed to silver sulfadiazine [212]. Morphological and histological data confirmed that treating the BWs with Ag NPs could modify the infiltration of leukocytes and reduce degeneration of collagen. The safety profile of the Ag NP-treated mice evidenced a significantly lower distribution of silver ions in different vital organs (i.e., liver, brain, and kidney) compared to those treated with silver-sulfadiazine. Thus, overall data suggested that Ag NPs promote burn wound healing by decreasing the local and systemic bacterial infection, while showing good safety profile [212].

Likewise, Mehrabani and co-researchers [228] fabricated a hybrid biocompatible and biodegradable scaffold composed of silk fibroin/chitins/Ag NPs for successful wound healing application. The silk fibroin/chitins/Ag NP nanocomposites showed good mechanical properties, high porosity, excellent swellability and water uptake capability, and good hemostatic property, all of which facilitate wound healing. Moreover, the antimicrobial efficacy of the fabricated nano-scaffolds was investigated and the resulting data showed that the developed formulations exerted a strong antimicrobial activity against a wide range of microbes such as E. coli, S. aureus, and C. albicans. Conclusively, the findings of this study revealed that the developed nanocomposite containing Ag NPs can be successfully used for wound dressing application [228]. The findings of this study were very similar to those of a study carried out by another research group [229]. They developed a transparent bacterial cellulose membrane that was then soaked with Ag NPs and tested for antimicrobial efficacy. Results showed a promising antibacterial efficacy of the fabricated Ag NP-impregnated cellulose membrane against the E. coli and S. aureus [229].

Similar to acute and chronic wounds, bacterial infections are one of the major challenges of burn injuries because burns cause drastic changes in the immune system that could lead to suppressed immune function as well as increased susceptibility to infection. Patients with severe burns (particularly involving third-degree burns over a larger TBSA) may die from septicemia due to an excessive discharge of inflammatory cytokines (i.e., TNF-α, IL-1b, IL-6, IL-8, and IFN-γ) [230–234]. Hence, to down-regulate the expression and release of pro-inflammatory cytokines, Dinescu et al. [235] fabricated a novel multiparticulate drug delivery system that was obtained by freeze drying a collagen matrix embedded with flufenamic acid (anti-inflammatory agent) to control over-inflammation on BWs. The developed multiparticulate system showed release of embedded drugs in a controlled manner for 48 hours compared to those of sponges with drugs incorporated in free form. Moreover, the developed formulation (i.e., collagen matrix microencapsulated with flufenamic acid) exhibited an efficient BW healing with minimal scar formation compared to other tested groups. Conclusively, they proposed that the flufenamic-acid–loaded collagen matrix system is an advanced and efficient therapy for management of BWs, soft tissue lesions, and other skin inflammatory conditions [235].

Apart from the Ag NPs, various other types of metal NPs (i.e., TiO_2 NPs, Al_2O_3 NPs, Fe_3O_4 NPs) have earned approval from the FDA for wound healing and tissue regeneration implications. Seisenbaeva et al. [236] synthesized titanium dioxide (TiO_2)-NPs and evaluated their BW healing efficacy. The application of prepared TiO_2 NPs on BWs in the experimental animal showed strong efficiency in eradication of bacterial bioburden on the wound bed as well as enhanced wound healing efficacy, which was evident from a greater wound closure rate compared to the control group (untreated). The strong wound healing efficacy of TiO_2 NPs was attributed to their potential to generate ROS on the wound bed via the photocatalytic effect to kill the invaded bacteria and hence promote wound healing. Furthermore, they demonstrated that application of TiO_2 NPs on wounded skin exhibited good hemostatic potential, which is an essential step in the wound healing mechanism. The data obtained from the histological analysis revealed that the healing area of the second-degree wounds treated with TiO_2 NPs demonstrated unchanged normal skin structure, unlike the untreated wounds (i.e., controls), in which significant alterations in the normal skin anatomy were observed, with thickened and tightened fibers in the papillary layer, fewer sweat glands, reduction in the size of sebaceous glands, flattened sweat epithelium and isolated hair follicles. Moreover, notable fibrosis was observed at the reticular layer, with fibroblasts activation and focal perivascular leukocyte infiltration. These results clearly indicate the superior antibacterial and wound healing ability of TiO_2 NPs on BWs [236]. Likewise, another research group developed titania-embedded cellulose nanofibers by loading two different types of antibiotics (i.e., tetracycline and phosphomycin) for controlled drug delivery to the wounds [237, 238]. The developed nanocomposites showed promising antimicrobial efficacy against a broad range of microbes.

11.4 CURRENT CHALLENGES TO NANOTHERAPEUTICS

The major aims for designing nanotherapeutics is to provide the best therapeutic outcomes in terms of efficient local delivery of drugs to burned skin tissues, prolonged retention in injured skin tissues, eradication of microbial bioburden (which can delay the wound healing process), and avoidance of systemic toxicity. Although, nanomedicines have been mainly employed as promising advanced therapies through the topical route to enhance the burn wound healing, they are also associated with a high risk of systemic absorption particularly after application on burned/inflamed skin with complete or partial loss of skin's barrier (stratum corneum). The systemic risks associated with nanotherapeutics can be minimized by making them biodegradable, biocompatible, non-immunogenic, non-toxic, and capable of releasing their therapeutic cargo in a slow or controlled fashion [162, 239]. Furthermore, the systemic absorption of nanomedicines can be minimized by optimizing their size, nature, and composition, which can potentially optimize the localization of nanoparticles in the burned tissues [240, 241]. Other challenges encountered with nanomedicines include unwanted biological interaction of nanomaterials with biological tissues causing local and/or systemic toxicity, high manufacturing cost, and requirement of extensive scale-up experimentation for uniformity of quality [242–244].

Another major hurdle faced by the nanotherapeutics, particularly after their systemic administration, is early clearance by reticuloendothelial system (RES), premature degradation due to interaction with immune players, early renal clearance, insufficient amount of drugs reaching injured skin tissues, and non-target accumulation of drugs, which may suggest various side effects. The interaction of nanomedicines with blood components leads to premature elimination [245–248]. On the other hand, damaged blood vessels, uneven vascularization, and irregular lymphatic vessel distribution in burn skin areas may also result in variations in blood flow to burn skin tissues and absence of efficient lymphatic drainage. Besides the aforementioned challenges, lack of sufficient knowledge of nanocarrier interactions with biological moieties as well as their drug release profiles also poses a great hurdle toward clinical translation of nanotherapeutics [249]. Additionally, large-scale production presents an issue of high importance, as the manufacturing of nanoformulations is a complex process that requires expensive raw materials and happens over multiple stages. Overall, the mass production of nanomedicines is time-consuming and costly, and the resulting nanotherapeutics often display inconsistency in physicochemical properties among various batches. Even after production, nanomedicine faces another key obstacle in getting the regulatory approval, as the FDA has not established rational and specific guidelines for development of nanotherapeutics. The regulatory approval for nanomedicine products is so far based on individual evaluation of benefits and risks [250].

11.5   SUMMARY AND FUTURE PROSPECTS

Skin wound healing is a highly specialized and intricate mechanism for replacing damaged/injured tissues with the newer healthy tissues. Owing to its complex pathophysiology, wound management is one of the challenging aspects of injuries to the skin and its substructures, particularly when involving secondary complications (i.e., microbial infection, immunosuppression, diabetes mellitus, cardiovascular diseases, etc.). Among various types of wounds, chronic wounds (including diabetic wounds, diabetic foot ulcers, and BWs) are of special concern, which significantly hampers the normal wound healing process. Though many conventional wound modalities are being used for the treatment of different types of wounds, an ideal and versatile modality is still lacking, particularly for BWs, due to various secondary complications associated with these chronic wounds. Due to co-occurrence of various underlying conditions, burn wound management requires aggressive and more efficient wound healing modalities, which not only keep the wound environment moist (for better healing) but also eradicate microbial infections (which happen due to immunosuppression) on the wounded area as well as systemically (sepsis and septicemia). Besides, burn wound healing requires special assistance for relieving various symptoms such as burn wound pain (by analgesic drugs), excessive inflammation (by anti-inflammatory agents), tissue regeneration (by growth factors), etc. These special circumstances associated with burn wound management require development of newer, advanced, and more-efficient wound healing modalities.

Nanotechnology-aided developments have been widely employed in various fields due to their unique features (i.e., ultra-small size ranging from 10–100 nm, high encapsulation efficiency, controlled release, and thermodynamic stability) and biopharmaceutical (i.e., protection of drug from premature, better, transmembrane permeability drug targeting, prolonged plasma circulation, etc.) and biomedical significance. Nanotherapeutics (nanodelivery systems used for treatment of certain diseases) have shown exceptional wound healing efficacy for the management of various types of wounds, including BWs. These advanced modalities not only keep the wound bed moist for improved wound healing and tissue regeneration but also prevent eschar formation and wound pain and preclude secondary complications (local and systemic microbial infections). The administration of a wide variety of bioactive molecules (i.e., natural, synthetic, biologicals) has been obtained via different types of nanotherapeutics (i.e., polymeric nanoparticles, liposomes, micelles, hydrogels, nanogels, metal NPs, ethosomes, carbon nanotubes, etc.). The application of drug-loaded nanotherapeutics has resulted in significant improvement in tissue regeneration (i.e., cell proliferation and differentiation, granulation tissue formation and maturation, recruitment of inflammatory cells, collagen deposition, etc.), anti-inflammation (i.e. via downregulating the pro-inflammatory cytokines, particularly at later stages of inflammatory phase), pain relief, antimicrobial efficacy (local wounded site and systemic), and improved wound healing efficacy.

Despite remarkable biopharmaceutical and wound healing efficacy of nanotherapeutics, they are also associated with several complications, including thermodynamic stability, premature drug leakage, unwanted interaction with biological tissues, prolonged accumulation, which may cause nanotoxicity, and short plasma half-life. These limitations in nanotherapeutics need further research to be carried out to improve their biopharmaceutical, pharmacokinetic, and pharmacodynamic properties.

ACKNOWLEDGMENTS

Authors would like to acknowledge the Department of Pharmaceutics and Pharmaceutical Technology, College of Pharmacy, University of Sharjah, Sharjah 27272, United Arab Emirates for support and incentives to accomplish this book chapter.

CONFLICT OF INTEREST

Authors reported no conflict of interest in the present work.

REFERENCES

1. Shao M, Hussain Z, Thu HE, Khan S, de Matas M, Silkstone V, Qin HL, Bukhari SNA. Emerging trends in therapeutic algorithm of chronic wound healers: recent advances in drug delivery systems, concepts-to-clinical application and future prospects. Crit Rev Ther Drug Carrier Syst. 2017;34(5):387–452.
2. Hussain Z, Thu HE, Shuid AN, Katas H, Hussain F. Recent advances in polymer-based wound dressings for the treatment of diabetic foot ulcer: an overview of state-of-the-art. Curr Drug Targets. 2018;19(5):527–550.
3. Colohan SM. Predicting prognosis in thermal burns with associated inhalational injury: a systematic review of prognostic factors in adult burn victims. J Burn Care Res. 2010;31(4):529–539.
4. Mofazzal Jahromi MA, Sahandi Zangabad P, Moosavi Basri SM, et al. Nanomedicine and advanced technologies for burns: preventing infection and facilitating wound healing. Adv Drug Deliv Rev. 2018; 123:33–64.
5. Douglas, HE, Dunne, JA, Rawlins, JM. Management of burns. Surgery. 2017;35:511–518.
6. Souto EB, Ribeiro AF, Ferreira MI, et al. New nanotechnologies for the treatment and repair of skin burns infections. Int J Mol Sci. 2020;21(2):393.
7. Tiwari VK. Burn wound: How it differs from other wounds? Indian J Plast Surg. 2012;45:364–373.
8. Peck M, Molnar J, Swart D. A global plan for burn prevention and care. Bull World Health Organ. 2009;87:802–803.
9. Rafla K, Tredget EE. Infection control in the burn unit. Burns. 2011;37:5–15.
10. Badía D, López-García S, Martí C, Ortíz-Perpiñá O, Girona-García A, Casanova-Gascón J. Burn effects on soil properties associated to heat transfer under contrasting moisture content. Sci Total Environ. 2017;601–602:1119–1128.
11. Hall C, Hardin C, Corkins CJ, Jiwani AZ, Fletcher J, Carlsson A, Chan R. Pathophysiologic mechanisms and current treatments for cutaneous sequelae of burn wounds. Compr Physiol. 2017;8(1):371–405.
12. Deodhar AK, Rana RE. Surgical physiology of wound healing: a review. J Postgrad Med. 1997;43(2):52–56.
13. Ethridge RT, Leong M, Phillips L. Wound healing. In: Touensend CM, Beauchamp RD, Evers BM, Mattox KL, editors. Sabiston Textbook of Surgery. 18th ed. Philadephia: Saunders; 2009. pp. 191–216.
14. Guo S, Dipietro LA. Factors affecting wound healing. J Dent Res. 2010;89:219–229.
15. Sanchez DA, Schairer D, Tuckman-Vernon C, Chouake J, Kutner A, Makdisi J, Friedman JM, Nosanchuk JD, Friedman AJ. Amphotericin B releasing nanoparticle topical treatment of Candida spp. in the setting of a burn wound. Nanomedicine. 2014;10:269–277.
16. Hu S, Che JW, Wang HB, Yu Y, Tian YJ, Sheng ZY. [Effects of early oral fluid resuscitation on organ functions and survival during shock stage in dogs with a 50% total body surface area full-thickness burn]. Zhonghua Yi Xue Za Zhi. 2008;88(44):3149–3152.
17. Vaughn L, Beckel N. Severe burn injury, burn shock, and smoke inhalation injury in small animals. Part 1: Burn classification and pathophysiology. J Vet Emerg Crit Care (San Antonio). 2012;22(2):179–186.
18. Jackson DM. [The diagnosis of the depth of burning]. Br J Surg. 1953;40(164):588–596.

19. Rowan MP, Cancio LC, Elster EA, Burmeister DM, Rose LF, Natesan S, Chan RK, Christy RJ, Chung KK. Burn wound healing and treatment: review and advancements. Crit Care. 2015;19:243.
20. Kowalske KJ. Burn wound care. Phys Med Rehab Clin North Am. 2011;22:213–227.
21. Martin NA, Falder S. A review of the evidence for threshold of burn injury. Burns. 2017;43(8):1624–1639.
22. Tan JQ, Zhang HH, Lei ZJ, Ren P, Deng C, Li XY, et al. The roles of autophagy and apoptosis in burn wound progression in rats. Burns. 2013;39:1551–1556.
23. Contassot E, Gaide O, French LE. Death receptors and apoptosis. Dermatol Clin. 2007; 25:487–501.
24. Rode H, Martinez R, Potgieter D, Adams S, Rogers AD. Experience and outcomes of micrografting for major paediatric burns. Burns. 2017;43(5):1103–1110.
25. Nielson CB et al. "Burns: Pathophysiology of Systemic Complications and Current Management." J Burn Care Res. 2017;38(1): e469–e481.
26. Jeschke MG, Bolder U, Finnerty CC, et al. The effect of hepatocyte growth factor on gut mucosal apoptosis and proliferation, and cellular mediators after severe trauma. Surgery. 2005; 138:482–489.
27. Rae L, Fidler P, Gibran N. The physiologic basis of burn shock and the need for aggressive fluid resuscitation. Crit Care Clin. 2016;32(4):491–505.
28. Cumming J, Purdue GF, Hunt JL, O'Keefe GE. Objective estimates of the incidence and consequences of multiple organ dysfunction and sepsis after burn trauma. J Trauma. 2001;50(3):510–515.
29. Baxter RM, Dai T, Kimball J, Wang E, Hamblin MR, Wiesmann WP, McCarthy SJ, Baker SM. Chitosan dressing promotes healing in third degree burns in mice: gene expression analysis shows biphasic effects for rapid tissue regeneration and decreased fibrotic signaling. J Biomed Mater Res A. 2013;101:340–348.
30. Satish L, Gallo PH, Johnson S, Yates CC, Kathju S. Local probiotic therapy with *Lactobacillus plantarum* mitigates scar formation in rabbits after burn injury and infection. Surg. Infect. 2017;18:119–127.
31. Hussain A, Dunn KW. Predicting length of stay in thermal burns: a systematic review of prognostic factors. Burns. 2013;39:1331–1340.
32. Edgar DW, Fish JS, Gomez M, Wood FM. Local and systemic treatments for acute edema after burn injury: a systematic review of the literature. J Burn Care Res. 2011;32(2):334–347.
33. Pham TN, Cancio LC, Gibran NS, American Burn Association. American Burn Association practice guidelines burn shock resuscitation. J Burn Care Res. 2008;29:257–266.
34. Shirani KZ, Vaughan GM, Mason AD, Jr, Pruitt BA, Jr. Update on current therapeutic approaches in burns. Shock. 1996;5:4–16.
35. Dries DJ. Management of burn injuries – recent developments in resuscitation, infection control and outcomes research. Scand J Trauma Resusc Emerg Med. 2009;17:14.
36. Porter C, Hurren NM, Herndon DN, Borsheim E. Whole body and skeletal muscle protein turnover in recovery from burns. Int J Burns Trauma. 2013;3:9–17.
37. Farina JA, Jr, Rosique MJ, Rosique RG. Curbing inflammation in burn patients. Int J Inflamm. 2013;2013:715645.
38. Cutting KF, White RJ. Criteria for identifying wound infection—revisited. Ostomy Wound Manage. 2005;51:28–34.
39. Ahrns KS. Trends in burn resuscitation: shifting the focus from fluids to adequate endpoint monitoring, edema control, and adjuvant therapies. Crit Care Nurs Clin North Am. 2004;16(1):75–98.
40. Wang PH, Huang BS, Horng HC, Yeh CC, Chen YJ. Wound healing. J Chin Med Assoc. 2018;81(2):94–101.

41. Coger V, Million N, Rehbock C. et al. Tissue concentrations of zinc, iron, copper, and magnesium during the phases of full thickness wound healing in a rodent model. Biol Trace Elem Res. 2019;191:167–176.
42. Krzyszczyk P, Schloss R, Palmer A, Berthiaume F. The role of macrophages in acute and chronic wound healing and interventions to promote pro-wound healing phenotypes. Front Physiol. 2018;9:419.
43. Li J, Zhang YP, Kirsner RS. Angiogenesis in wound repair: angiogenic growth factors and the extracellular matrix. Microsc Res Tech. 2003;60(1):107–114.
44. Eming SA, Hubbell JA. Extracellular matrix in angiogenesis: dynamic structures with translational potential. Exp Dermatol. 2011;20(7):605–613.
45. Schultz GS, Wysocki A. Interactions between extracellular matrix and growth factors in wound healing. Wound Repair Regen. 2009;17(2):153–162.
46. Calin MA, Coman T, Calin MR. The effect of low level laser therapy on surgical wound healing. Rom Rep in Phys. 2010;62:617–627.
47. Li J, Chen J, Kirsner R. Pathophysiology of acute wound healing. Clin Dermatol. 2007;25:9–18.
48. Enoch S, Leaper DJ. Basic science of wound healing. Surgery. 2008;26:31–37.
49. Chodorowska G, Roguś-Skorupska D. Cutaneous wound healing. Ann Univ Mariae Curie Sklodowska Med. 2004;59(2):403–407.
50. Everett J, Turner K, Cai Q, Gordon V, Whiteley M, Rumbaugh K. Arginine is a critical substrate for the pathogenesis of *Pseudomonas aeruginosa* in burn wound infections. mBio. 2017;8(2):e02160–16.
51. Alemdaroğlu C, Değim Z, Celebi N, Zor F, Oztürk S, Erdoğan D. An investigation on burn wound healing in rats with chitosan gel formulation containing epidermal growth factor. Burns. 2006;32(3):319–327.
52. Howell-Jones RS, Wilson MJ, Hill KE, Howard AJ, Price PE, Thomas DW. A review of the microbiology, antibiotic usage and resistance in chronic skin wounds. J Antimicrob Chemother. 2005;55:143–149.
53. Landis SJ. Chronic wound infection and antimicrobial use. Adv Skin Wound Care. 2008;21(11):531–540; quiz 541–2.
54. Dai T, Huang YY, Sharma SK, Hashmi JT, Kurup DB, Hamblin MR. Topical antimicrobials for burn wound infections. Recent Pat Antiinfect Drug Discov. 2010;5(2):124–151.
55. Hosseini SV, Tanideh N, Kohanteb J, Ghodrati Z, Mehrabani D, Yarmohammadi H. Comparison between Alpha and silver sulfadiazine ointments in treatment of Pseudomonas infections in 3rd degree burns. Int J Surg. 2007;5(1):23–26.
56. Li H, Binxu L, Ma J, Ye J, Guo P, Li L. Fate of antibiotic-resistant bacteria and antibiotic resistance genes in the electrokinetic treatment of antibiotic-polluted soil. Chem Eng J. 2018;337:584–594.
57. Gao W, Chen Y, Zhang Y, Zhang Q, Zhang, L. Nanoparticle-based local antimicrobial drug delivery. Adv Drug Deliv Rev. 2018;127:46–57.
58. Aoyagi S, Onishi H, Machida Y. Novel chitosan wound dressing loaded with minocycline for the treatment of severe BWs. Int J Pharm. 2007;330(1–2):138–145.
59. Cowling T, Jones S. Topical Antibiotics for Infected Wounds: A Review of the Clinical Effectiveness and Guidelines [Internet]. Ottawa (ON): Canadian Agency for Drugs and Technologies in Health; 2017 Mar 20. PMID: 29517882.
60. Lipsky, BA, Hoey, C. Topical antimicrobial therapy for treating chronic wounds. Clin Infect Dis. 2009;49:1541–1549.
61. Sevgi M, Toklu A, Vecchio D, Hamblin MR. Topical antimicrobials for burn infections - an update. Recent Pat Antiinfect Drug Discov. 2013;8:161–197.
62. Yin R, Dai T, Avci P, Jorge AE, de Melo WC, Vecchio D, Huang YY, Gupta A, Hamblin MR. Light based anti-infectives: ultraviolet C irradiation, photodynamic therapy, blue light, and beyond. Curr Opin Pharmacol. 2013;13(5):731–762.

63. Nisanci M, Eski M, Sahin I, Ilgan S, Isik S. Saving the zone of stasis in burns with activated protein C: an experimental study in rats. Burns. 2010;36:397–402.
64. Deniz M, Borman H, Seyhan T, Haberal M. An effective antioxidant drug on prevention of the necrosis of zone of stasis: N-acetylcysteine. Burns. 2013;39(2):320–325.
65. Zor F, Ozturk S, Deveci M, Karacalioglu O, Sengezer M. Saving the zone of stasis: is glutathione effective? Burns 2005;31:972–996.
66. Mahajan AL, Tenorio X, Pepper MS, Baetens D, Montandon D, Schlaudraff K, et al. Progressive tissue injury in burns is reduced by rNAPc2. Burns 2006;32:957–963.
67. Firat C, Samdanci E, Erbatur S, Aytekin AH, Ak M, Turtay MG, Coban YK. β-Glucan treatment prevents progressive burn ischaemia in the zone of stasis and improves burn healing: an experimental study in rats. Burns. 2013;39(1):105–112.
68. Singh V, Devgan L, Bhat S, Milner SM. The pathogenesis of burn wound conversion. Ann Plast Surg. 2007;59:109–115.
69. Medina A, Riegel T, Nystad D, Tredget EE. Modified Meek micrografting technique for wound coverage in extensive burn injuries. J Burn Care Res. 2016;37(5):305–13.
70. Chua AWC, Khoo YC, Truong TTH, Woo E, Tan BK, Chong SJ. From skin allograft coverage to allograft-micrograft sandwich method: A retrospective review of severe burn patients who received conjunctive application of cultured epithelial autografts. Burns. 2018;44(5):1302–1307.
71. Rajendran NK, Kumar SSD, Houreld NN, Abrahamse H. A review on nanoparticle based treatment for wound healing. J Drug Deliv Sci Technol. 2018;44:421–430.
72. Kranz I, Gonzalez JB, Dörfel I, Gemeinert M, Griepentrog M, Klaffke D, Knabe C, Osterle W, Gross U. Biological response to micron- and nanometer-sized particles known as potential wear products from artificial hip joints: Part II: Reaction of murine macrophages to corundum particles of different size distributions. J Biomed Mater Res A. 2009;89(2):390–401.
73. Malekzad H, Mirshekari H, Sahandi Zangabad P, Moosavi Basri SM, Baniasadi F, Sharifi Aghdam M, Karimi M, Hamblin MR. Plant protein-based hydrophobic fine and ultrafine carrier particles in drug delivery systems. Crit Rev Biotechnol. 2018;38(1):47–67.
74. Zhu X, Radovic-Moreno AF, Wu J, Langer R, Shi J. Nanomedicine in the management of microbial infection - overview and perspectives. Nano Today. 2014;9(4):478–498.
75. Hissae Yassue-Cordeiro P, Zandonai CH, Pereira Genesi B, Santos Lopes P, Sanchez-Lopez E, Garcia ML, Camargo Fernandes-Machado NR, Severino P, Souto EB, Ferreira da Silva C. Development of chitosan/silver sulfadiazine/zeolite composite films for wound dressing. Pharmaceutics. 2019;11:535.
76. Debone HS, Lopes PS, Severino P, Yoshida CMP, Souto EB, da Silva CF. Chitosan/Copaiba oleoresin films for would dressing application. Int. J. Pharm. 2019;555:146–152.
77. Md S, Kuldeep Singh JKA, Waqas M, Pandey M, Choudhury H, Habib H, Hussain F, Hussain Z. Nanoencapsulation of betamethasone valerate using high pressure homogenization-solvent evaporation technique: optimization of formulation and process parameters for efficient dermal targeting. Drug Dev Ind Pharm. 2019;45(2):323–332.
78. Hameed HA, Khan S, Shahid M, Ullah R, Bari A, Ali SS, Hussain Z, Sohail M, Khan SU, Htar TT. Engineering of naproxen loaded polymer hybrid enteric microspheres for modified release tablets: development, characterization, in silico modelling and in vivo evaluation. Drug Des Devel Ther. 2020;14:27–41.
79. Shah SMH, Shah SMM, Khan S, Ullah F, Ali Shah SW, Ghias M, Shahid M, Smyth HDC, Hussain Z, Sohail M, Elhissi A, Isreb M. Efficient design to fabricate smart Lumefantrine nanocrystals using DENA® particle engineering technology: Characterisation, in vitro and in vivo antimalarial evaluation and assessment of acute and sub-acute toxicity. J Drug Del Sci Technol. 2021;61:102228.

80. Rahim MA, Jan N, Khan S, Shah H, Madni A, Khan A, Jabar A, Khan S, Elhissi A, Hussain Z, Aziz HC, Sohail M, Khan M, Thu, HE. Recent advancements in stimuli responsive drug delivery platforms for active and passive cancer targeting. Cancers, 2021;13(4):670.
81. Safdar MH, Hussain Z, Abourehab MAS, Hasan H, Afzal S, Thu HE. New developments and clinical transition of hyaluronic acid-based nanotherapeutics for treatment of cancer: reversing multidrug resistance, tumour-specific targetability and improved anticancer efficacy. Artif Cells Nanomed Biotechnol. 2018;46(8):1967–1980.
82. Fang G, Zhang Q, Pang Y, Thu H, Hussain Z. Nanomedicines for improved targetability to inflamed synovium for treatment of rheumatoid arthritis: Multi-functionalization as an emerging strategy to optimize therapeutic efficacy. J Control Release. 2019;303:181–208.
83. Gao X, Guo L, Li J, Thu HE, Hussain Z. Nanomedicines guided nanoimaging probes and nanotherapeutics for early detection of lung cancer and abolishing pulmonary metastasis: Critical appraisal of newer developments and challenges to clinical transition. J Control Release. 2018;292:29–57.
84. Farooq MA, Aquib M, Khan DH. et al. Recent advances in the delivery of disulfiram: a critical analysis of promising approaches to improve its pharmacokinetic profile and anticancer efficacy. DARU J Pharm Sci. 2019;27:853–862.
85. Zhao YZ, Lu CT, Zhang Y, et al. Selection of high efficient transdermal lipid vesicle for curcumin skin delivery. Int J Pharm. 2013;454:302–309
86. Smith DM, Simon JK, Baker JR Jr. Applications of nanotechnology for immunology. Nat Rev Immunol. 2013;13(8):592–605.
87. Yah CS, Simate GS. Nanoparticles as potential new generation broad spectrum antimicrobial agents. Daru. 2015; 23:43.
88. Ayumi NS, Sahudin S, Hussain Z, Hussain M, Samah NHA. Polymeric nanoparticles for topical delivery of alpha and beta arbutin: preparation and characterization. Drug Deliv Transl Res. 2019;9(2):482–496.
89. Hussain Z, Katas H, Mohd Amin MC, Kumolosasi E, Buang F, Sahudin S. Self-assembled polymeric nanoparticles for percutaneous co-delivery of hydrocortisone/hydroxytyrosol: an ex vivo and in vivo study using an NC/Nga mouse model. Int J Pharm. 2013;444(1–2):109–119.
90. Hussain Z, Katas H, Mohd Amin MC, Kumolosasi E. Efficient immuno-modulation of TH1/TH2 biomarkers in 2,4-dinitrofluorobenzene-induced atopic dermatitis: nanocarrier-mediated transcutaneous co-delivery of anti-inflammatory and antioxidant drugs. PLoS One. 2014;9(11):e113143.
91. Hussain Z, Katas H, Mohd Amin MC, Kumolosasi E, Sahudin S. Downregulation of immunological mediators in 2,4-dinitrofluorobenzene-induced atopic dermatitis-like skin lesions by hydrocortisone-loaded chitosan nanoparticles. Int J Nanomedicine. 2014;9:5143–56.
92. Hussain Z, Pandey M, Choudhury H, Ying PC, Xian TM, Kaur T, Jia GW, Gorain B. Hyaluronic acid functionalized nanoparticles for simultaneous delivery of curcumin and resveratrol for management of chronic diabetic wounds: fabrication, characterization, stability and in vitro release kinetics. J Drug Deliv Sci Technol. 2020;57:101747.
93. Parisi OI, Scrivano L, Sinicropi MS, Puoci F. Polymeric nanoparticle constructs as devices for antibacterial therapy. Curr Opin Pharm. 2017;36:72–77.
94. Lam SJ, Wong EHH., Boyer C, Qiao GG. Antimicrobial polymeric nanoparticles. Prog Polym Sci. 2018;76:40–64.
95. Crucho CIC, Barros MT. Polymeric nanoparticles: a study on the preparation variables and characterization methods. Mater Sci Eng C Mater Biol Appl. 2017:80:771–784.

96. Bashir S, Aamir M, Muhammad Sarfaraz R, Hussain Z, Sarwer MU, Mahmood A, Akram M, Qaisar MN. Fabrication, characterization and in vitro release kinetics of tofacitinib-encapsulated polymeric nanoparticles: a promising implication in the treatment of rheumatoid arthritis. Int J Polym Mater Polym Biomater. 2020. DOI: 10.1080/00914037.2020.1725760.

97. Hussain Z. Nanotechnology guided newer intervention for treatment of osteoporosis: efficient bone regeneration by up-regulation of proliferation, differentiation and mineralization of osteoblasts, Int J Polym Mater Polym Biomater. 2021;70(1)1–13. DOI: 10.1080/00914037.2019.1683558.

98. Choi C, Nam J-P, Nah J-W. Application of chitosan and chitosan derivatives as biomaterials. J. Ind Eng Chem. 2016;33:1–10.

99. Ahsan SM, Thomas M, Reddy KK, Sooraparaju SG, Asthana A, Bhatnagar I. Chitosan as biomaterial in drug delivery and tissue engineering. Int J Biol Macromol. 2018;110:97–109.

100. Andreani T, Fangueiro JF, Severino P, Souza ALR., Martins-Gomes C, Fernandes PMV, Calpena AC, Gremiao MP, Souto EB, Silva AM. The influence of polysaccharide coating on the physicochemical parameters and cytotoxicity of silica nanoparticles for hydrophilic biomolecules delivery. Nanomaterials. 2019;9:1081.

101. Ferreira da Silva C, Severino P, Martins F, Santana MH, Souto EB. Didanosine-loaded chitosan microspheres optimized by surface-response methodology: a modified "Maximum Likelihood Classification" approach formulation for reverse transcriptase inhibitors. Biomed Pharm. 2015;70:46–52.

102. Ali A, Ahmed S. A review on chitosan and its nanocomposites in drug delivery. Int J Biol Macromol. 2018;109:273–286.

103. Kong M, Chen XG, Xing K, Park HJ. Antimicrobial properties of chitosan and mode of action: a state of the art review. Int J Food Microbiol. 2010;144(1):51–63.

104. Rossi S, Marciello M, Sandri G, et al. Wound dressings based on chitosan and hyaluronic acid for the release of chlorhexidine diacetate in skin ulcer therapy. Pharm Dev Technol. 2007;12(4):415–422.

105. Ding L, Shan X, Zhao X, Zha H, Chen X, Wang J, Cai C, Wang X, Li G, Hao J, Yu G. Spongy bilayer dressing composed of chitosan–Ag nanoparticles and chitosan–Bletilla striata polysaccharide for wound healing applications. Carbohydr Polym. 2017;157:1538–1547.

106. El-Feky GS, Sharaf SS, El Shafei A, Hegazy AA. Using chitosan nanoparticles as drug carriers for the development of a silver sulfadiazine wound dressing. Carbohydr Polym. 2017;158:11–19.

107. Blažević F, Milekić T, Romić MD, Juretić M, Pepić I, Filipović-Grčić J, Lovrić J, Hafner A. Nanoparticle-mediated interplay of chitosan and melatonin for improved wound epithelialisation. Carbohydr Polym. 2016;146:445–454.

108. Dai T, Tanaka M, Huang YY, Hamblin MR. Chitosan preparations for wounds and burns: antimicrobial and wound-healing effects. Expert Rev Anti Infect Ther. 2011;9:857–879.

109. Rabea EI, Badawy ME, Stevens CV, Smagghe G, Steurbaut W. Chitosan as antimicrobial agent: applications and mode of action. Biomacromolecules. 2003; 4(6):1457–1465.

110. Li P, Poon YF, Li W, Zhu HY, Yeap SH, Cao Y, Qi X, Zhou C, Lamrani M, Beuerman RW, Kang ET, Mu Y, Li CM, Chang MW, Leong SS, Chan-Park MB. A polycationic antimicrobial and biocompatible hydrogel with microbe membrane suctioning ability. Nat Mater. 2011; 10(2):149–156.

111. Tang H, Zhang P, Kieft TL, Ryan SJ, Baker SM, Wiesmann WP, Rogelj S. Antibacterial action of a novel functionalized chitosan-arginine against Gram-negative bacteria. Acta Biomater. 2010;6(7):2562–2571.

112. Burkatovskaya M, Tegos GP, Swietlik E, Demidova TN, P Castano A, Hamblin MR. Use of chitosan bandage to prevent fatal infections developing from highly contaminated wounds in mice. Biomaterials. 2006;27(22):4157–4164.

113. Dai T, Tegos GP, Burkatovskaya M, Castano AP, Hamblin MR. Chitosan acetate bandage as a topical antimicrobial dressing for infected burns. Antimicrob Agents Chemother. 2009;53:393–400.

114. Yagci A, Tuc Y, Soyletir G. Elastase and alkaline protease production by Pseudomonas aeruginosa strains: comparison of two procedures. New Microbiol. 2002;25(2): 223–229.

115. Burkatovskaya M, Castano AP, Demidova-Rice TN, Tegos GP, Hamblin MR. Effect of chitosan acetate bandage on wound healing in infected and noninfected wounds in mice. Wound Repair Regen. 2008;16(3):425–31.

116. Alsarra IA. Chitosan topical gel formulation in the management of BWs. Int J Biol Macromol. 2009;45(1):16–21.

117. Boucard N, Viton C, Agay D, Mari E, Roger T, Chancerelle Y, Domard A. The use of physical hydrogels of chitosan for skin regeneration following third-degree burns. Biomaterials. 2007;28(24):3478–3488.

118. Seyfarth F, Schliemann S, Elsner P, et al. Antifungal effect of high- and low-molecular-weight chitosan hydrochloride, carboxymethyl chitosan, chitosan oligosaccharide and N-acetyl-D-glucosamine against Candida albicans, Candida krusei and Candida glabrata. Int J Pharm. 2008;353(1–2):139–148.

119. Huang L, Dai T, Xuan Y, Tegos GP, Hamblin MR. Synergistic combination of chitosan acetate with nanoparticle silver as a topical antimicrobial: efficacy against bacterial burn infections. Antimicrob Agents Chemother. 2011;55:3432–3438.

120. Liu H, Du Y, Wang X, Sun L. Chitosan kills bacteria through cell membrane damage. Int J Food Microbiol. 2004;95(2):147–155.

121. Vimala K, Mohan YM, Sivudu KS, Varaprasad K, Ravindra S, Reddy NN, Padma Y, Sreedhar B, MohanaRaju K. Fabrication of porous chitosan films impregnated with silver nanoparticles: a facile approach for superior antibacterial application. Colloids Surf B Biointerfaces. 2010;76(1):248–258.

122. Thomas V, Yallapu MM, Sreedhar B, Bajpai SK. Fabrication, characterization of chitosan/nanosilver film and its potential antibacterial application. J Biomater Sci Polym Ed. 2009;20(14):2129–2144.

123. Hussain Z, Thu HE, Shuid AN, Kesharwani P, Khan S, Hussain F. Phytotherapeutic potential of natural herbal medicines for the treatment of mild-to-severe atopic dermatitis: a review of human clinical studies. Biomed Pharmacother. 2017;93:596–608.

124. Tumpang MA, Ramli NA, Hussain Z. Phytomedicines are efficient complementary therapies for the treatment of atopic dermatitis: a review of mechanistic insight and recent updates. Curr Drug Targets. 2018;19(6):674–700.

125. Hussain Z, Thu HE, Amjad MW, Hussain F, Ahmed TA, Khan S. Exploring recent developments to improve antioxidant, anti-inflammatory and antimicrobial efficacy of curcumin: a review of new trends and future perspectives. Mater Sci Eng C Mater Biol Appl. 2017; 77:1316–1326.

126. Dong J, Tao L, Abourehab MAS, Hussain Z. Design and development of novel hyaluronate-modified nanoparticles for combo-delivery of curcumin and alendronate: fabrication, characterization, and cellular and molecular evidences of enhanced bone regeneration. Int J Biol Macromol. 2018;116:1268–1281.

127. Khan S, Imran M, Butt TT, Shah SWA, Sohail M, Malik A, Das S, Thu HE, Adam A, Hussain Z. Curcumin based nanomedicines as efficient nanoplatform for treatment of cancer: new developments in reversing cancer drug resistance, rapid internalization, and improved anticancer efficacy. Trends Food Sci Technol. 2018;80:8–22.

128. Hussain Z, Thu HE, Ng SF, Khan S, Katas H. Nanoencapsulation, an efficient and promising approach to maximize wound healing efficacy of curcumin: a review of new trends and state-of-the-art. Colloids Surf B Biointerfaces. 2017;150:223–241.
129. Mirnejad R, Mofazzal Jahromi M, Al-Musawi S, Pirestani M, Fasihi Ramandi M, Ahmadi K, Rajayi H, Mohammad Hassan Z, Kamali M. Curcumin-loaded Chitosan Tripolyphosphate Nanoparticles as a safe, natural and effective antibiotic inhibits the infection of Staphylococcus aureus and Pseudomonas aeruginosa in vivo. Iran J Biotechnol. 2014;12(3):1–8.
130. Xie M, Fan D, Zhao Z, Li Z, Li G, Chen Y, He X, Chen A, Li J, Lin X, Zhi M, Li Y, Lan P. Nanocurcumin prepared via supercritical: improved anti-bacterial, anti-oxidant and anti-cancer efficacy. Int J Pharm. 2015;496:732–740.
131. Bhawana, Basniwal RK, Buttar HS, Jain VK, Jain N. Curcumin nanoparticles: preparation, characterization, and antimicrobial study. J Agric Food Chem. 2011;59: 2056–2061.
132. Chereddy KK, Her CH, Comune M, Moia C, Lopes A, Porporato PE, Vanacker J, Lam MC, Steinstraesser L, Sonveaux P, Zhu H, Ferreira LS, Vandermeulen G, Preat V. PLGA nanoparticles loaded with host defense peptide LL37 promote wound healing. J Control Release. 2014;194:138–147.
133. Sanchez-Lopez E, Guerra M, Dias-Ferreira J, Lopez-Machado A, Ettcheto M, Cano A, Espina M, Camins A, Garcia ML, Souto EB. Current applications of nanoemulsions in cancer therapeutics. Nanomaterials. 2019;9:821.
134. Uchechi O, Ogbonna JDN, Attama AA. Nanoparticles for dermal and transdermal drug delivery. In: Sezer AD, editor. Applications of Nanotechnology in Drug Delivery. London, UK: IntechOpen Limited; 2014. pp. 193–235.
135. Rai VK, Mishra N, Yadav KS, Yadav NP. Nanoemulsion as pharmaceutical carrier for dermal and transdermal drug delivery: Formulation development, stability issues, basic considerations and applications. J Control Release. 2018;270:203–225.
136. Singh Y, Meher JG, Raval K, Khan FA, Chaurasia M, Jain NK, Chourasia MK. Nanoemulsion: concepts, development and applications in drug delivery. J Control Release. 2017;252:28–49.
137. Dolgachev VA, Ciotti SM, Eisma R, Gracon S, Wilkinson JE, Baker JR Jr, Hemmila MR. Nanoemulsion Therapy for BWs Is Effective as a Topical Antimicrobial Against Gram-Negative and Gram-Positive Bacteria. J Burn Care Res. 2016;37(2):e104–14.
138. Song Z, Sun H, Yang Y, Jing H, Yang L, Tong Y, Wei C, Wang Z, Zou Q, Zeng H. Enhanced efficacy and anti-biofilm activity of novel nanoemulsions against skin burn wound multi-drug resistant MRSA infections. Nanomedicine. 2016;12(6):1543–1555.
139. Abbasi-Montazeri E, Khosravi AD, Feizabadi MM, Goodarzi H, Khoramrooz SS, Mirzaii M, Kalantar E, Darban-Sarokhalil D. The prevalence of methicillin resistant Staphylococcus aureus (MRSA) isolates with high-level mupirocin resistance from patients and personnel in a burn center. Burns. 2013;39(4):650–654.
140. Wearn CM, Hardwicke J, Moiemen N. Burns in the elderly: mortality is still a relevant outcome. Burns. 2015;41(7):1617–1618.
141. Eisenbeis J, Peisker H, Backes CS, Bur S, Hölters S, Thewes N, Greiner M, Junker C, Schwarz EC, Hoth M, Junker K, Preissner KT, Jacobs K, Herrmann M, Bischoff M. The extracellular adherence protein (Eap) of Staphylococcus aureus acts as a proliferation and migration repressing factor that alters the cell morphology of keratinocytes. Int J Med Microbiol. 2017;307(2):116–125.
142. Kirker KR, James GA, Fleckman P, Olerud JE, Stewart PS. Differential effects of planktonic and biofilm MRSA on human fibroblasts. Wound Repair Regen. 2012;20(2):253–261.

143. Thakur K, Sharma G, Singh B, Jain A, Tyagi R, Chhibber S, Katare OP. Cationic-bilayered nanoemulsion of fusidic acid: an investigation on eradication of methicillin-resistant Staphylococcus aureus 33591 infection in burn wound. Nanomedicine (Lond). 2018;13(8):825–847.

144. Hussain Z, Arooj M, Malik A, et al. Nanomedicines as emerging platform for simultaneous delivery of cancer therapeutics: new developments in overcoming drug resistance and optimizing anticancer efficacy. Artif Cells Nanomed Biotechnol. 2018;46(sup2):1015–1024.

145. Bonferoni MC, Sandri G, Rossi S, Dellera E, Invernizzi A, Boselli C, Cornaglia AI, Del Fante C, Perotti C, Vigani B, et al. Association of alpha tocopherol and Ag sulfa-diazine chitosan oleate nanocarriers in bioactive dressings supporting platelet lysate application to skin wounds. Mar Drugs. 2018;16:56.

146. Li D, van Nostrum CF, Mastrobattista E,Vermonden T, Hennink WE. Nanogels for intracellular delivery of biotherapeutics. J Control Release. 2017;259:16–28.

147. Mahinroosta M, Farsangi ZJ, Allahverdi A, Shakoori Z. Hydrogels as intelligent materials: a brief review of synthesis, properties and applications. Mater Today Chem. 2018;8:42–55.

148. Boateng JS, Matthews KH, Stevens HN, Eccleston GM. Wound healing dressings and drug delivery systems: a review. J Pharm Sci. 2008;97:2892–2923.

149. Rigo C, Roman M, Munivrana I, Vindigni V, Azzena B, Barbante C, et al. Characterization and evaluation of silver release from four different dressings used in burns care. Burns. 2012;38:1131–1142.

150. Teo EY, Ong SY, Chong MS, Zhang Z, Lu J, Moochhala S, et al. Polycaprolactonebased fused deposition modeled mesh for delivery of antibacterial agents to infected wounds. Biomaterials 2010;32:279–287.

151. Soni G, Yadav KS. Nanogels as potential nanomedicine carrier for treatment of cancer: a mini review of the state of the art. Saudi Pharm J. 2016;24:133–139.

152. Loo Y, Wong YC, Cai EZ, Ang CH, Raju A, Lakshmanan A, Koh AG, Zhou HJ, Lim TC, Moochhala SM, Hauser CA. Ultrashort peptide nanofibrous hydrogels for the acceleration of healing of Burn Wounds. Biomaterials. 2014;35(17):4805–4814.

153. Choi JS, Leong KW, Yoo HS. In vivo wound healing of diabetic ulcers using electrospun nanofibers immobilized with human epidermal growth factor (EGF). Biomaterials. 2008;29:587–596.

154. Yan H, Chen J, Peng X. Recombinant human granulocyte-macrophage colony stimulating factor hydrogel promotes healing of deep partial thickness BWs. Burns 2012;38:877–881.

155. Choi JS, Yoo HS. Pluronic/chitosan hydrogels containing epidermal growth factor with wound-adhesive and photo-cross-linkable properties. J Biomed Mater Res A. 2010;95:564–573.

156. Butcher M. Meeting the clinical challenges of burns management: a review. Br J Nurs 2011;20(S44):S46–51.

157. Arab WT, Niyas AM, Seferji K, Susapto HH, Hauser CAE. 2018. Evaluation of peptide nanogels for accelerated wound healing in normal micropigs. Front Nanosci Nanotech 4: DOI: 10.15761/FNN.1000173.

158. Soriano JL, Calpena AC, Rincón M, Pérez N, Halbaut L, Rodríguez-Lagunas MJ, Clares B. Melatonin nanogel promotes skin healing response in BWs of rats. Nanomedicine (Lond). 2020;15(22):2133–2147.

159. Hussain Z, Thu HE, Katas H, Bukhari SNA. Hyaluronic acid-based biomaterials: a versatile and smart approach to tissue regeneration and treating traumatic, surgical, and chronic wounds. Polym Rev. 2017;57(4)594–630.

160. Bukhari SNA, Roswandi NL, Waqas M, Habib H, Hussain F, Khan S, Sohail M, Ramli NA, Thu HE, Hussain Z. Hyaluronic acid, a promising skin rejuvenating biomedicine: a review of recent updates and pre-clinical and clinical investigations on cosmetic and nutricosmetic effects. Int J Biol Macromol. 2018;120(Pt B):1682–1695.

161. Pandey M, Choudhury H, Gunasegaran TAP, Nathan SS, Md S, Gorain B, Tripathy M, Hussain Z. Hyaluronic acid-modified betamethasone encapsulated polymeric nanoparticles: fabrication, characterisation, in vitro release kinetics, and dermal targeting. Drug Deliv Transl Res. 2019;9(2):520–533.

162. Zhuo F, Abourehab MAS, Hussain Z. Hyaluronic acid decorated tacrolimus-loaded nanoparticles: efficient approach to maximize dermal targeting and anti-dermatitis efficacy. Carbohydr Polym. 2018;197:478–489.

163. Chen LH, Xue JF, Zheng ZY, Shuhaidi M, Thu HE, Hussain Z. Hyaluronic acid, an efficient biomacromolecule for treatment of inflammatory skin and joint diseases: a review of recent developments and critical appraisal of preclinical and clinical investigations. Int J Biol Macromol. 2018;116:572–584.

164. Chen J, Cheng D, Li J, Wang Y, Guo JX, Chen ZP, Cai BC, Yang T. Influence of lipid composition on the phase transition temperature of liposomes composed of both DPPC and HSPC. Drug Dev Ind Pharm. 2013;39:197–204.

165. Mitragotri S, Burke PA, Langer R. Overcoming the challenges in administering biopharmaceuticals: formulation and delivery strategies. Nat Rev Drug Discov. 2014;13:655–672.

166. Sercombe L, Veerati T, Moheimani F, Wu SY, Sood AK, Hua S. Advances and challenges of liposome assisted drug delivery. Front Pharmacol. 2015;6:286.

167. Lombardo D, Calandra P, Barreca D, Magazù S, Kiselev MA. Soft interaction in liposome nanocarriers for therapeutic drug delivery. Nanomaterials (Basel). 2016;6(7):125.

168. Cheng R, Liu L, Xiang Y, Lu Y, Deng L, Zhang H, Santos HA, Cui W. Advanced liposome-loaded scaffolds for therapeutic and tissue engineering applications. Biomaterials. 2020;232:119706.

169. Pierre MB, Dos Santos Miranda Costa I. Liposomal systems as drug delivery vehicles for dermal and transdermal applications. Arch Dermatol Res. 2011;303(9):607–621.

170. Hou GR, Zeng K, Zhou ZG. The application and action mechanism of liposome in skin. J Dermatol Venereol. 2003;25(4):15.

171. Manca ML, Matricardi P, Cencetti C, Peris JE, Melis V, Carbone C, Escribano E, Zaru M, Fadda AM, Manconi M. Combination of argan oil and phospholipids for the development of an effective liposome-like formulation able to improve skin hydration and allantoin dermal delivery. Int J Pharm. 2016;505:204–211.

172. Bian DF, Liu M, Li Y, Xia Y, Gong Z, Dai Y. Madecassoside, a triterpenoid saponin isolated from Centella asiatica herbs, protects endothelial cells against oxidative stress. J Biochem Mol Toxicol. 2012;26(10):399–406.

173. Gallego A, Ramirez-Estrada K, Vidal-Limon HR, et al. Biotechnological production of centellosides in cell cultures of Centella asiatica (L) Urban. Eng Life Sci. 2014;14(6):633–642.

174. Li Z, Liu M, Wang H, Du S. Increased cutaneous wound healing effect of biodegradable liposomes containing madecassoside: preparation optimization, in vitro dermal permeation, and in vivo bioevaluation. Int J Nanomedicine. 2016;11:2995–3007.

175. Krishnamoorthy L, Morris HL, Harding KG. Specific growth factors and the healing of chronic wounds. J Wound Care. 2001;10(5):173–178.

176. Grazul-Bilska AT, Johnson ML, Bilski JJ, Redmer DA, Reynolds LP, Abdullah A, Abdullah KM. Wound healing: the role of growth factors. Drugs Today (Barc). 2003;39(10):787–800.

177. Xu HL, Chen PP, ZhuGe DL, Zhu QY, Jin BH, Shen BX, Xiao J, Zhao YZ. Liposomes with silk fibroin hydrogel core to stabilize bFGF and promote the wound healing of mice with deep second-degree scald. Adv Healthc Mater. 2017;6:1700344.

178. Değim Z, Çelebi N, Alemdaroğlu C, Deveci M, Öztürk S, Özoğul C. Evaluation of chitosan gel containing liposome-loaded epidermal growth factor on burn wound healing. Int Wound J. 2011;8(4):343–54.

179. Lu KJ, Wang W, Xu XL, Jin FY, Qi J, Wang XJ, Kang XQ, Zhu ML, Huang QL, Yu CH, You J, Du YZ. A dual deformable liposomal ointment functionalized with retinoic acid and epidermal growth factor for enhanced burn wound healing therapy. Biomater Sci. 2019;7(6):2372–2382. doi: 10.1039/c8bm01569d. PMID: 30916681.

180. Kiyohara Y, Komada F, Iwakawa S, Hirai M, Fuwa T, Okumura K. Improvement in wound healing by epidermal growth factor (EGF) ointment. II. Effect of protease inhibitor, nafamostat, on stabilization and efficacy of EGF in burn. J Pharmacobiodyn. 1991;14(1):47–52.

181. Grzybowski J, Ołdak E, Janiak MK. Miejscowe stosowanie cytokin G-CSF, GM-CSF oraz EGF w leczeniu ran [Local application of G-CSF, GM-CSF and EGF in treatment of wounds]. Postepy Hig Med Dosw. 1999;53(1):75–86.

182. Nunes PS, Rabelo AS, Souza JC, Santana BV, da Silva TM, Serafini MR, Dos Passos Menezes P, Dos Santos Lima B, Cardoso JC, Alves JC, Frank LA, Guterres SS, Pohlmann AR, Pinheiro MS, de Albuquerque RL Júnior, Araújo AA. Gelatin-based membrane containing usnic acid-loaded liposome improves dermal burn healing in a porcine model. Int J Pharm. 2016;513(1–2):473–482.

183. Jin J, Dong Y, He L. The study on skin wound healing promoting action of sodium usnic acid. ZhongYao Cai. 2005;28(2):109–111.

184. Nunes PS, Albuquerque RL Jr, Cavalcante DR, Dantas MD, Cardoso JC, Bezerra MS, Souza JC, Serafini MR, Quitans LJ Jr, Bonjardim LR, Araújo AA. Collagen-based films containing liposome-loaded usnic acid as dressing for dermal burn healing. J Biomed Biotechnol. 2011;2011:761593.

185. Chen R, Li R, Liu Q. et al. Ultradeformable liposomes: a novel vesicular carrier for enhanced transdermal delivery of procyanidins: effect of surfactants on the formation, stability, and transdermal delivery. AAPS PharmSciTech. 2017;18:1823–1832.

186. Cevc G. Rational design of new product candidates: the next generation of highly deformable bilayer vesicles for noninvasive, targeted therapy. J Control Release. 2012;160:135–146.

187. Choi JU, Lee SW, Pangeni R, Byun Y, Yoon IS, Park JW. Preparation and in vivo evaluation of cationic elastic liposomes comprising highly skin-permeable growth factors combined with hyaluronic acid for enhanced diabetic wound-healing therapy. Acta Biomater. 2017;57:197–215.

188. Manconi M, Manca ML, Caddeo C, Valenti D, Cencetti C, Diez-Sales O, Nacher A, Mir-Palomo S, Terencio MC, Demurtas D, Gomez-Fernandez JC, Aranda FJ, Fadda AM, Matricardi P. Nanodesign of new self-assembling core-shell gellan-transfersomes loading baicalin and in vivo evaluation of repair response in skin. Nanomedicine. 2018;14(2):569–579.

189. Kianvash N, Bahador A, Pourhajibagher M, Ghafari H, Nikoui V, Rezayat SM, Dehpour AR, Partoazar A. Evaluation of propylene glycol nanoliposomes containing curcumin on burn wound model in rat: biocompatibility, wound healing, and antibacterial effects. Drug Deliv Transl Res. 2017;7(5):654–663.

190. Elmoslemany RM, Abdallah OY, El-Khordagui LK, Khalafallah NM. Propylene glycol liposomes as a topical delivery system for miconazole nitrate: comparison with conventional liposomes. AAPS PharmSciTech. 2012;13:723–731.

191. El Maghraby GM, Barry BW, Williams AC. Liposomes and skin: from drug delivery to model membranes. Eur J Pharm Sci. 2008;34(4–5):203–222

192. Luo XS, Cen Y, Zhao JH. Therapeutic effect of liposome on II degree burn wound. Zhongguo Xiu Fu Chong Jian Wai Ke Za Zhi. 2000;14(6):358–360.

193. Hurler J, Sørensen KK, Fallarero A, Vuorela P, Škalko-Basnet N. Liposomes-in-hydrogel delivery system with mupirocin: in vitro antibiofilm studies and in vivo evaluation in mice burn model. BioMed Research International. 2013;2013:498485.

194. Gubernator J, Chwastek G, Korycinska M, Stasiuk M, Grynkiewicz G, Lewrick F, Suss R, Kozubek A. The encapsulation of idarubicin within liposomes using the novel EDTA ion gradient method ensures improved drug retention in vitro and in vivo. J Control Release. 2010;146:68–75.

195. Ran R, Middelberg APJ, Zhao CX. Microfluidic synthesis of multifunctional liposomes for tumour targeting. Colloids Surf B Biointerfaces. 2016;148:402–410.

196. Schröfel A, Kratošová G, Šafařík I, Šafaříková M, Raška I, Shor LM. Applications of biosynthesized metallic nanoparticles—a review. Acta Biomater. 2014;10:4023–4042.

197. Quester K, Avalos-Borja M, Castro-Longoria E. Biosynthesis and microscopic study of metallic nanoparticles. Micron. 2013;54–55:1–27.

198. Khodashenas B, Ghorbani HR. Synthesis of silver nanoparticles with different shapes. Arab. J. Chem. 2015;1–16.

199. Klasen HJ. A historical review of the use of silver in the treatment of burns. II. Renewed interest for silver. Burns. 2000;26:131–138.

200. Hussain Z, Thu HE, Elsayed I, Abourehab MAS, Khan S, Sohail M, Sarfraz RM, Farooq MA. Nano-scaled materials may induce severe neurotoxicity upon chronic exposure to brain tissues: A critical appraisal and recent updates on predisposing factors, underlying mechanism, and future prospects. J Control Release. 2020;328:873–894.

201. Hussain Z, Thu HE, Haider M, Khan S, Sohail M, Hussain F, Khan FM, Farooq MA, Shuid AN. A review of imperative concerns against clinical translation of nanomaterials: unwanted biological interactions of nanomaterials cause serious nanotoxicity. J Drug Deliv Sci Technol. 2020;59:101867.

202. Hussain Z, Thu HE, Sohail M, Khan S. Hybridization and functionalization with biological macromolecules synergistically improve biomedical efficacy of silver nanoparticles: reconceptualization of in-vitro, in-vivo and clinical studies. J Drug Deliv Sci Technol. 2019;54:101169.

203. Jones MC, Hoek EM. A review of the antibacterial effects of silver nanomaterials and potential implications for human health and the environment. J Nanopart Res. 2010;12:1531–1551.

204. Melaiye A, Youngs JW. Silver and its application as an antimicrobial agent. Expert Opin Ther Patents. 2005;15:125–130.

205. Bansal V, Li V, O'Mullane AP, Bhargava SK. Shape dependent electrocatalytic behaviour of silver nanoparticles. Crystengcomm. 2010;12:4280–4286

206. Andrade RM, Cho AT, Hu PG, Lee SJ, Deming CP, Sweeney SW, et al. Enhanced antimicrobial activity with faceted silver nanostructures. J Mater Sci. 2015;50:2849–2858.

207. Vukoje I, Lazic V, Vodnik V, Mitric M, Jokic B, Ahrenkiel SP, et al. The influence of triangular silver nanoplates on antimicrobial activity and color of cotton fabrics pretreated with chitosan. J Mater Sci. 2014;49:4453–4460.

208. Hackenberg S, Scherzed A, Kessler M, Hummel S, Technau A, Froelich K, et al. Silver nanoparticles: evaluation of DNA damage, toxicity and functional impairment in human mesenchymal stem cells. Toxicol Lett. 2011;201:27–33.

209. Lok CN, Ho CM, Chen R, He QY, Yu WY, Sun H, Tam PK, Chiu JF, Che CM. Proteomic analysis of the mode of antibacterial action of silver nanoparticles. J Proteome Res. 2006;5(4):916–24.

210. Durán N, Durán M, de Jesus MB, Seabra AB, Fávaro WJ, Nakazato G. Silver nanoparticles: a new view on mechanistic aspects on antimicrobial activity. Nanomedicine. 201612(3):789–799.

211. Tian J, Wong KK, Ho CM, Lok CN, Yu WY, Che CM, Chiu JF, Tam PK. Topical delivery of silver nanoparticles promotes wound healing. ChemMedChem. 2007;2(1):129–136.

212. Wasef LG, Shaheen HM, El-Sayed YS. et al. Effects of silver nanoparticles on burn wound healing in a mouse model. Biol Trace Elem Res. 2020;193:456–465.

213. Liu X, Hao W, Lok CN, Wang YC, Zhang R, Wong KK. Dendrimer encapsulation enhances anti-inflammatory efficacy of silver nanoparticles. J Pediatr Surg. 2014;49(12):1846–1851.
214. Zhang, S, Liu, X, Wang, H, Peng, J, Wong, KKY. Silver nanoparticle-coated suture effectively reduces inflammation and improves mechanical strength at intestinal anastomosis in mice. J Pediatr Surg. 2014;49:606–613.
215. Boucher W, Stern JM, Kotsinyan V, Kempuraj D, Papaliodis D, Cohen MS, Theoharides TC. Intravesical nanocrystalline silver decreases experimental bladder inflammation. J Urol. 2008;179(4):1598–602.
216. Hussain S, Ferguson C. Best evidence topic report. Silver sulphadiazine cream in burns. Emerg Med J. 2006;23:929–932.
217. Sondi I, Sondi SB. Silver nanoparticles as antimicrobial agent: a case study on E. coli as a model for Gram-negative bacteria. J Colloid Interface Sci. 2004;275:177–182.
218. Castanon M, Martinez NN, Gutierrez MF, Mendoza MJ. Synthesis and antibacterial activity of silver nanoparticles with different sizes. J Nanopart Res. 2008;10:1343–1348.
219. Pal S, Tak YK, Song JM. Does the antibacterial activity of silver nanoparticles depend on the shape of the nanoparticle? A study of the Gram-negative bacterium Escherichia coli. Appl Environ Microbiol. 2007;73:1712–1720.
220. Thiel J, Pakstis L, Buzby S, Raffi M, Ni C, et al. Antibacterial properties of silver-doped titania. Small. 2007;3:799–803.
221. Xiu ZM, Zhang QB, Puppala HL, Colvin VL, Alvarez PJ. Negligible particle-specific antibacterial activity of silver nanoparticles. Nano letters. 2012;12:4271–4275.
222. Taylor PL, Omotoso O, Wiskel JB, Mitlin D, Burrell, RE Impact of heat on nanocrystalline silver dressings. Part II: Physical properties. Biomaterials. 2005;26:7230–7240.
223. Paula MMD, Franco CV, Baldin MC, Silva. Synthesis, characterization and antibacterial activity studies of poly-{styrene-acrylic acid} with silver nanoparticles. Mater Sci Eng. 2009;29:647–650.
224. Lee BU, Yun SH, Ji JH, Bae GN. Inactivation of S. epidermidis, B. subtilis, and E. coli bacteria bioaerosols deposited on a filter utilizing airborne silver nanoparticles. J Microbiol Biotechnol. 2008;18:176–182.
225. Zhang Y, Peng H, Huang W, Zhou Y, Yan D. Facile preparation and characterization of highly antimicrobial colloid Ag or Au nanoparticles. J Colloid Interface Sci. 2008;325:371–376.
226. Flores CY, Diaz C, Rubert A, Benitez GA, Moreno MS, Lorenzo M, et al. Spontaneous adsorption of silver nanoparticles on Ti/TiO$_2$ surfaces. Antibacterial effect on Pseudomonas aeruginosa. J Colloid Interface Sci. 2010;350:402–408.
227. Zhang K, Lui VCH, Chen Y. et al. Delayed application of silver nanoparticles reveals the role of early inflammation in burn wound healing. Sci Rep. 2020;10:6338.
228. Mehrabani MG, Karimian R, Mehramouz B, Rahimi M, Kafil HS. Preparation of biocompatible and biodegradable silk fibroin/chitin/silver nanoparticles 3D scaffolds as a bandage for antimicrobial wound dressing. Int J Biol Macromol. 2018;114:961–971.
229. Jalili Tabaii M, Emtiazi G. Transparent nontoxic antibacterial wound dressing based on silver nano particle/bacterial cellulose nano composite synthesized in the presence of tripolyphosphate. J. Drug Deliv Sci Technol. 2018;44:244–253.
230. Meshulam-Derazon S, Nachumovsky S, Ad-El D, Sulkes J, Hauben DJ. Prediction of morbidity and mortality on admission to a burn unit. Plast Reconstr Surg. 2006;118:116–120.
231. Sabat R, Grutz G, Warszawska K, Kirsch S, Witte E, Wolk K, et al. Biology of interleukin-10. Cytokine Growth Factor Rev. 2010;21:331–344.
232. Albanesi C, Scarponi C, Giustizieri ML, Girolomoni G. Keratinocytes in inflammatory skin diseases. Curr Drug Targets Inflamm Allergy. 2005;4:329–334.
233. Accardo Palumbo A, Forte GI, Pileri D, Vaccarino L, Conte F, D'Amelio L. Analysis of IL-6, IL-10 and IL-17 genetic polymorphisms as risk factors for sepsis development in burned patients. Burns. 2012;38:208–213.

234. Sakallioglu AE, Basaran O, Karakayali H, Ozdemir BH, Yucel M, Arat Z, et al. Interactions of systemic immune response and local wound healing in different burn depths: an experimental study on rats. J Burn Care Res. 2006;27:357–366.
235. Dinescu S, Ignat SR, Lazar AD, Marin Ş, Danilă E, Marin MM, Udeanu DI, Ghica MV, Albu-Kaya MG, Costache M. Efficiency of multiparticulate delivery systems loaded with flufenamic acid designed for burn wound healing applications. J Immunol Res. 2019;2019, Article ID 4513108, 13 pages.
236. Seisenbaeva GA, Fromell K, Vinogradov VV. et al. Dispersion of TiO_2 nanoparticles improves burn wound healing and tissue regeneration through specific interaction with blood serum proteins. Sci Rep. 2017;7:15448. https://doi.org/10.1038/s41598-017-15792-w
237. Galkina OL, Ivanov VK, Agafonov AV, Seisenbaeva GA, Kessler VG. Cellulose nanofiber–titania nanocomposites as potential drug delivery systems for dermal applications. J Mater Chem B. 2015;3:1688–1698.
238. Galkina OL, Önneby K, Huang P, Ivanov VK, Agafonov AV, Seisenbaeva GA and Kessler VG. Antibacterial and photochemical properties of cellulose nanofiber–titania nanocomposites loaded with two different types of antibiotic medicines. J Mater Chem B. 2015;3:7125–7134.
239. Shao M, Hussain Z, Thu HE, Khan S, Katas H, Ahmed TA, Tripathy M, Leng J, Qin HL, Bukhari SNA. Drug nanocarrier, the future of atopic diseases: Advanced drug delivery systems and smart management of disease. Colloids Surf B Biointerfaces. 2016;147:475–491.
240. Chang EH, Harford JB, Eaton MA, Boisseau PM, Dube A, Hayeshi R, Swai H, Lee DS. Nanomedicine: past, present and future—a global perspective. Biochem Biophys Res Commun. 2015;468:511–517.
241. Schneider M, Stracke F, Hansen S, Schaefer UF. Nanoparticles and their interactions with the dermal barrier. Dermatoendocrinol. 2009;1:197–206.
242. Coty J-B, Vauthier C. Characterization of nanomedicines: A reflection on a field under construction needed for clinical translation success. J Control Release. 2018;275:254–268.
243. Severino P, Chaud MV, Shimojo A, Antonini D, Lancelloti M, Santana MH, Souto EB. Sodium alginate-cross-linked polymyxin B sulphate-loaded solid lipid nanoparticles: antibiotic resistance tests and HaCat and NIH/3T3 cell viability studies. Colloids Surf B Biointerfaces. 2015;129:191–197.
244. Shimojo AAM, Fernandes ARV, Ferreira NRE, Sanchez-Lopez E, Santana MHA, Souto EB. Evaluation of the influence of process parameters on the properties of resveratrol-loaded NLC using 2(2) full factorial design. Antioxidants. 2019;8:272.
245. Falagan-Lotsch P, Grzincic E, Murphy C. New advances in nanotechnology-based diagnosis and therapeutics for breast cancer: an assessment of active-targeting inorganic nanoplatforms. Bioconjug Chem. 2017;28(1):135–152.
246. Dadwal A, Baldi A, Kumar Narang R. Nanoparticles as carriers for drug delivery in cancer. Artif Cells Nanomed Biotechnol. 2018;46(sup2):295–305.
247. Sriraman S, Aryasomayajula B, Torchilin V. Barriers to drug delivery in solid tumors. Tissue Barriers. 2014;2(3):e29528.
248. Nie S. Understanding and overcoming major barriers in cancer nanomedicine. Nanomedicine. 2010;5(4):523–528.
249. Xue X, Liang X. Overcoming drug efflux-based multidrug resistance in cancer with nanotechnology. Chin J Cancer. 2012;31(2):100–109.
250. Soares S, Sousa J, Pais A, Vitorino C. Nanomedicine: principles, properties, and regulatory issues. Front Chem. 2018;6:360.

12 Nanomedicinal Materials for Diabetic Wound Healing and Tissue Regeneration

Kalpana Madgula
SAS Nanotechnologies LLC

Venkata Sreenivas Puli
Air Force Research Laboratory
Smart Nanomaterials Solutions LLC

CONTENTS

12.1 INTRODUCTION

Biomaterials have been utilized to effectively improve various aspects of healthcare and human life. Natural and synthetic materials have been utilized to derive biomaterials by chemical approaches involving metals, polymers, ceramics, or composite materials in applications involving hard and soft tissue Table 12.1 Illustrates some of the nanomaterials, their combination with other materials that are used in wound healing and skin regeneration. There has been an ongoing quest to find appropriate material systems that reduce infection at the wound site, to limit the exposure by efficient wound coverage. The matrix sometimes may support cell migration and growth but not necessarily act as a scaffold. The aim can be to provide the conditions or environment necessary for natural healing by preventing infection. Most of the time,

DOI: 10.1201/9781003140108-12

TABLE 12.1

Schematic Illustration of Nanomaterials and Other Combinations Used in Wound Healing and Skin Regeneration

Nanoparticles	Physical Characteristics or Scaffolds	Multi-Composite Materials	Other Materials (Micro or Nano)
Polymeric	Nanofibers	Nanofibers of metal or synthetic NPs	• Growth factors
• Natural			• Nucleic acids
• Synthetic			• Stem cells
Non-polymeric	Hydrogels	Films and membranes of metal or synthetic NPs	• Honey
• Metal			• Curcumin
• Ceramic			• Vegetable oils
• Lipid			
With suitable material combinations	Films and membranes	Hydrogels with metal or lipid NPs	
e.g., nanoparticle with bioactive component			
	Combination of above systems or materials	Multi-composite materials with natural NPs	

wound dressings require changing too often, whereas matrices provide a scaffold for the repair of tissue and hence persist in the wound for a sufficiently longer time [1]. In the context of wound healing, skin plays a major role.

Skin is the largest organ, which covers and protects the human body from the outside world. Injury to the epidermis (the outer protective layer of the skin) can be repaired; injury to the dermis would be triggered by wound healing mechanisms by which it can repair itself (as it contains blood vessels and infiltrating leukocytes) [2, 3] and which include the production of collagen, homeostasis, inflammation/proliferation with rebuilding the matrix with a combination of collagen and other extracellular matrix (ECM) materials. Most of the dermis made up of cells of fibroblasts, which produce collagen and elastin at the wound site, which could replace the damaged tissue with the connective skin tissue. However, the well-orchestrated events/stages can be impaired when there is considerable damage to dermis or epidermis due to injury or burns, which makes wound repair complex due to the destruction of cells and matrix involved in rebuilding and/or remodeling the skin. When there is a missing link among the order of events that occur during the healing, the wound may become chronic, potentially affecting the patient's progression to recover and therefore leading to a chain of collapsing events of wound care.

Figure 12.1 illustrates the timeline of events that are overlapped with wound healing stages after an injury or damage to the skin. When injury triggers wound healing, complex biological events kick in, creating four important steps: hemostasis and clotting, inflammation, proliferation, and tissue remodeling. Once hemostasis and clotting are achieved, healing of the wound advances to inflammation, proliferation, and remodeling in a few hours to days. Inflammation involves the removal of pathogenic bacteria from the wound site by the infiltration of immune cells, cytokine

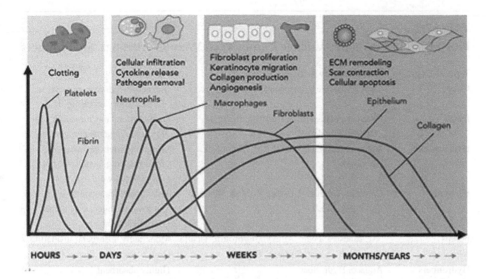

FIGURE 12.1 Depiction of interconnected phases in wound healing over the time line. After the preliminary phase of homeostasis and clotting the progress of wound through a period of inflammation, proliferation, and remodeling. Adapted with permission from Ref 4 Copyright 2013 and Elsevier.

release, and subsequently recruitment of other cells and production of ECM. After the inflammation stage, which persists for a couple of days, collagen is produced by the recruitment of fibroblasts and also endorsed by re-epithelialization and angiogenesis at this stage. The final stage of wound healing revolves around remodeling events: contracting scar, reworking the ECM, and apoptotic cell mechanisms [4].

Depending on the severity of injury, either cells or matrix needed for the skin restoration are in short supply or damaged, which further impedes the healing, which is slow, and increases the potential for scaring. The market has a broad range of treatments that manage wounds, and wound-care methods and are classified into standard or advanced [5], with a few examples of wound dressings listed in Table 12.2. In this direction, a vast number of significant research articles and reviews are available in the literature that detail fundamental aspects of wound healing [6] and mechanism [3]. There are also reports that comprise a variety of material classes or forms that claim the basis of what they intend to treat. However, efficiency toward the healing process remains the challenge. Various materials have been utilized to make wound dressings in the form of films and foam dressings, a few of them with biologics or with materials or properties such as antibacterial or components that can promote cell migration. Furthermore, commercially, there are treatments that include skin substitutes or the cells that are derived from the skin or tissue of de-epidermized dermis or the cells from fibroblasts and keratinocytes embedded in a biological matrix or delivery agent. Many wound-repair mechanisms are not completely clear, so the reader is directed to reviews [7–9] that could provide a comprehensive study of wound healing, for example, reviews on therapies involving gene and stem cells [10, 11], role of mechanical forces in wound healing [12–14], and immune response

TABLE 12.2

Illustration of Currently Available Commercial Wound Dressings and Products

Type of Dressing	Commercially Available Products	Notes
Gauge	Curity, Vaseline gauze, Xeroform	Inexpensive, drying, may cause further injury on changing
films	Bioclusive, Blisterfilm, Cutifilm, flexigrid, OpSite, Tegaderm	Occlusive, retains moisture, only for non-exudative compounds
Hydrocolloids	Aquacel, Comfeel, DuoDERM, Granuflex, Tegasorb	Long times between changes, fluid-trapping, occlusive, not for infected wounds
Hydrogels	Carrasyn, Curagel, NU-Gel, Purilon, Restore, SAF-gel, XCell	Rehydrates dry wounds, easy removal/changes, may cause over-hydration
Foams	3M Adhesive, Foam, Allevyn, Lyofoam, Ticelle	Moderately absorbent, insulating
Alginates	Algisite, Kaltostat, Sorbsan, Tegagen	Highly absorbent, hemostatic
Hydrofibers	Aquacel Hydrofiber	Highly absorbent
Tissue engineered skin substitutes	Alloderm, Apligraf, Biobrane, Bioseed, Dermagraft, Epicel, EZ Derm, Halograft, Integra Omnigraft, Laserskin, Myskin, TransCyte	Addresses deficient growth factors and cytokines, expensive, risk of infection, antigenicity

Source: Adapted from Ref 5; copyright 2017, https://creativecommons.org/licenses/by-nc/4.0/

to biomaterial implants [15]. A comprehensive list of nanocomposite materials, and their combinations for use in wound-healing antimicrobial materials is illustrated in Tables 12.3 and are categorized with respect to therapeutic uses based on NPs composition and properties, corresponding to the bacterial types [16].

Wounds are healed slowly or turn chronic due to various conditions related to the person's age (old people vs younger), obesity, diabetes, vascular disease, or high blood pressure [17]. Delayed wound healing is influenced by the type of bacteria on the wound surface (or infection by bacteria, fungi, or microbes that slow the healing), non-compliance with the therapies, poor control of blood sugar levels (especially in the case of foot ulcers), or wound care management. Injuries in people with diabetes commonly get infected, often leading to limb loss. Infections caused by these pathogens require multiple treatments and a broad spectrum of antibiotics. Most treatments are ineffective and expensive, due to most patients suffering from wounds with resistant microorganisms identified by the World Health Organization [18, 19]. Further, in developing countries, where a large proportion of patients are diabetic, the turnaround time for results, from the time of treatment to the wound being fully healed, can be matter of months, which aggravates the wound. This has raised a need for research, modification, and development of compounds that can treat antibiotic-resistant microorganisms in a low-cost, long-term manner. However, there is no single treatment option or modality for diabetic foot ulcer (DFU) management, and clinically a comprehensive treatment strategy is suggested and adopted by the diabetic wound physicians and surgeons [19].

TABLE 12.3

Schematic Representation of Nanocomposite Combinations as Wound Healing Antimicrobial Materials

NP Composite	Therapeutic Effects	Mechanism of Bactericidal Effects	Bacterial Species	NPs Properties	Remarks
Silver and gold NPs loaded into chitosan	Disinfection and keeping wound moist	Silver ion release	S. aureus, E. Coli	Gold NPs = <5 nm; silver = 10 nm space; lattice = 0.2122 and 0.2231 nm; chitosan pores size = 20–50 μm	Safe to mammalian cells
Solid lipid NP formulation	Disinfection, preventing inflammation, and increasing collagen-I deposition	LL37 and serpin have synergic toxic effects against gram-negative and gram-positive bacteria.	S. aureus, E. Coli	Size = 214.9±2.2 nm	Enhanced wound closure in BJ fibroblast cells and keratinocytes
Poly(N-isopropylacrylamide) (PNIAPM) inverse opal particles loaded with vancomycin	Disinfection and promoting angiogenesis and collagen deposition	Release of vancomycin in responded to temperature elevation caused by bacterial infection-induced inflammation	S. aureus	Silica colloidal crystal beads=250 nm	
Carbohydrate-coated gold-silver NPs	Disinfection and promoting tissue regeneration		S. aureus, E. Coli, Enterobacter cloacae	AuNP = 60.96 nm – 43.4 mV; Ag-NP = 216.8 nm – 54.2 mV; Au-AgNP = 147.0 nm – 31.5 mV	Showed no toxicity against skin keratinocytes or RBCs
Silver-incorporated nanocellulose fibers	disinfection	Silver ion release	E. Coli	Silver NPs = 12.578±3.34 nm	

(Continued)

TABLE 12.3 (Continued)
Schematic Representation of Nanocomposite Combinations as Wound Healing Antimicrobial Materials

NP Composite	Therapeutic Effects	Mechanism of Bactericidal Effects	Bacterial Species	NPs Properties	Remarks
Quaternized ammonium chitosan-Ce6	Disinfection, prevention of inflammation and induction of endothelial migration and proliferation	ROS production and bacterial membrane disruption under irradiation	S. aureus, E. Coli	250.6±4.03 nm; 20.5±0.42 mV; PDI = 0.148±0.016	Synergic chemical and photodynamic antibacterial impact
Hydrogel nanofibrous membrane	disinfection	Preventing biofilm growth, production of active oxygen species (O_2)	Bacillus subtilis, E. Coli	85±37 nm	High cytocompatibility
Hydrogel composed of PEP and Ag@rGO	Disinfection, prevention of inflammation and induction of re-epithelialization and collagen deposition	The antibacterial effect of hydrogel is related to Ag@rGO. The mechanism of toxicity was not investigated	Methicillin-resistant S. aureus	Ag@rGO nanosheets = 3–5 nm	thermoresponsive
Bimetallic Fe-Cu nanocomposite [26]	Disinfection, preventing inflammation	The antibacterial effect of hydrogel is related to Fe-Cu. The mechanism of toxicity was not investigated.	S. aureus, E. Coli	14.4±5.8 nm	Biocompatible and safe
Agarose matrix nanocomposite containing the cesium salt of phosphor-tungstic heteropolyacid	disinfection	Toxicity was not investigated. Acidifying the infected wound area	S. aureus, E. Coli, ATCC Candida albicans, Aspergillus fumigatus	21±4 nm	
Tigecycline NP incorporated chitosan-platelet-rich plasma (PRP) hydrogel	disinfection	Tigecycline release and damage bacterial membrane	S. aureus	97±18 nm, +37±15 mV; PDI< 0.3	
Nanocomposite consisted of gold-silver core and CuO2 shell	Disinfection, induction of re epithelialization and collagen deposition	Silver ion release under irradiation	S. aureus, E. Coli,	190 nm	Light responsive
AuNP@LL37 contained pro-angiogenic (VEGF) plasmids	Disinfection, promoting angiogenesis and tissue granulation	Disruption of bacterial membranes	S. aureus	80–130 nm, + 18.63±3.27 mV	

(Continued)

TABLE 12.3   (Continued)
Schematic Representation of Nanocomposite Combinations as Wound Healing Antimicrobial Materials

NP Composite	Therapeutic Effects	Mechanism of Bactericidal Effects	Bacterial Species	NPs Properties	Remarks
ssDNA-AgNP@GO	Disinfection, induction of re-epithelialization and collagen deposition	Silver ion release, ROS production, membrane disruption and interference with ATP production and metabolism	S. aureus, E. Coli, P. aeruginosa, B subtilis	50–200 nm; −27.5 mV	Effective against wide range of bacteria
Poly(vinyl alcohol) (PVA) – alginate (SA) hydrogel with Tb+2 and rGO	Disinfection, preventing inflammation and increasing collagen-1 deposition	Tb+2 and rGO destroyed the bacterial membrane in a synergic effect.	S. aureus, P aeruginosa		
Poly (vinyl alcohol) (PVA) – Melamine formaldehyde PVA-MFR/AgNP) films, sprays, and dressings [18]	Antimicrobial efficacy, keeping wound moist, reusability and long term storage	Silver ion release	S. aureus, P aeruginosa, Enterobacter Cloacae, B subtilis		Treating microorganisms from diabetic foot ulcers, in vitro studies
Hybrid hydrogel consisted of 3- (tri- methoxysilyl) propyl methacrylate and mesoporous silica modified CuS NP	Disinfection proliferation, angiogenesis, and tissue regeneration	Generation of ROS and disruption of bacterial membrane	S. aureus, E. Coli	25 nm	Under NIR irradiation, showed photothermal/ photodynamic properties
Ag/AgBr /MSNs	disinfection	Silver ion release, generation of ROS under irradiation, and triggering immune response	S. aureus, E. Coli	100 nm; ±34.1 mV	
Chitosan modified with AIMSOA and MPEG-COOH	disinfection	Disruption of bacterial membrane	S. aureus		Showed no cytotoxic or hemolytic effect
MoS$_2$@PDA-Ag nanosheets	disinfection	Silver ion release, disruption of biofilm and bacterial membrane	S. aureus	Size = 200-500 nm; thickness = 1.3 nm; −22mV	Photothermal therapy disrupted the biofilm and bacterial membrane and increased their permeability to NPs/ions

Source: Adapted with permission from Ref (16); copyright 2020

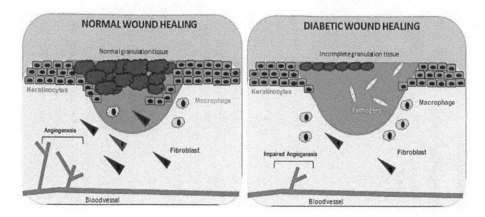

FIGURE 12.2 Schematic representation of the factors that affect wound healing in normal and diabetic conditions. Adapted with permission from Ref 20; Copyright 2020, MDPI (https://www.ncbi.nlm.nih.gov/pmc/articles/PMC7353122/) attribution to Creative Commons (CC BY 4.0).

There are number of biological factors that affect normal wound healing and in diabetic conditions [20], shown in Figure 12.2. The cells in diabetic wounds experience detrimental effects in their phenotype, which could undermine their ability to produce and react to the cytokine and growth factor cascade, which is the normal mechanism in wound healing. Within a diabetic wound, cells that get affected may include macrophages, fibroblasts, and keratinocytes, and hence the widely available methods are based on influencing the performance of these sets of cells. In contrast to normal wounds, DFUs are categorized by decreased response to cells and growth factors, weakened formation in the blood vessels, an overaccumulation of inflammatory macrophages along with large increase in fibroblast-cell and keratinocyte-cell apoptosis. In normal wounds, keratinocytes help in re-epithelialization by migrating and proliferating at the wound site, but at the ulcer site, keratinocytes lead to high levels of cell loss. Similarly, ulcer fibroblasts suffer untimely apoptosis or programmed cell death and generate excess collagen, which can avert the formation of healthy tissue by disassembling the enzymes in the matrix metalloproteinase family (MMPs). In the last phase, the macrophages facilitate controlled inflammation in normal wounds, which could boost the tissue regrowth through growth factor production (e.g., which can be associated with the ECM replaced by collagen type I, in place of collagen III) intermediated via PDGF and TGF-β. However, macrophages in wounds with diabetic conditions (in contrast to the normal conditions) would not evolve normally from the inflammatory stage to that of rebuilding the tissues or production of growth factors. The above-mentioned factors can contribute to dysregulation in cellular and molecular functions around wound environment, which creates an unfavorable response toward normal healing and ends up impairing the healing of ulcers in diabetics [21].

Currently available standard methods [22] of primary treatment in wounds consists of swabbing the infected area, cleaning the wound to remove tissue debris, and applying the dressing. However, to tackle advanced stages like extended skin abrasions, the use of skin autografts or allografts with the use of split thickness would be required, and these procedures deal with the safety issues associated with disease transmission and rejection of immune system.

When skin is undamaged and intact, there is a balanced colonization of bacteria. However, a wound jeopardizes this balance and may lead to infection. Further, the occurrence of infection-causing species such as *Staphylococcus aureus*, as in case of acute wounds and aerobic or facultative pathogens, can be key infective sources in the case of chronic wounds. Ulcers in chronic wounds require treatment of the aetiologic factors responsible for causing them and hence the occurrence of wound debridement also plays a part in healing the wound to prevent infection. If infection in the wound persists, alternative therapies with antimicrobials and antibiotics for the causative microbe are recommended. In the United States alone, the majority of chronic wound cases in clinics are 6 million per year, leading to the cost of 25 bn dollars per annum, and furthermore, they increase to a secondary injury stage due to rise of ailments such as diabetes in the general population. Hence this triggered intense research among academicians and companies for more advanced technologies with improved outcomes [23].

Table 12.1 lists various nanomaterials (metal, polymer, and both) combinations; some are currently used for wound healing and skin regeneration [24–29]. Das et al. [26] have reported an iron–copper nanocomposite (NC) powder alone or with iodine or as a cotton swab (or wound bed) treated with NC powder to study antimicrobial activity in vivo studies on diabetic wound healing in infected Wistar albino rats. Figure 12.3A presents the antimicrobial effectiveness of these composite materials

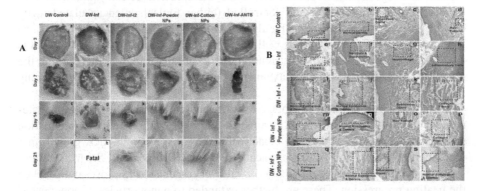

FIGURE 12.3   (A) Representative pictures of the results of in vivo study conducted after treating *S Aureus*–infected diabetic rats with wound healing materials; their progression from Day 3,7,14 & 21. (B) Schematic representation of dermal tissues (of rats) stained by Hematoxylin and Eosin. **DW Control (a–d)** of simple untreated diabetic wound, **DW-inf (e–h)**- untreated infected diabetic wound. **DW-inf-I2 (i–l)**- Infected diabetic wound treated with (0.2 M) iodine; **DW-inf-powder NPs (m–p)** and **DW-inf-cotton NPs (q-t)** infected diabetic wound treated with nanocomposite powder and infected diabetic wound treated with cotton impregnated with nanocomposite respectively. **DW-inf-ANTB (u–x)** Representative infected diabetic wound treated with topical antibiotic, Mupirocin (Fig A). Reprinted with permission from [26] https://doi.org/10.1021/acsabm.9b00870) Copyright (2019) American Chemical Society.

compared with traditional antibiotics (e.g., Mupirocin). As shown in the figure and reported by authors, on day 7 wounds were better with antibiotic, but by day 21 wounds healed with NCs were scarless and complete. Similarly, Figure 12.3B images display histopathological assessment and observations of diabetic wounds for control and treated tissue specimens making use of all the combinations of prepared NC materials that showed no inflammatory signs except minimal changes but with promoted healing.

The following sections provide a brief introduction to nanomedicinal materials and/or biomaterials that mimic the skin extracellular matrix or are employed as wound dressings in forms such as nanofibers, films, and hydrogels (either polymeric or non-polymeric combinations) along with techniques to incorporate and transport bioactive factors to improve the healing characteristics to attain smart, ideal wound dressings.

12.2   NANOTECHNOLOGY BASED MODALITIES FOR WOUND HEALING

Nanotechnology-based therapies are known to be one an effective treatment method for wounds and complications in diabetics. Nanomaterials offer advantages such as tuned sizes and physicochemical properties in addition to their versatile usage. Moreover, they offer efficient cell adhesion properties due to high surface area-to-volume ratio along with the flexibility to functionalize and encapsulate bioactive agents or drug components to facilitate specific functions including healing of the wounds and regeneration of tissues [30]. Thus, nanoparticle delivery platforms have been employed in sustained and controlled (either topical or encapsulated) drug delivery, with cell specificity in a regulated manner [31]. Though oral drug delivery has large potential and benefits as well as barriers [32], nanoparticles offer benefits such as better penetration and distribution at the site of wound, ability to tune the efficiency, and properties or quantity and delivery of drugs by encapsulation for long term or till the wound is healed.

Current clinical strategies embrace "smart nanoplatforms" derived from materials in fibrous forms, hydrogels, foams, and sponges fabricated in combination with nanoparticles or encapsulate bioactive agents such as antibiotics, growth factors, peptides, nucleic acids, and extracellular matrix components. Smart nanoplatforms provide synergetic combination as delivery agents to improve and quicken the healing progression. These are further extended to nanoparticles of polymerics/ inorganics/lipids, liposomes, and dendrimers with the morphological variabilities of nanofibers and nanohydrogels. Normally, nanoparticles are coated with drugs by absorption, dissolution, or dispersion and form an aqueous core or shell around the particles or make covalent linkages with the matrix on the surface of nanoparticles [33]. The nanoparticles release the drug, which gets diffused, dissolved, or reduced with the effective assimilation in the biological systems. The drugs or active components absorbed on the wound dressings or embedded/encapsulated in nanofibers, foams, films, or hydrogels result in multicomponent nanocomposite systems [34] and promote rapid wound healing due to the augmented porosity and increased volume with surface mimicking the morphology of endogenous extracellular matrix. These porous nanocomposite systems allow fibroblasts and keratinocytes attachment and spreading to enable the synthesis of collagen and wound re epithelialization [35].

Nanoparticles of gold [36–38] and silver nanoparticles (AgNPs) [39] in the form of nanocomposite containing ε-polylysine/silver nanoparticles (EPL-g-butyl@ AgNPs) have been found to be antimicrobial against both the Gram-negative (i.e., *Pseudomonas aeruginosa*) and Gram-positive (i.e., *Staphylococcus aureus*) bacteria, without having toxicity towards mammalian cells. AgNPs are known to alter the structure of fibroblasts by suppressing them and differentiating into myofibroblasts and thus reducing the expression of collagen type-1. This effect ultimately results in quick contraction of the wound and subsequent re-epithelialization [40]. Polyvinyl alcohol-based silver nanocomposite (PVA-MFR/AgNP) films, sprays, and dressings [18, 19, 41, 42] have been prepared and studied for their antimicrobial activity in vitro toward the microorganisms responsible for diabetic foot ulcers. The antimicrobial composites were cast into films, soaked to form polyvinyl foams, and coated on to Whatman paper. The antimicrobial efficacy of such prepared dressing materials was tested against the prepared AgNPs. The composites were reported to be stable and not lose their antimicrobial activity with time. In another report, PVA and multiwalled CNT (MWCNTs) scaffolds prepared by conjugation with glucose oxidase were reported for wound healing [43]. The potential effect of kaolin as a short-term material with blood-clotting efficiency and nanocellulose as a long-term material with water-adsorption ability was utilized to make Kaolin-cellulose nanocomposites for wound healing [44]. Recently, case studies were carried out to check the efficacy of topical administration of AgNPs (1.8mg/mL of metallic silver) along with conventional antibiotics employed for the treatment of diabetic foot ulcers of Wagner classification degrees II and III and other chronic ulcers [45].

Other combinations of polymeric nanoparticles with or without inorganic NPs have proved to be efficient in moisture retention (e.g., bacterial cellulose), fibroblasts proliferation (i.e., chitosan NPs loaded on to calcium alginate hydrogels) As in the case of Docetaxel-loaded gelatin nanoparticles, gelatin help control the fluids loss and release of the drug (docetaxel) by enzymatic action and sorption that increased the antibacterial activity, rapid skin wound healing and re-epithelialization indicating the efficient loading that controlled the release and its functionality as wound dressing in vivo [46–48, 49]. Bioactive components for slow and sustained release are also employed for skin tissue regeneration. For example, curcumin-loaded NPs or curcumin-loaded chitosan NPs in collagen alginate scaffolds quicken the wound healing and granulation tissue formation in diabetic mice as compared to pure curcumin, which has the limitation of poor antioxidative and antimicrobial activity [49, 51].

12.3   BIOMATERIAL COMBINATIONS USED FOR WOUND HEALING AND TISSUE REGENERATION

Inspired by the natural development of fully biodegradable materials with enhanced bioactive functionalities and sustainability, researchers moved toward developing a combination of matrices including natural and synthetic biomaterials as matrices or scaffolds for wound healing materials. Ancient medicine has evidence about the use of biomaterials available in nature such as honey, curcumin, and vegetable oils [51–53].

Biomaterials used for biomedical applications can be categorized [54, 55] under metals and ceramics (for stents, orthopedic, and dental implants) and a vast number of polymer devices and implants for applications not limited to sutures, vascular grafts, tissue, and tissue replacements. Over the past few years, biomaterials have played a major role in the development of wound care materials in the form of dressings, with innovative strategies for fabricating natural, synthetic, and hybrid biomaterials and with the inclusion of bioactive components in the form of nanoparticles (antimicrobial activity), stem cells, and growth factors (wound closure, with increased re-epithelialization, cellularity, and angiogenesis). PLGA (poly (lactic-co-glycolic acid)), hyaluronic acid, chitosan, polylactic acid (PLA), Pluronic F-127 [56] (Pluronic F-127 curcumin hydrogel–supported re-epithelization and angiogenesis), PGA, PVA, PEG, PCL, PEI, cellulose and alginate or their copolymerized forms (e.g., PEG-PCL) are some of the commonly used biomaterial systems for diabetic wound healing.

Natural polymers are usually protein based or polysaccharide in nature. These have advantages like mimicking the ECM and stimulating the cell environments and are known to undergo naturally controlled degradation. They are limited by factors such as heterogeneity based on source a d high cost (protein based) and cause infections when used as implants [57]. However, when they are combined with synthetic ones, they can be made feasible by varying the processing conditions suitable to the applications. The intricacy of skin structure and the number of components involved makes it difficult to imitate in the research laboratory and find one fit for all [58]. In this category, synthetic polymers such as poly(lactic-co-glycolic) acid, polyanhydrides, polyethylene glycol, and others have a broad range of cell therapeutic potentialities with precise physical and chemical features or functional entities that could facilitate precise tuning while creating a blend of biomaterials. However, it is to be noted that the most important features critical to the potential use of any polymer are bioactivity, biodegradability, and biocompatibility.

One such class considered consisted of products based on tissue engineering that may contain living cells (or cellular) or biologically inert cells (or acellular) or cells derived from biological tissue origin (e.g., equine/bovine/porcine), human tissue (e.g., cadaveric skin), or plant materials (e.g., containing oxidized regenerated cellulose/collagen). On the other hand, materials are also categorized as synthetic or composites (having two or more components that may be biological or synthetic). The terms "biological" (i.e., synthesized by nature), "synthetic" (i.e., derived from human-made materials) or "composite" (i.e., derived from a mix of materials of various origin) are normally preferred to general terms such as "natural," "organic," or "biomatrix."

In the following paragraphs, a brief introduction of physicochemical and biological properties of some polymers that are natural and biobased with particular attention towards skin tissue repair field is discussed, and a few are mentioned as future alternative materials for the development of a new generation of environmentally friendly and smart wound dressings.

A comprehensive review of chemical and physical characteristics of collagen has been explained in the literature [59]. Collagen dressings are dressings that are derived from animal sources, such as bovine (cattle), equine (horse), or porcine (pig). The unique mechanical properties, stimulated cell adhesion, and proliferation capabilities, along with highly biocompatible, biodegradable intrinsic endogenous collagenases occurrence in collagen, makes them the ideal choice of materials for most biomedical applications. The increased level of matrix metalloproteinases (or MMPs) degrades the viable collagen, leading to chronic wounds; in these conditions, fibroblasts are also not able to control the activity of MMPs in a chronic wound as they are not able to sufficiently secrete the tissue inhibitors of MMPs (TIMPs). In these situations, collagen-based wound dressings have significantly as act as sacrificial substrates to tackle and control elevated levels of MMPs in the wound [60] that can in turn control wound aggravation. At the wound site, fibroblasts produce collagen molecules that aggregate to form fibrils ranging in the sizes of 10–500 nm diameter and to support tissue repair [61] or cell passage they can also facilitate themselves into fibrous networks. Medscape reported dressings [62] that are capable of maintaining suitable temperatures at the microenvironments of the wound site.

The dressings based on collagen can be made with varying size of pores or with antimicrobial ingredients to control the aggravation of infection; sometimes they even need a secondary dressing (in the form of gels, powders, or paste or even sheets that are freeze dried) to cover the infected wounds. Most of the collagen dressings can last up to seven days and are replaced based on wound type. Collagen-based wound dressings are now available in various forms (i.e., hydrogels, fibers made from electrospinning, or scaffolds with nanocrystalline materials) and designed to treat wounds due to burns or ulcers in diabetics [63, 64], minimize scar or tissue tightening, and increase the rate of epithelization. Among collagen materials, the most promising ones are those made into sponges and membranes (fibrous) that have wetting strength and are capable of being sutured to soft tissue materials and those that behave as template materials for growth of new tissues.

In 1993, the US Food and Drug Administration (USFDA) recognized silk fibroin (SF) [65] along with other natural biopolymers, owing to its unique features that include mechanical, structural and biocompatible, biodegradable, and versatile functionalities [66, 67]. Silk fibers are produced from the epithelial cells of spiders and silkworms and contain amino acids arranged in sheets that are embedded in a matrix that is amorphous, tough, and elastic. Similarly, silk made from Bombyx mori, has been recently reported to have superior properties such as processability, biodegradability, biocompatibility, and efficient processing and mechanical capabilities. Yu et al. [68a] have reported diabetic wound (or antimicrobial) dressings based on silkworm cocoon–based wound film (SCWF) in a $CaCl_2$-ethanol-H_2O solution, where sericin wrapped around SF has reduced silver ion (Ag+) into silver NPs (in situ) linked by peptide bonds and considered to be a green method. SF is a natural protein fiber whose properties can be compared to those of synthetic polymers, collagen, and poly (L-lactic acid) (PLA), and it has been employed in the treatment of wounds as sutures and dressings [68b, 69 a, b] in varied morphologies from nanoparticles to fibers. There are two proteins in silkworms: fibroin and sericin fibroin. The main component of silk, is semi crystalline, tough, and strong acts as inner core that provide mechanical strength, and sericin is the outer coating which is amorphous or glue like with adhesive or binding properties to bind fibers of SF. Each silk fiber contains two SF filaments coated with sericin. SF has long been employed as scaffolds for reconstructing skin or encapsulating and releasing molecules that are bioactive due to their efficient cell adhesion or attaching capability [70, 71].

Matrices made of silk and polyvinyl alcohol (PVA) with a drug (e.g., ciprofloxacin) and active molecules (epidermal growth factors) [72, 73] improved adhesion/proliferation with human dermal cells in in vitro studies that favored conditions like closing the wound and depositing the collagen and repeated epithelialization in in vivo or in rabbit models. Similarly, Ju and coworkers reported nanomatrices of polyethylene oxide (PEO) with SF made by electrospinning, to study the inflammatory mechanism of cytokines in burn wounds of mouse models [74]. SF nanoparticles integrated into hydrocolloids have been studied by Lee et al. [75]. Sericin in silk fibers gets crosslinked in the presence of UV light to form a hydrogel that shows efficient mechanical and cell adhesion properties, promoting angiogenesis, regulation of growth factors, and recruitment of stem cells that heal the wounded site. Silk polymers based on genetic engineering have been used as scaffolds for (3D) cell culture in drug delivery or in tissue regeneration, which can be easily recovered or reproduced [76].

Another class of protein-based filament polymers is called Keratins, with rich features for biocompatible, biodegradable, hemostatic materials with potential applications in healing wounds, repairing tissue, and delivering drugs as well as in cosmetics [77, 78]. Keratin fibers also have been combined with other natural or synthetic polymeric systems as natural kertin has high molecular weight and low viscoelasticity e.g. keratin has been combined with PEO, PVA, SF or poly(3-hydroxybutyrate-co-3-hydroxyvalerate), chitosan, and gelatin to facilitate electrospinning into fibers. Moreover, keratin fibers lack intrinsic antimicrobial activity, they are incorporated with materials like silver NPs, antibiotics or bactericidal agents to render them antimicrobial.

Some of the naturally derived polysaccharide-based biopolymers are also utilized for wound healing and are discussed in the following paragraphs. Hyaluronic acid (HA) is a linear polysaccharide composed of alternating (1-4)-β linked D-glucuronic and (1-3)-β linked Nacetyl-D-glucosamine residues, having non-immunogenic response This glycosaminoglycan (GAG) is a component of the ECM of connective tissues [79]. Due to its prominent hygroscopicity, it can be used to construct hydrogels, which promote wound healing and controlled release of active compounds when encapsulated in three-dimensional HA networks [80, 81]. HA-based electrospun fibers, either pure or in combination with other biomacromolecules [82], have been proposed for tunable degradation and sustained release in vitro and in vivo.

Extensive literature can be found concerning exogenous applications of HA to wounds. Various HA sources, formulations, and delivery systems have been used in clinical trials. A rich natural source of HA is fetal membrane, especially the jelly substance from the umbilical cord and the amnion. The amniotic membrane has been used in traditional medicine and also in the form of a commercially available dressing in wound treatment. Studies have revealed that the amniotic membrane, even after various processing and preservation procedures, contains high amounts of HMWHA. This component of the amnion is one of the factors responsible for its beneficial actions observed in chronic wound therapy. An effective wound healing therapy remains one of the greatest challenges of modern clinical medicine.

Hyaluronic acid is a biologically active molecule that regulates tissue repair process on multiple levels should be considered a safe and effective option to be used in skin repair [83, 84].

Chitosan (CS), another polysaccharide, is linear and consists of β (1–4)-D-glucosamine and N-acetyl-D-glucosamine groups with random distribution. Due to its intrinsic antifungal, antibacterial, hemostatic, and muco-adhesive properties, chitosan has been widely exploited in the biomedical field for wound and burn treatments [85, 86]. Several dressing architectures have been proposed: CS-Aloe vera membranes, thyme oil-CS films, CS-gelatin sponges, CS-silk hydrogels, CS-cellulose films cinnamon oil-CS/polyethylene oxide nanofibers, and CS/poly(3-hydroxybutyrateco-3-hydroxyvalerate) scaffolds. Along with these, carboxymethyl CS and methacrylate glycol CS have been synthesized and reported to be water soluble derivatives for use in treating or healing wounds [87].

Alginate (Alg) is another polysaccharide-based biopolymer, abundantly found in algae or bacterial production. Due to its hydrophilic nature, it can absorb exudates from a wound to maintain moisture around the wound and provide biocompatibility [88, 89]. Alginate, when combined with other enzymes or antimicrobials, removes dead tissues or promotes new tissue formation. Alginate dressings are also useful as delivery platforms to provide controlled release of therapeutic substances to exuding wounds (e.g., pain-relieving, antibacterial, and anti-inflammatory agents). Biodegradable Na Alg/PVPI (povidone iodine complex) films and Ca-Alg/PVPI beads have displayed antimicrobial and antifungal activities. Moreover, Na-Alg/PVPI films have been shown to reduce the inflammatory response and accelerate the wound healing, providing a controlled release of PVPI [90].

Heparin polysaccharide-based biopolymer plays an important role in many biological processes, via its interaction with various proteins, and hydrogels. Nanoparticles comprising heparin exhibit attractive properties such as anticoagulant activity and growth factor binding as well as antiangiogenic and apoptotic effects, making them great candidates for emerging applications. Prospects are promising for heparin-containing polymeric biomaterials in diverse applications, ranging from cell carriers for promoting cell differentiation to nanoparticle therapeutics for cancer treatment [91]. These are being reviewed in the literature. Heparin has been identified since 1935 as an anticoagulant for blood because of its binding capability with serine protease inhibitor antithrombin, causing the inhibitor to inactivate thrombin.

12.4 REGENERATIVE THERAPIES FOR TISSUE FORMATION

Regenerative therapy, in general, is a combination of targeted genes, treatment with stem cells, molecules with solubility, and repeated programming with cells or tissue repair/engineering [92]. In all these techniques, basic principles of engineering are applied that enable natural wound healing in the presence of factors with physical/biochemical conditions. In all these a number of bioactive factors, such as growth factors and cytokines (extracellular signaling proteins secreted by immune cells) get involved in tissue repair mechanisms and promote dermal regeneration. Cytokines can be therapeutic targets whose intervention and modulation has gained significance in the wound healing process. Thus, the desired outcome can be achieved either by enhancing (recombinant cytokine, gene transfer) or inhibiting (cytokine or receptor antibodies, soluble receptors, signal transduction inhibitors, antisense) the particular cytokine and its response. On the other hand, growth factors, the signaling proteins that gets released at the wound site, are required for communication between cells such as smooth muscle cells (SMC), fibroblasts, myofibroblasts, keratinocytes, endothelial cells (EC) and immune cells [93, 100]. The all cells are angiogenic in nature with biologically relevant functions of new cells that are transplanted for organ substitution by supplying them with oxygen and nutrients [94]. Different studies on human patients have confirmed that growth factors such as platelet-derived growth factor (PDGF) are involved in enhancing the wound-healing rate in acute wounds and even provide complete healing in chronic wounds [95, 96]. Recent trends in regenerative medicine are focusing on alternate clinical methods for regenerating skin or tissue utilizing exogenously created growth factors.

12.5 CHALLENGES AND FUTURE PERSPECTIVES

Besides nanomedicinal materials and biomaterials, therapies based on stem cells have recently been found to be partially effective for tissue engineering applications; however, considering the potential [97] risks of malignant teratoma formation and long-term adverse effects of the stem cells, more extensive studies are required in this regard. Thus far, various procedures have been employed in the treatment of skin ulcers, among which cell-based therapy involving adult stem cells has emerged as a promising treatment to promote scarless wound healing. Due to their capability in immunomodulation and tissue regeneration, the human MSCs have received particular attention as compared to other stem cells. The sources for MSCs can be autologous or from young adult tissues, umbilical cord or placenta. Clinical data demonstrated that autologous MSC transplantation promoted healing in all wound-repair phases. However, it is difficult to harvest and isolate an optimum MSC pools in a highly pure state, and thus the application in novel therapeutic treatments are limited. It is necessary to understand underlying mechanisms of stem cell cellular and molecular behaviors for efficient applications in clinics, especially when used to treat wounds.

Similarly, immunotherapy treatments are also being considered for wound healing applications, but careful consideration needs to be taken when applied to clinical settings [98]. Inadequate immune responses and imbalance in immune signaling are common in diabetic and elderly patients, where high levels of the pro-inflammatory cytokine interleukin-1 (IL-1) play a central role [99], as an excess of IL-1β–driven inflammatory signals in wounds may trigger a cascade of events that delay wound closure. For example, an excess of IL-1β could slow down the removal of inflammatory cells from the wound bed, senescence of fibroblast cells, and degradation of repair-promoting growth factors and proteins of the extracellular matrix (ECM) because of increased levels of matrix metalloproteinases (MMPs). Hence blocking IL-1β or inhibiting the IL-1 receptor, and IL-1R1 signal may promote healing through receptor antagonists, selectively in low doses, which is not sustainable due to the short half -life period of proteins. Higher doses may help, and residual IL-1Ra may lead to adverse side effects or systemic devious infections. Tan et al. developed and reported a protein-engineering technique to locally block IL-1β and deliver an ECM-binding sequence that is derived from the heparin-binding domain of placental growth factor (e.g., IL-1Ra/PlGF$_{123-141}$) and well-known clinically approved platelet-derived growth factor for chronic wound treatment (and PDGF-BB/PlGF$_{123-141}$) without the need of biomaterial matrix, and it showed enhanced healing conditions and anti- inflammatory cells growth factors and cytokines in diabetic mice after 9 days of exposure. But again, immunotherapy treatments are proven to be risky, as reported in the case of cancer and autoimmune diseases [100]. In addition, there is a lack of information on long-term outcomes of skin wound treatment using such regenerative therapies. With the learnings and complexities involved in all cell-based engineering therapies, it is important to consider and improve the laboratory-based research when applied in clinical practice [101].

Becaplermin gel (Regranex®; Smith & Nephew, Inc., London, UK) is an early commercially available and approved wound gel or dressing by the USFDA to treat foot ulcers based on diabetic neuropathy. Becaplermin gel is a recombinant platelet-derived growth factor (PDGF)-BB produced by insertion of the gene into yeast Saccharomyces cerevisiae. It has also been warned recently that the use of Becaplermin gel can be carcinogenic and can cause the malignant conditions for diabetic populations. Further research is needed to compare the use of Becaplermin gel with other available biologics and skin substitutes. After a better understanding is reached regarding the risks, the patient and healthcare provider may decide whether the reward is worth the risks [102]. We maintain that these problems will certainly be resolved by developments in cell biology, tissue engineering, and regenerative medicine. According to a few advanced studies performed on traditional materials with novel functionalities as reported recently by researchers at Imperial College, London, a new molecule based on sponges made of collagen is believed to change the way traditional materials work with the body; also known as traction force-activated payloads (TrAPs), their method lets materials talk to the body's natural repair systems to drive healing [103].

Nanomedicinal treatments, i.e. therapies based on nanoparticles or NPs, NPs in some cases, believed to be toxic and cause damage to cells (or genes) or tissues due to their imbalanced distribution in free radicals and antioxidants (or that induce oxidative stress) and also raised a major concern in terms of their composition, particle size and varied shape. Yang et al. [104] reported comparative studies of nanoparticle toxicity in four different NPs of metal and carbon-based nanomaterials. For example, gold NPs are believed to trigger the rate of cell growth and cell differentiation in the case of keratinocytes that may pose cell toxicity when increased in doses. Similarly zinc oxide NPs can lead to cancer-causing conversions, and most of the NPs are believed to produce oxidative stress by generating reactive oxygen species along the membranes and further lead to cell death as well as depletion in glutathione. Unusually small NPs can lead to increased leakage of drugs or bioactive compounds before reaching the target or trigger undesirable entry into blood-brain barrier, and may initiate coagulation of blood, etc. [105]. Besides, when translated to clinical applications, the results may vary for the performance of nanomedicinal materials due to the slight differences in efficacy of NPs as compared to in vitro studies, or variation in the type of animal models or pathology of diseased site or tissue [106].

Considering the intricacy of pathological events in the wound, especially the ones with chronic conditions, surprisingly not enough methods or therapies are considered to get to the next stage of approval by the regulatory bodies (or USFDA) and further feasible application in clinics. There can be multiple reasons, such as insufficient data to understand various pathological and physiological events occurring when patient is being treated as well as other aspects, such as unpredictability with respect to age, population, or individual patient; multiple observations or symptoms; lack of awareness; cost associated with the treatment or clinical trials; and alternative strategies for treatment. No single treatment or a device can eliminate all the complexities that arise from DFUs [107]. There is insufficient data, not only in the academic research but in trials conducted at the clinical stage, such as standard data reports for variation in the wounds (e.g., full thickness, inherent conditions such as diabetic or infected, etc.) due to the lack of standardized wound models or procedures to study various stages of healing (identifying wound bioburden, changes in wound healing biomarkers, and their production e.g., cytokines or MMPs) and either biased or lack of comparative evidence among reported results. Societies like the American Association for the Advancement of wound care, European Wound Management Association (EWMA), and Canadian Association of Wound Care have recently initiated a set of proposals and comprehensive guidelines for a standard wound care management [19, 108–110].

12.6   CONCLUSIONS

The worldwide estimate of diabetes in 2015 was 8.8% and is projected to rise to 10.4% by 2040, raising a public health alarm. Diabetes is a chronic condition that involves a dysfunction of the pancreas, which impairs insulin production in the normal way and can lead to fluctuations or imbalance of blood glucose levels [111]. The severity of diabetes can lead to failure of kidneys, loss of sight, cardiovascular ailment, venous insufficiency, and peripheral neuropathy [112]. The last two conditions may lead to impaired or failed sensation or loss of limb sensitivity in patients with diabetes, also called diabetic foot ulcers (DFUs), leading to skin lesions or amputation of the limbs. To avoid long-term hospitalizations, it is always preferable to prevent DFUs or to use the best foot-based therapies and topical treatments (that promote natural healing) due to hard-to-heal wounds or most common ulcers in diabetic patients. In general, wounds get healed by a programmed and challenging task of cellular and molecular events occurring in a coordinated manner. Any imbalance in this coordination or harmony can lead to disturbance and delay in healing.

Researchers always explore nature-mimicking pathways to balance the irregularities of many diseases, including wound healing. In an effort to balance the demand and availability of natural resources, environmentally friendly, sustainable, biodegradable materials combinations and energy consumptions play a pivotal role in drug designing, packaging, and advanced manufacturing methods to meet human health needs while combating pollution. Taking inspiration from nature and finding ways to increase sustainable material development, these ongoing demands can be dealt with effectively by interdisciplinary and innovative research strategies in tissue engineering and regenerative medicine with the collaborative contribution from materials chemists, cell biologists, and researchers from other disciplines.

ACKNOWLEDGMENTS

One of the authors, KM acknowledges the support of her supervisor, Sumedh P Surwade, CEO and Founder, SAS Nanotechnologies LLC for working toward polymer nanocomposite self-healing materials. VSP acknowledges for National Research Council Senior Research Associate Fellowshp (National Academy of Science, Washington, DC, USA and Energy Directorate, Air Force Research Laboratory, Kirtland Air Force Base, NM and Materials and Manufacturing Directorate, Air Force Research Laboratory, Wright Patterson Air Force Base, OH, USA.

ABBREVIATIONS

AgNPs	silver nanoparticles
Alg	alginate
Ca-Alg/PVPI	calcium alginate/povidone iodine complex
CaCl$_2$	calcium Chloride
CNT	carbon nanotubes
CS	chitosan
DFUs	diabetic foot ulcers
EC	endothelial cells
ECM	extracellular matrix
EPL-g-butyl@AgNPs	ε-polylysine/silver nanoparticles
EWMA	European Wound Management Association
HA	hyaluronic acid
HMWHA	high molecular weight hyaluronic acid
IL-1	Cytokine interleukin-1
PCL	polycaprolactone
PDGF	platelet-derived growth factor
PEG	poly (ethylene glycol)
PEI	polyethylenimine
PEO	polyethylene oxide
PGA	poly(glycolic acid)
PIGF	placental growth factor
PLA	polylactic acid
PLGA	(poly (lactic-co-glycolic acid)),
PVA-MFR	polyvinyl alcohol- Melamine formaldehyde
MMPs	matrix metalloproteinase family
MSCs	mesenchymal stem cells
MWCNTs	Multiwalled carbon nanotubes
NC	Nanocomposite
SCWF	silkworm cocoon–based wound film
SF	Silk Fibroin

SMC	smooth muscle cells
Na Alg/PVPI	Sodium alginate /povidone iodine complex
TE	tissue engineering
TGF-β	Transforming growth factor beta
TrAPs	traction force-activated payloads
USFDA	US Food and Drug Administration
UV	ultraviolet

REFERENCES

1. International consensus. Acellular matrices for the treatment of wounds. An expert working group review. Wounds International: London, 2010.
2. https://advancedtissue.com/2015/09/the-6-steps-of-the-wound-healing-process/
3. Mandla, S., Huyer, L. D., and Radisic, Mi. (2018). Review- Multimodal bioactive material approaches for wound healing. APL Bioeng. 2, 021503; https://doi.org/10.1063/1.5026773
4. Shechter, R., and Schwartz, M. (2013). CNS sterile injury: just another wound healing? Trends Mol Med. 19(3), 135–143. doi: 10.1016/j.molmed.2012.11.007.
5. Han, G., Ceilley, R. (2017). Chronic wound healing: a review of current management and treatments. Adv Ther. 34(3), 599–610. doi: 10.1007/s12325-017-0478-y.
6. Stejskalová, A., and Almquist, B. D. (2017). Using biomaterials to rewire the process of wound repair. Biomater. Sci. 5, 1421.
7. Martin, P. (1997). Wound healing – aiming for perfect skin regeneration. Science. 276, 75–81. doi:10.1126/science.276.5309.75
8. Gurtner, G. C., Werner, S., Barrandon, Y., and Longaker, M. T. (2008). Wound repair and regeneration. Nature. 453, 314–321. doi: 10.1038/nature 07039.
9. Eming, S. A., Martin, P., and Tomic-Canic, M. (2014). Wound repair and regeneration: mechanisms, signaling, and translation. Sci Transl Med. 6, 265sr6. doi: 10.1126/scitranslmed.3009337.
10. Dehkordi, A. N., Babaheydari, F. M., Chehelgerdi, M. and Dehkordi, S. R. (2019). Skin tissue engineering: wound healing based on stem-cell-based therapeutic strategies. Stem Cell Res. Ther. 10, 111. https://doi.org/10.1186/s13287-019-1212-2.
11. Heublein, H., Bader, A., and Giri, S. (2015). Preclinical and clinical evidence for stem cell therapies as treatment for diabetic wounds. Drug Discov Today. 20, 703–717. doi: 10.1016/j.drudis.2015.01.005.
12. Agha, R., Ogawa, R., Pietramaggiori, G., and Orgill, D. P. (2011). A review of the role of mechanical forces in cutaneous wound healing. J Surg Res. 171, 700–708. doi: 10.1016/j.jss.2011.07.007.
13. Wong, V. W., Akaishi, S., Longaker, M. T., and Gurtner, G. C. (2011). Pushing back: wound mechanotransduction in repair and regeneration. J Invest Dermatol. 131, 2186–2196. doi:10.1038/jid.2011.212.
14. Wong, V. W., Longaker, M. T., and Gurtner, G. C. (2012). Soft tissue mechanotransduction in wound healing and fibrosis. Semin Cell Dev Biol. 23, 981–986. doi: 10.1016/j.semcdb.2012.09.010.
15. Franz, S., Rammelt, S., Scharnweber, D., and Simon, J. C. (2011). Immune responses to implants – a review of the implications for the design of immunomodulatory biomaterials. Biomaterials. 32, 6692–6709. doi:10.1016/j. biomaterials.2011.05.078.
16. Sharifi, S., Hajipour, M. J., Gould, L., and Mahmoudi, M. (2021) Nanomedicine in Healing Chronic Wounds: Opportunities and Challenges, Mol Pharmaceutics. 18 (2), 550–575. DOI: 10.1021/acs.molpharmaceut.0c00346.

17. Sen, C. K., Gordillo, G. M., Roy, S., Kirsner, R., Lambert, L., Hunt, T. K., Gottrup, F., Gurtner, G. C., and Longaker, M. T. (2009). Human skin wounds: a major and snow-balling threat to public health and the economy. Wound Repair and Regeneration. 17(6), 763–771. https://doi.org/10.1111/j.1524-475X.2009.00543.x.

18. Kakkar, R., Madgula, K., Saritha Nehru, Y. V., and Kakkar, J. (2015). Polyvinyl alcohol-melamine formaldehyde films and coatings with silver nano particles as wound dressings in diabetic foot disease. European Chemical Bulletin. 4(1–3), 98–105.

19. **The Diabetic Foot & Wound Care Clinic,** https://savelegs.com/ and; ePoster presentation in the International Conference European wound management Association (EWMA 2016), Bremen, Germany on research on the treatment and management of chronic wounds and diabetic foot problems, https://ewma.conference2web.com/#resources/nanosilver-coated-polymer-for-treatment-of-foot-infections-in-this-era-of-resistance-c9e43b05-5b2c-4042-a6f3-a6ccd87f4ded

20. Ezhilarasu, H., Vishalli, D., Dheen, S. T., Bay, B.-H., Srinivasan, D.K. (2020). Nanoparticle-based therapeutic approach for diabetic wound healing. Nanomaterials. 10, 1234.

21. Kasiewicz, L. N., and Whitehead, K. A. (2017). Recent advances in biomaterials for the treatment of diabetic foot ulcers. Biomater Sci. 5, 1962–1975. doi: 10.1039/C7BM00264E.

22. Dreifke, M. B., Jayasuriya, A. A., and Jayasuriya, A. C. (2015). Current wound healing procedures and potential care. Mater Sci Eng C. 48, 651–662, doi: 10.1016/j.msec.2014.12.068.

23. Suarato, G., Bertorelli, R., and Athanassiou, A. (2018). Borrowing from nature: biopolymers and biocomposites as smart wound care materials. Front Bioeng Biotechnol. 6, 137. doi: 10.3389/fbioe.2018.00137.

24. Ayuk, S. M., Abrahamse, H., Houreld, N. N. (2016). The role of matrix metalloproteinases in diabetic wound healing in relation to photobiomodulation. J Diabetes Res. 1–9.

25. Wang, S., Yan, C., Zhang, X., Shi, D., Chi, L., Luo, G., Deng, J. (2018). Antimicrobial peptide modification enhances the gene delivery and bactericidal efficiency of gold nanoparticles for accelerating diabetic wound healing. Biomater Sci. 6 (10), 2757–2772.

26. Das, M., Goswami, U., Kandimalla, R., Kalita, S., Ghosh, S. S., and Chattopadhyay, A. (2019). Iron–Copper bimetallic nanocomposite reinforced dressing materials for infection control and healing of diabetic wound. ACS Applied Bio Materials. 2 (12), 5434–5445.

27. Li, F., Shi, Y., Liang, J., Zhao, L. (2019). Curcumin-loaded chitosan nanoparticles promote diabetic wound healing via attenuating inflammation in a diabetic rat model. J Biomater Appl. 34 (4), 476–486.

28. Zgheib, C., Hilton, S. A., Dewberry, L. C., Hodges, M. M., Ghatak, S., Xu, J., Singh, S., Roy, S., Sen, C. K., Seal, S., Liechty, K. W. (2019) Use of cerium oxide nanoparticles conjugated with microRNA-146a to correct the diabetic wound healing impairment. J Am Coll Surg. 228 (1), 107–115.

29. Ren, X. Z., Han, Y. M., Wang, J., Jiang, Y. Q., Yi, Z. F., Xu, H., Ke, Q. F. (2018). An aligned porous electrospun fibrous membrane with controlled drug delivery - An efficient strategy to accelerate diabetic wound healing with improved angiogenesis. Acta Biomater. 70, 140–153.

30. Jackson, J. E., Kopecki, Z., Cowin, A. J. (2013) Nanotechnological Advances in Cutaneous Medicine. J Nanomater. 8, 808234

31. Goyal, R., Macri, L. K., Kaplan, H. M., Kohn, J. (2016). Nanoparticles and nanofibers for topical drug delivery. J Control Release. 240, 77–92.

32. Reinholz, J., Landfester, K., and Mailänder, V. (2018). The challenges of oral drug delivery via nanocarriers. Drug Deliv. 25, 1694–1705. doi: 10.1080/10717544.2018.1501119.

33. Auría-Soro, C, Nesma, T., Juanes-Velasco, P., Landeira-Viñuela, A., Fidalgo-Gomez, H., Acebes-Fernandez, V., Gongora, R., Almendral Parra, M. J., Manzano-Roman, R., Fuentes, M. (2019). Interactions of nanoparticles and biosystems: microenvironment of nanoparticles and biomolecules in nanomedicine. Nanomaterials (Basel). 9(10), 1365. doi: 10.3390/nano9101365.

34. Berthet, M., Gauthier, Y., Lacroix, C., Verrier, B., and Monge, C. (2017). Nanoparticle-based dressing: The future of wound treatment? Trends Biotechnol. 35, 770–784

35. Mordorski, B., Rosen, J., Friedman, A. (2015). Nanotechnology as an innovative approach for accelerating wound healing in diabetes. Diabetes Manag. 5, 329–332.

36. Chen, S. A., Chen, H. M., Yao, Y. D., Hung, C. F., Tu, C. S., Liang, Y. J. (2012). Topical treatment with anti-oxidants and Au nanoparticles promote healing of diabetic wound through receptor for advance glycation end-products. Eur J Pharm Sci. 47, 875–883.

37. Huang, Y.-H., Chen, C.-Y., Chen, P.-J., Tan, S.-W., Chen, C.-N., Chen, H.-M., Tu, C.-S., and Liang, Y.-J. (2014) Gas-injection of gold nanoparticles and anti-oxidants promotes diabetic wound healing. RSC Adv. 4, 4656–4662.

38. Ponnanikajamideen, M., Rajeshkumar, S., Vanaja, M., Annadurai, G. (2019). In vivo type 2 diabetes and wound-healing effects of antioxidant gold nanoparticles synthesized using the insulin plant chamaecostus cuspidatus in albino rats. Can J Diabetes. 43, 82–89.

39. Dai, X., Guo, Q., Zhao, Y., Zhang, P., Zhang, T., Zhang, X., Li, C. (2016). Functional silver nanoparticle as a benign antimicrobial agent that eradicates antibiotic-resistant bacteria and promotes wound healing. ACS Appl Mater Interfaces. 8, 25798–25807.

40. Liu, J., Sonshine, D. A., Shervani, S., and Hurt, R. H. (2010). Controlled release of biologically active silver from nanosilver surfaces. ACS Nano. 4, 6903–6913.

41. Kakkar, R., Sherly, E. D., Madgula, K., Devi, D. K., and Sreedhar, B. (2012). Synergetic effect of sodium citrate and starch in the synthesis of silver nanoparticles. J Appl Polym Sci. 126(S1), E154–E161. doi:10.1002/app.36727.

42. Kakkar, R., Madgula, K., Saritha Nehru, Y. V., Shailaja, R. M., and Sreedhar, B. (2014). Polyvinyl alcohol-melamine formaldehyde resin composite and nanocomposites with Ag, TiO_2, ZnO nanoparticles as antimicrobial films, coatings and sprays. Eur Chem Bull. 3(10–12), 1088–1097. DOI: http://dx.doi.org/10.17628/ecb.2014.3.1088-1097.

43. Santos, J. C. C, Mansur, A. A., Ciminell, V. S., Mansur, H. S. (2014). Nanocomposites of poly (vinyl alcohol)/functionalized-multiwall carbon nanotubes conjugated with glucose oxidase for potential application as scaffolds in skin wound healing. Int J Polym Mater Polym Biomater. 63, 185–196.

44. Wanna, D., Alam, C., Toivola, D. M., and Alam, P. (2013). Bacterial cellulose–kaolin nanocomposites for application as biomedical wound healing materials. Adv Nat Sci Nanosci Nanotechnol. 4, 045002.

45. Almonaci Hernández, C. A., Juarez-Moreno, K., Castañeda-Juarez, M. E., Almanza-Reyes, H., and Pestryakov, A., et al. (2017). Silver nanoparticles for the rapid healing of diabetic foot ulcers. Int J Med Nano Res. 4, 019. doi.org/10.23937/2378-3664/1410019.

46. Patel, H., Bonde, M., Srinivasan, G. (2011). Biodegradable polymer scaffold for tissue engineering. Trends Biomater Artif Organs. 1, 20–29.

47. Wen, X., Zheng, Y., Wu, J., Wang, L. N., Yuan, Z., Peng, J., and Meng, H. (2015). Immobilization of collagen peptide on dialdehyde bacterial cellulose nanofibers via covalent bonds for tissue engineering and regeneration. Int J Nanomedicine. 10, 4623–4637.

48. Wang, T., Zheng, Y., Shen, Y., Shi, Y., Li, F., Su, C., and Zhao, L. (2017). Chitosan nanoparticles loaded hydrogels promote skin wound healing through the modulation of reactive oxygen species. Artif Cells Nanomed Biotechnol. 46, 1–12.

49. Patel, A. K. (2017). In vitro and in vivo assessment of gelatin nanoparticles loaded doxocetal scaffolds. Int J Pharm Biol Sci Arch. 8, 40–51.

50. Cardoso, A. M., De Oliveira, E. G., Coradini, K., Bruinsmann, F. A., Aguirre, T., Lorenzoni, R., Barcelos, R. C. S., Roversi, K., Rossato, D. R., Pohlmann, A. R., and Guterres, S. S. (2018). Chitosan hydrogels containing nanoencapsulated phenytoin for cutaneous use: skin permeation/penetration and efficacy in wound healing. Mater Sci Eng C. 96, 205–217.

51. Krausz, A. E., Adler, B. L., Cabral, V., Navati, M., Doerner, J., Charafeddine, R. A., and Harper, S. (2015). Curcumin-encapsulated nanoparticles as innovative antimicrobial and wound healing agent. Nanomed: Nanotechnol Biol Med. 11, 195–206.

52. Molan P.C. Betts J. (2000). Using honey dressings: the practical considerations. Nurs Times. 96(49), 36–37. http://www.worldwidewounds.com/2001/november/Molan/honey-as-topical-agent.html.

53. Guidoni, M., Figueira, M. M., Ribeiro, G. P., Lenz, D., Grizotto, P. A., de Melo Costa Pereira, T., Scherer, R., Bogusz, S. Jr, and Fronza, M. (2019). Development and evaluation of a vegetable oil blend formulation for cutaneous wound healing. Arch Dermatol Res. 311(6), 443–452. doi: 10.1007/s00403-019-01919-8.

54. Vert, M., Doi, Y., Hellwich, K. H., Hess, M., Hodge, P., Kubisa, P., Rinaudo, M., and Schué, F. O. (2012). Terminology for biorelated polymers and applications (IUPAC Recommendations 2012). Pure Appl Chem. 84(2), 377–410. doi:10.1351/PAC-REC-10-12-04.

55. Williams, D. F. (1986). Definitions in Biomaterials: Proceedings of a Consensus Conference of the European Society for Biomaterials. Elsevier: Amsterdam.

56. Kant, V., Gopal, A., Kumar, D., Pathak, N. N., Ram, M., Jangir, B. L., Tandan S. K., and Kumar, D. (2015). J Surg Res. 193, 978–988

57. Song, R., Murphy, M., Li, C., Ting, K., Soo, C., and Zheng, Z. (2018). Current development of biodegradable polymeric materials for biomedical applications. Drug Des Devel Ther. 12, 3117–3145. doi:10.2147/DDDT.S165440.

58. Rognoni, E., and Watt, F. M. (2018). Skin cell heterogeneity in development, wound healing, and cancer. Trends Cell Biol. 28(9), 709–722.

59. Chattopadhyay, S. and Raines, R. T. (2014). Collagen based biomaterials for wound healing. Biopolymers. 101(8), 821–833. doi:10.1002/bip.22486.

60. Brett, D. (2008). A review of collagen and collagen based wound dressings. Wounds. 20(12), 347–356.

61. Baum, C. L, and Arpey, C. J. (2005). Normal cutaneous wound healing: clinical correlation with cellular and molecular events. Dermatol Surg. 31(6), 674–86. doi: 10.1111/j.1524-4725.2005.31612.x.

62. https://emedicine.medscape.com/article/1298129-overview.

63. Ghica, M. V., Albu Kaya, M. G., Dinu-Pîrvu, C. E., Lupuleasa, D., and Udeanu, D. I. (2017). Development, optimization and *in vitro/in vivo* characterization of collagen-dextran spongious wound dressings loaded with flufenamic acid. Molecules. 22, E1552. doi: 10.3390/molecules22091552.

64. Guo, R., Lan, Y., Xue, W., Cheng, B., Zhang, Y., and Wang, C. (2017). Collagen-cellulose nanocrystal scaffolds containing curcumin-loaded microspheres on infected full-thickness burns repair. J Tissue Eng Regen Med. 11, 3544–3555. doi: 10.1002/term.2272.

65. Melke, J., Midha, S., Ghosh, S., Ito, K., and Hofmann, S. (2016). Silk fibroin as biomaterial for bone tissue engineering. Acta Biomater. 31, 1–16.

66. Qi, Y., Wang, H., Wei, K., Yang, Y., Zheng, R.-Y., Soo Kim, I., and Zhang, K.-Q. (2017). A review of structure construction of silk fibroin biomaterials from single structures to multi-level structures. Int J Mol Sci. 18, 237; doi: 10.3390/ijms18030237.

67. Reimers, K., Liebsch, C., Radtke, C., Kuhbier, J. W., and Vogt, P. M. (2015). Silks as scaffolds for skin reconstruction. Biotechnol Bioeng. 112, 2201–2205. doi: 10.1002/bit.25654.

68. (a). Yu, K., Lu, F., Li, Q., et al. (2017). *In situ* assembly of Ag nanoparticles (AgNPs) on porous silkworm cocoon-based wound film: enhanced antimicrobial and wound healing activity. Sci Rep. **7**, 2107. https://doi.org/10.1038/s41598-017-02270-6; (b) Pollini, M., Paladini, F. (2020). Bioinspired materials for wound healing application: the potential of silk fibroin. Materials (Basel). 13(15), 3361. doi: 10.3390/ma13153361.

69. (a) Roh, D., Kang, S., Kim, J., Kwon, Y., Young Kweon, H., Lee, K., Park, Y., Baek, R., Heo, C., Choe, J., et al. (2006). Wound healing effect of silk fibroin/alginate-blended sponge in full thickness skin defect of rat. J Mater Sci Mater Med. 17, 547–552; (b) Long, D., Xiao, B., and Merlin, D. (2020) Genetically modified silk fibroin nanoparticles for drug delivery: preparation strategies and application prospects. Nanomedicine. 15(18), 1739–1742. DOI: https://doi.org/10.2217/nnm-2020-0182.

70. Meinel, L., Hofmann, S., Karageorgiou, V., Kirker-Head, C., McCool, J., Gronowicz, G.; Zichner, L., Langer, R., Vunjak-Novakovic, G., and Kaplan, D.L. (2005). The inflammatory responses to silk films in vitro and in vivo. Biomaterials. 26, 147–155.

71. Sun, W.; Gregory, D.A.; Tomeh, M.A.; Zhao, X. (2021) Silk Fibroin as a Functional Biomaterial for Tissue Engineering. Int. J. Mol. Sci 22, 1499. https://doi.org/10.3390/ijms2 2031499

72. Chouhan, D., Das, P., Thatikonda, N., Nandi, S. K., Hedhammar, M. Y., and Mandal, B. B. (2019). Silkworm silk matrices coated with functionalized spider silk accelerate healing of diabetic wounds. ACS Biomater Sci Eng. 5 (7), 3537–3548. https://doi.org/10.1021/acsbiomaterials.9b00514.

73. Mehrotra, S., Chouhan, D., Konwarh, R., Kumar, M., Jadi, P. K., Mandal, B. B. (2019). Comprehensive review on silk at nanoscale for regenerative medicine and allied applications. ACS Biomater Sci Eng. 5(5), 2054–2078. https://doi.org/10.1021/acsbiomaterials.8b01560.

74. Ju, H. W., JooLee, O., MinLee, J., Moon, B. M., Park, H. J., Park, Y. R., Lee, M. C., Kim, S. H., Ren, J., Ki, C. C. S., Park, C. H. (2016). Wound healing effect of electrospun silk fibroin nanomatrix in burn-model. Int J Biol Macromol. 85, 29–39.

75. Lee, O. J., Kim, J., Moon, B. M., Chao, J. R., Yoon, J., Ju, H. W., Lee, J. M., Park, H. J., Kim, D. W., Kim, S.J., et al. (2016). Fabrication and characterization of hydrocolloid dressing with silk fibroin nanoparticles for wound healing. Tissue Eng. Regen. Med. 13, 218–226.

76. Włodarczyk-Biegun, M. K., Farbod, K., Werten, M. W. T., Slingerland, C. J., de Wolf, F. A. (2016). Fibrous hydrogels for cell encapsulation: a modular and supramolecular approach. PLoS ONE. 11(7), e0159893. https://doi.org/10.1371/journal.pone.0159893.

77. Kelly, R. (2016). Wound healing biomaterials. Funct Biomater. 2, 353–365.

78. Arslan, Y. E., Arslan, T. S., Derkus, B., Emregül, E. (2017). Fabrication of human hair keratin/jellyfish collagen/eggshell-derived hydroxyapatite osteoinductive biocomposite scaffolds for bone tissue engineering: from waste to regenerative medicine products. Colloids Surfaces B Biointerfaces. 154, 160–170. doi: 10.1016/j.colsurfb.2017.03.034.

79. Mele, E. (2006). Electrospinning of natural polymers for advanced wound care: towards responsive and adaptive dressings. J Mater Chem B. 4, 4801–4812. doi: 10.1039/C6TB00804F.

80. Mogo, Sanu, G. D., and Grumezescu, A. M. (2014). Natural and synthetic polymers for wounds and burns dressing. Int J Pharm. 463, 127–136. doi: 10.1016/j.ijpharm.2013.12.015.

81. Maeda, N., Miao, J., Simmons, T. J., Dordick, J. S., and Linhardt, R. J. (2014). Composite polysaccharide fibers prepared by electrospinning and coating. Carbohydr Polym. 102, 950–955. doi: 10.1016/j.carbpol.2013, 10.038.

82. Dogan, G., Başal, G., Bayraktar, O., Özyildiz, F., Uzel, A., and Erdogan, I. (2016), Bioactive sheath/core nanofibers containing olive leaf extract. Microsc Res Tech. 79, 38–49. doi: 10.1002/jemt.22603.

83. Neuman, M. G., Nanau, R. M., Oruña-Sanchez, L., Coto, G. (2015). Hyaluronic acid and wound healing. J Pharm Pharm Sci. 18(1), 53–60. Litwiniuk, M., Grzela, T. (2014). Amniotic membrane: new concepts for an old dressing. Wound Repair Regen. 22(4), 451–456.

84. Litwiniuk, M., Bikowska, B., Niderla-Bielińska, J. et al. (2011). High molecular weight hyaluronan and stroma-embedded factors of radiation-sterilized amniotic membrane stimulate proliferation of HaCaT cell line in vitro. Cent Eur J Immunol. 36(4), 205–211.; and https://www.elenaconde.com/en/reasons-for-the-hyaluronic-acid-boom-in-wound-healing/

85. Norouzi, M., Boroujeni, S. M., Omidvarkordshouli, N., and Soleimani, M. (2015). Advances in skin regeneration: application of electrospun scaffolds. Adv Healthc Mater. 4, 1114–1133. doi: 10.1002/adhm.201500001.

86. Zhao, W., Liu, W., Li, J., Lin, X., and Wang, Y. (2015). Preparation of animal polysaccharides nanofibers by electrospinning and their potential biomedical applications. J Biomed Mater Res A. 103A, 807–818, doi: 10.1002/jbm.a.35187.

87. Romano, I., Mele, E., Heredia-Guerrero, J. A., Ceseracciu, L., Hajiali, H., Goldoni, L., et al. (2015b). Photo-polymerisable electrospun fibres of N-methacrylate glycol chitosan for biomedical applications. RSC Adv. 5, 24723–24728, doi: 10.1039/C5RA02301G.

88. Chiu, C. T., Lee, J. S., Chu, C. S., Chang, Y. P., and Wang, Y. J. (2008) Development of two alginate-based wound dressings. J Mater Sci Mater Med. 19, 2503–2513. doi: 10.1007/s10856-008-3389-2.

89. Setti, C., Suarato, G., Perotto, G., Athanassiou, A., and Bayer, I. S. (2018), Investigation of in vitro hydrophilic and hydrophobic dual drug release from polymeric films produced by sodium alginate-MaterBiR drying emulsions. Eur J Pharm Biopharm. 130, 71–82. doi: 10.1016/j.ejpb.2018.06.019.

90. Summa, M., Russo, D., Penna, I., Margaroli, N., Bayer, I. S., Bandiera, T., et al. (2018). A biocompatible sodium alginate/povidone iodine film enhances wound healing. Eur J Pharm. Biopharm. 122, 17–24. doi: 10.1016/j.ejpb.2017.10.004.

91. Liang, Y. and Kiick, K. L. (2014). Heparin-functionalized polymeric biomaterials in tissue engineering and drug delivery applications. Acta Biomater. 10(4), 1588–1600. doi: 10.1016/j.actbio.2013.07.031.

92. Park, U., Kim, K. (2017). Multiple growth factor delivery for skin tissue engineering applications. Biotechnol Bioprocess Eng. 22, 659–670.

93. Werner, S., Grose, R., and Rosenthal, N. (2008). Regulation of wound healing by growth factors and cytokines. Physiol Rev. 83(3), 835–870.

94. Tabata, Y. (2003). Tissue regeneration based on growth factor release. Tissue Eng. 9, 5–15.

95. Berlanga-Acosta, J., Gavilondo-Cowley, J., Barco-Herrera, D. G., Martín-Machado, J., Guillen-Nieto, G. (2011). Epidermal growth factor (EGF) and platelet-derived growth factor (PDGF) as tissue healing agents: clarifying concerns about their possible role in malignant transformation and tumor progression. J Carcinog Mutagen. 02, 1–14.

96. Pierce, G. F., Mustoe, T. A., Altrock, B. W., Deuel, T. F., Thomason, A. (1991). Role of platelet-derived growth factor in wound healing. J Cell Biochem. 45(4), 319–326. doi: 10.1002/jcb.240450403.

97. Ng, W. L., Wang, S., Yeong, W. Y., Naing, M. W. (2016). Skin bioprinting: impending reality or fantasy? Trends Biotechnol. 34, 689–699.

98. Satyanarayana, M. (2021). IL-2 treatment can be dangerous. Here's how drug firms are trying to fix it. 99(12). https://cen.acs.org/magazine/99/09912.html

99. Rea, I. M. et al. (2018). Age and age-related diseases: role of inflammation triggers and cytokines. Front Immunol. 9, 586.

100. Tan, J. L., Lash, B., Karami, R. et al. (2021). Restoration of the healing microenvironment in diabetic wounds with matrix-binding IL-1 receptor antagonist. Commun Biol. 4, 422. https://doi.org/10.1038/s42003-021-01913-9.

101. De Pieri, A., Rochev, Y. & Zeugolis, D. I. (2021). Scaffold-free cell-based tissue engineering therapies: advances, shortfalls and forecast. Npj Regen Med. 6, 18. https://doi.org/10.1038/s41536-021-00133-3.

102. Blume, P., Bowlby, M., Schmidt, B., Donegan, R. (2014). Safety and efficacy of Becaplermin gel in the treatment of diabetic foot ulcers. Chronic Wound Care Management and Research. 1, 11–14. https://doi.org/10.2147/CWCMR.S64905.

103. Stejskalová, A., Oliva, N., England, F. J., Almquist, B. D. (2018). Biologically inspired, cell-selective release of aptamer-trapped growth factors by traction forces. Adv Mater. DOI: 10.1002/adma.20180638.

104. Yang, H., Liu, C., Yang, D., Zhang, H., and Xi, Z. (2009). Comparative study of cytotoxicity, oxidative stress and genotoxicity induced by four typical nanomaterials: the role of particle size, shape and composition. J Appl Toxicol. 29(1), 69–78. doi:10.1002/jat.1385.

105. Zhou, Y., Peng, Z., Seven, E. S., and Leblanc, R. M. (2017). Crossing the blood-brain barrier with nanoparticles. J Control Release. 270, 290–303. doi: 10.1016/j.jconrel.2017.12.015.

106. Mitchell, M. J., Billingsley, M. M., Haley, R. M. Marissa, Wechsler, E., Peppas, N. A., and Langer, R. (2021). Engineering precision nanoparticles for drug delivery. Nat Rev Drug Discov. 20, 101–124. https://doi.org/10.1038/s41573-020-0090-8.

107. Game, F. L., Jeffcoate, W. J. (2016). Dressing and diabetic foot ulcers: a current review of the evidence. Plast Reconstr Surg. 138, 158S–164S.

108. Zenilman, J., Valle, M. F., Malas, M. B., Maruthur, N., Qazi, U., Suh, Y., Wilson, L. M., Haberl, E. B., Bass, E. B., and Lazarus, G. (2013). Chronic Venous Ulcers: A Comparative Effectiveness Review of Treatment Modalities. Rockville, MD: Agency for Healthcare Research and Quality (US). AHRQ Comparative Effectiveness Reviews.

109. Lantis, J. C. Paredes, J. A. Topical Wound Care Treatment and Indications for Their Use, 4th ed.; Springer International Publishing AG, 2018.

110. EWMA - European Wound Management Association – https://ewma.org, and [18] [The Nanomed Zone. https://www.nanomedzone.com/willthe-lessons-learned-from-cancer-nanomedicine-facilitate-the-clinicaltranslation-of-nanomedicine-beyond-cancer/

111. Gomes, A., Teixeira, C., Ferraz, R., Prudêncio, C., and Gomes, P. (2017). Review-wound-healing peptides for treatment of chronic diabetic foot ulcers and other infected skin injuries. Molecules. 22, 1743. doi:10.3390/molecules22101743.

112. International Diabetes Federation. IDF Diabetes Atlas, 7th ed.; IDF: Brussels, Belgium, 2015.

13 Novel Biologicals and Technological Platforms for Dental Clinical Use

*Vasudha Bakshi, Mounika Nerella,
and Narender Boggula*
Anurag University

CONTENTS

DOI: 10.1201/9781003140108-13

13.1 INTRODUCTION: TOOTH MORPHOLOGY, PHYSIOLOGY, AND PATHOLOGY

Dentistry is also known as oral medicine or dental medicine. It is the field of medical science concerned with the evaluation, detection, avoidance, and intervention of various dental abnormalities. Understanding the morphology of the tooth and anatomy has immense use in dental clinical practices [1]. Oral health starts with tooth hygiene and good oral habits. Dental health is defined by World Health Organization as "a state of being free from chronic mouth and facial pain, oral and throat cancer, oral infection and sores, periodontal (gum) disease, tooth decay, tooth loss, and other diseases and disorders that limit an individual's capacity in biting, chewing, smiling, speaking and psychogenic wellbeing" [2].

A tooth is defined as, a hard, calcified mineral-rich structure derived and formed by the ectoderm and ectomesenchyme in mammals. These are the hardest substances in the human body; they help in masticating food, give shape to the face, and play a key role in speech [3]. The development and growth of teeth is a complex process that involves the interaction among the soft tissues, connective tissues, nerves, and blood vessels along with various types of hard tissues. All teeth are anatomically made up of the same substances, irrespective of their shapes and sizes. The tooth is made up of the two basic parts—dental crown and dental root—and is associated with supporting structures such as periodontal ligaments, alveolar bone, and gingival. The chemical composition and some functional parameters of the inorganic phases of the human calcified tissues are shown in Table 13.1 [4].

The primary function of teeth is to break down, tear, chew, mix with saliva, and grind the ingested food and form it into a soft food mass before it enters the alimentary canal. Apart from the mastication process, the teeth have an important role in speech. The teeth are also involved in mineral exchange, such as bone, as the innermost membrane of the tooth is near to the vascular supply and dental soft tissue [5]. According to "The Global Burden of Disease Study 2017," about 3.5 billion people worldwide live with caries in permanent teeth, while more than 530 million juveniles experience tooth decay in their deciduous teeth. Dental health diseases are among the most prevalent diseases worldwide and have severe health and financial burdens that reduce the quality of life of affected individuals [6].

13.2 NOVELTY IN CURRENT DENTAL TECHNOLOGIES: FROM DENTAL COMPONENTS TO RESTORATION

Prominent advances in computing applied technologies and substances have augmented the possibilities for alternative dental therapies that offer more reliable detection tools and treatment plans [7–8]. A great number of improvements have been made with the invention of novel imaging approaches, namely CAD/CAM software, requisite intraoral imaging, X-ray–sensitive digital radiography, and computer-mediated dental implant surgery. Aside from its use as a diagnostic tool, imaging technology is the backbone that has contributed to the advancement of the general dental practitioner, because treatment is assisted by high-powered microscopes that allow the precise perception of the dentistry [9].

TABLE 13.1

Relative Compositions and Structural Parameters of Dentin, Hydroxyapatite, and Enamel

Composition	Dentin	Hydroxyapatite	Enamel
Calcium (wt. %)	35.1	39.6	36.5
Phosphorus (wt. %)	16.9	18.5	17.7
Ca/P (molar ratio)	1.61	1.67	1.63
Carbonate (CO_3^{2-}) (wt. %)	5.6	-	3.5
Sodium (wt. %)	0.6	-	0.5
Magnesium (wt. %)	1.23	-	0.44
Potassium (wt. %)	0.05	-	0.08
Fluoride (wt. %)	0.06	-	0.01
Chloride (wt. %)	0.01	-	0.30
Pyrophosphate ($P_2O_7^{4-}$) (wt.%)	0.1	-	0.022
Total inorganic (wt. %)	70	100	97
Total organic (wt. %)	20	-	1.5
Water	10	-	1.5
a axis (nm)	0.9421	0.9430	0.9441
c axis (nm)	0.6887	0.6891	0.6880
Crystallinity Index (HA -100)	33–37	100	70–75
Crystalline size (nm)	$35 \times 25 \times 4$	200–600	$100 \times 90 \times 30$
Ignition products (800 °C)	β-TCP + HA	HA	β-TCP + HA
Elasticity modulus (GPa)	15	10	80
Compressive strength (MPa)	100	100	10

Material engineering sciences have shown the way for the expansion of therapeutic interventions with the aim to reconstruct destroyed or lost natural dental structures. Although there are limitations in performance and durability, biomaterials are currently in use in dental practices because nano-dentistry has tremendously improved their medical performance and exhibits new clinical dental procedures with clinical outcomes [10]. The combination of nanomaterials with sophisticated and innovative strategies has enhanced replacement and aesthetic dentistry, which are dental science fields addressing effective, functional, and aesthetic appearance of dentition. 3D bioprinting is popularly known as additive manufacturing and has become a tremendous strategy to develop bioengineered tissues. The process includes bio-inks that form target tissues into 3D bioprinted tissue structures that replicate the functioning of organ [11]. 3D bioprinting technology has been applied to several fields, including surgical planning, tissue engineering, regenerative medicine, therapeutic devices, instrumentation, transplantation, and clinics to prove that new discoveries are ready for patient use. 3D cell tissue spheroids are fantastic lead molecules to mimic physiological environments within the living organ that can be reconstituted to regenerate tissue complexes; moreover, co-cultured substances can be used as bio-fabricating materials [12].

Dental-pain management has progressed enormously since the advent of alternative and novel technological approaches. To reduce the perception of pain, low-energy laser-beam therapy and light-emitting diode therapy have been clinically used. These therapeutic approaches relieve pain, provide dental tissue healing, and minimize the swelling by activating the inflammatory cell response. Their effectiveness has been already determined for the treatment of orthodontic pain management, orofacial surgeries, neuralgic pain, and dentin immune reactions [13].

However, the most prominent advancement that has recently been introduced into the dental discipline is the stem cell regeneration approach, which is based on the ability of undifferentiated cells to specialize and to restore or regenerate structural dental defects. Stem-cell–based regenerative medicine is connected to nanotechnology and highly sophisticated tissue engineering, which have developed innovative therapeutic strategies toward the physiological repair and reproduction of destroyed dental tissues [14].

13.3 NANOTECHNOLOGY-COMBINED STEM CELL BIOLOGY FOR DENTAL TISSUE RECONSTRUCTION

Stem cells are non-differentiated, immature cells that have the potential to self-renew and specialize to develop into many cell lineages by differentiation [15]. Stem cells are primarily categorized into embryonic and adult cell populations, later stem cells are situated in human tissues such as bone marrow, cutaneous tissue, dental pulp, adipose tissue, peripheral blood, liver, retina, brain, and muscle tissues. Adult stem cells can self-renew to a limited differentiation potential to other cell lineages [16]. The stem cells present in the orofacial region have been divided into adult, tissue, and mesenchymal stem cells. A variety of skeletal mesenchymal cells have been commonly extracted from permanent dental pulp (DPSC) and human exfoliated deciduous tooth (SHED), extensively described, and investigated for their dental applications in regenerative dentistry [17]. In addition, periodontal stem cells (PDLSC), apical papilla stem cells (SCAP), adipose-derived MSCs (ADMSCs), and dental follicle cells (DFCs) have been discovered as attractive cell sources for osseous and dental restoration approaches because of their relative availability and ease of accessibility. Among different stem cells, adult DMSCs located in periodontal tissue and dental pulp regulate human tooth homeostasis and regeneration; therefore they are optimal dental clinical tools for the dental tissue repair process [18].

Research efforts are focused toward impaired dental pulp and periodontal tissue restoration, where these damaged tissue structures can be held and regenerated by novel dental tissue engineering approaches either by transplantation of stem cells alone or in collaboration with functionalized scaffolds. More challenging and problematic, however, is the reconstruction of tooth enamel because neither dental epithelial stem cells (DESCs) nor ameloblasts are found in the tooth crown of permanent functional teeth [19]. More exciting, but immensely perplexing, is the effort to create entire damaged dental structures by using both DESCs and DMSCs. Although this is currently beyond our reality, numerous preclinical research attempts have been investigated, and there will be revolutionary change in regenerative dentistry in clinical practice.

The effectiveness and significance of stem-cell–based therapy can be analyzed by current nanotechnology devices, because the tools facilitate tracking

TABLE 13.2
Applications of Common Nanomaterials in Dentistry

Nanomaterials	Applications
Carbonate hydroxyapatite nanocrystals	Mouthwashes, toothpastes, and composite resins for
Amorphous calcium phosphate nanoparticles	prevention of cavities and periodontal disorders
Silver and zinc oxide nanoparticles	
Calcium carbonate nanoparticles	
Calcium PHOSPHATE nanoparticles	Dental adhesives for mineralization
Gold nanoparticles	Diagnosis of cancer and pre-cancerous oral diseases
Semiconductor nanocrystals	
Nanostructured hydroxyapatite	Promotion of bone regeneration/repair/
Carbon nanotubes	remineralization
Polymeric nanofibrous scaffold	
PLLA/MWNTs/HA, PLLA/HA, PCL/gelatin/HA	Entire-tooth regeneration
nanofibrous scaffolds	

the mobility, fate, and proliferation capability of stem cells in vivo. For instance, stem cells that have been transplanted can be monitored and tracked for longer duration with imaging approaches using fluorescent dyes and with nanoparticles that can be traced by MRI and elucidate required information about their movements and fate during tooth regeneration. This profound knowledge could be utilized for remodeling appropriate scaffolds that will anchor stem cells before grafting procedure. Additionally, it will permit estimating the treatment efficacy of unambiguous dental stem cell lineages that have been unveiled to specific ambient environments. In fact, unnatural microenvironments, which may govern stem cells in regard to a precise destination and physiology, can be attained through nanotechnology [20].

A substantial variety of nanosize decomposable or biodegradable molecular components with specific size, shape, and surface chemistry can be utilized for the design of microenvironments that are modified for the necessity of regenerative dentistry. Table 13.2 shows nanomaterials and their applications in dentistry. Such biodegradable scaffolds, once transplanted, may mimic short-term niches that regulate stem cell properties and direct dental tissue repair. It is evident that the scope of dental disciplines that can gain from the recent improvements of stem cell biology, nanotechnology, and material sciences is exceptional all the way. This chapter covers current and future therapeutic approaches for controlling tooth crown damage, tooth loss, oral sarcomas, and periodontal injuries [21].

13.4 DENTAL CROWN DESTRUCTION

13.4.1 Current Therapeutic Interventions in Endodontic Dentistry

The outer hard impervious layer of enamel and insulating dentine coverage under the enamel of the tooth crown are usually the prime tissues damaged following dental injuries or caries. Proficient healing of enamel and/or dentin is cardinal to arrest infection and damage expanding toward soft dental tissues (i.e., periodontium, pulp) and alveolar bone. The typical procedure for managing enamel and dental problem is the replacement and restoration of the damaged or lost dental hard tissues by advanced composite materials. Nevertheless, conventional cohesive systems are unstable and go wrong over a period of time, thus leading to marginal leakiness and poor confinement of the restoration of the tooth [22–23]. Accordingly, a considerable task of nanoscience in odontics is to produce and improve novel long-lasting molecular components and adhesive systems with enriched enamel and/or dentin-interaction performance in order to enhance the durability of the restorations and restrict multiple treatments. Doubtless, the launching of innovative materials like mono methacrylate diluents and phosphine oxide initiators has given way to dental composites with acceptable and adequate properties [24]. The development and improvement of nanomaterials and nanofillers led to even more noticeable advances in enhancing composite properties and performance. These innovative nanotechnology-mediated approaches utilizing crosslinking materials and calcium- and phosphorous-releasing modes, which resemble the natural process of dentin mineralization, have also minimized the depletion of the dentin-resin bonded interface.

Ceramic-mediated materials are in use by dental physicians for the redesign of destroyed tooth crowns, predominantly because of their high-quality aesthetic appearance and compatibility with living tissues. To counter the reality that ceramic materials are fragile and prone to brittleness propagation, various hardening/transformation mechanisms have emerged, contributing to superior aging-resistant ceramics like zirconia with unusual toughness and strength [25].

Nanomodified substances could be also remodeled for regulating oral microbial environment and the emergence of dental plaque, and, moreover, for intensifying the mineralization procedure in the case of enamel erosion and/or dentin exaggerated immune reaction due to excessive intake of acidic drinks. In fact, the use of artificial nano hydroxyapatite particles and other calcium-containing modified nanomaterials in dentifrices may provide a defensive nanostructured coating on dental surfaces that concurrently restores the minerals that have been lost from enamel [26].

The conservation of the dental pulp living tissue, ensuring tooth function, is of chief importance throughout the treatment of a destroyed tooth crown. In severe dental injury, the dental pulp may be damaged and could lose its functionality. Hence, dental therapy (i.e., dental pulp removal) is imposed to protect from microbial contamination and damage of the nearby alveolar bone. This is superseded by sterilization of the root canals and the restoration of the dental pulp with inorganic components. The vitality loss are more brittle than natural teeth and therefore are exposed to postoperative fractures [27].

13.4.2   CHALLENGES IN CLINICAL APPLICATIONS OF DENTAL PULP REGENERATION

Regenerative dentistry focused on redesigning the actual pulp tissue structure and function depends on principles of tissue engineering [28–29]. Nanomaterials can be utilized either singly or combined with stem cells and growth factors in order to trigger and increase the regenerative ability of dental pulp tissue. Modification of biomaterials for specific dental procedures would need adjustments at a nanoscale level, thus contributes to multiple physiological activities within limited small surfaces, that can be enhancing the quality of targeting, and better controlling biologically active molecules delivery. Nanomaterials developed for dental procedures can target antimicrobial and anti-inflammatory molecules in addition to growth factors that will govern the behavior (e.g., cell relocation, multiplication, and differentiation) of the many dental pulp cell lineages (e.g., endothelial cells, dental pulp fibroblasts, neuronal cells, immune cells). Biosimilar scaffolds consisting of natural components, such as hyaluronic acids, type-I collagen, and chitosan, together with nano-organized substances acquiring anti-inflammatory abilities, have been created to encourage pulp-tissue regeneration and to eliminate inflammation [30–32]. Even though such microporous and nanofibrous integuments have imparted optimistic results, remarkable improvements are quite required to generate scaffolds that upgrade proper pulp regeneration.

A great number of efforts using human DMSCs have been created in diverse animal models in attempts to accomplish complete pulp rejuvenation, a procedure that also needs angiogenesis and nerve supply of this tissue. Investigations have revealed that human DMSCs have the ability to transform into odontoblasts and to generate dentin-like armature when grafted along with a ceramic powder in immune deficient mice ex vivo [33–34]. Comparable experiments have shown that human DMSCs embedded on L-lactide/glycol and poly-D scaffolds are capable to rejuvenate vascularized dental tissue when implanted into an unoccupied mouse tooth root canal. Over the past few years, new investigational protocols have been unfolded, where DMSC-embedded scaffolds associated with bioactive materials satisfy the vacant pulp chamber instantly after pulp decimation. Exploratory studies in humans have validated the safety and efficacy of DMSCs for full pulp restoration and original dentin constitution. Bone morphogenetic proteins (BMPs) have been commonly utilized for expanding and increasing the development of dentin in the course of pulp regeneration. In spite of these stem-cell–mediated processes to ameliorate pulp tissue regeneration, their effectiveness for achieving precise, proper, and long-standing therapeutic approaches is still ambiguous [35].

In actual fact, a lot of procedures directed at dental pulp regeneration showed the emergence of fibroblast tissues that can experience deterioration over time or to replace with bone cells. The potential to decellularize healthy human tooth pulp unlocks a new outlook in regenerative dental discipline because these decellularized tissues could provide natural scaffolds for guiding transplanted homologous DMSCs. Decellularized pulp tissue appears to be a perfect biomaterial for anchoring stem cells and supporting new blood vessels and neuron supply within the rejuvenating tissues. Furthermore, innovative 3D printing approaches have been established to engineer pre-vascularized dental pulp-like hydrogel tissue fabricates in the entire root canals. Although notable attempts have been developed so far, regenerative strategies have to be additionally investigated in order to eventually furnish evidence of physiological dental pulp regeneration in vivo [36].

13.4.3   Challenges in Enamel Reconstruction

A new generation of the outermost enamel layer in humans is one of the main challenges in regenerative odontics, because amelogenesis is a complicated procedure and DESCs that could recreate enamel are very infrequent in human permanent teeth. Very limited dental epithelial cells along with stem cell characteristics have been segregated from the periodontal tissue (i.e., epithelial rests of Malassez ERM). Investigational studies on porcine ERM have demonstrated that these cells can transform into ameloblasts when co-cultured in vitro with dental pulp cells and can generate enamel morphological compounds after their implantation in vivo [37]. Even though ERM is a possible stem cell source for enamel rejuvenation, accessibility of these cells in human dental structures is limited, thus it is recommended for the identification of other epithelial stem cell populations from other non-dental sources that could transform into enamel-developing ameloblasts.

Another important concern in regenerating enamel is time. The complete generation of proper dental enamel depends upon longer duration, a time frame certainly inappropriate with scientific needs. However, mild interruptions throughout the process could be able to generate abnormal enamel [38]. Hence, any approach and procedure that will appreciably hasten the process of amelogenesis will be advantageous to dental patients and the clinical dental practice community.

13.5 PERIODONTAL DISEASES

13.5.1 POTENTIAL APPLICATIONS IN PERIODONTAL TREATMENTS

Periodontal infections are common diseases that affect both the morphology of the surrounding tissues (i.e., alveolar bone and dental root) and physiology of the dental tissue. Severe host immune response to the periodontium contributes to notable changes in not only the structure but also the amount of the alveolar bone, an approach that ultimately may lead to tooth removal. Current periodontal therapeutic approaches contain a broad range of incision procedures together with the use of bone transplants as tissue replacements, barrier membranes for covering the wound healing area from unwanted epithelial cell mass, and growth factors for improving the alleviating capacity of the damaged tissues [39]. Bone transplanting materials, directs to trigger bone enhancement and gum tissue restoration, consists of freeze dried and fresh frozen allografts, extraoral or intra oral autografts, animal-based bone non-proteinised xenografts, and hydroxyapatite and beta-tricalcium phosphate alloplasts [40–41]. These transplanting materials could be utilized alone or in combination with variety of growth factors. It has been shown that utilization of these restoration methods in dental clinics permitted the generation of new osseous tissues with biosimilarity to natural bone properties. Anyway, these techniques do not consistently verify a predictable and beneficial outcome of periodontal regeneration and repeatedly result in palliating with epithelial membrane rather than new gum tissue formation [42].

13.5.2 CHALLENGES IN PERIODONTAL TISSUE RENEWAL

The primary aim in regenerative endodontics is to redesign a physiological periodontium including novel cementum, alveolar bone, and periodontal ligament surrounding the area of the damaged tooth root. DMSCs secluded from the gum space (i.e., periodontal ligament stem cells and dental follicle stem cells) of adult teeth can transform into the different cell types of the periodontium in vitro when associated with various dentin matrix or scaffolds [43–46]. These stem cell lineages have been revealed to enhance periodontal rejuvenation when grafted into immunodeficient animals ex vivo, showing their immense capability for future stem cell mediated treatment strategies in dentistry [47]. Numerous growth factors have been also utilized for developing the restorative efficacy of stem cells in the periodontium. Several investigations have illustrated that platelet-derived growth factors (PDGFs) initiate periodontal tissue regeneration, although BMPs intensify alveolar bone and cementum production [48–49]. However, uncontrolled bone production induces tooth ankylosis and can be a recurrent unwanted effect with the use of BMPs since these fragments aid and guide stem cell transformation approaching osteogenic destination. The supreme way to confirm the dispatch of a huge quantity of growth factors is to utilize the blood constructs as platelet-rich plasma (PRP) merged with various natural and artificial transplants [50]. It is anticipated that PRP will immensely stimulate tissue regeneration, being that the recovery process is promoted by the factors found in PRP. Certainly, clinical investigations have revealed that periodontal regeneration was stimulated by the utilization in association with PRP and stem cells [89]. However, there are still significant key issues to be considered related to the consistency of constructs formulation, the effectiveness of their target distribution, and specific immune responses of the patient [51–52].

Clinical trials have revealed that enamel matrix replicas also favor and stimulate periodontal tissue regeneration [53–54]. Modern sophisticated novel bone transplantation materials with enhanced physicochemical characteristics have been utilized as transporters of enamel protein products to additionally enrich their clinical outcome [55]. Regardless, in spite of encouraging clinical performance, the mode of action of the enamel matrix components is ambiguous. In recent times, many efforts to attain quick and effective periodontal regeneration have been conducted using 3D printed and micropatterned biomaterials that furnish architectural support for cell alignment and encouraged during tissue healing [56].

13.6 DENTAL LOSS

13.6.1 Current Concepts in Dental Implant Technology

The design, development, and use of dental implants are among the biggest technological advancements in dentistry in the past few decades for dental pathology, injury, and hereditary disorders. Dental implants are the most popular, effective, and improved dental practice therapy for extracted teeth or missing teeth due to periodontal disease [57]. A normal dental implant contains a metal screw that incorporates and interfaces with the alveolar bone and has another part where the dental crown replacement is placed [58]. The retention of a tooth implant depends upon its intimate contact with the alveolar bone, a procedure called osseointegration. Even though they are routinely handled in dental unit, implants further need substantial improvements, distinctly in their ability to trigger cellular processes at the transplantation region that would assure their long-lasting integration and retention [59–60]. The application of nanotechnology has developed the osseointegration of dental implants by altering their surfaces, thus decreases repairing time [61–62].

Undoubtedly, nanohydroxyapatite-blasted facets, nanotextured blasted titanium surfaces, zinc-altered calcium silicate coatings, and with gold nanoparticle-coated surfaces have significantly improved the adhesive characteristics of dental implants and thus their osseointegration [63–64].

However, there is a significant risk of microbial infection around implanted tissues, a condition called peri-implantitis [65–66]. In vivo and in vitro experiments have revealed that the integration of antimicrobial agents (e.g., silver nanoparticles) with implants could partially stop the proliferation of bacteria and hence reduce the rate of implant failure [67]. It has been also illustrated that poly (acrylic acid) bilayer/gallium-modified chitosan coatings may enhance implant performance of titanium by restricting bacterial attachment and growth [68–69]. Dental implants have also gained from restorative strategies, utilizing stem cells, scaffolds, and growth factors committed to improve osseointegration and host tissue response..

Despite a considerable number of preclinical investigations in animal models for directed periodontal and bone regeneration surrounding implants utilizing growth factors and protein transporting systems, and the perceptible clinical benefits, well-organized human randomized clinical trials that will apparently verify these technologies are still inadequate. To date, very few randomized human studies have been conducted, and therefore it is essential to have more large clinical studies [70–72].

13.6.2 CHALLENGES IN WHOLE-TOOTH REGENERATION

Regeneration of complete dental structures for the restoration of missing or lost teeth is the fundamental aim in regenerative dentistry and calls for the use and recombination of mesenchymal and dental epithelial stem cells. DMSCs can generate all mesenchymal structures of the teeth and the nearby tissues like cementum, dentin, and alveolar bone; however, DESCs are necessary for the creation of enamel. Since a great number of dental epithelial cells vanish shortly after tooth destruction and DESCs are fewer in permanent teeth, current knowledge on DESCs has been procured chiefly from rodents, which favor the regeneration of enamel in the continuously proliferating incisors [73–74].

Two important technologies have been demonstrated for regenerating entire new teeth. One procedure consists in combining and culturing DESCs and DMSCs in vitro until they develop a tooth pathogen that eventually will be implanted into the alveolar bone. It is contemplated that this tooth pathogen will still grow and develop, erupt, and lastly transform into a functional tooth. Another strategy depends on tooth-structured polymeric bio decomposable scaffolds that are profuse with both DMSCs and DESCs and, transplanted into the alveolar bone will ultimately transform to functional teeth. The tri-dimensional structure of the scaffolds should initiate the differentiation of the grafted stem cells into odontoblasts and ameloblasts [75].

Indeed, many studies utilizing biologically engineered procedures in mice have shown that functional dental structures with suitable dental pulp covers, dental roots, and periodontal ligaments can be generated subsequent to their transplantation in mandibles [76]. However, the same solutions have not yet been attained with adult human cells because of the merger number of DESCs and mainly extended time duration that is essential for actual tooth growth. Insufficiency of DESCs within permanent teeth might be successfully resolved by transforming patient-oriented inducible pluripotent stem cells (iPSCs) to DESCs. Certain protocols have revealed that iPSCs technique could be used in regenerative endodontics, since recombination of human iPSC-based mesenchymal cells and mice dental epithelium preceded generation of whole teeth ex vivo [77]. Despite promising advances, this technology also requires additional investigation, as effective experimental procedures for the differentiation of human cells DESCs from iPSCs are unavailable yet.

13.7   INNOVATIVE TECHNOLOGIES FOR DENTAL DESIGN, DRUG DEVELOPMENT, AND DIAGNOSTICS

13.7.1   APPLICATION OF ORGANOIDS AND ORGANS ON CHIP DEVICES IN DENTISTRY

Applicable systems for designing human tissues describe a persistent need in all fields of biomedical research and practice, along with dentistry. Preclinical models and two-dimensional adult human cell-culture techniques have been conventionally utilized for most animal models focused on the improvement of new cell-mediated and pharmaceutical treatment strategies. However, shifting of animal data into effective therapeutic procedures remains unsatisfactory, featuring the demand for appropriate human-emulation methods [78]. In these circumstances, considerable predictions are associated with the current developments on organoids, micro fluidics, spheroids, and organ-on-chip approaches.

Organoids and spheroids are three-dimensional culture procedures, procured by primary stem cells, which are flourishingly utilized to model and acknowledge the specific-tissue function. The two systems permit initiation of complicated cell–cell interconnections and alteration of nutrients, oxygen, and soluble signals that produce tissue-specific different cell types. In contrast to spheroids, organoids illustrate additional properties, as they are capable of self-organization, show similar design and construction to the tissue origin, and exhibit specific-tissue complicate functions [79].

Dentospheres or tooth spheroids have been generated from animal and human dental mesenchymal (e.g., periodontium and pulp) and epithelial tissues. Epithelial dental spheroids produced from mice incisors and molars, upon attenuation of their growth medium requirements, have likewise manifested robust stem cell abilities or produced differentiated gradients. Human adult mesenchymal dentospheres steadily exhibited higher interpretation of odontoblast and periodontal tissue specific differentiation markers when correlated to two-dimensional culture systems [80–84]. These conditions make dentospheres expensive tools for analyzing cell differentiation events in human dental tissues in vitro and might be considered a source of stem cells for individualized tooth renewal approaches. However, inherited disorders are generally accompanied by dental abnormalities [85–86], which can be conveniently designed and researched in disease-specific dentospheres. Similarly, such spheroids serve as innovative tools for examining the performance of distinct dental cell lineages to new materials and active ingredients. In spite of despite their obvious benefits, it is uncertain to what degree organoids and spheroids could truly demonstrate the in vivo dental condition. Both the spheroids and organoids in general lack a lot characteristics that are crucial for any organ function, such as neovascularization, innervations, immune, and mechanical responses [87].

These restrictions are the foundation for the improvement of micro fluidic "organ-on-chip" systems. These devices contain different chambers where tissue-specific components like epithelial, mesenchymal, neuronal, and endothelial cells and/or cell mass are cultured [88]. Permeable membranes permit the passage of molecular signals between various chambers while blood flow is simulated by the controlled circulation of enhanced and specific media. The above-mentioned tools can integrate mechanical pressures to regenerate functional movements and stresses, along with electrical motive, permitting the designing and evaluation of organ-specific functional and diseased processes. Significantly, moving immune cells and even microbes can be incorporated in these instruments to resemble higher organ-level responses [88].

Micro fluidic tools comprising dental tissues have been utilized for the first time for evaluating the crosslinking of tooth pathogens and DMSCs with trigeminal nerve innervations [89–90]. These exploratory studies have revealed that micro fluidics can truly mimic and regenerate the in vivo dental condition and thus strengthen the choices to investigate dental tissues in "organ-on-chip" systems. Data derived from these tools assist in successfully reproducing human and patient-specific dental tissues in vitro. The main aim of these micro fluidic devices is the designing of the physiological interlinkage between various human organs In general, "organ-on-chip" tools could be intercommunicated via micro fluidic tubes, which mimic systemic blood supply. Through such emulated blood vessels, molecular signals and immune responses can transmit to all body parts, permitting the detection of body-level reactions to organ-specific events. This technology was formerly used and improved for modeling pharmacokinetics and pharmacodynamics of systemic responses to drug in human [91].

By means of these platforms, it will be possible to investigate body-level reactions to the different dental diseases. Dental pathologies are vigorously associated with several systemic abnormalities, which comprising stroke, atherosclerosis and infections, the pathological mechanisms underlying these disorders and thus their treatment application are far from being known [92]. A human "body-on-chip" system would ultimately permit interpretation of how tooth and systemic health are interconnected, thus assessing how the therapeutic strategy of dental disorders affects normal function.

Microfluidic tools can be also engaged for the determination of specific bacterial species and particular metabolites that are employed in chronic diseases [93]. In the dental field, microfluidic devices have been utilized for identification of infectious bacteria that causes gum inflammation and dental cavity diseases. Advanced technological improvements allowed a remarkable decrease in the length of this procedure through enhancement of labor-saving and DNA-incorporated extraction, multiplex PCR pre-amplification, and strain-specific actual PCR [94–95]. These procedures allow quick processing of samples, without lack of sensitivity and complicated laboratory equipment.

Current nanotechnology devices allow the determination of single oral pathogens in situ through grapheme-biosensors integrated with electrodes and antennae, which were imprinted onto enamel as "temporary tattoos." These wearable tools are thus capable of regulating bacteria existing in the oral cavity and more particularly on the dental surface

[96]. A similar working principle has been adapted very recently for determination and identifying engulfed food components. These are embedded onto enamel nanotools and can be improved to sense a broad range of features of drinks, like salt content, alcohol amount, sugars, temperature, and pH [97]. Although still in their investigational trials, such sensors promise to be excellent devices for the refined regulation and recognizing of oral circumstances that will immensely favor the discipline of preventive dentistry.

13.8 ORAL CANCERS

13.8.1 CURRENT TREATMENT APPROACHES IN MOUTH-CANCER–AFFECTED TISSUE REGENERATION

Malignancy is the second most common cause of morbidity and mortality. The incidence of oral sarcoma is increasing in several regions of the world, where oropharyngeal cancer is an important part of global burden of cancer [98]. Depending on the cancer treatment approach, the side effects most commonly seen in the oral cavity include dryness of mouth, oral mucositis, osteoradionecrosis (ORN), trismus, and infections. During treatment procedures, normal cells that maintain body homeostasis may also be affected [99]. For xerostomia, carboxymethylcellulose, mucin, glycerin, or water-based saliva substituents may be used; salivary stimulants like pilocarpine and cevimeline are recommended. Stannous fluoride gel is highly recommended to reduce caries. Fluoride-releasing glass ionomers and or amalgam restorations are more predictable when compared to composite restorations. Tooth extraction is recommended for ORN; therefore, invasive dental approaches existed [100]. Periodontal strategies like deep scaling and flap surgery are not used in heavily irradiated patients. Instead, more conservative approaches like endodontic treatment or coronal restorations are preferable. Antibiotics may relieve pain. If possible, it is highly encouraged to remove any sources of dental diseases, including advanced caries, periapical infection, and pathologic periodontal bone loss before treating with radiation therapy. New alternatives to Hyper Baric Oxygen (HBO) treatments are being introduced, such as the use of pentoxifylline and/or tocopherol [101]. Medication-related osteonecrosis of the jaw (MRONJ) invasive dental procedures should be avoided, but conservative approaches are recommended. It is important to know whether cancer patients are taking aforementioned medications, because dental treatment options are significantly limited due to increased risk of having MRONJ after invasive dental treatment [102].

13.9 CONCLUSION

Dentistry has followed an advanced path historically with innovative developments in understanding the pathophysiological changes and technologies. Research over the past three decades has given us an opportunity and renewed enthusiasm for dental clinical care. The novel technological platforms in dentistry have resulted in several research innovations being put into practice and used on a daily basis. Most of the treatment approaches are yet to be applicable in dental clinics. This chapter attempted to explore and elaborate on some of the novel biological and technological advancements in dental clinical care.

REFERENCES

1. Albrektsson T, Zarb G, Worthington P, Eriksson AR. The long-term efficacy of currently used dental implants: a review and proposed criteria of success. Int J Oral Maxillofac Implants. 1986;1:11–25.
2. Dhage VS, Chougule P. Importance of oral hygiene in oro-dental diseases: a review study. International Journal of Research and Review. 2019;6(12):69–74.
3. Balic A. Biology explaining tooth repair and regeneration: a mini-review. Gerontology. 2018;64, 382–388.
4. Dorozhkin SV, Epple M. Biological and Medical Significance of Calcium Phosphates. *Angew. Chem. Int.* 2002;41:3130–3146.
5. Peyron MA, Sante-Lhoutellier V, François O, Hennequin M. Oral declines and Mastication deficiencies cause alteration of food bolus properties. *Food Funct.* 2018;9(2):1112–1122.
6. Heller D, Helmerhorst EJ, Oppenheim FG. Saliva and Serum Protein Exchange at the Tooth Enamel Surface. *J. Dent. Res.* 2017;96(4):437–443.
7. Beuer F, Schweiger J, Edelhoff D. Digital dentistry: an overview of recent developments for CAD/CAM generated restorations. *Br. Dent. J.* 2008;204:505–511.
8. Levato CM, Farman AG, Miles DA. The "inevitability" of digital radiography in dentistry. *Compend. Contin. Educ. Dent.* 2015;36:238–240.
9. Hammerle CH, Stone P, Jung RE, Kapos T, and Brodala N. Consensus statements and recommended clinical procedures regarding computer-assisted implant dentistry. *Int. J. Oral Maxillofac. Implants.* 2009;24(Suppl.):126–131.
10. Zhang S. Fabrication of novel biomaterials through molecular self-assembly. *Nat. Biotechnol.* 2003;21:1171–1178.
11. Wiersma DS. The physics and applications of random lasers. *Nature Phys.* 2008;4:359–367.
12. Sweeney C, Coluzzi DJ, Sulewski JG, White JM. Laser safety in dentistry: a position paper. *J Laser Dent.* 2009;17(1):39–49.
13. Carroll JD, Milward MR, Cooper PR, Hadis M, Palin WM. Developments in low level light therapy (LLLT) for dentistry. *Dent. Mater.* 2014;30:465–475.
14. Kathuria V, Dhillon JK, Kalra G. Low level laser therapy: a panacea for oral maladies. *Laser Ther.* 2015;24:215–223. doi: 10.5978/islsm.15-RA-01
15. Gronthos S, Brahim J, Li W, Fisher LW, Cherman N, et al. Stem cell properties of human dental pulp stem cells. *J. Dent. Res.* 2002;81:531–535.
16. Mitsiadis TA, Graf D. Cell fate determination during tooth development and regeneration. *Birth Defects Res. C Embryo Today.* 2009;87:199–211.
17. Lymperi S, Ligoudistianou C, Tarasila V, et.al. Dental stem cells and their applications in dental tissue engineering. *Open Dent. J.* 2013;7:76–81.
18. Lee JS, Hong JM, Moon GJ, et.al. A long term follow up study of intravenous and autologous mesenchymal stem cell transplantation in patients with ischaemic stroke. *Stem Cells.* 2010;28 (6):1099–1106.
19. Jamal M, Chogle S, Goodis H, Karam SM. Dental stem cells and their potential role in regenerative medicine. *J Med Sci.* 2011;4(2):53–61.
20. Seki T, Fukuda K, Methods of induced pluripotent stem cells for clinical application. *World J Stem Cells.* 2015;7(1):116–125.
21. Bluteau G, Luder HU, De Bari C, Mitsiadis TA. Stem cells for tooth engineering. *Eur. Cell Mater.* 2008;16:1–9.
22. Mitsiadis TA, Harada H. Regenerated teeth: the future of tooth replacement. *Regen. Med.* 2015;10:5–8. doi: 10.2217/rme.14.78.
23. Perdigão J. Dentin bonding-variables related to the clinical situation and the substrate treatment. *Dent Mater.* 2010;26:e24–37.

24. Vaidyanathan TK, Vaidyanathan J. Recent advances in the theory and mechanism of adhesive resin bonding to dentin: a critical review. *J. Biomed. Mater. Res. B Appl. Biomater.* 2009;88:558–578.

25. Breschi L, Maravic T, Cunha SR, Comba A, Cadenaro M, Tjaderhane L, et al. Dentin bonding systems: from dentin collagen structure to bond preservation and clinical applications. *Dent. Mater.* 2018;34:78–96. doi: 10.1016/j.dental.2017.11.005.

26. Kilambi H, Cramer NB, Schneidewind, LH, Shah, P, Stansbury, JW, Bowman CN. Evaluation of highly reactive mono-methacrylates as reactive diluents for BisGMA-based dental composites. *Dent. Mater.* 2009;25:33–38.

27. Ilie N, Kessler A, Durner J. Influence of various irradiation processes on the mechanical properties and polymerisation kinetics of bulk-fill resin based composites. *J. Dent.* 2013;41, 695–702.

28. Monterubbianesi R, Orsini G, Tosi G, Conti C, Librando V, Procaccini M, et al. Spectroscopic and mechanical properties of a new generation of bulk fill composites. *Front. Physiol.* 2016;7:652.

29. Guazzato M, Albakry M, Ringer SP, Swain MV. Strength, fracture toughness and microstructure of a selection of all-ceramic materials. Part II. Zirconia-based dental ceramics. *Dent. Mater.* 2004;20:449–456. doi: 10.1016/j.dental.2003.05.002.

30. Lelli M, Putignano A, Marchetti M, Foltran I, Mangani F, Procaccini M, et al. Remineralization and repair of enamel surface by biomimetic Zn- carbonate hydroxyapatite containing toothpaste: a comparative in vivo study. *Front. Physiol.* 2014;5:333.

31. DeRosa TA. A retrospective evaluation of pulpotomy as an alternative to extraction. *Gen. Dent.* 2006;54:37–40.

32. Diogenes A, Hargreaves KM. Microbial modulation of stem cells and future directions in regenerative endodontics. *J. Endod.* 2017;43:S95–S101.

33. Murray PE, Garcia-Godoy F. The outlook for implants and endodontics: a review of the tissue engineering strategies to create replacement teeth for patients. *Dent. Clin. North Am.* 2006;50:299–315.

34. Fioretti F, Mendoza-Palomares C, Avoaka-Boni MC, Ramaroson J, Bahi S, Richert L, et al. Nano-odontology: nanostructured assemblies for endodontic regeneration. *J. Biomed. Nanotechnol.* 2011;7:471–475.

35. Gronthos S, Mankani M, Brahim J, Robey PG, and Shi S. Postnatal human dental pulp stem cells (DPSCs) in vitro and in vivo. *Proc. Natl. Acad. Sci. U.S.A.* 2000;97:13625–13630.

36. Li X, Hou J, Wu B, Chen T, Luo A. Effects of platelet-rich plasma and cell coculture on angiogenesis in human dental pulp stem cells and endothelial progenitor cells. *J Endod.* 2014;40, 1810–1814.

37. Diogenes A, and Ruparel NB. Regenerative endodontic procedures: clinical outcomes. *Dent. Clin. North Am.* 2017;61:111–125.

38. Shinmura Y, Tsuchiya S, Hata K, Honda MJ. Quiescent epithelial cell rests of Malassez can differentiate into ameloblast-like cells. *J. Cell. Physiol.* 2008;217:728–738.

39. Lynch SE, De Castilla GR, Williams RC, Kiritsy CP, Howell TH, Reddy MS, et al. The effects of short-term application of a combination of platelet-derived and insulin-like growth factors on periodontal wound healing. *J. Periodontol.* 1991;62:458–467.

40. Pilipchuk SP, Plonka AB, Monje A, Taut AD, Lanis A, Kang B, et al. Tissue engineering for bone regeneration and osseointegration in the oral cavity. *Dent. Mater.* 2015;31:317–338.

41. Sheikh Z, Hamdan N, Ikeda Y, Grynpas M, Ganss B, Glogauer M. Natural graft tissues and synthetic biomaterials for periodontal and alveolar bone reconstructive applications: a review. *Biomater. Res.* 2017;21:9.

42. Lynch SE. Methods for evaluation of regenerative procedures. *J. Periodontol.* 1992;63:1085–1092.

43. Takahashi K, Yamanaka S. Induction of pluripotent stem cells from mouse embryonic and adult fibroblast cultures by defined factors. *Cell*. 2006;126:663–676.
44. Washio K, Iwata T, Mizutani M, Ando T, Yamato M, Okano T, et al. Assessment of cell sheets derived from human periodontal ligament cells: a pre-clinical study. *Cell Tissue Res*. 2010;341:397–404.
45. Yang B, Chen G, Li J, Zou Q, Xie D, Chen Y, et al. Tooth root regeneration using dental follicle cell sheets in combination with a dentin matrix - based scaffold. *Biomaterials*. 2012;33:2449–2461.
46. Arakaki M, Ishikawa M, Nakamura T, Iwamoto T, Yamada A, Fukumoto E, et al. Role of epithelial-stem cell interactions during dental cell differentiation. *J. Biol. Chem.* 2012;287:10590–10601.
47. Seo BM, Miura M, Gronthos S, Bartold PM, Batouli S, Brahim J, et al. Investigation of multipotent postnatal stem cells from human periodontal ligament. *Lancet*. 2004;364:149–155.
48. Caton J, Bostanci N, Remboutsika E, De Bari C, Mitsiadis TA. Future dentistry: cell therapy meets tooth and periodontal repair and regeneration. *J. Cell Mol. Med*. 2011;15:1054–1065.
49. Howell TH, Fiorellini JP, Paquette DW, Offenbacher S, Giannobile WV, Lynch SE. A phase I/II clinical trial to evaluate a combination of recombinant human platelet-derived growth factor-BB and recombinant human insulin-like growth factor-I in patients with periodontal disease. *J. Periodontol*. 1997;68:1186–1193.
50. Clark D, Rajendran Y, Paydar S, Ho S, Cox D, Ryder M, et al. Advanced platelet-rich fibrin and freeze-dried bone allograft for ridge preservation: a randomized controlled clinical trial. *J. Periodontol*. 2018;89:379–387.
51. Fernandes G, Yang S. Application of platelet-rich plasma with stem cells in bone and periodontal tissue engineering. *Bone Res*. 2016;4:16036.
52. Dhillon RS, Schwarz EM, Maloney MD. Platelet-rich plasma therapy - future or trend? *Arthritis Res. Ther*. 2012;14:219.
53. Miron RJ, Sculean A, Cochran DL, Froum S, Zucchelli G, Nemcovsky C, et al. Twenty years of enamel matrix derivative: the past, the present and the future. *J. Clin. Periodontol*. 2016;43:668–683.
54. Miron RJ, Zucchelli G, Pikos MA, Salama M, Lee S, Guillemette V, et al. Use of platelet-rich fibrin in regenerative dentistry: a systematic review. *Clin. Oral Investig*. 2017;21:1913–1927.
55. Miron RJ, Chandad F, Buser D, Sculean A, Cochran DL, Zhang Y. Effect of enamel matrix derivative liquid on osteoblast and periodontal ligament cell proliferation and differentiation. *J. Periodontol*. 2016;87:91–99.
56. Pilipchuk SP, Monje A, Jiao Y, Hao J, Kruger L, Flanagan CL, et al. Integration of 3D printed and micropatterned polycaprolactone scaffolds for guidance of oriented collagenous tissue formation in vivo. *Adv. Healthc. Mater*. 2016;5:676–687.
57. Albrektsson T, Wennerberg A. Oral implant surfaces: Part 1 - review focusing on topographic and chemical properties of different surfaces and in vivo responses to them. *Int J Prosthodont*. 2004;17(5):536–543.
58. Variola F, Brunski JB, Orsini G, Tambasco De Oliveira P, Wazen R, Nanci A. Nanoscale surface modifications of medically relevant metals: state-of-the art and perspectives. *Nanoscale*. 2011;3:335–353.
59. Variola F, Vetrone F, Richert L, Jedrzejowski P, Yi J-H, Zalzal S, et al. Improving biocompatibility of implantable metals by nanoscale modification of surfaces: an overview of strategies, fabrication methods, and challenges. *Small*. 2009;5:996–1006.
60. Barbucci R, Pasqui D, Wirsen A, Affrossman S, Curtis A, Tetta C. Micro and nanostructured surfaces. *J. Mater. Sci. Mater. Med*. 2003;14:721–725.
61. Mendonca G, Mendonca DB, Aragao FJ, Cooper LF Advancing dental implant surface technology–from micron- to nanotopography. *Biomaterials*. 2008;29:3822–3835.

62. Coelho PG, Zavanelli RA, Salles MB, Yeniyol S, Tovar N, and Jimbo R. Enhanced bone bonding to nanotextured implant surfaces at a short healing period: a biomechanical tensile testing in the rat femur. *Implant Dent.* 2016;25:322–327.

63. Bezerra F, Ferreira MR, Fontes GN, Da Costa Fernandes CJ, Andia DC, Cruz NC, et al. Nano hydroxyapatite-blasted titanium surface affects pre-osteoblast morphology by modulating critical intracellular pathways. *Biotechnol. Bioeng.* 2017;114:1888–1898.

64. Yu J, Xu L, Li K, Xie N, Xi Y, Wang Y, et al. Zinc-modified calcium silicate coatings promote osteogenic differentiation through TGF-beta/Smad pathway and osseointegration in osteopenic rabbits. *Sci. Rep.* 2017;7:3440.

65. Singh P. Understanding peri-implantitis: a strategic review. *J. Oral Implantol.* 2011;37:622–626.

66. Godoy-Gallardo M, Manzanares-Cespedes MC, Sevilla P, Nart J, Manzanares N, Manero JM, et al. Evaluation of bone loss in antibacterial coated dental implants: an experimental study in dogs. *Mater. Sci. Eng. C Mater. Biol. Appl.* 2016;69:538–545.

67. Pokrowiecki R, Zareba T, Szaraniec B, Palka K, Mielczarek A, Menaszek E, et al. In vitro studies of nanosilver-doped titanium implants for oral and maxillofacial surgery. *Int. J. Nanomedicine.* 2017;12:4285–4297.

68. Bonifacio MA, Cometa S, Dicarlo M, Baruzzi F, De Candia S, Gloria A, et al. Gallium-modified chitosan/poly(acrylic acid) bilayer coatings for improved titanium implant performances. *Carbohydr. Polym.* 2017;166:348–357.

69. Selvig KA, Sorensen RG, Wozney JM, Wikesjo UM. Bone repair following recombinant human bone morphogenetic protein-2 stimulated periodontal regeneration. *J. Periodontol.* 2002;73:1020–1029.

70. Alvarez P, Hee CK, Solchaga L, Snel L, Kestler HK, Lynch SE, et al. Growth factors and craniofacial surgery. *J. Craniofac. Surg.* 2012;23:20–29.

71. Larsson L, Decker AM, Nibali L, Pilipchuk SP, Berglundh T, Giannobile WV. Regenerative medicine for periodontal and peri-implant diseases. *J. Dent. Res.* 2016;95:255–266.

72. Kaigler D, Avila-Ortiz G, Travan S, Taut AD, Padial-Molina M, Rudek I, et al. Bone engineering of maxillary sinus bone deficiencies using enriched CD90+ stem cell therapy: a randomized clinical trial. *J. Bone Miner. Res.* 2015;30:1206–1216.

73. Kaigler D, Pagni G, Park CH, Braun TM, Holman LA, Yi E, et al. Stem cell therapy for craniofacial bone regeneration: a randomized, controlled feasibility trial. *Cell Transplant.* 2013; 22:767–777.

74. Otsu K, Kumakami-Sakano M, Fujiwara N, Kikuchi K, Keller L, Lesot H, et al. Stem cell sources for tooth regeneration: current status and future prospects. *Front. Physiol.* 2014;5:36.

75. Mitsiadis TA, Papagerakis P. Regenerated teeth: the future of tooth replacement? *Regen. Med.* 2011;6:135–139.

76. Huang GT, Yamaza T, Shea LD, Djouad F, Kuhn NZ, Tuan RS, Shi S. Stem/progenitor cell-mediated de novo regeneration of dental pulp with newly deposited continuous layer of dentin in an in vivo model. *Tissue Eng Part A.* 2010;16:605–615.

77. Jimenez-Rojo L, Granchi Z, Graf D, Mitsiadis TA. Stem cell fate determination during development and regeneration of ectodermal organs. *Front. Physiol.* 2012;3:107.

78. Breslin S, O'Driscoll L. Three-dimensional cell culture: the missing link in drug discovery. *Drug Discov Today.* 2013;18:240–249.

79. Weeber F, Ooft SN, Dijkstra KK, and Voest EE. Tumor organoids as a pre-clinical cancer model for drug discovery. *Cell Chem. Biol.* 2017;24:1092–1100.

80. Skardal A, Shupe T, and Atala A. Organoid-on-a-chip and body-on-a- chip systems for drug screening and disease modeling. *Drug Discov. Today.* 2016;21:1399–1411.

81. Yin X, Mead BE, Safaee H, Langer R, Karp JM, Levy O. Engineering stem cell organoids. *Cell Stem Cell.* 2016;18:25–38.

82. Berahim Z, Moharamzadeh K, Rawlinson A, and Jowett AK. Biologic interaction of three-dimensional periodontal fibroblast spheroids with collagen-based and synthetic membranes. *J. Periodontol.* 2011;82:790–797.

83. Bonnamain V, Neveu I, Naveilhan P. In vitro analyses of the immunosuppressive properties of neural stem/progenitor cells using anti- CD3/CD28-activated T cells. *Methods Mol. Biol.* 2011;677:233–243.

84. Miquel A. In the 11- M terrorist tragedy in Madrid. *Rev. Clin. Esp.* 2011;211:158–162.

85. Natsiou D, Granchi Z, Mitsiadis TA, Jimenez-Rojo L. Generation of spheres from dental epithelial stem cells. *Front. Physiol.* 2017;8:7.

86. Mitsiadis TA, Luder HU. Genetic basis for tooth malformations: from mice to men and back again. *Clin. Genet.* 2011;80:319–329.

87. Klein C, Le Goff C, Topouchian V, Odent S, Violas P, Glorion C, et al. Orthopedics management of acromicric dysplasia: follow up of nine patients. *Am. J. Med. Genet. A.* 2014;164A:331–337.

88. Ingber DE. Reverse engineering human pathophysiology with organs-on-chips. *Cell.* 2016;164:1105–1109.

89. Bhatia SN, Ingber DE. Microfluidic organs-on-chips. *Nat. Biotechnol.* 2014;32:760–772.

90. Pagella P, Miran S, Mitsiadis T. Analysis of developing tooth germ innervation using microfluidic co-culture devices. *J. Vis. Exp.* 2015;102:e53114.

91. Pagella P, Neto E, Jimenez-Rojo L, Lamghari M, Mitsiadis TA. Microfluidics co-culture systems for studying tooth innervation. *Front. Physiol.* 2014;5:326.

92. Prantil-Baun R, Novak R, Das D, Somayaji MR, Przekwas A, Ingber DE. Physiologically based pharmacokinetic and pharmacodynamic analysis enabled by microfluidically linked organs-on-chips. *Annu. Rev. Pharmacol. Toxicol.* 2018;58:37–64.

93. Slavkin HC, Baum BJ. Relationship of dental and oral pathology to systemic illness. *JAMA.* 2000;284:1215–1217.

94. Wu J, Dong M, Santos S, Rigatto C, Liu Y, and Lin F. Lab-on-a- chip platforms for detection of cardiovascular disease and cancer biomarkers. *Sensors.* 2017;17:E2934.

95. Chen Z, Mauk MG, Wang J, Abrams WR, Corstjens PL, Niedbala RS, et al. A microfluidic system for saliva-based detection of infectious diseases. *Ann. N. Y. Acad. Sci.* 2007;1098:429–436.

96. Czilwik G, Messinger T, Strohmeier O, Wadle S, Von Stetten F, Paust N, et al. Rapid and fully automated bacterial pathogen detection on a centrifugal-microfluidic LabDisk using highly sensitive nested PCR with integrated sample preparation. *Lab. Chip.* 2015;15:3749–3759.

97. Tseng P, Napier B, Garbarini L, Kaplan DL, Omenetto FG. Functional, RF-trilayer sensors for tooth-mounted, wireless monitoring of the oral cavity and food consumption. *Adv. Mater.* 2018; 30:e1703257.

98. Otoh EC, Johnson NW, Danfillo IS, Adeleke OA, Olasoji HA. Primary head and neck cancers in North Eastern Nigeria. *West Afr J Med.* 2004;23:305–313.

99. Le QT, Kim HE, Schneider CJ, et al. Palifermin reduces severe mucositis in definitive chemoradiotherapy of locally advanced head and neck cancer: a randomized, placebo-controlled study. J. *Clin. Oncol.* 2011;29(20):2808–2814.

100. Marx RE A new concept in the treatment of osteoradionecrosis. *J. Oral Maxillofac. Surg.* 1983;41(6):351–357.

101. Hayashi M, Pellecer M, Chung E, Sung E. The efficacy of pentoxifylline/tocopherol combination in the treatment of osteoradionecrosis. *Spec. Care Dentist.* 2015;35(6):268–271.

102. Khan AA, Morrison A, Hanley DA, et al. Diagnosis and management of osteonecrosis of the jaw: a systematic review and international consensus. *J. Bone Miner. Res.* 2015;30(1):3–23.

14 Surgical Nanomaterials for Spinal Deformities

Design of Materials and Their Investigations

Dilip Kumar Patel and Roohi Kesharwani
Sam Higginbottom University of Agriculture,
Technology and Sciences

Surendra Tripathy
Northeast Frontier Railway Hospital

S.N. Singh
Ayurvedic Services

Vikas Kumar
Sam Higginbottom University of Agriculture,
Technology and Sciences

CONTENTS

DOI: 10.1201/9781003140108-14

14.1 INTRODUCTION

The present revolutionary change because of the developing interest of the aged people and the high action level in the old aged people. Techniques of the therapy have been adjusted; the objective has moved from decreasing the agony in patients with spine-related infection to enhancing the mobility of sufferers and keeping a level of activity (Genitiempo 2019). Around the world it was estimated that 2.5 million individuals are living with a spinal injury that more than one lac thirty thousand new wounds revealed on an annual basis. It's a health-related crisis that requires investigative restorative techniques to focus on spinal cord injuries (Ramezani, Nasirinezhad, and Abotaleb 2016; Silva et al. 2014; Thuret, Moon, and Gage 2006).

The spine has a connection with tissues, muscle, and bones, all of which create problems for recovery. For example, the modulus of the flexibility of the spinal unit should be contemplated (Genitiempo 2019; Mameren et al. 1990). Accessible treatments of spinal cord injury (SCI) have included drugs, medical procedures, foundational microorganism trans-estate, sub-atomic treatment, and tissue designing. Until this point there is not any accessible solid clinical treatment for patients with spinal injury that re-establishes the injury instigated loss of capacity to arrive at a degree that a free life can be ensured. In the past decade, nanotechnology has risen as an evolution in medicine (Muheremu, Peng, and Ao 2016). The beginning of nanotechnology can be followed back to 1959, when physicist Richard Feynman (Richard Feynman 1960) perceived the capability of controlling each particle and molecule at the nanometer scale and recommended that substances at this scale have one of a kind actual property (Gilmore et al. 2008; Feynman 2018). Nanotechnology conveys the development of the active three-dimensional nano atmosphere or nano scaffolds with designed nanostructures and diverse bioactive substrates of atomic grade for conservation, multiplication, and separation of immature microorganisms needed to get the progression of tissue engineering (Pan et al. 2017). Interest in the investigation for nano range material for regenerative medication is increasing day by day. For example, from a material property perspective, nonmaterial can be manufactured from metals, polymers, natural materials, and composites. In the designing of nano scaffolds, nanomaterials incorporate nanocrystals, nanotubes, nanofibers, nanofilms, nanoclusters, nanowires, nanoparticles, nanorods, and so forth (Kesharwani et al. 2016; Zhang and Webster 2009; Singh et al. 2016). Because of the potential for the treatment of neural tissue, research is exploring the utilization of nanomaterials for spinal injury. In treating this type of physical issue, cell-based treatment has indicated promising outcomes (Figure 14.1) (Nakamura and Okano 2013; Tsuji et al. 2010; Amezcua, Vimbela, and Stout 2017).

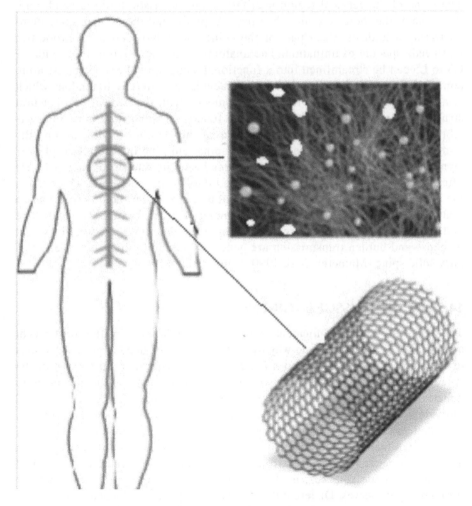

FIGURE 14.1 Approaches to treating spinal injury using nanoparticles as drug delivery systems and carbon nanotubes.

14.2   SPINAL ANATOMY

The Spinal anatomy should consistently be thought about, to comprehend the complex communication among inserts and the science of the spine. The spine comprises five parts:

1. The cervical spine, comprising of 7 vertebrae (C1–C7), is separated into the upper spine (C0–C2), the subaxial spine (C2–C5), and the lower spine (C5–T1).
2. The thoracic spine, comprising 12 vertebrae, is isolated into the upper (T1–T4), the center (T4–T8), and lower (T8–L1) thoracic spine.
3. The lumbar spine, comprises 5 vertebrae (L1–L5).
4. The sacrum and the coccyx also comprise 5 combined vertebral bodies.

The spine of the cervical region manifests a characteristic lordotic bend, with the spine of the thoracic region framing a kyphosis and the lumbar spine demonstrating a lordosis. Each part of the spine shows biomechanical properties and needs specific examination. The anatomy of the spine from the region of C3 to L5 can be streamlined into a functional spinal unit (FSU) demonstrating comparative mechanical properties. Movement is permitted by 10 tendons which is associated with FSU and limit developments, with the protection of neural structures. Another significant part of the functional spinal unit is an intervertebral circle that is linked to the endplates of the vertebral bodies around the fringe. In the pathology of the functional spinal unit, the intervertebral plate is significant for its inclusion; the circle begins losing its fine sustenance per year after birth. Hence beginning of a moderate inflexible degeneration, which alters the biomechanics of entire functional spinal unit (FSU) We should remember so that methodologies of inserts and utilized materials in the healthcare department and should be molded as per requirements of the deteriorated spine, in which response and burden transmission are genuinely not quite the same as an ordinary solid spine (Mameren et al. 1990; Genitiempo 2019).

14.3   NEURAL TISSUE ENGINEERING

The aging and improved financial conditions have driven over the most recent couple of years to an alternate way to deal with treating degenerative infections of the spine. What's a more, constant exploration of the normal history of the spine has prompted a wide range of approaches. Innovation and advances in materials have likewise permitted broad medical procedures in more seasoned individuals with improved outcomes, diminished agony, and boosted mobility. In spinal injury, nerve repair is a troublesome and significant issue in tissue regeneration medication, and further exploration is needed in material science and nerve science (Pan et al. 2017). Tissue engineering is a multidimensional field in which life sciences, medicine and design cooperate to create options for recovery of nerves. Different directions are implicated alongside design and surgical and diagnostic techniques to fix nerve deficits and advance recovery of nerve damage. listed signs and symptom incorporate the utilization of help and

TABLE 14.1
Merits and Demerits of Conventional Therapies Used for SCI Treatment

S.No.	Therapy	Demerits	Merits
1.	Medications: Intravenous methylprednisolone	Immune suppression is followed by increased susceptibility to infections (pneumonia, infection, etc.).	Decreasing inflammation near the site of injury.
		Increasing the risk of gastrointestinal abnormalities (ulcers, bleeding, and bowel obstruction), hyperglycemia, adult respiratory distress syndrome, deep vein thrombosis, and pulmonary embolism.	Reducing damage to nerve cells.
2.	Surgery	Surgery cannot reverse damage to the nerve cell and spinal cord.	Remove fragments of bones and foreign objects, avoid pain and spinal deformities in the future.
3.	Molecular therapy	These treatment methods are usually not sufficient alone and are used in combination with other methods.	Control axonal growth using activator and inhibitor molecules and moderate the inflammatory responses.
4.	Stem cell	Ethical concerns.	Self-renewal.
		Human neural stem cell tendency to generate more glial cells, especially astrocytes, than neurons in natural states.	Ability to become any cell in the body.

undeveloped cells, trophic and development factors and natural and synthetic biomaterials (Table 14.1). They are actualized on stages known as frameworks. The scaffold configuration is significant in nerve recovery as its direction signals may imitate the microenvironment of the extracellular matrix and advance connection, multiplication, development, relocation, separation, and endurance of the cells, and offer empowering results and other helpful options. The basic principles involved in tissue engineering and regeneration is summarized are Figure 14.2 (Marti et al. 2013; Langer and Vacanti 1993).

14.4 INNOVATIVE NANOSCAFFOLD DESIGN TECHNIQUES

In the regeneration of nerves, nanotechnology could be helpful by advancing neurotrophic elements and cell presentation impeding inhibitory variables, and connecting a physiologic cavity by giving a proper framework (Yiu and He 2006). The structure and geometry of nanostructure frameworks are significant in advancing improved cell movement for neural recovery. In this way, innovation to deliver these substances is basic for acquiring ideal surface properties and mechanical strength for the recovery. By giving a framework/underlying scaffolding for an injured spinal cord, nanomaterials can give axonal outgrowth. A few methodologies may potentially be uses

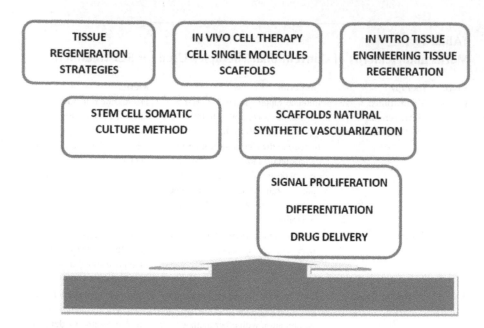

FIGURE 14.2 The basic principles of tissue engineering and regeneration (Mariappan 2019).

to form nanostructure scaffolds, such as electro spinning, self-assembled and stage partition (Cunha, Panseri, and Antonini 2011; Marti et al. 2013).

14.4.1 ELECTROSPINNING

Electrospinning refers to an appealing strategy for the handling of polymeric biomaterials into nanorange from synthetic and natural polymers. This strategy offers an open door to command excessive thickness and nanofiber development, alongside pores of the nanofiber networks, utilizing a generally straightforward test arrangement. The arrangement is first done via spinneret, with the utilization of higher voltage to charge the arrangement at basic voltage supply, regularly N200 volt per meter (Tan et al. 2005; Lyons, Li, and Ko 2004).

Nanofibers rising out of the spinneret are then gathered in an same direction utilizing a pivoting authority. The last can be a drum or a circle just like a plate. Arrangement properties (for example, fixation, conductivity, consistency, and flexibility) and cycle boundaries (for example temperature, voltage, needle shape, and distance from target) could be changed to manufacture different sorts of strands for different applications. Polymer arrangement makes it conceivable and not command its direction, empowering the creation of situated nanofibers that could be helpful to plan frameworks in tissue engineering. Electrospun NFs have appeared to improve and quicken cell exercises, for example, expansion, axon recovery, development, and relocation utilized in the application of nerve tissue engineering (Kijeńska et al. 2012; Dong et al. 2006; Liu et al. 2012a; Wang et al. 2011).

14.4.2 SELF-ASSEMBLY

Self-assembly methodology recently arose as another methodology in designing counterfeit scaffold materials that copy common extracellular mix (ECM) both fundamentally and practically (Viswanathan et al. 2019). It is the unconstrained and reversible development of a stable ordered structure, from disordered elements through different weak interactions (Toksöz and Guler 2009). The distinct peptide groupings show the ability to self-assemble toward different structures, going from β-sheets assembly through hydrogen clinging to round and hollow micelles utilizing lipophilic connections. This sort of self-assembling peptide frameworks incorporate self-assembling peptide nanofiber scaffolds and diblock polypeptide hydrogels (Tysseling-Mattiace et al. 2008). The glycine spacer adds up to improve the highlights of peptides having self-assembled property for a particular tissue reaction having adjustable and sufficient property for the introduction of the function to the tissues, regardless of hindering the limit of the biomaterials to self assemble. (Taraballi et al. 2009; Taraballi et al. 2010). The repeating units of hydrophobic and hydrophilic amino acids are used to prepare amphiphilic oligopeptides and framed stable β - sheet structures in water and utilized to create frameworks for recovery of nerve injury.

14.4.3 PHASE SEPARATION

One more strategy for the development of nanofibers (NFs) is the phase separation technique. This is utilized due to the immiscibility of the polymers and solvent. At first, the breakdown of the polymer occurs in the solvent, and the subsequent arrangement is retained at the gelation temperature for the development of advanced gel at the polymer stage. Subsequently, the dissolvable can be separated from the gel to recover the permeable nanofibrous skeleton. Different sorts of phase separation techniques are used for planning nanofibers, for example, synthetically and thermally actuated phase separation (Marti et al. 2013). Another method is called thermally actuated fluid stage division to develop materials with nanofibrous property. The nanofibrous froths delivered utilizing the stage partition procedure are fundamentally the same as in measurement to the characteristic collagen present in the extracellular matrix (Ma and Zhang 2001). In thermally actuated phase separation, solvent-rich and polymer-rich stages are delivered by reducing the polymer arrangement temperature. The phase having solvent is eliminated from the arrangement via extraction, giving up a strong, skeletal-like polymer grid with pores (Marti et al. 2013). Phase separation can be actuated through the addition of nonsolvent and varying temperatures to the polymeric system, this is called warm incited or non-dissolvable initiated Phase separation, individually. Polymer scaffolds acquired by the stage detachment technique normally have sponge-like permeable morphology along with circular pores of micro-scale. The nanostructured exceptionally permeable framework created by Yang et al. is made up of biodegradable polymer by the phase separation technique. This Phase separation process develop nanoscale fibers with diameters of 50–500 nanometers. The up side of the stage division measure is that it is a moderately straightforward strategy and the prerequisites are exceptionally negligible regarding gear contrasted and the recently examined strategies, electrospinning, and self-assembly (Cunha, Panseri, and Antonini 2011; Yang et al. 2004; Hua et al. 2002).

14.5   NANOMATERIAL SCAFFOLDS FOR NEUROREGENERATION

Nanotechnology contains various nanostructures having a size range of 1–100 nanometers. The consequence of their small size has various primary and useful properties these materials, for example, electrical conductance, chemical reactivity, optical impacts, attraction. The utilization of nanotechniques provides the potential to treat hopeless illness such as SCI (Pitkethly 2004; Krishnamoorti 2006). Various approaches used in the treatment of spinal cord injury are summarized in Figure 14.3. The most significant nanoscaffolds are nanoparticle nanogels, specifically, nanofibers and nanotubes as these can mirror the cylindrical structures found inside tissues and cells (Gilmore et al. 2008).

14.5.1   Magnetic Nanoparticles

Magnetic nanoparticles are mainly composed of a core made up of inorganic magnetic material. This magnetic core might have biocompatible surface coatings for improving stability in physiological conditions and utilized in the field of biomedicine. The three main applications for the MNPs have the following applications:

1. Magnetic drug targeting (MDT)
2. Hyperthermia treatment
3. Medical imaging

Nanoparticles are being researched extensively for treatment of spinal cord lesions due to spinal cord injury (SCI), with emphasis on preventing secondary injury at the

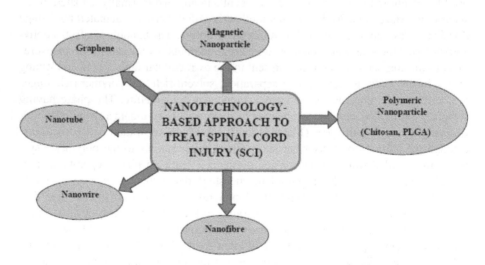

FIGURE 14.3   Nanotechnology-based approach for SCI treatment.

affected site. In the first application of drug targeting, drug-loaded MNPs are administered into a body fluid, and external magnetic fields guide and localize the particles in specific diseased areas of the body and ultimately release the loaded drug at the affected area. The significant advantages of using MNPs over viral approaches for gene delivery for treating SCIs were studied by Jeffery et al. In this, they suggested that a therapeutic window of opportunity opens post-SCI during which the Blood Brain Barrier is compromised and MNPs can be used for gene delivery to the trauma site. Magnetic nanoparticles could be selectively heated by applying a high-frequency alternating externally applied magnetic field, at which the magnetic moment of the MNPs align and realign with the applied field. This generates heat, which degrades tumor tissue. Electromagnetic field (EMF) simulations are used to encourage nerve cell regeneration after SCI. Specifically, these nanoparticles are utilized to improve the therapeutic efficacy of SCI treatment by applying magnetic fields (Sharma et al. 2007; Venugopal, Mehta, and Linninger 2020; Zhang and Webster 2009).

14.5.2 NANOTUBES

Nanotubes are cylindrical-shaped structures with a span in the 1–100 nanometer range; they are made out of a concentric computation of a single-walled or multi-walled as appears in Figure 14.4. These nanostructures highlight conductive and mechanical properties ideal for neural disorders, notwithstanding demonstrating an alluring effect on neuronal cell morphology and volatility (Balasubramanian and Burghard 2005). Single-walled carbon nanotubes (SWNTs) have conductive

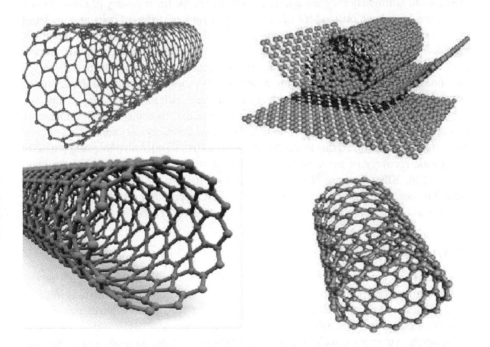

FIGURE 14.4 Schematic figure of the structure of the nanotube.

properties that might be utilized to advance nerve repair after spinal cord injury (Lee and Parpura 2009). Extension in one dimension can offer greater help and direction to the regeneration of axons (Liu et al. 2012b). The main use of the nanotubes comprising carbon in the investigation of neuroscience depicted by Mattson et al. who develop multiwall carbon nanotubes on neurons of rodent brain. These are used along with various nanocomposites for the restoration of damaged tissue. In this study after experimental spinal cord injury, organization of the nanotubes in a rodent model showed advance axon's recovery into the injury pit and useful recuperation of the rear appendages (Zagari et al. 2016).

14.5.3 Nanofibers

Nanofibers are described as strands with measurements under 100 nanometers that are incorporated under specific procedures, for example, interfacial polymerization and electrospinning (Venugopal, Mehta, and Linninger 2020). By setting engineered polymer set as center material and characteristic polymer, for example, collagen as shell material, nanofibers with solid mechanical strength and surface with greater biocompatibility could be acquired. This may take care of the issue of manufactured polymer nanofibers' biocompatibility. Nanofibers have been indicated not exclusively to be viable along with tissues and cells, however likewise to advance, development, cell connection separation, and long haul endurance of neurons. (Mazzatenta et al. 2007; Elias, Price, and Webster 2002).

Nanofiber materials are regularly joined in conjunction with bioactive materials or medication. Ultimately they are utilized as platforms for the recovery of tissue. Novel nanofibers have been utilized for helping the recovery of different cells and axons in the spine for the therapy of spinal cord injury. A few exceptionally intriguing nanofiber materials have been created to treat injuries related to the spine. As peptide amphiphile atoms were combined that self assembled material converted in barrel-shaped nanofibers at the time of infusion into a string of bunnies of the spine at the damaged site. Nanofibers comprised of polyhydroxyalkanoate which has to be seen to advance neural undeveloped cell connection, CNS recovery and neurotransmitter developments (Xu et al. 2010; Tysseling-Mattiace et al. 2008). The nanofibers network tube containing chitosan immobilized due to electrical charged Beta tricalcium phosphate particles to upgrade recovery of nerve with the expansion of thickness and zone of the axon (Wang et al. 2010). The use of nanofibers as a substrate builds the neuron's development. Further it was noticed expanded pace of NSC separation on adjusted nanofiber. (Yang et al. 2004; Ramezani, Nasirinezhad, and Abotaleb 2016).

14.5.4 Nanowires (NW)

Nanowires are outrageous slim shapes with a diameter in the 2-nm range, having multiple times longer length. The nanowire encounters quantum constraint impacts by electrons and photons due to this structure and furthermore particular optical and electrical properties. (Rahong et al. 2016). These nano-type wires are found in numerous structures, including semiconductors, metals, natural mixes and covers (Berthing et al. 2009). The organization could be adjusted to make hetero-type structures and fabricate them in a conceivable manner to tailor the structure of the band and the wire electronic properties. In 2012 Bechara and associates grew polymeric frameworks with the surface of these wires of nano range that were bio-functionalized via electroconductive polymers that were ready to give physiological degrees of electrical stimulation to NSCs. The report demonstrated that these nanowire surfaces upgrade NSC attachment, separation, and proliferation for as long as 7 days of culture (Hällström et al. 2007; Von Ahnen, Piret, and Prinz 2015; Bechara, Wadman, and Popat 2011). Drug-stacked nanowires are additionally being created to treat spinal cord injury. Another researcher labeled three mixes, one from Acure Pharma and the other two from Uppsala and Sweden, demonstrating TiO2 nanowires having the capability of neuroprotection. The labeled nanowires are employed topically on the site of spinal injury in creatures. Compared with the use of medications alone, the medication-stacked NWs further lessened conduct segregation and upgraded spinal cord pathology (cell injury, edema development). Nonetheless, when these NWs were used alone, no constructive outcomes were noticed (Sharma et al. 2007; Sharma et al. 2009).

14.5.5 GRAPHENE

Graphene is a two-dimensional sheet of carbon atoms arranged in a hexagonal grid, which makes for the thinnest, most electrically and thermally conductive material in the world with flexibility, transparency, and super strong features. Its electrical conductivity can be applied to organs with properties such as nerve tissue and spinal elements. It has been utilized in SCI treatment as a scaffold for neural cell growth. Li et al. in 2013 utilized graphene foam (a three-dimensional porous structure) as a novel scaffold for neuronal stem cells for the first time. It was revealed that three-dimensional graphene foams not only can support neuron stem cell growth but also, in comparison with two-dimensional graphene films, keep cells at an active proliferation state better than that of two-dimensional graphene films. Sahni and colleagues in 2013 studied the biocompatibility of graphene for interface with cortical neurons of a rat. Serrano et al found in his investigation that novel, free-standing, porous, and flexible scaffolds of 3D graphene oxide having potential for neural tissue regeneration (Ramezani, Nasirinezhad, and Abotaleb 2016; Amezcua, Vimbela, and Stout 2017).

14.5.6 POLYMERIC NANOPARTICLES

Various polymers are used in the treatment of spinal injury. Some are discussed below with their properties and function:

14.5.6.1 Chitosan Nanoparticles

Chitosan is widely used in the synthesis of nanoparticles due to its ability to enhance the penetration of large molecules across mucosal surfaces. Here we discuss a few examples of the use of chitosan in spinal injury. Chen et al. observed that chitosan nanoparticles could restore transmission of nerve impulses through the spinal cord of an adult guinea pig that had undergone severe injury. The animals were subcutaneously injected with the nanoparticles at the nape of the neck, which was able to effectively restore nerve impulse transmission through the spinal cord after severe injury. Some self-assembled nanoparticles that are used for SCI treatment, such as ferulic acid-modified glycol chitosan nanoparticles for their neuroprotective effects were researched by Wu and team.(Deng, Chang, and Wu 2019; Chen et al. 2016).

14.5.6.2 Poly(Lactide-Co-Glycolide) Nanoparticles (PLGA Nanoparticles)

PLGA nanoparticle indicated that having a safe, biocompatible, and biodegradable feature which is widely used in many nanoparticle-based drug delivery systems. In spine treatment it is utilized for sustained delivery of flavopiridol, a CDK inhibitor as observed by Hao Ren et al. Being a broad-spectrum inhibitor, flavopiridol shows adverse effects when administered systemically. Therefore, targeted local delivery of flavopiridol via nanoparticles has potential for SCI treatment. The glial cell line–derived neurotrophic factor (GDNF) encapsulated in PLGA nanoparticles for intraspinal delivery at the lesion site of an SCI rat model utilized by Wang et al. showed hind limb locomotor recovery and efficient preservation of neuronal fibers (Wang et al. 2010; Wang et al. 2011).

14.6 PROPERTIES OF BIOMATERIALS APPLIED TO SPINAL SURGERY

In spine-related medical procedures, biomaterials have to upgrade the achievement of adjustment at the spinal site. Whereas re-creating bone imperfections isn't the essential expectation of exploration in spine-related medical procedures, to get fragment adjustment, bone combinations speaks to the main objective. The best material that we have available to permit combination is our bone, and for quite a long time the standard method to meld sections of the anatomy has been bone transfer. Currently the spine-related medical procedure depends on the advancement of novel materials that decrease the rate of pseudoarthrosis, in this way lessening the factor site a medical procedure expansion and conceivably related entanglements. The material should be a combination of osteoinductive and osteoconductive. Indeed, for treatment and diagnosing purposes, for a long time a mix of osteoinductive frameworks with osteoconductive tissue was utilized to build the achievement pace of combination for spinal surgery. (Ambrosio and Tanner 2012; Ramezani, Nasirinezhad, and Abotaleb 2016).

14.6.1 Osteoconductive Materials

Osteoconductive materials are basically materials whose involvement in structural activities is such that they allow bone ingrowth and the orthotopic migration of osteogenic cells in the site, but alone they cannot promote osteogenesis or induce bone formation. The preferable materials in this category are calcium phosphate, ceramics, and porous metal. The best osteoconductive material remains autologous bone; it shows the best properties, though allografts have also been extensively utilized. Because primary stability represents a weak point, they have been utilized in combination with the hollow metal of polyetheretherketone (PEEK) cages, showing better response at the fusion area.

14.6.2 Osteoinductive Materials

Osteoinductive materials exhibit bone-forming properties with improved characteristics. In 1968 Friedstein explained osteoinduction as "the induction of undifferentiated inducible osteoprogenitor cells that are not yet committed to the osteogenic lineage to form osteoprogenitor cells." In various studies it was observed that both bone morphogenetic protein and demineralized bone matrix (DBM) induce heterotopic bone formation as they are the initiators of an events cascade, the so-called endochondral model, namely chemotaxis of mesenchymal cells and differentiation of cells in the specific lineage of chondroblasts and chondrocytes ultimately responsible for formation of a collagen II-rich cartilaginous matrix. The process of osteoprogenitor cells reaching the site with absorption in the cartilage and new bone formation occurs due to maturation of the chondrocytes and is then followed by vessel growth and proliferation. Usually bone formation is induced by BMP, although some researchers proposed a direct bone formation model. Calcium phosphate type of material also has osteoinductive properties and is observes by various researchers in their research activity. It was observed that the bone proliferation due to calcium phosphate was always intramembranous, so it is called the intramembranous model and showed a slower reactivity of bone formation in comparison to BMP. Precipitation of the carbonated apatite together with organic compounds by calcium phosphate, which able to liberate in the form of Ca^{2+} and PO_4^{3-} in the solution by supersaturation of the site and allowing therefore mineralization of the tissue. The main concern with these materials is the inability to grow vessels and therefore undergo remodeling.

14.6.3 Osteogenic Tissue

Currently research has focused on the activity and application of activated osteoprogenitors defining bone tissue engineering. It has been defined by the use of specific principles to design, produce, grow, and replicate living cells and tissue. The most promising tissue engineering has been the implant of acellular osteoconductive scaffolds, combined with osteoinductive factors, and the isolation of mesenchymal stem cells activated and implanted with growth factors to induce differentiation and grow on an osteoconductive scaffold in orthopedics. Osteogenic human cells can be obtained from fetuses, infants, and adults. Bone marrow aspiration in adults can provide mesenchymal stem cells, which can then be amplified and produce osteogenic cells, reticular cells, and fibroblastic lineage. It is also rich in growth factors, which seem to stimulate bone growth by helping mesenchymal stem cells to differentiate, such as the vascular endothelial growth factor. Currently, the use of adipose tissue stem cells has become thought-provoking, thanks to the better understanding of the chemistry of regulation. Due to abundance of donor sites, some authors have reported a clinical role in helping to regenerate bone tissue in adults. Embryonic stem cells show potential to differentiate in every cell lineage, having the capability to form any tissue, but ethical considerations about the implant of such cells, as well as the possibility of transmitting pathologies, restrain the clinical use of such technology. Bone engineering is influenced by many different growth factors, which can lead to the differentiation of the osteogenic lineage of the mesenchymal stem cells; most research is concentrated on the BMP family, vascular endothelial growth factor, core binding factor alpha1, and fibroblast growth factor-2 (Genitiempo 2019).

14.7 NANOTECHNOLOGY-ENHANCED PEEK-BASED SPINAL IMPLANTS

Nowadays Polyether-ether-ketone (PEEK) has been gaining attention as it acts as a high-strength polymer with favorable imaging compatibility and stiffness that closely matches bone, rendering it suitable for spinal implant applications. PEEK has many merits, such as excellent mechanical properties, chemical inertness, ease of processing, biocompatibility, and low toxicity utilized for spinal implants. PEEK and PEEK-based composites are commonly used for fabricating spinal fusion cages. However, PEEK deals with the issue of lacking osteointegrative capacity, and the normal arrangement of adding HA to PEEK experiences drastically diminished mechanical strength. To tackle this issue, nanophase HA has been joined with PEEK and showed better mechanical properties because of the solid grip of HA fillers to the PEEK network. The nanocomposite showed enhanced mechanical properties, with tensile strength increased from 92 MPA to 98 MPa and hardness increased from 23 HV to 27 HV when the HA content increased from 0 vol% to 5 vol% as revealed in one of the review. The investigation additionally uncovered that scattered HA nanoparticles reinforced firmly to PEEK, and no debonding was noticed, proposing that utilizing nanoparticles is a potential answer for the debonding issue experienced with current PEEK-HA composites. In any case, the rigidity diminished from 98 MPa to 24 MPa as the HA content expanded from 5 vol% to 10 vol% because of broad agglomeration of HA nanoparticles. In a further endeavor to stay away from agglomeration of HA nanoparticles, a novel PEEK/HA nanocomposite was created by in situ process. (Gilmore et al. 2008)

14.8 SAFETY CONCERNS WITH NANOTECHNOLOGY

Nanotechnology offers potential for huge improvement in the field of orthopedic repair and regeneration, although concerns regarding safety are as yet an issue in regard to execution of nanotechnology in muscular health. The clinical pertinence of SCI treatment that mistreat the improved material properties of nanotechnology relies intensely upon whether specialists can affirm non-toxic impacts on the patient. This subject has been intensely debated for a long while now, particularly as a result of the huge number of associated factors when utilizing nanostructures in an biological system. For instance, there exists critical inconstancy in the assembling techniques, crude materials, and response scaling to make uniform nanomaterials. Moreover, a few material properties influence their association with the biological system, such as size, shape, surface territory, synthetic creation, grid structure, surface science, surface charge, and accumulation state. Carbon-based nanomaterials (CBNs) are exceptionally questionable. There have been reports of unfriendly impacts through inward breathwork of CBNs, cell passing, and repressed cell expansion. To dodge this issue, functionalization of CBNs is a standard methodology that straightforwardly influences the level of cytotoxicity.

Subsequently, the impacts of CBNs in natural frameworks should be satisfactorily evaluated prior to offering any viable clinical treatment. Further dangers and harmfulness of nanotechnology are important to be assessed before being broadly utilized clinically. Harmfulness of nanosilver particles and silver particles, which radiate from nanocomposites, is a significant matter of concern. Comparable well-being concerns in regard to barium particles delivered from barium sulfate nanoparticles have likewise been talked abou.. In this manner, the impacts of CBNs in biological frameworks should be satisfactorily measured prior to offering any clinical treatment (Amezcua, Vimbela, and Stout 2017; Wang et al. 2011; Viswanathan et al. 2019).

14.8.1 TOXICITY OF CARBON NANOTUBES (CNTS)

In neural tissue design, the findings on the utilization of nanomaterials have not been entirely positive. Multi-walled carbon NTs were found to hinder the regenerative limit of axons of DRG neurons without causing the passing of cells. An electrically directing hydrogel containing single-walled carbon nanotubes (SWCNTs) was appeared to diminish SC multiplication in a 2D microenvironment without influencing cell reasonability. Nonetheless, a comparable hydrogel imitating a 3D climate appeared to have no critical impact on SC development. Impacts of SWCNTs appeared to diminish the DNA substance of cells taken from early stage avian spinal rope. The SWCNTs diminished the number of glial cells in both PNS and the CNS, prompting a decrease of tangible neurons and improving the resting layer capability of refined DRG neurons when contrasted with controls observed by Belyanskaya et al. The CNTs have special ingestion in the close infrared area, which empowers its utility for biological sensing. CNTs can possibly interface with macromolecules like proteins and DNA because of their nano size. The close- infrared optical retention of carbon nanotubes being utilized for laser warming malignant growth treatment and the surprising one-measurement empty nanostructure especially makes CNTs helpful as novel medication and quality conveyance tools. As a result of the rich electronic properties of CNTs, they have been investigated for the advancement of profoundly sensitive and explicit nanoscale biosensors. In another investigation, detailed that unbiased and negative charged MWCNTs were nontoxic to cell lines at a centralization of up to 100 mg/L, yet the positive charged ones were discovered to be toxic to cells at 10 mg/L. Some examinations on rodents and mice have shown that SWCNT and MWCNT instigate oxidative pressure, irritation, granulomas, and fibrosis in the lungs (Marti et al. 2013; Lee and Parpura 2009).

14.8.2 TOXICITY OF QUANTUM DOTS

Quantum dots are round nanocrystals from 1 to 10 nm in breadth They have remarkable electronic, optical, attractive, and reactant properties and show explicit quantal impact, which is measurement subordinate. Disregarding having wide applications in various fields, these ENPs also exhibit some toxicity. The cytotoxicity of CdSe quantum dots was observed by in an in vitro study. The viability of hepatocytes incubated in a solution containing quantum dots diminished as per its conc (0.0625 < 0.25 < 1 mg/ml). They additionally recommended that the quantum dots that had been exposed to UV radiations for 8 hours diminished the cellular feasibility essentially.

14.8.3 Toxicity of Iron/Iron Oxide Nanoparticles

Nanostructured iron oxides permit a wide scope of possible applications in nano-technology-related fields. Hematite-containing nanoparticles were found to diminish cell viability. A decrease in the activity of antioxidative enzymes induced by oxidative stress in cells may happen

Because of such cytotoxicity a few specialists examined the near harmfulness of nano and miniature particles of some metal oxides like Fe_2O_3, Fe_3O_4, TiO_2, and CuO. They detailed cell demise, mitochondrial harm, DNA harm, and oxidative DNA injuries when the human cell line was presented to these nano and micropar-ticles. This investigation showed that CuO nanoparticles were considerably more harmful when contrasted with the CuO microparticles. Bregoli et al. noticed that Sb_2O_3 and cobalt (Co) NPs were more poisonous than others. They likewise inferred that Sb_2O_3 NPs hinder the proliferation of erythroid progenitors.

14.8.4 Toxicity of Chitosan/Gold/Silica Nanoparticles

Necrotic or autophagic cell death was seen in a study of chitosan nanoparticles (1% w/v) in the cell nucleus after 4 hrs exposure. It might be because of damage of the cell membrane and resultant enzyme spillage. It was tracked down that the PEG-covered NPs can prompt intense aggravation and apoptosis in the liver. It was accounted for that the PEG-covered NPs were caught in liver Kupffer cells and spleen macrophages. Monodisperse polypyrrole (PPy) nanoparticles with five unique measurements (20, 40, 60, 80, and 100 nm) were created through oxida-tion polymerization to assess size dependent cytotoxicity (Wang et al. 2011; Deng, Chang, and Wu 2019).

14.9 THE PROMISING APPLICATION OF NANOMATERIAL IN NEURAL TISSUE ENGINEERING

As well as supporting in muscular and vascular tissue recovery, nanomaterials are additionally assisting to heal damaged nerves. Specifically, sensory system wounds, sicknesses, and issues happen unreasonably frequently. About 250,000–400,000 patients experience a spinal cord injury every year in the US. Even though differ-ent cell treatments and inserts have been researched, repairing damaged nerves and accomplishing full recovery and yet considering about nervous system com-plexity. For instance, of the 1.4 million Americans who suffer horrible traumatic injuries yearly, almost 50,000 patients die. By and large, the sensory system can be separated into the two main parts: the one containing brain and the spinal cord—i.e., the central nervous system (CNS)—and the other one containing spinal and autonomic nerves—i.e. the peripheral nervous system (PNS). They have different strategies to repair injuries. For the PNS, the damages axons generally recover a through multiplying Schwann cells, phagocytosing myelin by macrophages or monocytes, framing groups of Bünger by the packaging of Schwann cells, and growing axons in the distal portion. Notwithstanding, it is hard to re-stretch and re-innervate axons to recover capacities in the CNS because of the shortfall of Schwann cells. More significantly, because of the impact of astrocytes, meningeal cells, and oligodendrocytes, the thick glial scar tissue regularly conformed to the present neural biomaterials will forestall proximal axon development and repress neuron recovery. Consequently, CNS wounds may cause serious practical harms and are considerably harder to fix than PNS wounds. Ideal materials for neural tissue design ought to have amazing cytocompatible, mechanical, and electrical properties. Without great cytocompatibility properties, materials may fail to improve neuron development and simultaneously may inspire serious irritation or contamination. Without adequate mechanical properties, the platform may not keep going long enough to truly uphold neural tissue recovery. Furthermore, major electrical properties of platforms are needed to help invigorate and control neuron conduct under electrical incitement, subsequently, more viably controlling neural tissue repair.

Until this now, different characteristics and manufactured materials have been used as nerve unions to fix seriously harmed nerves by crossing over nerve holes and directing neuron outgrowth. Nonetheless, there are still numerous weaknesses for these neural biomaterials including the following. For autografts, it is normally hard to gather adequate contributor nerves from patients, and it is conceivable that benefactor site nerve capacities might be weakened; and for allografts, inflammation, rejection, and transmission of diseases may often happen, prompting collapse of implants. Other conventional biomaterials (for example, silicon tests utilized in neuroprosthetic gadgets and polymers utilized as nerve conductors) used for neural tissue repair have been restricted by the broad development of glial scar tissue around the material for regrowth of nerve as non-ideal mechanical and electrical properties.

Nanotechnology provided a wide stage to create novel and improved neural tissue design materials and treatment, including planning nanofiber/nanotube platforms with remarkable cytocompatibility and conductivity properties to help neuron exercises. Nanomaterials have likewise been utilized to embody different neural undifferentiated organisms and Schwann cells into biomimetic nanoscaffolds to improve nerve repair. Because carbon nanotubes/filaments have electrical conductivity, solid mechanical properties, and comparative nanoscale measurements to neurites, they have been utilized to direct axon recovery and improve neural action as biomimetic platforms at the portion of neural tissue injury. Additionally, CNT/CNF lattices or unattached nanotube films have been created for neural tissue design applications. For example, Gheith et al. explored the biocompatibility of a detached clearly charged SWCNT/polymer slender film arranged in layer-by-layer assembly. They saw that 94–98% of neurons were feasible on the SWCNT/polymer films following a multi-day hatching. The SWCNT/polymer films effectively initiated neuronal cell separation, guided neuron expansion, and coordinated more intricate branches than controls (Zhang and Webster 2009; Cunha, Panseri, and Antonini 2011; Venugopal, Mehta, and Linninger 2020).

14.10 CONCLUSION AND FUTURE PERSPECTIVES OF BIOMATERIALS APPLIED TO SCI

In this chapter, we discussed the nanotechnology involvement in the surgery of spinal cord injury. Nanotechnology has advanced in all clinical areas. It participated in treatment, diagnosis, and surgeries related to spinal injury. Furthermore, research is moving toward stem cell study and regeneration for various applications. Nanoscaffolds (nanotubes, nanowires, nanofibers) are involve in spinal treatment and utilized in advancements to serve humankind and improve human life. Additionally, nanomaterials used in designing scaffolds demonstrate remarkable potential in the future to design custom-tailored serviceability and customized implants utilized in the delivery of medication in surgery or regeneration. These materials can be designed as a scaffold utilizing 3D printing technology to simulate the host environment and provide more up-gradation in regeneration. It also enhanced the improvement in healthcare via utilizing nanomaterials in spinal treatment and they become capable not exclusively to incorporate with the host, yet additionally to coordinate cell adjustment as per the need of the situation improving recuperation and patients' satisfaction.

ABBREVIATIONS

BMP	bone morphogenetic protein
CBNs	carbon-based nanomaterials
CDK	cyclin-dependent kinase
CNS	central nervous system
DBM	demineralized bone matrix
GDNF	glial cell line-derived neurotrophic factor
MDT	magnetic drug targeting
NFs	nanofibers
NSCs	neural stem cells
NWs	nanowires
PEEK	polyetheretherketone
PLGA	poly(Lactide-Co- Glycolide)
PNS	peripheral nervous system
PPy	polypyrrole
SCI	spinal cord injury
SWNTs	single-walled carbon nanotubes

REFERENCES

Ambrosio, L., and E. Tanner. 2012. *Biomaterials for Spinal Surgery.* Woodhead Publishing 2012

Amezcua, R., G. Vimbela, and D.A. Stout. 2017. Nanomaterials for Spinal Cord Injury Recovery. *Spine Research.*

Balasubramanian, K., and M. Burghard. 2005. Chemically Functionalized Carbon Nanotubes. *Small.*

Bechara, S., L. Wadman, and K.C. Popat. 2011. Electroconductive Polymeric Nanowire Templates Facilitates in Vitro C17.2 Neural Stem Cell Line Adhesion, Proliferation and Differentiation. *Acta Biomaterialia.*

Berthing, T., C.B. Sørensen, J. Nygård, and K.L. Martinez. 2009. Applications of Nanowire Arrays in Nanomedicine. *Journal of Nanoneuroscience.*

Chen, F.-M., X. Liu, P. Polym, and S. Author. 2016. Advancing Biomaterials of Human Origin for Tissue Engineering HHS Public Access Author Manuscript. *Prog Polym Sci.*

Cunha, C., S. Panseri, and S. Antonini. 2011. Emerging Nanotechnology Approaches in Tissue Engineering for Peripheral Nerve Regeneration. *Nanomedicine: Nanotechnology, Biology, and Medicine.*

Deng, C., J. Chang, and C. Wu. 2019. Bioactive Scaffolds for Osteochondral Regeneration. *Journal of Orthopaedic Translation.*

Dong, W., T. Zhang, M. McDonald, C. Padilla, J. Epstein, and Z.R. Tian. 2006. Biocompatible Nanofiber Scaffolds on Metal for Controlled Release and Cell Colonization. *Nanomedicine: Nanotechnology, Biology, and Medicine.*

Elias, K.L., R.L. Price, and T.J. Webster. 2002. Enhanced Functions of Osteoblasts on Nanometer Diameter Carbon Fibers. *Biomaterials.*

Feynman, R. 2018. There's Plenty of Room at the Bottom. In *Feynman and Computation.*

Genitiempo, M. 2019. Biomaterial in Spinal Surgery. In *Bone Repair Biomaterials.* Woodhead Publishing 2019.

Gilmore, J.L., X. Yi, L. Quan, and A.V. Kabanov. 2008. Novel Nanomaterials for Clinical Neuroscience. *Journal of NeuroImmune Pharmacology.*

Hällström, W., T. Mårtensson, C. Prinz, P. Gustavsson, L. Montelius, L. Samuelson, and M. Kanje. 2007. Gallium Phosphide Nanowires as a Substrate for Cultured Neurons. *Nano Letters.*

Hua, F.J., G.E. Kim, J.D. Lee, Y.K. Son, and D.S. Lee. 2002. Macroporous Poly(L-Lactide) Scaffold 1. Preparation of a Macroporous Scaffold by Liquid-Liquid Phase Separation of a PLLA-Dioxane-Water System. *Journal of Biomedical Materials Research.*

Kesharwani, S., P.K. Jaiswal, R. Kesharwani, V. kumar, and D.K. Patel. 2016. Dendrimer: A Novel Approach for Drug Delivery. *Journal of Pharmaceutical & Scientific Innovation.*

Kijeńska, E., M.P. Prabhakaran, W. Swieszkowski, K.J. Kurzydlowski, and S. Ramakrishna. 2012. Electrospun Bio-Composite P(LLA-CL)/Collagen I/Collagen III Scaffolds for Nerve Tissue Engineering. *Journal of Biomedical Materials Research - Part B Applied Biomaterials.*

Krishnamoorti, R. 2006. Extracting the Benefits of Nanotechnology for the Oil Industry. *JPT, Journal of Petroleum Technology.*

Langer, R., and J.P. Vacanti. 1993. Tissue Engineering. *Science.*

Lee, W., and V. Parpura. 2009. Wiring Neurons with Carbon Nanotubes. *Frontiers in Neuroengineering.*

Liu, M., G. Zhou, W. Song, P. Li, H. Liu, X. Niu, and Y. Fan. 2012. Effect of Nano-Hydroxyapatite on the Axonal Guidance Growth of Rat Cortical Neurons. *Nanoscale.*

Liu, T., J. Xu, B.P. Chan, and S.Y. Chew. 2012. Sustained Release of Neurotrophin-3 and Chondroitinase ABC from Electrospun Collagen Nanofiber Scaffold for Spinal Cord Injury Repair. *Journal of Biomedical Materials Research - Part A.*

Lyons, J., C. Li, and F. Ko. 2004. Melt-Electrospinning Part I: Processing Parameters and Geometric Properties. *Polymer.*

Ma, P.X., and R. Zhang. 2001. Microtubular Architecture of Biodegradable Polymer Scaffolds. *Journal of Biomedical Materials Research.*

Mameren, H. V., J. Drukker, H. Sanches, and J. Beursgens. 1990. Cervical Spine Motion in the Sagittal Plane (I) Range of Motion of Actually Performed Movements, an X-Ray Cinematographic Study. *European Journal of Morphology.*

Mariappan, N. 2019. Recent Trends in Nanotechnology Applications in Surgical Specialties and Orthopedic Surgery. *Biomedical and Pharmacology Journal.*

Marti, M.E., A.D. Sharma, D.S. Sakaguchi, and S.K. Mallapragada. 2013. Nanomaterials for Neural Tissue Engineering. In *Nanomaterials in Tissue Engineering: Fabrication and Applications.* Elsevier 2013.

Mazzatenta, A., M. Giugliano, S. Campidelli, L. Gambazzi, L. Businaro, H. Markram, M. Prato, and L. Ballerini. 2007. Interfacing Neurons with Carbon Nanotubes: Electrical Signal Transfer and Synaptic Stimulation in Cultured Brain Circuits. *Journal of Neuroscience.*

Muheremu, A., J. Peng, and Q. Ao. 2016. Stem Cell Based Therapies for Spinal Cord Injury. *Tissue and Cell.*

Nakamura, M., and H. Okano. 2013. Cell Transplantation Therapies for Spinal Cord Injury Focusing on Induced Pluripotent Stem Cells. *Cell Research.*

Pan, S., H. Yu, X. Yang, X. Yang, Y. Wang, Q. Liu, L. Jin, and Y. Yang. 2017. Application of Nanomaterials in Stem Cell Regenerative Medicine of Orthopedic Surgery. *Journal of Nanomaterials.*

Pitkethly, M.J. 2004. Nanometerials - The Driving Force. *Materials Today.*

Rahong, S., T. Yasui, N. Kaji, and Y. Baba. 2016. Recent Developments in Nanowires for Bio-Applications from Molecular to Cellular Levels. *Lab on a Chip.*

Ramezani, F., F. Nasirinezhad, and N. Abotaleb. 2016. A Review of Nanotechnology Strategies for Neuron Regeneration after Spinal Cord Injury. *Journal of Medical Physiology.*

Sharma, H.S., S.F. Ali, W. Dong, Z.R. Tian, R. Patnaik, S. Patnaik, A. Sharma, et al. 2007. Drug Delivery to the Spinal Cord Tagged with Nanowire Enhances Neuroprotective Efficacy and Functional Recovery Following Trauma to the Rat Spinal Cord. In *Annals of the New York Academy of Sciences.* Wiley Online 2007.

Sharma, H.S., D.F. Muresanu, A. Sharma, R. Patnaik, and J.V. Lafuente. 2009. Nanoparticles Influence Pathophysiology of Spinal Cord Injury and Repair. *Progress in Brain Research.*

Silva, N.A., N. Sousa, R.L. Reis, and A.J. Salgado. 2014. From Basics to Clinical: A Comprehensive Review on Spinal Cord Injury. *Progress in Neurobiology.*

Singh, N., A. Tiwari, R. Kesharwani, and D.K. Patel. 2016. Pharmaceutical Polymer in Drug Delivery: A Review. *Research Journal of Pharmacy and Technology.*

Tan, S.H., R. Inai, M. Kotaki, and S. Ramakrishna. 2005. Systematic Parameter Study for Ultra-Fine Fiber Fabrication via Electrospinning Process. *Polymer.*

Taraballi, F., M. Campione, A. Sassella, A. Vescovi, A. Paleari, W. Hwang, and F. Gelain. 2009. Effect of Functionalization on the Self-Assembling Propensity of β-Sheet Forming Peptides. *Soft Matter.*

Taraballi, F., A. Natalello, M. Campione, O. Villa, S.M. Doglia, A. Paleari, and F. Gelain. 2010. Glycine-Spacers Influence Functional Motifs Exposure and Self-Assembling Propensity of Functionalized Substrates Tailored for Neural Stem Cell Cultures. *Frontiers in Neuroengineering.*

Thuret, S., L.D.F. Moon, and F.H. Gage. 2006. Therapeutic Interventions after Spinal Cord Injury. *Nature Reviews Neuroscience.*

Toksöz, S., and M.O. Guler. 2009. Self-Assembled Peptidic Nanostructures. *Nano Today.*

Tsuji, O., K. Miura, Y. Okada, K. Fujiyoshi, M. Mukaino, N. Nagoshi, K. Kitamura, et al. 2010. Therapeutic Potential of Appropriately Evaluated Safe-Induced Pluripotent Stem Cells for Spinal Cord Injury. *Proceedings of the National Academy of Sciences of the United States of America.*

Tysseling-Mattiace, V.M., V. Sahni, K.L. Niece, D. Birch, C. Czeisler, M.G. Fehlings, S.I. Stupp, and J.A. Kessler. 2008. Self-Assembling Nanofibers Inhibit Glial Scar Formation and Promote Axon Elongation after Spinal Cord Injury. *Journal of Neuroscience.*

Venugopal, I., A.I. Mehta, and A.A. Linninger. 2020. Drug Delivery Applications of Nanoparticles in the Spine. In *Methods in Molecular Biology.* Springer nature 2020.

Viswanathan, V.K., S.R. Rajaram Manoharan, S. Subramanian, and A. Moon. 2019. Nanotechnology in Spine Surgery: A Current Update and Critical Review of the Literature. *World Neurosurgery.*

Von Ahnen, I., G. Piret, and C.N. Prinz. 2015. Transfer of Vertical Nanowire Arrays on Polycaprolactone Substrates for Biological Applications. *Microelectronic Engineering.*

Wang, C.Y., K.H. Zhang, C.Y. Fan, X.M. Mo, H.J. Ruan, and F.F. Li. 2011. Aligned Natural-Synthetic Polyblend Nanofibers for Peripheral Nerve Regeneration. *Acta Biomaterialia*.

Wang, W., S. Itoh, N. Yamamoto, A. Okawa, A. Nagai, and K. Yamashita. 2010. Enhancement of Nerve Regeneration along a Chitosan Nanofiber Mesh Tube on Which Electrically Polarized β-Tricalcium Phosphate Particles Are Immobilized. *Acta Biomaterialia*.

Xu, X.Y., X.T. Li, S.W. Peng, J.F. Xiao, C. Liu, G. Fang, K.C. Chen, and G.Q. Chen. 2010. The Behaviour of Neural Stem Cells on Polyhydroxyalkanoate Nanofiber Scaffolds. *Biomaterials*.

Yang, F., R. Murugan, S. Ramakrishna, X. Wang, Y.X. Ma, and S. Wang. 2004. Fabrication of Nano-Structured Porous PLLA Scaffold Intended for Nerve Tissue Engineering. *Biomaterials*.

Yiu, G., and Z. He. 2006. Glial Inhibition of CNS Axon Regeneration. *Nature Reviews Neuroscience*.

Zagari, Z., S.R. Zarchi, M. Jorjani, N. Sima, S. Imani, and F. Lotfi. 2016. Functional Recovery of Carbon Nanotube/Nafion Nanocomposite in Rat Model of Spinal Cord Injury. *Artificial Cells, Nanomedicine and Biotechnology*.

Zhang, L., and T.J. Webster. 2009. Nanotechnology and Nanomaterials: Promises for Improved Tissue Regeneration. *Nano Today*.

15 Future Directions of Nanomaterials in Artificial Organ Transplantation

Hemant Borase
Uka Tarsadia University

Satish Patil
Kavayitri Bahinabai Chaudhari North Maharashtra University

Gopal Jee Gopal and Bhairavi Rathod
Uka Tarsadia University

CONTENTS

DOI: 10.1201/9781003140108-15

15.1 INTRODUCTION

A group of various eukaryotic cells leads to formation of tissue; tissues give rise to an organ. The organ is an internal or external part of an organism that is typically self-contained and has a specific vital function for the ultimate survival of the organism. Quality of life is dependent on dynamic tasks such as blood circulation, breathing, absorption, metabolism, and detoxification, which are performed by multiple organs. Numerous factors, such as stroma, lifestyle, aging, surgery, sepsis, etc., lead to malfunction and failure of major organs such as the heart, kidneys, liver, lungs, pancreas, and intestine (Go et al., 2019; Arnhold et al., 2019). Organ failure leads to immediate death of the individual if organ replacement is not made on a priority basis (Jones, 2005). The discovery of antibiotics, vaccines, and organ transplantation technology are considered major medical milestones that significantly improved the life expectancy of the human population. Among the above three miracles of medicine, organ transplantation has its own importance.

Organ transplantation is a specific medical procedure in which an entire, functionally active organ is removed from a donor and incorporated into a recipient's body. Organ transplantation can occur between members of same species or between two different species (Platt, 1998; WHO, 2020).

Credit for the first successful organ (kidney) transplantation surgery goes to Dr. Joseph Murray and his colleagues working at Peter Bent Brigham Hospital in Boston in 1954. Because of this contribution, Dr. Murray was awarded the Nobel Prize in physiology or medicine in 1990. The successful transplantation of kidney proved that organ transfer is possible, and this led to thousands of other successful kidney transplants and ultimately prepared the road for transplantation of other organs (Nobel Prize Organization, 2020; Platt, 1998; Watson and Dark, 2012).

Transplantation represents a very effective way to treat organ failure; however, shortage of human organs is a major factor limiting the availability of transplantation (Krishna, 2007). Apart from this, costly immunosuppressive drugs (having serious side effects) are administered for elimination of immunorejection (Jones, 2005). Efficiency of natural organs decrease once it is transplanted, the kidney is reported to have a rejection rate of around 18% (Malchesky, 2014). Financially, it is very difficult for most developing countries to bear the very high cost of transplantation. It costs about US $220,002dollars for a heart transplant in Brazil (Barreto et al., 2019). In traditional organ transplantation, graft viability is dependent on the medical status of donor, such as age, brain death, metabolism, and multiple factors forcing the recipient to consider before going ahead with such risky treatment.

Kidney transplantation is most frequent, followed by liver, heart, lungs, pancreas, and small bowel (Grinyó, 2013). But that number of transplants is much lower than the actual requirements. Moreover, there is drastic difference between transplantation activities in different parts of the world; it ranges from more than 70 per million population in developed countries to 0–2.4 per million population in developing countries. In the United States alone, 109,000 patients are on the national organ transplant waiting list as of September, 2020, and 17 people die each day due to organ shortage (HRSA, 2020). Overall survival rate of patient and transplanted kidney were 52% and 35%, respectively and the viability of the transplanted kidney decreased with increasing in the age of transplant (Go et al., 2019). Due to developments in diagnostics and therapeutics, the elderly population is increasing, and an alternative to traditional organ transplantation is required to fulfill demand of organs. Considering the above figures and facts, there is an urgent need to find a sustainable and affordable alternative to traditional organ transplantation procedure.

Xenotransplantation is an alternative to human-to-human organ transplantation. Xenotransplantation involves an organ transplant from a non-primate animal to human and has been presented as a useful strategy to meet increased organ demand. But there are several issues before xenotransplantation appears in routine clinical practice, such as religious concerns, ethical-legal complexity, psychological considerations, and the high rate of graft failure. The above shortcomings have created clouds around xenotransplantation procedure (Splendiani et al., 2003; Fraux et al., 2020).

15.2 ARTIFICIAL ORGANS

An artificial organ is a human-made device that is implanted inside the body to mimic the function of a natural organ, and it is a promising alternative to natural organs. Use of artificial organs is a relatively new technology (Malchesky, 2014). The life expectancy of millions of people has been prolonged and improved by artificial organ technology. In the total global medical device market, artificial organs are a major player, with about $415 billion in 2016, compared with $322 billion in 2011, and the US artificial implant market is expected to increase by an annual rate of 8% (Malchesky, 2014).

Different kinds of artificial substitutes and artificial replacement technologies are available, such as synthetic lenses, pacemakers, mechanical and synthetic heart valves, false teeth, artificial limbs and joints, and renal dialysis machines. Artificial organs are reported to be produce by stem cells and three-dimensional (3D) printing methods; both of these technologies are revolutionizing the area of organ transplantation. 3D printing of tissue/organ is used to make the internal cellular structure and is used in the treatment of bone defects and heart disease. 3D printing is able to produce the desired organ in one process, using scaffold and desired cells. Bones and trachea types of structural tissues are reported to be produced by 3D printing. However, for creating more complex organs, such as liver and kidney, which require a specific combination of more than 40 cells, is challenge for this method (Jeong et al., 2020; Javaid and Haleem, 2020).

There are several recently developed artificial tissue and organ manufacturing technologies such as artificial kidney, artificial heart, two-nozzle 3D bio printing, multi-nozzle rapid prototyping (MNRP), partially automated additive combined molding, and decellularized matrix regeneration (Marga et al., 2012; Xu and Wang, 2015). Combinations of different advanced technologies are also used to create new artificial organs; these include combined MNRP technologies, decellularized matrices, computer-aided design modeling, and additive combined molding (Wang, 2019). For the treatment of airway cancer, the first artificial trachea was fabricated from stem cells seeded on a nanocomposite (Teoh et al., 2015). Two bioartificial devices—artificial placenta and renal assist devices—were developed by integrating arrays of numerous organs on chip platforms. This has an potential to develop novel bioartificial organ support systems. This support system can help in healing damaged organs before the main transplantation (Ashammakhi et al., 2019). Readily available artificial organs will save the lives of patients by decreasing the wait list and facilitating rapid transplantation.

Currently, artificial organs such as heart, lungs, liver, kidney, and pancreas are at different stages of development (Wang, 2019). There are a few hurdles to establishing artificial organs as a commercial success. Manufacturing and implanting artificial organs is a time- and research-intensive process. Several problems that exist in traditional organ transplantation still continue with artificial organs. Concerns regarding patient stratification and allocation criteria still exist (Splendiani et al., 2003). Transplant rejection due to immune response to transplanted organ as a foreign material (antigen) leading its destruction is still a problem with artificial organs. Immunosuppressant medication is required to overcome the risk of artificial-organ rejection (Jones, 2005; Yambe, 2009). With artificial organs, the chances of mechanical or process-related failures are expected to be high. If any device has a problem during the continuous transplantation process, there are higher chances of failure. In such a situation the patient who needs the transplantation or receives the artificial organ may require further additional transplantation, thus increasing the financial and health burden.

According to several reports, the post-transplantation cost per year is very high (ranging from \$20,000 to \$150,000 in case of kidney, heart, and liver) compared to the main transplantation procedure. It means that if we use any technology related to organ transplantation or artificial substitutes it becomes more and more expensive. If such a high cost is not covered by public funds, medical insurance, or charity, it will be out of reach for the general population (Flaman, 1994).

15.3   NANOTECHNOLOGY AND ARTIFICIAL ORGANS

Nanotechnology is recognized as a branch of science and technology working on synthesis, characterization, and applications of materials having a size range of around 100 nm (ec.europa.eu, 2007; FDA, 2014). The pioneering works of several physicists, biologists, and material scientists make nanotechnology a highly interdisciplinary dynamic field. Nanotechnology has been a most attractive research field for the past three decades (Borase et al., 2014, Khan et al., 2019a, Weissig et al., 2014, Wang et al., 2014). At nanodimensions, materials acquire useful properties such as strength, reactivity, dispersibility, conductivity, and surface functionalization, to name few (Soares et al., 2018; Khan et al., 2019b). Several types of nanomaterials, such as organic (polymers, liposomes, peptides) and inorganic (metal nanoparticles, metal oxides, quantum dots), continue to exhibit superior properties in different disciplines, leading to entry of nanoproducts into the consumer market (Table 15.1). Newer types of nanomaterials of natural, organic, and inorganic nature are constantly added into assets of nanotechnology. Diverse products of nanotechnology, such as graphene, nanoemulsion, metal nanoparticles,

TABLE 15.1

Different Types of Nano Forms of Materials for Artificial Organ Transplantation

Sr. No.	Category of Nanomaterials	Nanomaterials	Applications in Transplantation	References
1.	Carbon based	Carbon nanotubes (CNTs)	Beneficial for cardiac tissue engineering approach	Amin et al., 2020
2.	Carbon based	Graphene	Used in different tissue engineering applications	Bai et al., 2019
3.	Carbon based	Carbon nanotubes	Artificial bone replacement	Khan et al., 2019
4.	Metal oxide	Zinc oxide nanoparticles	Artificial tissue engineering	laurenti et al., 2017
5.	Fluorescent Nanoparticles	Quantum dots	Suitable for deep cell or tissue imaging	Voura et al., 2004
6.	Metal oxide	Titanium dioxide (TiO_2)	Prepared for cell imaging through fluorescent analysis or magnetic resonance imaging (MRI)	Yin et al., 2013
7.	Metal	Gold nanoshells	Muscle tissue engineering	Marino et al., 2017
8.	Metal	Gold nanoparticles	Used in scaffolds for enhancing bone regeneration	Zhang et al., 2014
9.	Nanocomposite	Silicate-doped nano-hydroxyapatite/ graphene oxide composite	Used for reinforcement of fibrous scaffolds	Dalgic et al., 2018
10.	Magnetic	Iron oxide NPs, (usually Fe_3O_4 or Fe_2O_3)	Monitoring of transplanted tissues and imaging cancer cells	Li et al., 2016
11.	Magnetic	Superparamagnetic magnetite nanocrystal clusters	Utilized for cell imaging	Li et al., 2016
12	Magnetic	Iron oxide NPs $(Fe_3O_4$ or $Fe_2O_3)$	Bioprinting of skin, cartilage and bone, biofabrication of robotic and automated 3D human tissues and organs	Rezende et al., 2012

nanocomposites, and quantum dots, have established themselves as major players in electronics, medicine, water purification, cosmetics, aviation, catalysis, agriculture, food, and many more (Borase et al., 2014, Braza et al., 2018, Lee et al., 2011, Bondarenko et al., 2013).

In the field of medicine, nanotechnology is moving from its traditional use as a biocidal agent to advanced applications such as thermal tumor destruction, gene therapy, cancer cures, vaccines, ultrasound contrast agents, and in artificial organs preparation (Anselmo and Mitragotri, 2016; Tasciotti et al., 2016). Many nanotechnology-based therapeutic products are already approved by various drug regulatory agencies and are commonly termed "nanopharmaceuticals" (Weissig et al., 2014; Anselmo and Mitragotri, 2016).

In the area of artificial organ development, several nanotechnology-based items, such as carbon nanotubes, nanosensors, nanocomposites, and nanoparticles, have contributed immensely, and diverse properties of nanomaterials are playing a pivotal role in the process of transplantation as well as the performance of artificial organs (Teoh et al., 2015). Unique properties of nanomaterials, such as size, easy surface modification, positive interactions with host molecules, and targeted and sustained drug delivery, are now found to be useful in transplantation of artificial organs (Tasciotti et al., 2016, Yao and Martins, 2020). Apart from this, nanomaterials are emerging as promising materials in transplantation due to their use in imaging and diagnosis to precisely monitor the performance of transplants (Yao and Martins, 2020).

For artificial organs, there is limited space inside the body. Therefore, the smaller the artificial organ, the better it will be. Nanotechnology can be helpful to reduce size of the organ (Yambe, 2009). Nanopores are useful for adsorption and growth of cells for sustained release of useful biomolecules. Before involving nanomaterials in artificial organs, several aspects needed to be verified, including modification of nanomaterials to escape the immune system clearance, effect of nanomaterials size and composition on interactions with biomolecules, and intracellular fate of nanomaterials. The basic science aspect of natural organs, such as composition, anatomy, physiology, and pathophysiology, must correlate in details with artificial organ structure, materials, function, and tissue interface in order to mimic the natural organ function as closely as possible (Bartlett et al., 2002).

Increased understanding of surface interactions between an implant and the molecules normally present in living system makes the entry of nanotechnology in the field of artificial organ transplantation feasible. Nanotechnological products can sense/control the operation of artificial organs. Nanocomposite scaffolds promote tissue growth. Nanomaterials are known to protect organs from pathogens and reduce immunological responses. Imaging techniques can be useful to monitor the fate of an artificial organ inside the body for management purposes (Busque et al., 2004; Yao and Martins, 2020).

Multiple complex sequences of events occur after a patient receives a transplant; many of them are the cause of organ transplant failure. Shortage of suitable donors, side effects of immunosuppressive drugs, microbial infections, behavioral changes, and malignancy are unwanted results of traditional organ transplantation. Researchers are working on different aspects to be able to circumvent such transplantation-associated problems and present artificial organs as a more promising alternative. Different reports have ascertained that nanomaterials can be useful for both graft and patient, they can make the graft less immunogenic and increase delivery of immunosuppressive drugs (Solhjou et al., 2017; Braza et al., 2018; Yao and Martins, 2020)

For the enhancement of efficiency during transplantation, another approach is to use nanosensors for higher precision (Shafiee et al., 2019). To overcome the problems of biocompatibility and microbial infections, biocompatible nanopolymers and metal nanoparticles having excellent antibacterial, antiviral, and anti-inflammatory properties have been introduced into the hydrogel matrix to form nanoparticle-hydrogel composite scaffolds for the enhancement of physical and biological properties (Tan et al., 2019).

In this chapter, we explore and discuss the challenges faced during artificial organ transplantation and correlated nanotechnology with present and future applications of artificial organ development and transplantation. There is discussion of selective properties of diverse nanomaterials as a major player for success of artificial organ transplantation technology. Advantages are explained about introducing nanotechnology for development of scaffolds and artificial organs. Introductory and application-based information on nanotechnology and artificial organs will empower readers about this emerging area for nanotechnology research. Apart from this, light is thrown on interactions between nanomaterials and biomolecules that is vital before applying nanomaterial in transplantation science.

15.4 NANOMATERIALS USED IN ARTIFICIAL ORGAN TRANSPLANTATION

Nanotechnology is reported to play a major role in the development of artificial organs and regenerative medicine (Teoh et al., 2015). Nanomaterials can cause a manifold increase in the imaging, tracking, and tissue growth inside the body. Nanocomposites fabricated using biocompatible materials can be used for more superior scaffolds. Antimicrobial properties of nanomaterials (silver, gold, zinc oxide nanoparticles) are already established and can be utilized to prevent infection and promote wound healing (Teoh et al., 2014). These properties of nanomaterials are highly beneficial to develop "intelligent artificial organs" that are not only comparable to but perform better than natural organs.

Due to lack of kidney donors, clinical dialyzers are playing an important part in end stage renal failure. The next step in the treatment of renal failure is a fabrication of device that will mimic the functions of a real kidney. Progress in nanotechnology is improving synthesis of the dialysis membrane with high efficiency. A polysulfonate membrane synthesized from a nanocontrol spinning procedure can be fine-tuned for preventing leakage of useful molecules such as β2-microglobulin serum albumin (Busque et al., 2004).

Nobakht et al (2012) created an implantable device having pump, sensors, display, and cartridge. The size of the entire assembly is like that of a natural kidney. They used nanotechnology for synthesizing a series of chiral macrocyclic molecules functioning as semi specific ion channels. The filtration capacity of this device is equivalent to a glomerular filtration rate. Apart from filtration, the kidney also has several metabolic functions. The renal tubule assist device (RAD), together with filtration, is reported to perform transport, metabolic, and endocrine functions of the kidney in the animal model (bioartificial kidney) (Humes et al., 1999). The use of a bioartificial kidney, along with advanced nanofabrication membrane, may be an early step in the development of a complete artificial kidney (Fissell et al., 2003).

The liver is the largest organ of the body. It consists of hepatocytes. It is the site for biomolecule metabolism and detoxification of toxic compounds. Loss of liver function leads to kidney failure, encephalopathy, cerebral edema, and pathogenesis. Demand for liver transplantation has significantly increased in recent times, but owing to the complexity and multiple roles, the development of artificial liver is far more complex then kidney (Busque et al., 2004). Nanomaterials are used to stimulate in vitro hepatic stem cell differentiation and liver extracellular matrix. A hydrogel made up of polyethylene glycol-linked multi-walled carbon nanotube-coated poly-acrylamide (CNT-PA) has been found to differentiate human amniotic epithelial cells (hAECs) into functional hepatocyte-like cells (HLCs) in in vitro. CNT-PA exhibits a hepatocytic role, such as secretion and enzymatic function (Zhao et al., 2018). CNT-PA can be optimized to match natural deformation and nanosurface in liver cells. Similar types of findings are important milestones for manufacturing an efficient artificial liver.

The pancreas plays an important role in the maintenance of glucose levels by secreting insulin. In most cases, pancreas transplantation is done along with kidney transplantation. Separate pancreas transplantation suffers with high graft rejection, critical surgery, morbidity, and mortality (Robertson, 2004). Construction of an artificial pancreas required beta cells with integration of three entities, including a glucose sensor, insulin delivery system, and a system to release optimal insulin dose. Currently available in vitro glucose sensors are not applicable to in vivo due to compatibility and selectivity, but construction of biocompatible nanomaterials are useful for glucose sensing. An electrochemical nanosensor for glucose made using glucose oxidase, platinum nanoparticles, and single-wall carbon nanotubes has been reported for higher sensitivity and rapid response (Hrapovic et al., 2004).

Heart failure is a major cause of death worldwide. Twelve million deaths per annum are expected by 2030 due to heart attack and atherosclerosis only (Mahmoudi et al., 2017). The repair after cardiac injury includes cardiomyocyte generation (angiogenic). Despite advances in cardiac treatment, 50% of heart patients died within a span of five years. Around 2000 annual heart transplantation were performed versus 5,50,000 new cases that need transplants in the USA (Dunlay and Roger, 2014). Currently nanofibers and nanoporous scaffolds are engineered for maximum cardiomyocyte and cellular-molecular interaction. Alginate biopolymer incorporated with gold nanowires improved cell alignment, tissue integration, and electrical communication and is useful as cardiac patches to treat heart injuries and reduce risk of patch-associated cardiac arrhythmias (Liau et al., 2012). Nano-bioengineering products can help to sense regeneration and condition of cardiac tissue. Heart valves play important role in regulation of blood flow. Heart valve malfunctioning is corrected by replacement surgeries involving prosthetic and mechanical valves having severe limitations (Hasan et al., 2016). Nanofibres and nanopolymers (chitosan, collagen, poly L lactic acid etc.) based scaffolds are reported for development of heart valves, cardiovascular tissue sheet with higher biocompatibility, enhanced mechanical properties, complete patch degradation, and regeneration of endothelial tissue and extracellular matrix (Hasan et al., 2016).

Cardiac tissue engineering using cell-dependent approaches struggles with viability, stability, and regulatory challenges, but use of non-cellular biomaterials is attractive for not only cellular regeneration but also precise delivery of therapeutics. Cardiac patches prepared from nano-fibrillar collagen were able to regenerate adult mammalian heart tissue following myocardial infarction (Mahmoudi et al., 2017).

Scaffolds are used as hosts and carriers, supporting cellular growth and differentiation. They provide the required dimensions for new tissue formation. Several methods, including electrospinning, solvent casting, and 3D printing, are used for scaffold preparation (Luo et al., 2019). Tissue engineering based on growing cells on a scaffold provides a favorable environment like natural extracellular matrix for natural functioning of cells. Scaffolds produced using nanomaterials are used in multiple applications such as regeneration of skin and ophthalmic and muscles tissue.

The strength and rigidity of polyurethane composite is enhanced many times after adding nanofibrillated cellulose (NFC) and has been found useful in tissue implants such as heart valves and vascular grafts (Cherian et al., 2011). Nanocellulose has active hydroxyl groups, superior hydrophobicity, and biocompatibility; this has attracted attention for tissue healing, scaffold development, hydrogel, and in drug delivery (Luo et al., 2019).

An artificial trachea (windpipe) produced from a nanocomposite containing POSS-PCU (polyhedral oligomericsilsesquioxane [POSS]) covalently bonded to poly-[carbonate-urea] urethane [PCU]) is seeded with autologous bone-marrow mononuclear cells. This nanocomposite was successfully used in treatment of airway cancer and defects (Jungebluth et al., 2011). Scaffolds are prepared using electrospun polystyrene support growth and organization of skin fibroblast, keratinocytes, and endothelial cell. Keratinocytes colonize on upper surface of the scaffold as continuous layer while the remaining two cells are grown below the keratinocytes (Sun et al., 2005).

15.5   NANOMATERIALS FOR IMMUNOSUPPRESSION

Immunological rejection is one of the prominent reasons behind the failure of organ transplantation. Intake of immunosuppressive agents has been found to be effective in graft survival (Ngobili and Daniele, 2016). Diverse drugs such as mycophenolic acid, calcineurin inhibitors, and rapamycin are successful in masking immunoresponse to transplant. However, immunosuppressive drugs are associated with nephrotoxicity, neurotoxicity, serum sickness, and other side effects (McDermott, 2020). Sometimes the recipient is at higher risk not because of graft failure but due to higher toxicity of immunosuppressive drugs to avoid graft rejection. Successful organ transplant largely depends on the interplay of organ survival and immunosuppression.

Research efforts in nanotechnology and material science lead to development of multiple targeted drug delivery approaches that are more effective for immunosuppression (Hubbell et al., 2009; Look et al., 2014). A diverse consortium of nanomaterials discussed in literature has tremendous potential to for direct and indirect use as well as selective binding and release of therapeutic molecules to modulate the immune response (Ngobili and Daniele, 2016). Nanomaterials can direct expression and production of immulogical cells and molecules, cellular uptake, targeting, and functioning. Accordingly, researchers are modifying nanomaterials' physicochemical properties to control immune responses.

Poly(L-lactic acid) (PLA) particles coated with polyethylene glycol (PEG) have been found to deliver a high amount of radioactive antigen to the lymphatic system due to more particle hydrophobicity after PEG coupling (Balmert and Little, 2012). The conjugation of cyclosporine (CsA) to PLA-PEG nanoparticles (84 nm) reduced T cell proliferation. Nanoparticles treated dendritic cells are also capable to do the same as compared to untreated dendritic cells (Azzi et al., 2010).

Mycophenolic acid (MMF) is used to weaken immune response. (Look et al., 2014). No toxicity signs were reported in patients after treatment of mycophenolic acid with nanoparticles; on the other hand, recipients taking mycophenolic acid alone developed symptoms of toxicity (iatrogenic cytopenias). Mycophenolic acid mixed with cyclodextrins nanoparticles in a lipid bilayer (nanogel) increases survival in a mouse model of lupus as compared with drug alone (mycophenolic acid). Direct uptake of nanogel by the dendritic cells is a major reason behind reduced inflammation by nanogels. Transportation of interleukin (IL) 10 gene with cationic liposomes is found to be very beneficial to increase organ survival after heart transplantation due to overexpression of IL-10 gene and decrease in response of lymphocytes. The liver transplant survived for longer periods when administered with liposomal tacrolimus as compared with intravenous administration of tacrolimus only (Ko et al., 1995).

Apart from organic nanomaterials, metal and metal oxide nanoparticles are being tested for immunosuppression purpose (Ngobili and Daniele, 2016). In mice models, gold nanoparticles coated by citrate have been found to inhibit activity of interleukin 1 beta (IL-1β), an inflammatory cytokine vital for innate and adaptive immune response. Interestingly, the effect was size dependent; that is, 5 nm gold nanoparticles completely inhibits the IL-1β pathway, while larger particles (10 nm) exhibit less activity; and finally the 35-nm gold nanoparticles were ineffective to stop the IL-1β pathway (Sumbayev et al., 2013).

The humoral immune response, along with B cells, is associated with the identification of antigens, and xenobiotics present in blood cell. Ovalbumin antigen was injected into sensitive mice followed by a dose of nanoparticles of iron oxide; the production of ovalbumin-specific antibodies was found to be decreased. The iron oxide nanoparticles prevent the activity of T-helper cells and macrophages as well as expression of interleukin-6 and tumor necrosis factor-a (Shen et al., 2011). Polystyrene nanoparticles (50 nm) inhibited inflammation of lungs due to shrinkage of dendritic cells in the lungs; on the other hand, opposite results (dendritic cells maturation and enhanced T cell activity) were obtained by change in surface charge of polystyrene nanoparticles (Hardy et al., 2012; Frick et al., 2012).

Detailed study of interaction of nanomaterials size, structure, and composition is vital before clinical introduction. On the other hand, attractive properties of nanomaterials, such as direct immunosuppressive, anti-inflammatory, and targeted delivery, are key factors in the development of artificial organ transplantation as a more acceptable technology. Nanomaterial-based approaches represent a rapidly growing and promising field for drug delivery in order to modulate immunoresponse, and

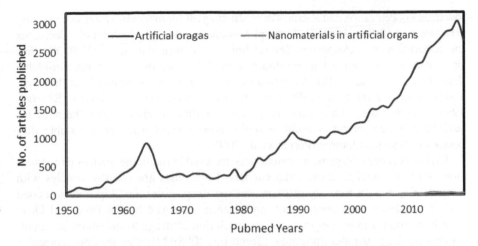

FIGURE 15.1 Use of nanomaterials on artificial organ is still in infancy. (PubMed database on number of articles produced per year on artificial organs and use of nanomaterials in artificial organs [https://pubmed.ncbi.nlm.nih.gov/, accessed on 22 Dec. 2020].)

this will ultimately a be major factor for the future of transplantation (Figures 15.1 and 15.2).

Targeted delivery is important to send drugs to a desired location, whereas sustained release involves the release of drugs at specific time at a desired concentration. Several studies have demonstrated the potential of nanocarriers for sustained, targeted drug delivery leading to decreases in dose, toxicity, and side effects associated with conventional drug delivery system (Grattoni et al., 2012). Iron oxide nanoparticles (40 nm) loaded with mycophenolic acid were able to deliver this immunosuppressant at peripheral blood mononuclear cells. It was found that this nanoconjugate of drug and nanomaterial effectively inhibits cytokines interleukin 2 and tumor necrosis factor at a

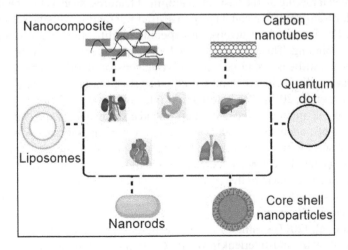

FIGURE 15.2 Use of different nanomaterials in organ transplantation.

low drug concentration and also acts as contract agent for magnetic resonance imaging (Hwang et al., 2016). After renal transplant, consumption of a high-fat diet decreases the adsorption of cyclosporine. Several lipid-based formulations, such as micelles, liposomes, and nanoemulsion, are attractive candidates for delivery of water-insoluble drugs (Tasciotti et al., 2016). Reformulation of cyclosporine as an emulsion (less than 150 nm) was thermodynamically stable, with improved pharmacokinetics (Ritschel, 1996). Another drug, rapamycin encapsulated within micelles, avoids the need for surfactant and co-solvent to solubilize highly concentrated drug, and it is stable after contact with serum albumin (Forrest et al., 2006).

Different types of organic nanomaterials are used in medicine, such as nanoemulsions with potential to act as drug carriers. Liposomes are circular vesicles with a lipid bilayer with capacity to carry diverse drug molecules. Liposomes loaded with doxorubicin (anticancer agent) are already approved by the Food and Drug Administration. Liposomes increase accumulation of drugs to the tumor site compared with drugs without liposomes. (Torchilin, 2005). Micelles are lipid molecules that arrange themselves in a spherical form in aqueous solutions.

15.6   NANOTECHNOLOGY APPLICATIONS IN TRANSPLANTATION MEDICINE AND GENE DELIVERY

The ability to show effects at low concentration, high manipulability, sustained release of drugs, low immunogenicity, and toxicity make nanomaterials ideal for drug delivery, sensing, and diagnostics, and the utility of nanomaterials as drug and genetic agents can be useful in transplantation medicine (Yao and Martins, 2020). Nanomaterials can be administered via intravenous, oral, local, and topical methods for active or passive targeting. Organic nanomaterial, such as nanoforms of lipid, chitosan, and alginate, as well as inorganic nanomaterials, such as silver, gold, and silica, show promising applications as transplantation medicine (Yao and Martins, 2020). Multiple approaches are used in delivery and targeting of nanomaterials. First, there is targeting on the basis of anatomical features, such as the specific organ intended for transplantation and its response after interaction with the selected nanomaterials. Passive targeting involves no specific modifications with nanomaterials for receptor binding. This type of approach depends on enhanced permeability and poor drainage, while active targeting involves extensive modifications of nanomaterials so that it will specifically bind with the target cell/organ receptor (Cheng et al., 2015; Tietjen et al., 2018). The binding and interactions are affected by several factors, such as the amount of receptors and ligands, shape and size of nanomaterials, and the fate of nanomaterials (internalization, accumulation etc.). The traditional approach of successful transplantation management involves the use of immunosuppressive drugs, but there is need to pay attention to increasing graft viability because lowering immune damage to the graft is vital in preventing rejection (Martins et al., 2006). Thus, side effects due to immunosuppressive drugs can be decreased by graft treatment before the process of organ transplantation.

Solhjou et al. (2017) synthesized poly(lactic-co-glycolic acid) (PLGA) nanoparticles loaded with anti-Interleukin-6 (IL-6) antibody with average size of 100 nm. This nanodelivery of PLGA-anti IL6 greatly reduced chronic rejection of a transplanted ischemic heart in mice. The experiment involves perfusion with control and nanoparticles in the heart before transplantation. Use of nanoparticles was found to reduce tissue necrosis and cellular infiltration at very small dose as compared with control. More precise control on synthesis and characterization of materials at nanoscale holds great promise in transplantation. A synergistic combination of two nano immunotherapeutics were checked in mice heart (Tietjen et al., 2018): first, mammalian target for rapamycin (mTOR) inhibitor with high-density lipoprotein mTORi-HDL and second tumor necrosis factor receptor (TNFR)-associated factor 6 inhibitor (TRAF6) CD40-TRAF6-specific nanobiologic (TRAF6i-HDL). It was found that the mTORi-HDL avert trained immunity and CD40 action was masked by TRAF6i-HDL, leading to transplant acceptance up to a hundred days after transplantation. Such a strategy offers control over inflammatory immune response, leading to higher immunological tolerance.

Reactive oxygen species (ROS) are formed during normal metabolism and are kept under control by enzymatic and non-enzymatic systems of the body. However abnormal increase in ROS affects important biomolecules such as DNA and proteins. Generation of ROS is characteristic of liver ischemia/reperfusion (I/R) injury. Delivery of antioxidant genes (superoxide dismutase and catalase) using lipid polycationic nanoparticles (PLNP) were performed in mice. It was found that PLNP-mediated antioxidant gene delivery significantly increases expression of superoxide dismutase and catalase genes in liver (He et al., 2006). Moreover overexpression of those genes also reduced I/R-induced serum alanine aminotransferase levels and reestablished reserve glutathione. The above approach proves that he nanomaterials' role in delivery of important genes is responsible for uplifting graft functioning and post-transplantation survival.

The ideal candidate for gene delivery must be able to prevent nuclease degradation of the gene of interest and facilitate entry inside the cell membrane and nucleus in active from. Viral vectors used for gene delivery have good potential but suffer from mutations, immunological response, and inability to carry big genes, emphasizing the need for more research exploring nanomaterials as targeted delivery vehicle of therapeutic genes (Li and Loh, 2008). Apart from peptides, lipids, and polymers, inorganic nanoparticles are also emerging as effective material for gene delivery purposes (Dobson, 2006). Nanomaterials with a surface positive charge can noncovalently bind with DNA and RNA by electrostatic attraction. Similarly, covalent binding is also possible between gene and nanomaterial that can be separated from each other by stimulus within the system or from outside (Loh et al., 2016).

Gold nanoparticles have an easy synthesis protocol and good biocompatibility and are tunable for molecular imaging. The synthesis of gold nanoparticles coated with polyethyleneimine was reported for small interfering (si) RNA (siRNA) delivery. The above gene delivery method was found to be effective in gene silencing in cancer cells with low cytotoxicity (Lee et al., 2011). Apart from gold nanoparticles, different inorganic metal nanoparticles, such as magnetic nanoparticles, carbon nanotubes, graphene, quantum dot, and silica nanoparticles, have been reported for targeted delivery of oligo antisense DNA, plasmid DNA, and siRNA. This area of research is in the infant stage and researchers are working on some questions, such as the fate of nanoparticles inside the body after gene release and how to tackle different moieties generated during delivery event. Optimization of nanosize binding properties and transfection ability will further clarify utilization of nanomaterials in transplantation medicine and gene delivery (Loh et al., 2016).

15.7   NANOPARTICLES AS CONTRAST AGENTS AND IN CELLULAR, MOLECULAR IMAGING

In vivo methods of cell and molecule imaging are particularly important in transplantation as these methods yield very useful information about metabolic activity, cell viability in artificial scaffold, distribution, and overall status of artificial organ functioning. Ultrasound, optical imaging, computed tomography (CT), single-photon emission computed tomography (SPECT), and magnetic resonance imaging (MRI) are common imaging tools available. Several dyes and reagents called contrast agents are used for in vivo imaging; they are helpful to see the internal situations of organs. There are many contrast agents based on gadolinium, barium sulfate, and iodine currently used in diagnostic imaging. These traditional contrast agents suffer from shorter half-life, toxicity at high dose, and low accumulation at the site of interest (Achilefu, 2010).

Nanoparticles are good alternatives for higher image resolution and better contrast. Tissue enriched with these nanoparticles appears darker due to protons decaying from excited states more effectively via energy transfer to neighboring nuclei (Hahn et al., 1990; Lavik and Recum, 2011). Coating or encapsulation of the imaging agent (polymeric nanomaterials) has been found to increase circulation time inside the body and provide high accumulation and better contrast (Fathi-Achachelouei et al., 2019). With the help of nanotechnology, it is possible to image a cell within the artificial organ scaffold for migration, tissue healing, and differentiation purpose (Lalwani et al., 2014; Zolata et al., 2015; Fathi-Achachelouei et al., 2019).

Mesenchymal stem (stromal) cells (MSCs) of bone marrow generate and repair tissue and bone. MSCs are useful in treatment of graft-versus-host disease and myocardial infarction. MSCs could be used in artificial organs as they lead to habitation of cells at the site of injury. The United States Food and Drug Administration (FDA) approved the use of iron oxide nanoparticles for labeling MSCs, leading to tracking up to 6 months (Lavik and Recum, 2011). In the case of artificial organs having matrix harboring cellular population, it is important to trace proliferation and journey as well as death of cells. Nanomaterials could be developed in such a way that they would continue to function as contrast agents as long as the cell was alive and would be removed from the system if the cells containing them died. Apart from this, care needs to be taken if the nanomaterials in absence of attached moiety are showing uncontrolled distribution and cellular and molecular damage. Functionalization of nanoparticles was developed by Choi et al. (2007), involving preparation of quantum dots of cadmium selenide and zinc sulfide nanoparticles coated with different molecules such as cysteine, cysteamine, dihydrolipoic acid, and dihydrolipoic acid and connected with polyethylene glycol. The diameter of quantum dots is about 5.5 nm, resulting in urinary excretion and removal from body. Coating quantum dots with cysteine keeps the size small, increases solubility, and acts as a barrier in binding of serum proteins.

Nanoparticles have a long blood circulation time and can be used as contrast agents in magnetic resonance imaging (MRI). Functionalization of biodegradable poly(lactic-co-glycolic acid) (PLGA) nanoparticles was developed with gadolinium (a widely used MRI contrast agent) and ligation of DTPA (diethylene triamine penta acetic acid). A high amount of gadolinium (236 micro gram/mg PLGA) was immobilized uniformly. That nanomaterial was found to be a superior MRI contrast agent (Ratzinger et al., 2010). A dual contrast agent (suitable for both MRI and PET imaging) with very high imaging was prepared by manganese and graphene sheets functionalized with iodine (average size of 200 nm). Further, lactate dehydrogenase (LDH) and calceine in an in vitro cytotoxicity assay performed on human kidney epithelial cell and mouse fibroblasts indicated a cytocompatible property of the above nanomaterial. Such nanotechnology-based contrast agents will give rise to multimodal, more effective, and less toxic contrast agents (Lalwani et al., 2014).

The use of nanomaterials as theranostic (therapeutic and diagnostic) agents holds a lot of promise for the future. Magnetic iron oxide nanoparticles (MIONs) are an active candidate in MRI studies, and binding of MIONs with drugs, antibodies, dyes, and aptamers have high chances to develop theranostic agents. On the other hand, liposomes are extensively used for sustained targeted delivery of imaging and therapeutic agent. Liposomes conjugated with magnetic iron oxide nanoparticles (MRI contrast agent) and mitoxantrone (antineoplastic drug) have been found to be effective not only in inhibition of cancerous cell but also acting as contrast agents. The above formulation successfully delivered mitoxantrone to tumor cells and real-time non-invasive monitoring (He et al., 2014). Superparamagnetic iron oxide NPs (SPIONs) with size of 16 nm were functionalized with different chemicals to use in imaging, targeting, and drug delivery. The SPION surface was activated by 3-Aminopropyltriethoxy silane and functionalized with olyethylene glycol. Trastuzumab (antibody), Indium-111 (contrast agent), and Doxorubicin (chemotherapeutic agent) were conjugated on SPIONs. SPIONs maintain magnetic potential, high accumulation in tumor and enhanced circulation time (Zolata et al., 2015).

15.8 PHYSICOCHEMICAL PROPERTIES OF NANOMATERIALS VITAL FOR TRANSPLANTATION

Physiochemical properties of nanomaterials, such as size, shape, surface charge, stability, surface area, roughness, and chemical composition, are significantly important for using nanomaterials in transplantation (Gatoo et al., 2014).

15.9 SIZE

The size and the surface area of nanomaterials to be used in artificial organ transplantation will become a determining factor for interactions with host biological systems and biomolecules (Nel et al., 2006). Alteration in size of the nanomaterials can either upregulate or downregulate not only the desired therapeutic potential but also the undesired toxicity issues (Sumbayev et al., 2013; Borase et al., 2019). In general, decrease in size of nanomaterials increases the reactivity and toxicity. Important biological mechanisms such as enzymatic response, phagocytosis, cellular uptake, inflammation, and endocytic pathways are dependent on the size of nanomaterials (Aillon et al., 2009). The size of nanomaterials is possible to adjust with optimization in synthesis protocols. In the case of nanomaterials the smaller the size, the higher the surface-to-volume ratio compared to macro particles. Therefore, more molecules with medicinal importance can be attached on the nanosurface for new grafts/scaffold systems, regenerative medicine, and targeted drug delivery purposes (Chaudhury et al., 2014).

Microbial contamination of artificial organs and implants needs to be addressed as different scaffold used may be prone to microbial attack (Johnson et al., 2018). Most nanoparticles are already reported to have antimicrobial activity; therefore further research is needed to optimize the combination of nanomaterial and organ to be transplanted. Conjugate of silica nanoparticles (15 nm) and penicillin-G have been found to have strong biocidal potential against methicillin-resistant *Staphylococcus aureus* (Hwang et al., 2016).

Engels et al. (2011) investigated the relationship between increased frequencies of cancer among transplant recipients. According to the author, a transplant saved the life of patient with organ failure, but it also put the patient at high risk of cancer development; the drugs used for immunosuppression to prevent graft rejection are one of the main reasons for the carcinoma.

Surface attachment of gold nanoparticles with paclitaxel derivatives, tumor necrosis factor alpha, and thiolated polyethylene glycol were used in targeted delivery at tumor site (Paciotti et al., 2016).

In another experiment, gold nanoparticles of spherical and star shape with sizes of 50 and 40 nm enhanced the ability of small interfering RNA to enter into eukaryotic cells, compared with 13 nm spherical gold nanoparticles. Gold nanoparticles of two sizes (2 and 15 nm) were coated with an anticancer drug (tiopronin), and as expected, the 2-nm gold nanoparticles were more localized and accumulated in breast cancer cells more than 15-nm gold nanoparticles (Navya et al., 2019).

For successful utilization of nanomaterials in artificial organ manufacturing and transplantation, there needs to be deep understanding of size effect with respect to miniaturization, sustained release, and scaffold strength. Multiple reports clearly mentioned that alteration in nanoparticle size resulted in positive or negative impact on cellular functions such as blood circulation, breathing, and digestion, which are directly related to organ functioning. (Bondarenko et al., 2013, Borase et al., 2019; Holmes et al., 2020).

15.10 SHAPE

Nanomaterials with different shapes (rod, tube, porous, spherical, triangular, hexagonal) are synthesized by diverse physicochemical methods. Very few studies have elaborated on the effect of nanomaterial shape with desired applications (Tasciotti et al., 2008; Huang et al., 2017; Nyoka et al., 2020). Cerium oxide nanoparticles (nanoceria) have the ability to switch between valency states, allowing them to function like some antioxidant enzymes present in body. Cube-shaped cerium oxide nanoparticles are safer on RAW 264.7 cells than rod-shaped cerium oxide (Forest et al., 2017). Rod-shaped iron oxide nanoparticles are more toxic than spherical shaped nanoparticles; they exhibit high cytotoxicity by producing a high level of lactate dehydrogenase leakage, inflammatory response, reactive oxygen species production, and necrosis (Lee et al., 2014).

15.11   EFFECT OF SURFACE COATING AND SURFACE ROUGHNESS

Apart from shape and size, the toxicity of nanomaterials largely depends on its synthesis methods. Chemical and physical methods used for nanosynthesis utilized harmful chemicals such as sodium borohydrate and hydrazine (Gatoo et al., 2014). Therefore eco-friendly green nanosynthesis methods by utilizing living organisms (bacteria, fungi, and plants) or biomolecules can be safer for biomedical applications (Singh et al., 2016). The surface properties of particles, such as charge, roughness smoothness, and ligand bindin, are important factors influencing the properties (affinity, magnetic, electrical, stability) of nanomaterials as well as biological responses such as distribution, pharmacokinetics, accumulation, and penetration (Yin et al., 2005). Inflammatory reaction may developed due to presence of oxygen radicles or ozone on the surface of nanomaterials, leading to unwanted consequences during transplantation (Donaldson and Stone, 2003). Adsorption of proteins on a nanosurface is competitive and depends on the affinity of individual proteins and different immunological components such as macrophages. Platelets will identify and attach, leading to inflammation and fibrosis (Collier and Anderson, 2002). Diversity of chemicals, such as antibodies, peptides, drugs, and anticoagulants, can be attached on a nanosurface to make it bioactive and biocompatible (Teoh et al., 2015).

15.12   UNWANTED INTERACTIONS OF NANOPARTICLES WITH BIOMOLECULES PRESENT IN THE HUMAN BODY

The major advantage of nanomaterials is the extremely small size, but that same characteristic can also be the biggest disadvantage when we translate laboratory findings to the human system (bench-to-bed concept), such as transplantation of an artificial organ containing nanomaterials into the host. Consider an example that 5-nm nanoparticles developed for multiple desirable properties helpful in transplantation (immunosuppression, contrast agent, cell viability, etc.) may not exhibit same properties if the size of nanoparticles during large-scale manufacturing or inside the body increases or decreases. Apart from size, shape, and type of nanomaterial, other factors will give variable results. Reproducibility, high yield, low cost, and expected biological behavior need to be kept in mind from the first day. Despite this, compared to xenotransplantation, the use of artificial organs looks more acceptable with respect to patient preference and religious and ethical point of view. However, nanomaterials have been reported to cross biological barriers and enter into vital organs. Binding to nanoparticles with serum proteins forms protein corona, which affects the intended application. New nanomaterial may lead to formation of reactive oxygen species (Zeng et al., 2019).

Nanoparticles can cause higher toxicity on the surface of cellular membrane, which is a complex and dynamic network of proteins and extracellular polymeric materials. Interaction between the surface properties—namely hydrophobicity and hydrophilicity of nanomaterial and cellular membrane—can induce oxidative stress, with increasing levels of ROS in the cell (Chen et al., 2017). Nanoparticles can damage components of the cytoskeleton, DNA, mitochondria, and lysosomes. It can also disturb intracellular transport and cell division. Quantum dots can exhibit various toxic effects for health in both in vitro and in vivo experiments (Ajdary et al., 2018). An experiment done by Korani et al (2013) showed that higher concentration of silver nanoparticles can cause cardiocyte deformity and inflammation. In chronic obstructive pulmonary disease, high reactivity of nanoparticles has been found to generate free radicals, which induce oxidative stress and inflammation (MacNee and Donaldson, 2003). The unwanted effects of nanoparticles on cells depends on the dose. The dosage level of nanoparticles determines lower or higher toxicity on the surface protein, nucleic acids, glycoproteins, and other macromolecules. Toxicity also depends on the surface–to-volume ratio. The surface area and concentration appear to be more reasonable parameters for dose determination. If the surface area is high, it can induce intrinsic toxicity. According to one report, very low concentration of titanium dioxide nanoparticles (TiO_2) can lead to a very severe inflammation in the lungs (Donaldson et al., 2004). The effect of carbon black on the lungs has been shown to be more severe than TiO_2, which can also lead to epithelial damage (Renwick et al., 2004). Single-wall carbon nanotubes (SWCNTs) can cause lung granulomas (Warheit et al., 2004). Nanoparticles are also reported to induce pro-inflammatory activity and effects on the immune and inflammatory systems, such as reduction in function and mobility of macrophages, phagocytosis, and induction of cytokines (Donaldson et al., 2004). Nanoparticles can also modify the activity of cellular uptake, protein and DNA binding, translocation from entry to target site, and eventual production of reactive oxygen species (ROS) during their interaction (Nel et al., 2006; Piao et al., 2011; von Moos and Slaveykova, 2014).

There are different types of nanoparticles, such as Silica nanoparticles, silver nanoparticles, titanium dioxide nanoparticles, carbon nanoparticles, and zinc oxide (ZnO). Each of them has a different toxicity effect; some can induce autophagy and autophagic cell death in human hepatocellular carcinoma (HepG2) cells (Yu et al., 2014), triggered cellular responses, and induced pulmonary inflammation in human (Wiesner et al., 2006).

According to the study, gold nanoparticles and titanium dioxide nanoparticles induce conformational changes in the structure of bovine serum albumin (Wangoo et al., 2008; Liu et al., 2012), while there are no changes visible through the use of carbon C60 fullerene nanoparticles and zinc oxide-nanoparticles (Bardhan et al., 2009). Variable cell proliferation and cytotoxicity effects were exhibited by carbon nanofibers, carbon black, and carbon nanotubes on human lung-tumor cell lines (Magrez et al., 2006). Experiments on normal human lung fibroblast cells by the use of zinc oxide nanoparticles showed that the morphology and physicochemical properties of this nanomaterials influences the toxicity (Park et al., 2011). Different types of nanoparticles, such as copolymer, ceria, carbon nanotubes, and quantum dots, can also induce fibrillation of β2-microglobulin, and this protein can cause Parkinson's and Alzheimer's diseases (Mikecz and Schikowski, 2020).

The major issues in artificial organ transplantation (similar to that of natural organ) are low success rate in comparison with financial risk and physical and mental stress to the patient. Host acceptance of a transplant is gradually increasing due mostly to the use of immunosuppressants and increase in experience of the transplanting experts, but it still needs a lot of improvement. Nanomaterials have been reported to assist in transportation and accumulation of useful agents (therapeutic, imaging), therefore minimizing toxicity by lowering the doses (Tasciotti et al., 2016). Artificial organs have been quite costly (average cost of around $20,000). Although incorporation of nanotechnology will improve the overall quality and acceptance of artificial organs, cost is also expected to rise (Malchesky, 2014).

15.13 CONCLUSIONS

High cost and high rejection rate are major problems associated with organ transplantation technology, and there is an urgent need to find a promising alternative. Nanomaterials have many useful properties including small shape, ability to conjugate different molecules having therapeutic and diagnostic value, and variable biocidal potential. The above properties are indispensable for not only development but also successful transplantation of artificial organs. With the increase in our understanding about physical and chemical reactions at the interface of cells, nanomaterials, and scaffold, nanotechnology is finding many potent applications in organ transplantation. Involvement of nanomaterials for development of robust and cell-growth–supporting scaffolds has future potential for mimicking functions of complex multicellular organs, such as liver. Extensive research efforts are needed for up scaling nanomaterials synthesis. Good results obtained in the laboratory should replicate in the patient also. To achieve that milestone, the continuous flow of funds, experienced personnel, and interdisciplinary collaboration is most important. The field of nanotoxicology is still in its infancy, and several reports suggest removal of nanomaterials from the biological system; but still its impact on biological networks needs more clarification. In conclusion, nanotechnology harbors tremendous potential for sustainable transplantation of artificial organs.

ACKNOWLEDGMENT

Authors are thankful to the Uka Tarsadia University and Kavayitri Bahinabai Chaudhari North Maharashtra University for providing necessary facilities.

DECLARATION OF COMPETING INTEREST

All authors declare no conflicts of interest.

REFERENCES

Achilefu, Samuel. Introduction to concepts and strategies for molecular imaging. *Chemical Reviews* 110(5), (2010): 2575–2578.

Aillon, Kristin L., Yumei Xie, Nashwa El-Gendy, Cory J. Berkland, and M. Laird Forrest. Effects of nanomaterial physicochemical properties on in vivo toxicity. *Advanced Drug Delivery Reviews* 61(6), (2009): 457–466.

Ajdary, Marziyeh, Mohammad Amin Moosavi, Marveh Rahmati, Mojtaba Falahati, Mohammad Mahboubi, Ali Mandegary, Saranaz Jangjoo, Reza Mohammadinejad, and Rajender S. Varma. Health concerns of various nanoparticles: a review of their in vitro and in vivo toxicity. *Nanomaterials* 8(9), (2018): 634–662.

Anselmo, Aaron C., and Samir Mitragotri. Nanoparticles in the clinic. *Bioengineering & Translational Medicine* 1(1), (2016): 10–29.

Arnhold, Jurgen, Organ damage and failure. Arnhold, Jurgen, eds. *Cell and Tissue Destruction: Mechanisms, Protection, and Disorders.* (2019) Academic Press.

Ashammakhi, Nureddin, Elmahdi Elkhammas, and Anwarul Hasan. Translating advances in organ on a chip technology for supporting organs. *Journal of Biomedical Materials Research Part B: Applied Biomaterials* 107(6), (2019): 2006–2018.

Azzi, Jamil, Li Tang, Robert Moore, Rong Tong, Najib El Haddad, Takurin Akiyoshi, Bechara Mfarrej et al. Polylactide cyclosporin A nanoparticles for targeted immunosuppression. *The FASEB Journal* 24(10), (2010): 3927–3938.

Balmert, Stephen C., and Steven R. Little. Biomimetic delivery with micro- and nanoparticles. *Advanced Materials* 24(28), (2012): 3757–3778.

Bardhan, Munmun, Gopa Mandal, and Tapan Ganguly. Steady state, time resolved, and circular dichroism spectroscopic studies to reveal the nature of interactions of zinc oxide nanoparticles with transport protein bovine serum albumin and to monitor the possible protein conformational changes. *Journal of Applied Physics* 106(3), (2009): 1–6.

Barreto, Maynara Fernanda Carvalho, Mara Solange Gomes Dellaroza, Karen Barros Parron Fernandes, Paloma de Souza Cavalcante Pissinati, Maria José Quina Galdino, and Maria do Carmo Fernandez Lourenço Haddad. Cost and factors associated with the hospitalization of patients undergoing heart transplantation. *Transplantation Proceedings* 51(10), (2019) 3412–3417.

Bartlett, Adam S., Ravi Ramadas, Sue Furness, Ed Gane, and John L. McCall. The natural history of acute histologic rejection without biochemical graft dysfunction in orthotopic liver transplantation: a systematic review. *Liver Transplantation* 8(12), (2002): 1147–1153.

Bondarenko, O., K. Juganson, A. Ivask, K. Kasemets, M. Mortimer, A. Kahru, Toxicity of Ag, CuO and ZnO nanoparticles to selected environmentally relevant test organisms and mammalian cells in vitro: a critical review. *Archives of Toxicology* 87, (2013): 1181–1200.

Borase, Hemant P., Bipinchandra K. Salunke, Rahul B. Salunkhe, Chandrashekhar D. Patil, John E. Hallsworth, Beom S. Kim, and Satish V. Patil. Plant extract: a promising biomatrix for ecofriendly, controlled synthesis of silver nanoparticles. *Applied Biochemistry and Biotechnology* 173 (1), (2014): 1–29.

Borase, Hemant P., Satish V. Patil, and Rekha S. Singhal. *Moina macrocopa* as a non-target aquatic organism for assessment of ecotoxicity of silver nanoparticles: Effect of size. *Chemosphere* 219, (2019): 713–723.

Braza, Mounia S., Mandy MT van Leent, Marnix Lameijer, Brenda L. Sanchez-Gaytan, Rob JW Arts, Carlos Pérez-Medina, Patricia Conde. Inhibiting inflammation with myeloid cell-specific nanobiologics promotes organ transplant acceptance. *Immunity* 49(5), (2018): 819–828.

Busque, Stephan, Hootan Roozrokh, and Minnie Sarwal. 19 nanotechnology in organ transplantation. *Nanoscale Technology in Biological Systems* (2004): 427–432.

Chaudhury, Koel, Vishu Kumar, Jayaprakash Kandasamy, and Sourav Roy Choudhury. Regenerative nanomedicine: current perspectives and future directions. *International Journal of Nanomedicine* 9, (2014): 4153–4160.

Chen Gan, Hongzhang Deng, Xiang Song, Mingzi Lu, Lian Zhao, Sha Xia, Guoxing You et al. Reactive oxygen species-responsive polymeric nanoparticles for alleviating sepsis-induced acute liver injury in mice. *Biomaterials* 144, (2017): 30–41.

Cheng, Christopher J., Gregory T. Tietjen, Jennifer K. Saucier-Sawyer, and W. Mark Saltzman. A holistic approach to targeting disease with polymeric nanoparticles. *Nature Reviews Drug Discovery* 14(4), (2015): 239–247.

Cherian, Bibin Mathew, Alcides Lopes Leão, Sivoney Ferreira de Souza, Ligia Maria Manzine Costa, Gabriel Molina de Olyveira, M. Kottaisamy, E. R. Nagarajan, and Sabu Thomas. Cellulose nanocomposites with nanofibres isolated from pineapple leaf fibers for medical applications. *Carbohydrate Polymers* 86(4), (2011): 1790–1798.

Choi, Hak Soo, Wenhao Liu, Preeti Misra, Eiichi Tanaka, John P. Zimmer, Binil Itty Ipe, Moungi G. Bawendi, and John V. Frangioni. Renal clearance of nanoparticles. *Nature Biotechnology* 25 (10), (2007): 1165–1170.

Collier, T. O., and J. M. Anderson. Protein and surface effects on monocyte and macrophage adhesion, maturation, and survival. *Journal of Biomedical Materials Research* 60(3), (2002): 487–496

Dobson, J. Gene therapy progress and prospects: magnetic nanoparticle-based gene delivery. *Gene therapy* 13 (4) (2006) 283–287.

Donaldson, Ken, and Vicki Stone. Current hypotheses on the mechanisms of toxicity of ultra-fine particles. *Annali Dell'Istituto Superiore Di Sanità* 39(3), (2003): 405–410.

Donaldson, Ken, Vicki Stone, C. L. Tran, Wolfgang Kreyling, Paul J. A. Borm. Nanotoxicology. *Occup Environ Med* (2004): 727–728.

Dunlay, Shannon M., and Véronique L. Roger. Understanding the epidemic of heart failure: past, present, and future. *Current Heart Failure Reports* 11(4), (2014): 404–415.

ec.europa.eu. (2007) https://ec.europa.eu/health/scientific_committees/opinions_layman/en/nanotechnologies/l-3/1-introduction.htm

Engels, Eric A., Ruth M. Pfeiffer, Joseph F. Fraumeni, Bertram L. Kasiske, Ajay K. Israni, Jon J. Snyder, Robert A. Wolfe et al. Spectrum of cancer risk among US solid organ transplant recipients. *Jama* 306(17), (2011): 1891–1901.

Fathi-Achachelouei, Milad, Helena Knopf-Marques, Cristiane Evelise Ribeiro da Silva, Julien Barthès, Erhan Bat, Aysen Tezcaner, and Nihal Engin Vrana. Use of nanoparticles in tissue engineering and regenerative medicine. *Frontiers in Bioengineering and biotechnology* 7, (2019): 113–117.

FDA. *Guidance for Industry Considering Whether an FDA-Regulated Product Involves the Application of Nanotechnology.* Food and Drug Administration, (2014).

Fissell, William H., Liandi Lou, Simin Abrishami, Deborah A. Buffington, and H. David Humes. Bioartificial kidney ameliorates gram-negative bacteria-induced septic shock in uremic animals. *Journal of the American Society of Nephrology* 14(2), (2003): 454–461.

Flaman, Paul. Organ and tissue transplants: Some ethical issues. *Topics in Bioethics for Science and Religion Teachers: Readings and Study Guide* (1994): 31–46.

Forest, Valérie, Lara Leclerc, Jean-François Hochepied, Adeline Trouvé, Gwendoline Sarry, and Jérémie Pourchez. Impact of cerium oxide nanoparticles shape on their *in vitro* cellular toxicity. *Toxicology in Vitro* 38, (2017): 136–141.

Forrest, M. Laird, Chee-Youb Won, A. Waseem Malick, and Glen S. Kwon. In vitro release of the mTOR inhibitor rapamycin from poly (ethylene glycol)-b-poly (ε-caprolactone) micelles. *Journal of Controlled Release* 110(2), (2006): 370–377.

Fraux, Cécile, Maria Teresa Muñoz Sastre, Lonzozou Kpanake, Paul Clay Sorum, and Etienne Mullet. French people's views regarding xenotransplantation. *Transplantation Proceedings.* 5(2), (2021): 529–438.

Frick, Stefanie U., Nicole Bacher, Grit Baier, Volker Mailänder, Katharina Landfester, and Kerstin Steinbrink. Functionalized polystyrene nanoparticles trigger human dendritic cell maturation resulting in enhanced CD4+ T cell activation. *Macromolecular Bioscience* 12(12), (2012): 1637–1647.

Gatoo, Manzoor Ahmad, Sufia Naseem, Mir Yasir Arfat, Ayaz Mahmood Dar, Khusro Qasim, and Swaleha Zubair. Physicochemical properties of nanomaterials: implication in associated toxic manifestations. *BioMed Research International* 2014, (2014): 1–9.

Go, Jin, KyungJai Ko, Dami Jun, Su-kyung Kwon, Sanghyeop Han, Young Hwa Kim, Mi-Hyeong Kim et al. A half-century 3000 cases of kidney transplant experiences in a single hospital: the longest registry in Korea. *Transplantation Proceedings* 51(8), (2019) 2559–2567.

Grattoni, Alessandro, Ennio Tasciotti, Daniel Fine, Joseph S. Fernandez-Moure, Jason Sakamoto, Ye Hu, Bradley Weiner, Mauro Ferrari, and Scott Parazynski. Nanotechnologies and regenerative medical approaches for space and terrestrial medicine. *Aviation, Space, and Environmental Medicine* 83(11), (2012): 1025–1036.

Grinyó, Josep M. Why is organ transplantation clinically important? *Cold Spring Harbor Perspectives in Medicine* 3(6), (2013): a014985.

Hahn, Peter F., David D. Stark, Jerome M. Lewis, Sanjay Saini, G. Elizondo, R. Weissleder, C. J. Fretz, and J. T. Ferrucci. First clinical trial of a new superparamagnetic iron oxide for use as an oral gastrointestinal contrast agent in MR imaging. *Radiology* 175(3), (1990): 695–700.

Hardy, Charles L., Jeanne S. LeMasurier, Gabrielle T. Belz, Karen Scalzo-Inguanti, Jun Yao, Sue D. Xiang, Peter Kanellakis et al. Inert 50-nm polystyrene nanoparticles that modify pulmonary dendritic cell function and inhibit allergic airway inflammation. *The Journal of Immunology* 188(3), (2012): 1431–1441.

Hasan, Anwarul, John Saliba, Hassan Pezeshgi Modarres, Ahmed Bakhaty, Amir Nasajpour, Mohammad RK Mofrad, and Amir Sanati-Nezhad. Micro and nanotechnologies in heart valve tissue engineering. *Biomaterials* 103, (2016): 278–292.

He, Song Qing, Yan Hong Zhang, Senthil K. Venugopal, Christopher W. Dicus, Richard V. Perez, Rajen Ramsamooj, Michael H. Nantz, Mark A. Zern, and Jian Wu. Delivery of antioxidative enzyme genes protects against ischemia/reperfusion–induced liver injury in mice. *Liver Transplantation* 12(12), (2006): 1869–1879.

He, Yingna, Linhua Zhang, Dunwan Zhu, and Cunxian Song. Design of multifunctional magnetic iron oxide nanoparticles/mitoxantrone-loaded liposomes for both magnetic resonance imaging and targeted cancer therapy. *International Journal of Nanomedicine* 9, (2014): 4055–4062.

Holmes, Amy M., Lorraine Mackenzie, and Roberts, Michael S. Disposition and measured toxicity of zinc oxide nanoparticles and zinc ions against keratinocytes in cell culture and viable human epidermis. *Nanotoxicology* 14(2), (2020): 263–274

Hrapovic, Sabahudin, Yali Liu, Keith B. Male, and John HT Luong. Electrochemical biosensing platforms using platinum nanoparticles and carbon nanotubes. *Analytical Chemistry* 76(4), (2004): 1083–1088.

HRSA. (2020) https://www.organdonor.gov/statistics-stories/statistics.html

Huang, Yue-Wern, Melissa Cambre, and Han-Jung Lee. The toxicity of nanoparticles depends on multiple molecular and physicochemical mechanisms. *International Journal of Molecular Sciences* 18(12), (2017): 1–13.

Hubbell, Jeffrey A., Susan N. Thomas, and Melody A. Swartz. Materials engineering for immunomodulation. *Nature* 462 (7272), (2009): 449–460.

Humes, H. David, Deborah A. Buffington, Sherrill M. MacKay, Angela J. Funke, and William F. Weitzel. Replacement of renal function in uremic animals with a tissue-engineered kidney. *Nature Biotechnology* 17(5), (1999): 451–455.

Hwang, Jangsun, Eunwon Lee, Jieun Kim, Youngmin Seo, Kwan Hong Lee, Jong Wook Hong, Assaf A. Gilad, Hansoo Park, and Jonghoon Choi. Effective delivery of immunosuppressive drug molecules by silica coated iron oxide nanoparticles. *Colloids and Surfaces B: Biointerfaces* 142, (2016): 290–296

Javaid, Mohd, and Abid Haleem. 3D printed tissue and organ using additive manufacturing: an overview. *Clinical Epidemiology and Global Health* 8(2), (2020): 586–594.

Jeong, Hun-Jin, Hyoryung Nam, Jinah Jang, and Seung-Jae Lee. 3D bioprinting strategies for the regeneration of functional tubular tissues and organs. *Bioengineering* 7(2), (2020): 32–38.

Johnson, Christopher T., James A. Wroe, Rachit Agarwal, Karen E. Martin, Robert E. Guldberg, Rodney M. Donlan, Lars F. Westblade, and Andrés J. García. Hydrogel delivery of lysostaphin eliminates orthopedic implant infection by Staphylococcus aureus and supports fracture healing. *Proceedings of the National Academy of Sciences* 115(22), (2018): E4960–E4969.

Jones, Julian, Artificial organs. Hench, Larry and Jones Julian, eds. *Biomaterials, Artificial Organs and Tissue Engineering.* (2005) CRC press.

Jungebluth, P., E. Alici, and S. Baiguera. Tracheobronchial transplantation with a stem-cell-seeded bioartificial nanocomposite: a proof-of-concept study. *Lancet* (11), (2011): 61715–61717.

Khan, Fahad Saleem Ahmed, N. M. Mubarak, Mohammad Khalid, and Ezzat Chan Abdullah. Functionalized Carbon nanomaterial for artificial bone replacement as filler material. *Sustainable Polymer Composites and Nanocomposites* (2019b): 783–804.

Khan, Ibrahim, Khalid Saeed, and Idrees Khan. Nanoparticles: Properties, applications and toxicities. *Arabian Journal of Chemistry* 12(7), (2019a): 908–931.

Ko, Saiho, Yoshiyuki Nakajima, Hiromichi Kanehiro, Masato Horikawa, Atsushi Yoshimura, Junichiro Taki, Yukio Aomatsu, Tatsuya Kin, Kazuaki Yagura, and Hiroshige Nakano. The enhanced immunosuppressive efficacy of newly developed liposomal FK506 in canine liver transplantation. *Transplantation* 59(10), (1995): 1384–1388.

Korani, Mitra, Seyed Mahdi Rezayat, and Sepideh Arbabi Bidgoli. Sub-chronic dermal toxicity of silver nanoparticles in guinea pig: Special emphasis to heart, bone and kidney toxicities. *Iranian Journal of Pharmaceutical Research* 12, (2013): 511–519.

Krishna V.S., *Bioethics and Biosafety in Biotechnology.* (2007) New Age international Limited.

Lalwani, Gaurav, Joe Livingston Sundararaj, Kenneth Schaefer, Terry Button, and Balaji Sitharaman. Synthesis, characterization, in vitro phantom imaging, and cytotoxicity of a novel graphene-based multimodal magnetic resonance imaging-X-ray computed tomography contrast agent. *Journal of Materials Chemistry B* 2(22), (2014): 3519–3530.

Lavik, Erin, and Horst von Recum. The role of nanomaterials in translational medicine. *ACS Nano* 5(5), (2011): 3419–3424.

Lee, Jang Han, Jae Eun Ju., Byung Il Kim, Pyo June Pak, Eun-Kyung Choi, Hoi-Seon Lee, and Namhyun Chung. Rod-shaped iron oxide nanoparticles are more toxic than sphere-shaped nanoparticles to murine macrophage cells. *Environmental Toxicology and Chemistry* 33(12), (2014): 2759–66.

Lee, Yuhan, Soo Hyeon Lee, Jee Seon Kim, Atsushi Maruyama, Xuesi Chen, and Tae Gwan Park. Controlled synthesis of PEI-coated gold nanoparticles using reductive catechol chemistry for siRNA delivery. *Journal of Controlled Release* 155(1), (2011): 3–10.

Li, Jun, and Xian Jun Loh. Cyclodextrin-based supramolecular architectures: syntheses, structures, and applications for drug and gene delivery. *Advanced Drug Delivery Reviews* 60 (9), (2008): 1000–1017.

Liau, Brian, Donghui Zhang, and Nenad Bursac. Functional cardiac tissue engineering. *Regenerative Medicine* 7(2), (2012): 187–206.

Loh, Xian Jun, Tung-Chun Lee, Qingqing Dou, and G. Roshan Deen. Utilising inorganic nanocarriers for gene delivery. *Biomaterials Science* 4(1), (2016): 70–86.

Look, Michael, W. Mark Saltzman, Joe Craft, and Tarek M. Fahmy. The nanomaterial-dependent modulation of dendritic cells and its potential influence on therapeutic immunosuppression in lupus. *Biomaterials* 35 (3), (2014): 1089–1095.

Luo, Huize, Ruitao Cha, Juanjuan Li, Wenshuai Hao, Yan Zhang, and Fengshan Zhou. Advances in tissue engineering of nanocellulose-based scaffolds: A review. *Carbohydrate Polymers* 224, (2019): 115–144.

MacNee, W., and K. Donaldson. Mechanism of lung injury caused by PM10 and ultrafine particles with special reference to COPD. *European Respiratory Journal* 21 (40) (2003): 47–51.

Magrez, Arnaud, Sandor Kasas, Valérie Salicio, Nathalie Pasquier, Jin Won Seo, Marco Celio, Stefan Catsicas, Beat Schwaller, and László Forró. Cellular toxicity of carbon-based nanomaterials. *Nano Letters* 6, (2006): 1121–1125

Mahmoudi, Morteza, Mikyung Yu, Vahid Serpooshan, Joseph C. Wu, Robert Langer, Richard T. Lee, Jeffrey M. Karp, and Omid C. Farokhzad. Multiscale technologies for treatment of ischemic cardiomyopathy. *Nature Nanotechnology* 12(9), (2017): 845–855.

Malchesky, Paul S., Are artificial organs still needed? *Artificial Organs* 38(10), (2014): 827–828.

Marga, Francoise, Karoly Jakab, Chirag Khatiwala, Benjamin Shepherd, Scott Dorfman, Bradley Hubbard, Stephen Colbert, and Gabor Forgacs. Toward engineering functional organ modules by additive manufacturing. *Biofabrication* 4(2), (2012): 022001.

Martins, Paulo NA, Anil Chandraker, and Stefan G. Tullius. Modifying graft immunogenicity and immune response prior to transplantation: potential clinical applications of donor and graft treatment. *Transplant International* 19(5), (2006): 351–359.

McDermott JK. Complications of Immunosuppression. Bogar, L., Stempien-Otero A. (eds) *Contemporary Heart Transplantation. Organ and Tissue Transplantation.* (2020) Springer Publications 205–222.

Navya, P. N., Anubhav Kaphle, S. P. Srinivas, Suresh Kumar Bhargava, Vincent M. Rotello, and Hemant Kumar Daima. Current trends and challenges in cancer management and therapy using designer nanomaterials. *Nano Convergence* 6(1), (2019): 1–30.

Nel, Andre, Tian Xia, Lutz Mädler, and Ning Li. Toxic potential of materials at the nanolevel. *Science* 311(5761), (2006): 622–627.

Ngobili, Terrika A., and Michael A. Daniele. Nanoparticles and direct immunosuppression. *Experimental Biology and Medicine* 241(10), (2016): 1064–1073.

Nobakht Niloofar, Anjay Rastogi, Ann Hernandez, and Allen Nissenson. Nanotechnology. In Todd S. Ing, Mohamed A. Rahman, and Carl M. Kjellstrand, eds. *Dialysis: History, Development and Promise.* (2012) World Scientific 829–836.

Nyoka, Mpumelelo, Yahya E. Choonara, Pradeep Kumar, Pierre Kondiah, and Viness Pillay. Synthesis of cerium oxide nanoparticles using various methods: Implications for biomedical applications. *Nanomaterials* 10(2), (2020): 1–21.

Paciotti, Giulio F., Jielu Zhao, Shugeng Cao, Peggy J. Brodie, Lawrence Tamarkin, Marja Huhta, Lonnie D. Myer, Jay Friedman, and David GI Kingston. Synthesis and evaluation of paclitaxel-loaded gold nanoparticles for tumor-targeted drug delivery. *Bioconjugate Chemistry* 27 (11), (2016): 2646–2657.

Park, Soo Jin, Young Chan Park, Sang Won Lee, Min Sook Jeong, Kyeong-Nam Yu, Haksung Jung, Jin-Kyu Lee, Jun Sung Kim, and Myung-Haing Cho. Comparing the toxic mechanism of synthesized zinc oxide nanomaterials by physicochemical characterization and reactive oxygen species properties. *Toxicological Letters* 207, (2011): 197–203.

Piao, Mei Jing, Kyoung Ah Kang, In Kyung Lee, Hye Sun Kim, Suhkmann Kim, Jeong Yun Choi, Jinhee Choi, and Jin Won Hyun. Silver nanoparticles induce oxidative cell damage in human liver cells through inhibition of reduced glutathione and induction of mitochondria-involved apoptosis. *Toxicology Letters* 201(1), (2011): 92–100.

Platt, Jeffrey L. New directions for organ transplantation. *Nature* 392(6679 Suppl), (1998): 11–17.

Ratzinger, Gerda, Prashant Agrawal, Wilfried Körner, Julia Lonkai, Honorius MHF Sanders, Enzo Terreno, Michael Wirth, Gustav J. Strijkers, Klaas Nicolay, and Franz Gabor. Surface modification of PLGA nanospheres with Gd-DTPA and Gd-DOTA for high-relaxivity MRI contrast agents. *Biomaterials* 31(33), (2010): 8716–8723.

Renwick, L. C., D. Brown, A. Clouter, and K. Donaldson. Increased inflammation and altered macrophage chemotactic responses caused by two ultrafine particle types. *Occupational and Environmental Medicine* 61(5), (2004): 442–447.

Ritschel, Wolfgang. Microemulsion technology in the reformulation of cyclosporine: the reason behind the pharmacokinetic properties of Neoral. *Clinical Transplantation* 10(4), (1996): 364–373.

Robertson, R. Paul. Islet transplantation as a treatment for diabetes—a work in progress. *New England Journal of Medicine* 350(7), (2004): 694–705.

Shafiee, Ashkan, Elham Ghadiri, Jareer Kassis, and Anthony Atala. Nanosensors for therapeutic drug monitoring: implications for transplantation. *Nanomedicine* 14 (20), (2019): 2735–2747.

Shen, Chien-Chang, Chia-Chi Wang, Mei-Hsiu Liao, and Tong-Rong Jan. A single exposure to iron oxide nanoparticles attenuates antigen-specific antibody production and T-cell reactivity in ovalbumin-sensitized BALB/c mice. *International Journal of Nanomedicine* 6, (2011): 1229–1235.

Singh, Priyanka, Yu-Jin Kim, Dabing Zhang, and Deok-Chun Yang. Biological synthesis of nanoparticles from plants and microorganisms. *Trends in Biotechnology* 34(7), (2016): 588–599.

Soares, Sara, João Sousa, Alberto Pais, and Carla Vitorino. Nanomedicine: principles, properties, and regulatory issues. *Frontiers in Chemistry* 6, (2018): 360–365.

Solhjou, Zhabiz, Mayuko Uehara, Baharak Bahmani, Omar H. Maarouf, Takaharu Ichimura, Craig R. Brooks, Wanlong Xu et al. Novel application of localized nanodelivery of anti–Interleukin 6 protects organ transplant from Ischemia–reperfusion injuries. *American Journal of Transplantation* 17(9), (2017): 2326–2337.

Splendiani, G., S. Cipriani, A. Vega, C.U. Casciani, Artificial organs and transplantation. *Artificial Cells, Blood Substitutes, and Biotechnology* 31(2), (2003): 91–96.

Sumbayev, Vadim V., Inna M. Yasinska, Cesar Pascual Garcia, Douglas Gilliland, Gurprit S. Lall, Bernhard F. Gibbs, David R. Bonsall, Luca Varani, François Rossi, and Luigi Calzolai. Gold nanoparticles down regulate interleukin1β induced proinflammatory responses. *Small* 9(3), (2013): 472–477.

Sun, Tao, Shaoming Mai, David Norton, John W. Haycock, Anthony J. Ryan, and Sheila Macneil. Self-organization of skin cells in three-dimensional electrospun polystyrene scaffolds. *Tissue engineering* 11(7), (2005): 1023–1033.

Tan, Hui-Li, Sin-Yeang Teow, and Janarthanan Pushpamalar. Application of metal nanoparticle–hydrogel composites in tissue regeneration. *Bioengineering* 6(1), (2019): 1–17.

Tasciotti, Ennio, Fernando J. Cabrera, Michael Evangelopoulos, Jonathan O. Martinez, Usha R. Thekkedath, Malgorzata Kloc, Rafik M. Ghobrial, Xian C. Li, Alessandro Grattoni, and Mauro Ferrari. The emerging role of nanotechnology in cell and organ transplantation. *Transplantation* 100(8), (2016): 1629–1638.

Tasciotti, Ennio, Xuewu Liu, Rohan Bhavane, Kevin Plant., Ashley D. Leonard, Katherine Price, Mark Ming-Cheng. Mesoporous silicon particles as a multistage delivery system for imaging and therapeutic applications. *Nature Nanotechnology* 3(3), (2008): 151–157.

Teoh, G. Z., P. Klanrit, M. Kasimatis, and A. M. Seifalian. Role of nanotechnology in development of artificial organs in development of artificial organs. *Minerva Medica* 106, (2015): 17–33.

Tietjen, Gregory T., Laura G. Bracaglia, W. Mark Saltzman, and Jordan S. Pober. Focus on fundamentals: achieving effective nanoparticle targeting. *Trends in Molecular Medicine* 24(7), (2018): 598–606.

Torchilin, Vladimir P. Recent advances with liposomes as pharmaceutical carriers. *Nature Reviews Drug Discovery* 4(2), (2005): 145–160.

von Mikecz, Anna, and Tamara Schikowski. Effects of airborne nanoparticles on the nervous system: Amyloid protein aggregation, neurodegeneration and neurodegenerative diseases. *Nanomaterials* 10(7), (2020): 1–10.

von Moos, Nadia, and Vera I. Slaveykova. Oxidative stress induced by inorganic nanoparticles in bacteria and aquatic microalgae–state of the art and knowledge gaps. *Nanotoxicology* 8(6), (2014): 605–630.

Wang, Lei, Yung Pin Chen, Kristen P. Miller, Brandon M. Cash, Shonda Jones, Steven Glenn, Brian C. Benicewicz, and Alan W. Decho. Functionalised nanoparticles complexed with antibiotic efficiently kill MRSA and other bacteria. *Chemical Communications* 50(81), (2014): 12030–12033.

Wang, Xiaohong. Bioartificial organ manufacturing technologies. *Cell Transplantation* 28(1), (2019): 5–17.

Wangoo, Nishima, C. Raman Suri, and G. Shekhawat. Interaction of gold nanoparticles with protein: a spectroscopic study to monitor protein conformational changes. *Applied Physics Letters* 92(13), (2008): 1–3.

Warheit, David B., Brett R. Laurence, Kenneth L. Reed, David H. Roach, and Tom R. Webb. Comparative pulmonary toxicity assessment of single-wall carbon nanotubes in rats. *Toxicological Sciences* 77(1), (2004): 117–125.

Watson, C.J.E. and J.H. Dark, Organ transplantation: historical perspective and current practice. *British Journal of Anaesthesia* 108(1), (2012): i29–i42.

Weissig, Volkmar, Tracy K. Pettinger, and Nicole Murdock. Nanopharmaceuticals (part 1): products on the market. *International Journal of Nanomedicine* 9, (2014): 4357

Wiesner, Mark R., Greg V. Lowry, Pedro Alvarez, Dianysios Dionysiou, and Pratim Biswas. Assessing the risks of manufactured nanomaterials. *Environment Science and Technology*. 40, (2006): 4336–4345.

WHO. (2020) https://www.who.int/topics/transplantation/en/ (accessed on 15 Nov., 2020)

Xu, Y, D. Li, and X. Wang. Current trends and challenges for producing artificial hearts. Wang, X., eds. *Organ Manufacturing*. (2015) *Nova Science Publishers Inc.: Hauppauge, NY, USA*. 101–125.

Yambe, Tomoyuki. Artificial Organs with nano-technology and development of the new diagnosis tool. *Annals NanoBME* 2, (2009): 1–10.

Yao, Christine G., and Paulo N. Martins. Nanotechnology applications in transplantation medicine. *Transplantation* 104(4), (2020): 682–693.

Yin, H., H. P. Too, and G. M. Chow. The effects of particle size and surface coating on the cytotoxicity of nickel ferrite. *Biomaterials* 26(29), (2005): 5818–5826.

Yu, Yongbo, Junchao Duan, Yang Yu, Yang Li, Xiaomei Liu, Xianqing Zhou, Kin-fai Ho, Linwei Tian, and Zhiwei Sun. Silica nanoparticles induce autophagy and autophagic cell death in HepG2 cells triggered by reactive oxygen species. *Journal of Hazardous Materials* 270, (2014): 176–186.

Zeng, Li, Jiejun Gao, Yanna Liu, Jie Gao, Linlin Yao, Xiaoxi Yang, Xiaolei Liu et al. Role of protein corona in the biological effect of nanomaterials: Investigating methods. *Trends in Analytical Chemistry* 118, (2019): 303–314.

Zhao, Chunyan, Jamie Siqi Lin, Mahesh Choolani, Yock Young Dan, Giorgia Pastorin, and Han Kiat Ho. Enhanced hepatic differentiation of human amniotic epithelial cells on polyethylene glycolinked multiwalled carbon nanotube coated hydrogels. *Journal of Tissue Engineering and Regenerative Medicine* 12(7), (2018): 1556–1566.

Zolata, Hamidreza, Fereydoun Abbasi Davani, and Hossein Afarideh. Synthesis, characterization and theranostic evaluation of Indium-111 labeled multifunctional superparamagnetic iron oxide nanoparticles. *Nuclear Medicine and Biology* 42(2), (2015): 164–170.

Index

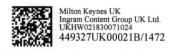

9 780367 690335